Complications
of
Gynecologic
and Obstetric
Management

Michael Newton, M.D.

Professor of Obstetrics and Gynecology
Northwestern University Medical School
Chicago, Illinois

Edward R. Newton, M.D.

Assistant Professor of Obstetrics and Gynecology
Division of Maternal-Fetal Medicine
University of Texas Health Science Center at San Antonio
San Antonio, Texas

1988 87-8157
W.B. SAUNDERS COMPANY
Harcourt Brace Jovanovich Inc.
Philadelphia London Toronto
Montreal Sydney Tokyo

W. B. SAUNDERS COMPANY
Harcourt Brace Jovanovich, Inc.

West Washington Square
Philadelphia, PA 19105

Library of Congress Cataloging-in-Publication Data

Newton, Michael, 1920–

Complications of gynecologic and obstetric management.

1. Gynecology, Operative—Complications and sequelae.
   2. Obstetrics—Surgery—Complications and sequelae.
   3. Pregnant women—Surgery—Complications and
   sequelae.   4. Generative organs, Female—Diseases—
   Treatment—Complications and sequelae.   5. Genitourinary organs—Diseases—Treatment—Complications and
   sequelae.   6. Gynecology—Moral and ethical aspects.
   7. Obstetrics—Moral and ethical aspects.
   I. Newton, Edward R.   II. Title. [DNLM: 1. Genitalia,
   Female—surgery.   2. Intraoperative Complications.
   3. Postoperative Complications.   4. Pregnancy
   Complications.   5. Surgery, Operative—adverse
   effects.   6. Therapeutics—adverse effects.   WP 660
   N565c]

RG104.2.N48 1988   618   87–12696

ISBN 0–7216–6769–4

Editor: W. B. Saunders Staff
Designer: Terri Siegel
Production Manager: Carolyn Naylor
Manuscript Editor: Susan Short
Illustration Coordinator: Walt Verbitski
Indexer: Barbara Farabaugh

Complications of Gynecologic and Obstetric Management   ISBN 0–7216–6769–4

Last digit is the print number: 9   8   7   6   5   4   3   2   1

To Niles and Karen

CONTRIBUTORS

ROBERT BOUER, M.D.

Assistant Professor, Department of Obstetrics and Gynecology, Northwestern University Medical School; Chairman, Department of Obstetrics and Gynecology, St. Joseph Hospital, Chicago, Illinois

Legal and Ethical Considerations

TERRENCE J. BUGNO, M.D.

Attending Staff, St. Joseph Hospital, Elgin, Illinois; St. Joseph Hospital, Joliet, Illinois; Sherman Hospital, Elgin, Illinois

Radiation Reactions and Complications: Etiology, Prevention, Diagnosis and Management

HARRY COHEN, M.D.

Professor of Clinical Anesthesia, Department of Obstetrics and Gynecology, Northwestern University Medical School; Attending Staff, Northwestern Memorial Hospital, Chicago, Illinois

Anesthesia Considerations and Complications in Obstetric and Gynecologic Surgery

JOHN R. LURAIN, M.D.

Head, Section of Gynecologic Oncology, Associate Professor, Department of Obstetrics and Gynecology, Northwestern University Medical School; Chief, Gynecologic Oncology Service, Prentice Women's Hospital and Maternity Center of Northwestern Memorial Hospital, Chicago, Illinois

Complications of Radical Oncologic Operations

WARREN P. NEWTON, M.D.

Robert Wood Johnson Clinical Scholar, Department of Family Medicine, University of North Carolina at Chapel Hill; Staff, North Carolina Memorial Hospital, Chapel Hill, North Carolina

Historical Aspects of Complications in Gynecology and Obstetrics

RICHARD J. PEIRCE, M.D.

Associate Professor of Clinical Anesthesia, Department of Obstetrics and Gynecology, Northwestern University Medical School; Associate, Obstetrics, Gynecology, and Anesthesia Services, Northwestern Memorial Hospital, Chicago, Illinois

Anesthesia Considerations and Complications in Obstetric and Gynecologic Surgery

RAMANANDA M. SHETTY, M.D.

Assistant Professor of Radiation Oncology, Department of Radiology, Northwestern University Medical School; Attending Staff, Northwestern Memorial Hospital, Chicago, Illinois

Radiation Reactions and Complications: Etiology, Prevention, Diagnosis and Management

PREFACE

The complications of operations, procedures and medications used in gynecology and obstetrics have traditionally been thought to be due to the progress of the disease itself. Recently, the uneasy medicolegal situation has put emphasis on the unfavorable results of physicians' actions. However, it is often difficult to decide which sequelae are normal or inevitable and which are compensable. Therefore, knowledge concerning the prevention, assessment and management of complications becomes essential for all who provide health care for women. This book concentrates on these issues.

Complications may occur during diagnostic procedures and before, during or after treatment. Many are general and apply to several different operations and procedures; these are covered in Chapters 2, 3 and 4. Others relate to specific procedures and are described in subsequent chapters. Medical (drug) therapy, radiotherapy and anesthesia are integral parts of gynecology and obstetrics. A separate chapter on each is included.

Broader issues are also covered. A brief historical overview is given in Chapter 1. Social, psychological and sexual effects are included throughout the book, since these are important aspects of women's reproductive function and well-being. The final chapter deals with some of the legal and ethical issues that surround current gynecologic and obstetric management.

With regard to specific therapies we have generally outlined the primary procedure or treatment and followed this with a review of the incidence, diagnosis and management of the more common complications. Selected references are supplied for readers who wish further information.

MICHAEL NEWTON
EDWARD R. NEWTON

ACKNOWLEDGMENTS

We are greatly indebted to our secretaries, illustrators and editors. Our specific thanks go to Donna Moore, who typed repeated versions of the majority of the manuscript. We are also grateful to Drs. Douglas Kosa, Harold Michelwitz, Tariq Murad, Ramona Slupik and Robert Vogelsang, who contributed valuable material for illustrations.

MICHAEL NEWTON
EDWARD R. NEWTON

CONTENTS

HISTORICAL ASPECTS OF COMPLICATIONS IN GYNECOLOGY AND OBSTETRICS

1

WARREN P. NEWTON

In current medical usage, the term "complications" has two distinct meanings. It may imply progression of disease, as ureteral obstruction may be a complication of cervical cancer. Alternatively, it may imply a condition that is iatrogenic, as a severed ureter may be a complication of hysterectomy. This book focuses on iatrogenic complications.

EARLY CONCEPTS

Old medical writings and recent histories of medicine usually overlook iatrogenic complications. There are several reasons for this. First, documentary evidence of medical treatments, even those used as little as 200 to 300 years ago, is scanty, particularly with respect to women and their diseases. Second, birth and women's diseases were traditionally managed by women. Knowledge of treatment and complications was handed down orally from woman to woman and seldom reached even the few recorded medical treatises. Third, the focus on complications of therapy is itself a modern concern; older writers emphasized different issues. Fourth, historians of medicine have traditionally concentrated on the men and discoveries that anticipated or made major breakthroughs; more recently they have tended to stress the context and rationale of past medical thinkers.

Occasional references to women's problems and their management are found in early Egyptian, Mesopotamian, Chinese and Indian writings. Although complications of therapy that affected the patient were poorly understood and defined, those involving the physician were recognized, and the principle that physicians were liable for failure to cure dates from this period. Under the code of Hammurabi in Babylon, a physician could lose his life if his patient died. This penalty presumably depended upon the importance of the patient. Less severe penalties may have been imposed in other cultures, particularly if the patient were a slave or a member of an unaccepted

1

racial group, but there is no record of them having been codified. In the case of obstetrics and gynecology, there was less likelihood of punishment for failure, since women were generally regarded as being of less importance than they are at the present time, and, in addition, much of the therapy was in the hands of "wise" women and did not come to the attention of the men or the rulers.

As with many aspects of medicine, however, a fundamental contribution to the understanding of complications was made in the works attributed to Hippocrates. The hallmark of these writings was the accurate description of the natural history of disease. An account of puerperal sepsis provides an excellent example: "The wife of Dromeates, having been delivered of a female child and all other matters going on properly, on the second day after was seized with rigor and acute fever. Began to have pain about the hypochondrium on the first day; had nausea and incoherence and for some hours afterwards had no sleep. Respiration rare, large and suddenly interrupted." Knowledge of the natural history of disease is essential to understanding the complications of therapy. The physician who is familiar with the course and crises of a particular disorder is then able to gauge the effects, both beneficial and adverse, of his therapy.

Another cardinal feature of Hippocratic medicine was therapeutic minimalism. The Hippocratic writings were imbued with a non-invasive spirit. The emphasis was on the body's ability to heal itself. The therapeutics were, for the most part, gentle, with mild herbal medicines, diet, limited physical therapies and, in selected cases, surgery. Closely related was the insistence that physicians do no harm. The Hippocratic oath mandated this, and Hippocrates stated "The physician must meditate these things and have two special objects in view with regard to disease—namely to do good or to do no harm."

Soranus' *Gynecology* provides an excellent example of the attitude of an ancient gynecologist toward complications. Soranus flourished in Rome in the 2nd century A.D., during the reigns of Hadrian and Trajan. His book contained an extraordinary amount of clinical acumen, based on the theories of the Methodist School of Medicine. Methodism provided an alternative to the traditional schools of Dogmatism and Empiricism. The Dogmatist or Alexandrian school emphasized the necessity and

possibility of rational investigations as the basis of medicine. Observation and experimentation were necessary to discover the hidden causes of disease. By contrast the Empiricists rejected the attempt to learn the processes of disease as impossible and emphasized the development of therapeutics based on efficacy. The Methodists, the third and youngest sect, rejected both etiologic research and mere experience as guides for physicians. Heavily influenced by Epicurean atomism, they had in common an understanding of the body as a collection of atoms, traversed by pores, which carried bodily fluids and pneuma. Health and disease depended upon the size, shape, number and movement of the particles and the condition of the pores. It was, therefore, possible to classify diseases according to phenomena, that is, whether the symptoms represented constriction, laxity or a mixed condition of the fundamental pores. Therapy was based on this classification.

Soranus' description of what we understand as dysmenorrhea gives some insight into his understanding of treatment and complications. Dysmenorrhea was construed as a disease caused by a "constricted state." "When a constricted state develops in the region of the uterus, the menstrual flow is sometimes retained completely, sometimes it becomes difficult and painful; now colic is present and pains in the groins, loins and pubic region, now in the head, the tendons of the neck, the eyes, the hips and thighs; the breasts are swollen, appetite is lacking, the genitals are hot and dry—all of which in the woman so disposed occurs at about the time of menstruation."

Therapy was usually conservative and directed toward relaxation of the uterus. "One should put the woman to bed in a room which is moderately warm and bright and should see that she is quiet but awake and fasts completely; and one should lightly press her extremities and those parts that offer excessive pain." First line treatment, then, emphasizes gentle environmental therapy and massage. For more serious or unremitting pain, more drastic action is necessary, including venesection, vaginal packs with relaxing materials, leeches and cupping with or without scarification.

For Soranus, as for many historical authors, it is difficult to assess the attitude taken toward complications. *Gynecology* is incomplete, and there is variation in available manuscripts. More importantly, the author's purpose was not to write an exposition of complications. Rather, the book seems to have been a textbook, directed to midwives and general practitioners, which instructs from generalities rather than particulars. No case histories are given. Finally, the text follows a Methodist philosophy, and so it is difficult to generalize easily to ancient medicine as a whole.

It is apparent, however, that Soranus was aware that some treatments had bad side-effects. He warned, "The ancients were wrong in prescribing so-called blood-drawing suppositories for bringing the blood down and draughts producing the same result. They did not realize that the draughts upset the stomach while corroding suppositories ulcerate the uterus, and thus produce deep ulcerations of an evil character which heal poorly, while over the ulcerations a scar forms which is thicker than any normal flesh so that the menstrual catharsis may be retained." Acknowledgment that his treatments might cause bad effects is lacking. For Soranus, complications are conditions that follow others' therapies. The decision to give treatment was seldom the result of a calculation of risks and benefits, and the dangers of a given treatment are rarely discussed.

TECHNICAL AND THERAPEUTIC ADVANCES (1400 to 1900 A.D.)

Little new knowledge or skill was infused into gynecology and obstetrics between the 2nd and 15th centuries A.D. Although famous physicians such as Oribasius (ca 325–403), Aetius of Ameda (502-575), Trotula (11th century) and Maimonides (1135–1204) wrote on gynecologic and obstetric subjects, the theories of Galen and Hippocrates continued to dominate concepts of disease and guide therapy. In Rowland's translation of an English medieval guide to women's health, published in the early 1400s, therapy for most obstetric and gynecologic conditions consisted of a variety of complex potions, the use of suppositories, venesection or external treatments of various sorts. The possible ill effects of therapy are not mentioned.

As this epoch progressed, knowledge of anatomy (starting with Vesalius and Fallopius) became somewhat more common, and obstetric maneuvers began to be used in attempts primarily to save the mother's life but later to obtain a living child. Prominent among these were podalic version (introduced by Paré in 1549), the use of a hook (crochet) or fillet (bandage tied around part of the infant and used for traction), obstetric forceps (Chamberlen) and the first report of cesarean section. Smellie describes in detail the use of the obstetric forceps and the effects of difficult labor on the genital tract, including lacerations of the perineum and uterus, but he does not definitively connect the operative procedures with untoward consequences.

The 19th century saw the beginning of major technical advances, which greatly expanded the scope of diagnostic and therapeutic procedures and, as a result, the possibility of complications. Chief among these advances was the development of anesthesia and antisepsis/asepsis. Morton first popularized the use of ether for tooth extractions and operations in the late 1840s, and acceptance of anesthesia was rapid. Less quickly accepted was the insight of Lister that suppuration was much less likely if the operation was performed and the dressings were applied in an antiseptic fashion.

The combination of innovations made the specialty of obstetrics and gynecology possible. Cesarean sections had been performed at least as early as the 16th century, but had always been desperate measures, of great risk to the mother and undertaken only in unusual circumstances. By the end of the 19th century, however, operative obstetrics was becoming more common. Similarly, operative gynecology received a major impetus from these discoveries. Abdominal procedures such as excision of ovarian tumors became feasible. Vaginal surgery was shown by Sims to be possible and successful. Gynecologic surgery began to have its own specialists and the first modern texts of gynecology were published. Specialty journals began, and women's hospitals opened.

With new techniques came new problems. Anesthesia brought with it a whole set—the dangers of too little or too much anesthetic drug, the flammability of the ether derivatives commonly used and the dangers of emesis and aspiration of vomitus. Similarly, the interventions made possible by anesthesia and antisepsis increased the scope of operations and thus the rate of operative complications, for example, iatrogenic hemorrhage and bowel or bladder injury.

Associated with the new technical advances were the beginnings of change in the attitude taken toward the recognition of complications—the critical approach to practices, one's own and those of the past. In 1861 Semmelweis published his thesis on puerperal fever. Foreshadowed by White, Gordon and Holmes, Semmelweis proposed that major vectors for the spread of puerperal fever were physicians themselves who came to patients directly from pathology dissections. He also demonstrated that disinfection, the washing of hands prior to examining parturient or puerperal women, dramatically reduced the incidence of puerperal fever.

The response to Semmelweis was violent and hostile. Gradually, however, the bacteriologic discoveries of Pasteur and Koch took hold and the medical world began to accept his concepts. Recognition that one's own actions may be dangerous for patients is difficult at any time, no matter how complicated the technology, and the experience of Semmelweis was not new. What was new was that his ideas marked the beginning of an increased concern about iatrogenic complications.

The story of Semmelweis also underscores the importance of medical journals. Medical theories and argumentation had been present for a long time. In the latter part of the 19th century, however, modern medical journals began to develop. They were published regularly and became widely available. The growth of medical literature as a forum for debate, with a permanent record made available to a large number of people, was essential for the development of an understanding of the complications of therapy.

MODERN PERSPECTIVES

The trend begun in the 19th century has continued in the 20th. Major technical advances, radiology, antibiotics, blood banking, ultrasound and new pharmacotherapy, have greatly expanded the possibility for diagnostic and therapeutic intervention and consequently have increased the potential for complications.

The workup and therapy of an ovarian tumor dramatizes this explosive growth. In 1809, the first successful laparotomy for an ovarian tumor was performed by Ephraim McDowell in Danville, Kentucky. The diagnostic workup consisted of a history and physical examination. Therapy consisted of an operation lasting about 25 minutes without anesthesia and involving

removal of a tumor weighing 22½ pounds. No mention was made of the exact pathologic diagnosis, whether the tumor was malignant or benign, of any follow-up examinations, additional medicines to counteract fever or other difficulties.

By contrast, a woman in the 1980s, just 180 years later, who has an ovarian tumor, may undergo an extensive diagnostic and therapeutic course. Her tumor may present as an adnexal mass found on routine internal (pelvic) examination. Diagnostic studies may include ultrasonography of the pelvis and, preoperatively, an intravenous pyelogram, barium enema and various chemical tests. Exploratory laparotomy is performed and, if frozen section pathologic studies establish that the tumor is malignant, the cancer is aggressively excised at the operation. If appropriate, triple-agent chemotherapy is used for a period of time and finally a second-look laparotomy may be performed. Further treatment depends upon the progress of the disease.

At every step of diagnosis and treatment, current practices expose the patient to risk. The dye used for the preoperative intravenous pyelogram may cause an allergic reaction. Anesthetic drugs may have varied toxic effects. Intubation of the trachea may injure the vocal chords. Wide excision of the tumor may result in injury to neighboring vital structures such as the bladder, ureter or bowel. Postoperatively, chemotherapeutic drugs carry the danger of life-threatening myelosuppression and other side effects. The list of possible risks is almost endless.

Similarly in obstetrics, the transition from home to hospital and the varied operative and therapeutic techniques used in pregnancy and for delivery has saved the lives of countless mothers and babies. However, drugs to delay labor have significant cardiovascular effects. The use of oxytocin carries the risk of uterine hypertonicity. Forceps can damage the baby. Cesarean section involves the danger of infection, while the antibiotics used to counteract this have their own side effects, such as allergy to penicillin and renal damage from aminoglycosides. Resuscitation of the immature newborn may carry the risk of permanent lung damage. An important concomitant of the change in the obstetric environment and of modern technological medicine has been the emotional shock to which the woman and her partner and baby are exposed when she is subjected to a strange hospital environment and to the many different people who, for all their good will, intrude upon her person and her privacy.

In both gynecology and obstetrics, technology has also vastly increased our ability to detect complications of therapy. For example, rising blood urea nitrogen and creatinine may be the only signs of otherwise asymptomatic aminoglycoside renal toxicity. Ultrasonography of the neonate can demonstrate the intraventricular hemorrhage that may result from traumatic delivery. Moreover, changes in the delivery of care have increased the possibility of detecting complications. Patients are seen more frequently and over longer periods of time and, as a result, the physician has more opportunity to observe complications of therapy.

The scope of iatrogenic complications has grown with better understanding of the natural history of disease. Whereas, formerly, complications were viewed primarily as acts of commission, that is, the direct result of physicians' actions, now it is recognized that complications may also follow acts of omission, that is, physicians' failure to act in situations in which disease is preventable. An example is screening for Down's syndrome. The association between advanced maternal age and an increased incidence of Down's syndrome is now well established. The development of amniocentesis makes second trimester diagnosis of Down's syndrome possible, and abortion is now feasible in these cases. In a woman over 35 years of age who would choose to abort, the birth of a child with Down's syndrome has come to represent a complication of medical therapy—the omission of amniocentesis.

Malpractice litigation also represents a complication of medical therapy, and the incidence of malpractice suits has increased markedly. The belief that the patient who suffers a bad result is entitled to financial compensation has become widespread. In elaborate gynecologic as well as in other operations there is always a chance that something will go wrong. In obstetrics, the extension of possible injury and expensive disability for many years after birth while the child is a minor and incompetent increases the parents' desire for recompense. Concomitantly, recourse to the law as a method of deciding fault and the amount of recompense involved in a bad result has added enormously to the cost of medical practice. Although the liability problem applies to many enterprises, both public and private, medicine, and obstetrics and gynecology in particular, have been greatly affected by it. This is shown by the fact that many obstetrician-gynecologists are currently (1987) limiting or abandoning their obstetric practices, and other personnel, such as nurse-midwives, who might provide more obstetric care, are finding it increasingly difficult to meet the expenses of liability insurance.

Fear of malpractice as well as the explosion of diagnostic and therapeutic interventions have combined to push the cost of medical care to very high levels. At this time, expense represents a very serious complication of therapy. This is especially important in obstetrics, because the patients are young and often have limited resources. In the past, expenses had been paid primarily by the individual patient and her family. Starting in the 1930s and 1940s insurance programs began to be available whereby for the payment of a regular monthly or annual fee, part or all of the health care costs were reimbursed. With rapidly escalating expenses, however, insurance payments, never satisfactory for obstetric patients, have, in many instances, become quite inadequate. In the case of indigent patients, the government now provides partial payment. Health maintenance organizations, involving regular monthly payments and covering most medical bills, are spreading rapidly throughout the United States. The finances of medicine are in flux. In the next two decades we will see great changes in the financial complications of obstetric and gynecologic care.

In conclusion, it seems unlikely that the pace of technologic developments will slow down. The need to cope with their complications will continue. For the near future, issues of greatest concern appear to be:

1. Adequate and thorough trial of new instruments and techniques before they are put into general use.

2. Development and use of new measures to prevent side-effects of treatment.

3. Earlier recognition and management of complications.

4. Solutions to the medicolegal dilemma of whether fault is present or not and to the standardization of recompense for complications.

5. Methods of dealing with the financial, legal and ethical complications implicit in the availability and limitation of resources.

6. Understanding that the Hippocratic precept "to do no harm" must be modified to the effect that "rarely is there cure without the chance of harm."

Selective Bibliography

Adams F: *The Genuine Works of Hippocrates (translated)*. Baltimore, Williams & Wilkins, 1939.

Carter K (translation): *Ignaz Semmelweis. The Etiology, Concept and Prophylaxis of Childbed Fever*. Madison, University of Wisconsin Press, 1983.

Cianfrani T: *A Short History of Obstetrics and Gynecology*. Springfield, IL, Charles C Thomas, 1960.

McDowell E: Three cases of extirpation ovarii. *Eclectic Rep. Anal. Rev.* 7:242, 1817.

Rowland B: *Medieval Woman's Guide to Health*. Kent, OH, Kent State University Press, 1981.

Smellie W: *A Treatise on the Theory and Practice of Midwifery—Facsimile Printing*. London, Scolar Press, 1974.

Speert H: *Obstetric and Gynecologic Milestones*. New York, The MacMillan Co., 1958.

Speert H: *A Pictorial History of Gynecology and Obstetrics*. Philadelphia, FA Davis Co., 1973.

Steinberg W, Muntner S: Maimonides' views on gynecology and obstetrics. *Am. J. Obstet. Gynecol.* 91:443, 1965.

Temkin O: *Soranus' Gynecology (translated with an Introduction)*. Baltimore, Johns Hopkins Press, 1956.

PRETREATMENT AND PREOPERATIVE COMPLICATIONS

2

MICHAEL NEWTON

EVALUATION OF RISK

Any operation, procedure or treatment in gynecology and obstetrics carries some risk to the patient. The extent of the risk depends not only on the type and severity of the therapy but also on the health status of the individual woman. The purposes of this chapter are to outline a standard pretreatment evaluation and to describe the further management of specific problems in the various organs that must be resolved before therapy. The primary emphasis will be on the gynecologic patient; the special problems of pregnant and puerperal women are considered in Chapters 8 to 11.

Any patient for whom an operation, procedure or treatment is recommended should have a thorough evaluation, including a history, a physical examination, indicated laboratory studies and relevant consultation with appropriate specialist(s). How complete and detailed should this evaluation be? There is no easy answer. It is clear, however, that on the initial visit to the office or clinic a detailed history (subjective assessment), including past history, family history and social history, should be obtained. This can be done by the physician himself, by having the patient complete a check list after which the positive findings can be explored further by the nurse or the physician, or by computer, with data being supplied by the patient assisted by an office worker. Special aspects of the history that need to be included are sexual history, nutritional status and presence of allergies. General and pelvic examinations (objective assessment) should be complete and performed by the physician or by a nurse-practitioner with physician backup. A good idea of the risk status of the patient and the procedures that may be necessary to optimize her pretreatment condition will then already have been developed.

Laboratory studies are not usually included in this initial assessment because the results are not immediately available. When specific tests and consultations are indicated, a final opinion regarding risk status may have to await reports. Even if the picture is clear, however, certain routine laboratory studies should precede full assessment. Opinion regarding these varies with the practice of the individual gynecologist and the procedure to be performed. As a minimum, the initial workup should probably include a complete blood count and urinalysis. A pregnancy test is often indicated if there is doubt about the menstrual pattern. In women over the age of 40, blood chemistry surveys, a chest x-ray and an electrocardiogram should be added. Once these baseline assessments have been made, they should be updated later if another operation or procedure is contemplated. Formal listing of risk factors on the patient's chart is helpful.

Finally, and most importantly, the operation or procedure (and alternative therapies) and the known or expected risks and complications must be discussed with the patient. Often this can be done at the first visit, but further discussion at another visit may be required. Information should be as complete as a reasonable person would expect, and it must be expressed in language that the patient can understand, not in medical jargon. When possible a significant family member should be present at this interview. Questions should be answered simply and directly (see page 33).

AGE

Childhood

In children the history, physical examination and operative and postoperative management sometimes present problems. For the prepubertal child (under 11 years of age) the historical data must usually be obtained from the parent, commonly the mother. Problems with birth, major congenital anomalies and childhood illnesses should be identified. Examination is limited by the child's size and unfamiliarity with the procedure. Younger children are best examined while held on their mothers' laps. A simple explanation of the technique of examination is often understood at a younger age than one expects. It should never be omitted in the child who is over six months of age. Use of a doll may be effective. It is often helpful to know the particular family word used for the female genitalia or for functions such as urination and defecation. Nevertheless, the examiner should

use ordinary anatomic terms as well as the vernacular. In the pelvic examination the external genitalia may easily be inspected if cooperation and rapport have been established. Vaginal examination is not usually feasible in the prepubertal child. Recto-abdominal examination is almost always possible, usually with the examiner's index finger. When the vagina has to be inspected because of bleeding, discharge, congenital anomaly or the possible presence of a foreign body, a pediatric speculum or vaginoscope, as described by Huffman (1981), can be used. If the examination is difficult but crucial to the diagnosis, anesthesia may be necessary.

When operations upon children are contemplated the gynecologist should be aware that anesthetic difficulties may be encountered if the anesthesiologist is not familiar with techniques appropriate for children. Operating instruments need to be of the proper size. The postoperative recovery of children may present a problem to staff unaccustomed to dealing with them. They may, therefore, be better managed in a children's hospital or in a specific children's unit. For example, facilities for parents to stay with their young children are essential.

Adolescence

Adolescents are sometimes embarrassed and reluctant to discuss gynecologic problems and to be examined, and this behavior may be exaggerated by their mothers' reactions. When possible it is best to talk to the girl without the mother, at least for some part of the consultation, and to treat her as an intelligent adult woman who is capable of understanding the reason for the examination. Actually, inspection of the vagina and cervix is usually possible in adolescents with a small Graves or Pedersen speculum, particularly if the girl has started to menstruate and has used tampons. Adolescents can usually be handled operatively and postoperatively on an adult gynecologic floor, provided that visiting privileges are liberal and the staff is sensitive to their needs.

Reproductive Years

Between the ages of 12 and 45 (menarche to perimenopause) preoperative complications are most likely to be due to coincidental diseases rather than to any characteristic of age itself.

However, the major preoperative concern in women of this age group is reproductive function—its preservation, enhancement or termination. This concern means that the patient's menstrual and reproductive histories are very important as well as her sexual involvements and expectations for future pregnancies. The effect of the proposed procedure on these must be fully discussed. For example, the extent of an operation for leiomyomata must be limited, if possible, to myomectomy if the patient is very anxious to conceive; if the patient has completed her family and is in her 40's, hysterectomy may be appropriate. The reaction of the patient's partner to any procedure must also be carefully considered in patients in this and in older age groups.

Perimenopausal Years

Between the ages of 45 and 55 preservation of reproductive potential is less important to the patient. To many women cessation of menstruation by hysterectomy presents no concerns. In the past 10 years public question about the necessity of hysterectomy has made many patients anxious to preserve uterine function and to have their ovaries conserved unless to do so represents a threat to their lives. These considerations demand careful preoperative evaluation.

Postmenopausal Years

With the average life expectancy of women now at 75 years, gynecologic procedures on women over the age of 80 and even 90 are becoming more common. Preoperative and pretreatment conditions that add risks to the operation or procedure are more common in older women (Adkins and Scott, 1984). Thus, more thorough evaluation is necessary. Ultraradical operations (exenteration or extensive debulking for ovarian cancer) are not well tolerated by the older woman. Postoperative recovery from an operation or procedure is likely to be slower. For example, there may be a greater likelihood of respiratory difficulties because the lung has less reserve capacity, and intestinal function may return to normal more slowly than in the younger woman. Most importantly, the change from home to hospital puts a greater stress on the older woman. This stress is exaggerated when she requires convalescent care by family or friends away from her usual surroundings.

METABOLISM

Fluid, Electrolyte and Nutritional Deficiencies

Metabolic alterations include acute fluid and electrolyte changes, chronic nutritional inadequacies and specific disorders such as diabetes or endocrinologic abnormalities. The majority of gynecologic and obstetric patients are relatively healthy and will not be undergoing life-threatening procedures. For other than minor procedures they need screening for electrolyte and fluid balance and for the specific diseases described in the following sections. Screening is generally best done by obtaining a blood chemistry survey (SMA 6, 12 or 20). Laboratory values listed in this section should be regarded as representative only, since they vary from hospital to hospital. A general estimate of nutritional status should also be made, but a detailed nutritional evaluation is not usually necessary. Women with more serious problems such as cancer or major pelvic infections require, in addition to screening, a thorough assessment of nutritional status.

FLUID AND ELECTROLYTE IMBALANCE

Assessment. Changes in body fluid concentrations (dehydration or overhydration), in acid-base balance and in serum electrolyte levels are rarely due to specific dietary and metabolic alterations or malnutrition. They are most likely to be caused by the patient's disease. These changes often occur together, but frequently one may predominate. Fluid volume deficit, i.e., dehydration, can be recognized clinically by the patient's thirst, dry mouth and loss of skin turgor; it is frequently associated with vomiting and inadequate intake of fluids. Fluid volume overload is seldom seen preoperatively, except in patients with heart disease and from iatrogenic causes, and it is characterized clinically by edema, particularly in the feet, sacrum and face.

Common causes of acid-base imbalance, particularly in gynecologic patients with cancer, are vomiting, sequestration of fluid (third space) or renal disease. Vomiting due to gastric, duodenal or high jejunal obstruction leads to loss of chloride and potassium, resulting in excess bicarbonate and metabolic alkalosis (bicarbonate concentration over 35 mEq/liter), and the blood pH is generally high. In obstruction of the lower jejunum and ileum with vomiting, the electrolytes lost are similar to those in plasma, and all plasma levels may be lower. Some sequestration of fluid in the intestine may also occur under these circumstances, exaggerating the fluid volume deficit. In renal disease, severe diarrhea and some enterocutaneous fistulas, excess chloride and bicarbonate are lost, leading to metabolic acidosis and a fall in blood pH to less than 7.35.

Electrolyte disorders may be summarized as follows:

Hyponatremia (blood sodium concentration less than 125 mEq/liter) is characterized by excess water or water intoxication. It is commonly due to fluid replacement without salt, renal disease, metabolic oxidation of food, mobilization of water from cellular breakdown or low total body sodium. Hyponatremia is accompanied by weight gain and may be associated with weakness, confusion, nausea and vomiting and, rarely, convulsions.

Hypernatremia (blood sodium concentration more than 155 mEq/liter) is accompanied by a decrease in the fluid in the intracellular compartment because increased osmolality of the extracellular space draws fluid from inside the cells. It may be due to sepsis, renal disease, central nervous system injury or disease or nonketotic hyperosmolar dehydration caused by diabetes or high glucose concentrations associated with intravenous hyperalimentation. Thirst and disorientation are the chief symptoms.

Hypokalemia (blood potassium concentration less than 3.0 mEq/liter) is usually due to continued loss of potassium and inadequate replacement; prolonged use of diuretics may also be responsible. Neuromuscular weakness, paresthesia and paralysis may be noted. The most important effect is on the heart; bradycardia and arrhythmias may be seen, and the toxic effects of digitalis are exaggerated.

Hyperkalemia (blood potassium concentration more than 5.0 mEq/liter) is seen primarily in renal failure. Cardiac effects—bradycardia, ventricular fibrillation and cardiac arrest—are important.

Hypocalcemia (blood calcium concentration less than 7.5 mEq/liter) may occur when other electrolyte levels fall due to vomiting or renal disease or in association with parathyroid disorders. Since 45% of the calcium is bound to albumin, a low calcium value must be corrected upward if the albumin is also low (0.8 mEq for each 1.0 gm of serum albumin below 4.5 gm/100 ml). Muscular irritability and twitching are noted. A positive Chvostek's sign (tapping the

facial nerve anterior to the ear produces twitching of the facial muscles) may be elicited; this sign is not always pathognomonic.

Hypercalcemia (blood calcium concentration greater than 11.0 mEq/liter) may occur in malignancy when there is considerable bone destruction or may be associated with excessive use of a diuretic or with parathyroid disease. It is characterized by muscular weakness, depression and confusion, even simulating organic brain syndrome.

Hypomagnesemia (blood magnesium concentration less than 1.5 mEq/liter) occurs in prolonged vomiting as other salts are lost or in renal disease, especially that due to chemotherapy with cisplatin. Weakness is a characteristic symptom.

Treatment. Restoration of fluid volume changes, electrolyte levels and acid-base alterations to normal is urgent and should certainly be undertaken before operation, since the stress of anesthesia and the procedure may further alter them and lead to more dangerous levels. It is important to remember the following points:

1. The normal daily requirements (Table 2–1) of fluid and electrolytes must be maintained. Over the short term these needs can be met by intravenous administration of the equivalent of two units of 1000 ml 5% dextrose in water, with 20 mEq of potassium chloride, and 500 ml of normal saline. This solution should maintain a urine output of 1000 ml or more daily.

2. Continuing losses, for example, from gastric or intestinal suction, must be replaced as they occur.

3. Additional fluid and electrolyte deficits can be calculated from the blood chemistry data, and the patient's needs should be supplied accordingly.

Table 2–1. Daily Fluid and Electrolyte Losses*†

	Water (ml)	Sodium (mEq)	Potassium (mEq)
Urine	1500	10–40	40
Feces	200	0–20	2–3
Insensible			
Lungs	400	–	–
Skin	400	10–60	1–2
Total	2500	50–90	40–45

*Loss varies with ambient temperature, age and loss from other organs.

†Adapted from Proctor HJ: Fluid and electrolyte management. In Hardy JD (ed.): *Textbook of Surgery.* Philadelphia, JB Lippincott, 1983, p. 27.

4. Restoration of deficits to normal should be carried out over 24 to 48 hours, not hastily within the first few hours.

5. A multivitamin preparation should be added daily to the intravenous fluid to avoid deficiencies and to improve postoperative wound healing.

6. Plans for fluid and electrolyte replacement cannot be laid out for 48 or even 24 hours in advance. They must be determined every six to 12 hours, depending upon the patient's clinical condition and urine output and the results of blood chemistry studies.

7. Fluid and electrolyte replacements are temporary measures. No fat or protein is supplied, and the amount of calories is limited. Either the problem needs prompt correction within five to seven days with return to oral feeding or intravenous hyperalimentation should be considered.

Specific electrolyte deficiencies are managed as follows. Hyponatremia may often be controlled simply by restriction of fluid, use of normal saline and rarely, but not in older patients, the use of hypertonic (3%) saline. Hypernatremia may be corrected by intravenous 5% dextrose in water or oral fluids, together with treatment of the underlying pathologic process. Hypokalemia is corrected by intravenous potassium chloride in amounts of 40 mEq/ liter of intravenous fluids given over at least four hours. Oral intake of potassium is important (Table 2–2). Hyperkalemia is treated by discontinuing all obvious sources of potassium. Prompt but temporary reversal of hyperkalemia may be obtained by hypertonic glucose (50 ml of 50% solution) with 10 to 25 units of regular insulin or (if the patient is not receiving digitalis) intravenous calcium, 5 to 10 ml of a 10% solution of calcium gluconate. Over the longer term a cation-exchange resin, which binds potassium in the intestine in exchange for sodium, can be given by mouth or by enema, e.g., sodium polystyrene sulfonate (Kayexalate), 40 to 80 gm daily. Hypocalcemia can be corrected promptly by intravenous infusion of 10 to 20 ml of a 10% solution of calcium gluconate. Oral calcium gluconate (1 gm every two to four hours) may also be given. Additional therapy such as vitamin D may be needed if a diagnosis of hypoparathyroidism is made. Hypercalcemia is managed initially by hydration with normal saline together with furosemide, 40 to 100 mg every six to 12 hours. Oral phosphate, 2 gm per day, or calcitonin, 3 to 8 MRC units per kg intramuscularly every six hours, are useful if

Table 2–2. Foods High in Potassium

Food	Portion	Potassium (mEq)
Cantaloupe	half, small	13.0
Squash, baked	half cup	12.0
Banana	one, small	9.0
Radishes	ten	8.0
Cauliflower, cooked	one cup	7.6
Broccoli	half cup	7.0
Tomatoes	half cup	6.5
Strawberries	one cup	6.3
Peach	one, medium	6.2
Orange juice	half cup	5.7
Orange	one, medium	5.1

hydration fails. In patients with malignancy, mithramycin 25 mg/kg intravenously (repeated weekly) may be of help. Hypomagnesemia is treated by intravenous magnesium sulfate (2 mE/kg every four hours) and/or oral magnesium oxide, 600 to 1200 mg/day.

NUTRITIONAL DEFICIENCIES

Assessment. General evaluation of nutritional status should be a part of any history taken prior to the performance of an operation or procedure. Criteria of deficiency used for screening include:

1. History of debilitating illness, e.g., cancer, prolonged infection, intestinal disorder such as ulcerative colitis or terminal ileitis or anorexia nervosa.

2. History of inadequate intake of food, especially proteins and vitamins. If this is not easily ascertained, a standard 24- or 48-hour dietary history may be helpful (Jain et al, 1982).

3. Excessive intake of tobacco, alcohol or other harmful substance.

4. Weight 10% under or 20% over that expected for the patient's age and bone structure (Table 2–3).

Specific evaluation of the potentially undernourished individual identified by screening is usually advisable if the patient is to undergo a major operative procedure. Unfortunately, nutritional assessment is not yet a precise science. Details of current methods and standards are given by Blackburn and co-workers (1977) and Orr and Shingleton (1984). Among the methods used are the following:

GENERAL APPEARANCE. The greatly undernourished (starving) individual appears gaunt and wasted with deepset eyes and hollow cheeks, muscular atrophy and weakness.

Table 2–3. Metropolitan Height-Weight Tables for Women (1983)*†

Height (Ft & In)	Small Frame	Medium Frame	Large Frame
4–10	102–111	109–121	118–131
4–11	103–113	111–123	120–134
5–0	104–115	113–126	122–137
5–1	106–118	115–129	125–140
5–2	108–121	118–132	128–143
5–3	111–124	121–135	131–147
5–4	114–127	125–138	134–151
5–5	117–130	127–141	137–155
5–6	120–133	130–144	140–159
5–7	123–136	133–147	143–163
5–8	126–139	136–150	146–167
5–9	129–142	139–153	149–170
5–10	132–145	142–156	152–173
5–11	135–148	145–159	155–176
6–0	138–151	148–162	158–179

*Weight according to frame (ages 25–59) for women with indoor clothing weighing 3 pounds and shoes with 1-inch heels.

†Adapted from Metropolitan Life Insurance Company, New York, 1983.

WEIGHT CHANGES. Involuntary loss of 5 to 10% of body weight during the preceding three months is a warning sign. A loss of more than 10% of body weight is evidence of a serious problem.

LOSS OF MUSCLE MASS. This can be appreciated by noting the size of the arms and legs; often loss of muscle mass is best perceived by a spouse or close friend. Measurements of mid-arm circumference for triceps skinfold thickness are useful, particularly if prior measurements are available for comparison.

HEMATOLOGIC DATA. A low hemoglobin level (less than 11.5 gm) may be indicative of poor nutrition as well as loss of blood.

BLOOD CHEMISTRIES. Serum albumin is a good marker for nutrition. Standards vary in different laboratories. A value of less than 3.5 gm/100 ml is indicative of decreased protein synthesis, increased loss or turnover of protein or both. Determination of levels of transferrin, a major iron-binding protein, may be helpful in determining nutritional status. Normal levels are 180 to 260 mg/ml, but lower figures are found in patients with anemia. If the hemoglobin level is normal, the transferrin levels may be helpful. Retinol-binding protein and prealbumin may also be helpful in the future, but it is difficult to measure their concentrations accurately because of their short half-lives. These tests are expensive, but they may help in following the progress of nutritional status.

NITROGEN EXCRETION. The amount of creatinine excreted in urine measures muscle mass and its metabolism. The normal excretion for women is 16 to 20 mg/kg over 24 hours, determined from a carefully collected 24-hour specimen of urine. With a normal plasma creatinine level, 24-hour excretion below the expected normal range indicates hypometabolism of muscle and suggests a diminished skeletal muscle mass. Nitrogen balance may also be important. The 24-hour excretion of urea in urine +3 gm (for women) equals the total nitrogen excreted. If the intake is known, positive or negative nitrogen balance can be calculated.

IMMUNOLOGIC ASSAYS. Decreased immunocompetence is a sign of nutritional deficiency and impairs the body's response to infection. Immunocompetence is a complex process involving a number of host defences only some of which can be measured. Total lymphocyte count has been used as one index. Less than 1000 lymphocytes/mm^3, calculated from total and differential white blood cell counts, may indicate deficiency in nutrition and immunocompetence. Delayed hypersensitivity (DH) has been used extensively to determine immunocompetence; 0.1 mg of recall skin antigens such as *Candida albicans*, mumps, streptokinase-streptodornase, dermatophytin or intermediate strength PPD (purified protein derivative) is injected intradermally in the forearm, and the area is inspected at 24 to 48 hours. A 5 mm area of induration is considered positive, and a positive reaction to one or more antigens is considered to demonstrate immunocompetence.

Treatment. If the diagnosis of severe nutritional deficiency is made, preoperative correction, at least partial, is indicated (Girtanner, 1985). This consists of an attempt for several days and probably no longer than a week to give sufficient protein and calories. If the oral route and sufficient time are available, a high protein diet can be supplemented by high protein snacks, some of which contain specific amino acids, so as to give a daily protein intake of 100 to 125 gm with 2500 to 3000 calories. The assistance of a dietitian to select appropriate supplements and to exhort and help the patient is essential.

In patients with an intact intestinal tract but inability to ingest the required additional food, enteral feeding may be given through a nasogastric tube. A No. 8 French pediatric (or smaller) feeding tube is inserted and a constant infusion (pump) of dietary solution is given over

16 or 24 hours. There are many nutritional low residue diets available; all contain simple sugars, l-amino acids, electrolytes, minerals and trace elements. The concentration of the solution can be varied. The diet should be started slowly and increased gradually up to, if necessary, 4000 calories/day. Complications of tube feeding include nausea, vomiting, diarrhea, abdominal cramps, distention, fluid and electrolyte imbalance and aspiration. The last may be a special potential problem in older patients and may require discontinuing the infusion at night and when the patient is sleeping, even though night-time feeding allows the patient more normal mobility during the day.

Total parenteral nutrition (TPN) may be used when the enteral route is not available. This does not occur very frequently in obstetric-gynecologic patients except in those with marked prenatal malnutrition or with severe infections or cancer. In the last situation malabsorption may occur because of intestinal obstruction, major bowel resection, small bowel fistula, radiation enteritis or severe nausea and vomiting, especially with chemotherapy. TPN is not a technique to be used lightly, since it is expensive and there are significant complications.

Total parenteral nutrition must be given through a central venous line because of the hyperosmolality of the solution and the consequent danger of venous inflammation and thrombosis. The subclavian vein is most commonly used, the right in preference to the left so as to avoid injuring the thoracic duct. The external or internal jugular veins can be used but are less comfortable for the patient. Various techniques of catheter insertion have been described (Peters, 1983). A single (or double) lumen catheter, best inserted over a guide wire, is satisfactory.

There are certain technical requisites for central venous catheters. Insertion should be done or supervised by someone with experience. Once inserted for hyperalimentation, a single lumen catheter should only be used for that purpose. Preferably, blood should not be given nor withdrawn through a single-lumen central line, nor should antibiotics or other medication be administered through it. The less the catheter is manipulated, the better. Use of an occlusive plastic dressing avoids the need for frequent changing; once a week is often sufficient. Usually the catheter does not need to be replaced unless it becomes occluded or is thought to be infected. A guide wire should be

used for replacement. A double lumen catheter is more difficult to insert, but may avoid the use of a peripheral vein for other needed venous access. A subclavian catheter may be left in place for an indefinite time. If access is required for many months, such as for repeated courses of chemotherapy or home hyperalimentation, a more permanent tunnelled catheter is preferable. For this a Hickman, Broviac or similar catheter is inserted and brought out lower on the chest wall through a subcutaneous tunnel; this is a full surgical procedure and is more complicated than the simple insertion of the subclavian line.

Complications of TPN are related to (1) the catheter (see previous discussion and Chapter 12), (2) the solution used, (3) infection and (4) metabolic changes. Continuing supervision by an experienced nutrition team provides the best care for the patient with a catheter. Most major hospital pharmacies now make up sterile hyperalimentation solutions. They should be freshly prepared and used within 24 hours. These solutions should contain amino acids and 50% dextrose in sufficient amounts to provide a minimum of 2000 calories per day together with electrolytes (sodium, potassium, chloride, phosphate, magnesium and calcium) and vitamins sufficient for daily requirements, and weekly additives that include folate, vitamin K, zinc, copper, manganese, chromium and fat in the form of a fat emulsion (Rayburn et al, 1986).

Infections related to the central line are a cause for concern. Patients receiving hyperalimentation may have many reasons for fever. If the temperature is over 101°F on two occasions four hours apart, a search should be made for the source, i.e., pulmonary, urinary tract, intraperitoneal or pelvic infection or tumor necrosis. Often catheter sepsis is diagnosed by exclusion, although it is suggested by pain, redness or swelling at the site of catheter entry. If the evidence points to the catheter being responsible, it should be removed by using a guide wire, and a new catheter inserted if there is need for TPN to be continued. Appropriate antibiotics should be given (see Chapter 12).

Metabolic complications are related to the hypertonic glucose used and to electrolyte imbalance or to deficiencies of trace elements. The individual response to glucose infusion varies. Therefore, the solution should be started slowly and increased to the full amount over 48 to 72 hours. In the first three to four days the concentration of sugar in the urine should be followed closely, and the blood sugar level should be tested two to four times daily. A blood chemistry survey should be done every two days and later twice a week. Hyperalimentation solutions often do not maintain hemoglobin at an adequate level, and transfusion of packed cells may be needed every two to four weeks, especially if other factors leading to anemia are present.

The duration of hyperalimentation varies with the circumstances. For preoperative preparation a maximum of seven days is usually sufficient. Postoperatively, to aid healing, one to two weeks may be adequate if the patient's gastrointestinal tract returns to normal function. Long-term hyperalimentation (at home) may be continued for months or even years, but is seldom necessary in obstetrics and gynecology unless the gastrointestinal tract is permanently without function. Continued hyperalimentation in patients with cancer may be useful in those receiving chemotherapy in the expectation of cure, but when the disease is progressing it serves to feed the cancer rather than the patient.

Diabetes

Diabetes is an important complication prior to and after gynecologic operations of any sort. Patients with diabetes are prone to develop arteriosclerosis, renal disease and neurologic disorders, especially if the disease was first manifest in childhood or has existed for a long time. Uncontrolled diabetes may of itself lead to ketoacidosis, hyperosmolar coma, intracellular dehydration and subsequent delayed wound healing and impaired response to infection. Stress and alterations in food intake and activity that are associated with even minor procedures must always be taken into account.

Diabetes may be discovered for the first time prior to operation. A history of diabetes in the family, large babies (over nine pounds) in a woman of average size or excessive thirst or urination may be important. A screening fasting blood sugar (normal 72 to 110 mg/dl), or one hour (greater than 170 mg/dl) or two hour (greater than 120 mg/dl) blood sugar determination after a glucose load of at least 100 gm is the first step in diagnosis. If these figures are only slightly elevated, i.e., less than 200, 250 or 200 mg/dl, respectively, then one can proceed with the planned operation and monitor the patient as indicated in the following discussion. Later the diabetes may need to be more carefully controlled. If the blood sugar levels are moderately high (up to 250, 350 or 250 mg/dl), the patient needs careful monitoring, and she may require subcutaneous insulin if glycosuria is present or the blood sugar level rises above 350 mg/dl. If the blood sugar levels are high (greater than 350 mg/dl in any specimen), the diabetes needs to be brought under reasonable control before the operation. This can usually be done satisfactorily and within two to three days by giving small doses of insulin (5 to 10 units) subcutaneously on a regular six-hour basis, prior to meals, and varying the dose according to blood (or urine) sugar concentrations.

If it is known that the patient has diabetes (growth-onset or adult-onset type), an accurate history of the medication taken should be obtained. For diabetes that is under fair control with diet alone or with oral antidiabetic agents, management should be along the lines discussed before. If the patient is insulin-dependent and the diabetes is under at least fair control (blood sugar level less than 250 mg/dl), the dose of long-acting insulin needs to be adjusted so that the patient receives half of it in the morning prior to operation, and additional regular insulin is given subcutaneously in small amounts as determined by blood or urine sugar determinations. The usual dose of long-acting insulin can then be resumed when the patient has adequate oral intake of food. The patient's inactivity after operation must be taken into account when ordering diet and insulin. Many patients with growth-onset diabetes and those with either type who are taking large amounts of insulin or whose blood sugar levels appear to rise and fall precipitously will require more precise management. It is generally better for the responsible surgeon to manage the orders for a diabetic patient, using an internist as a consultant if necessary, since the surgeon or his housestaff is likely to see the patient with the frequency necessary for proper management.

HEMATOPOIETIC SYSTEM

Evaluation

Assessment of the patient's hematopoietic status helps the obstetrician-gynecologist to ascertain and correct preoperative blood loss or poor nutritional status and also to predict and take precautions against excess intraoperative or postoperative bleeding. A thorough history is most important. It includes inquiries about familial bleeding tendencies, the patient's experience with prolonged bleeding from previous procedures or minor injuries, easy bruisability and the ingestion of prescription or over-the-counter medications that may have hematologic consequences. Among the more important of these drugs are oral contraceptives (increased coagulability), aspirin (decreased platelet thromboxane B_2 levels or abnormal template bleeding times) (Ferraris and Swanson, 1983), indomethacin (myelosuppression), warfarin (anticoagulation) or chemotherapeutic agents (myelosuppression). Many other drugs have been implicated in hematologic problems. On physical examination the skin may show bruises and evidence of minor injuries; these may indicate a bleeding tendency and remind the patient of previous bleeding episodes. If the history and physical examination do not suggest a hematologic disorder, elaborate laboratory studies are of little help. However, a complete blood count, sickle cell test and hemoglobin electrophoresis may give a clue to unsuspected anemia or another disorder. More detailed tests are valuable primarily in providing a baseline for intraoperative and postoperative tests, especially when large blood loss is anticipated, many replacement transfusions are likely or prophylactic anticoagulants are to be given.

Many factors are involved in the coagulation process. When a blood vessel is injured, platelet adhesion occurs with release of various platelet factors, causing vasoconstriction and forming a platelet plug in small vessels. At the same time, as a result of various factors (extrinsic and intrinsic systems), prothrombin is converted to thrombin, which then changes fibrinogen to fibrin with the aid of Factor XIII and calcium. Combined with the platelet plug, fibrin produces the hemostatic plug. Figure 2–1 shows a simplified schema of the mechanism of hemostasis. For a more detailed account of hemorrhagic disorders see Salzman (1983).

Although it is possible to identify specific coagulation factors, practically speaking, two tests, one-stage prothrombin time (PT) and partial thromboplastin time (PTT), are most useful in identifying a general coagulation problem. PT is prolonged in deficiencies of Factors I (fibrinogen), II (prothrombin), V, VII and X, whereas PTT is prolonged in deficiencies of Factors I, II, V, VIII, IX, X, XI and XII. Determination of bleeding time or deficient platelet function (adhesiveness) may identify von Willebrand's disease or toxicity due to drugs such as aspirin. Measurement of fibrinogen levels and fibrin split products may be important, particularly in disseminated intravascular coagulation (DIC) syndromes.

Anemia

Anemia of any degree implies a decrease in the oxygen carrying power of the blood. It puts stress on the cardiovascular and respiratory systems and magnifies the expected operative blood loss, thus increasing the risks of the procedure. Anemia is evidence of a chronic

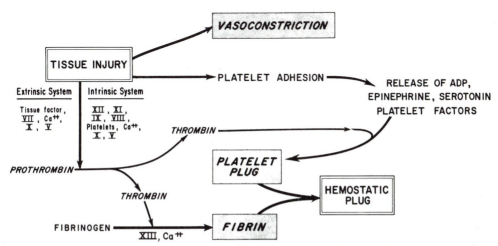

Figure 2–1. Mechanism of hemostasis. (Reprinted with permission from Salzman EW: Hemorrhagic disorders. In American College of Surgeons: Manual of Preoperative and Postoperative Care. Philadelphia, W. B. Saunders Co., 1983.

deficiency. In acute blood loss fluid shifts do not occur immediately, and the anemia is not apparent until 12 hours to as long as four days after the loss.

Borderline anemia is present when a patient's hemoglobin level is 10 gm/dl or more but less than 13 gm/dl or her hematocrit is 30% or more but less than 40%. In frank anemia the hemoglobin level is less than 10 gm/dl and the hematocrit is less than 30%. Borderline anemia usually does not require treatment prior to minor operations, although its cause and management should be a matter of concern. Before major procedures patients with borderline anemia may need therapy, depending upon the likelihood of major blood loss and the extent of the procedure, e.g., radical hysterectomy or exenteration. Frank anemia usually requires treatment prior to major procedures and may require it before minor operations.

If treatment for anemia is indicated and the operation is elective, there is often time to build up the patient's hemoglobin concentration by diet and supplementary oral iron. When the anemia is marked (hemoglobin level less than 8 gm/dl) or the need for the operation is urgent, transfusion with two or more units of packed red cells is appropriate. For complications of transfusions of blood or the use of other blood products see Chapter 3.

Sickle Cell Syndromes

Persons who are heterozygous for hemoglobin S have sickle cell trait. About 8% of black Americans are in this category (usually less than 50% HbS). They have few clinical problems. No special preoperative preparation is needed, but anoxia during anesthesia should be minimized because of the remote danger of sickle cell crisis or damage to the renal medulla.

Sickle cell anemia (homozygosity for hemoglobin S) occurs in 0.15% of black children in the United States. Because of decreased life expectancy of persons with sickle cell anemia, its incidence is lower in adults. The clinical picture is characterized by impairment of growth, vaso-occlusive phenomena in many organs with painful crises and anemia. The last is usually severe with hematocrits between 18 and 30% and a short mean red cell survival of 10 to 15 days. Infection and folic acid deficiency can induce acute hemolytic crises. Women with sickle cell disease are at high risk for operations and procedures, since complications such as stress, anoxia and infection predispose to hemolytic crises. Transfusions so that over 50% of the patient's red blood cells are of donor origin may be helpful temporarily.

Other Hematologic Disorders

The treatment of specific blood dyscrasias or coagulopathies is outside the scope of this book. When an offending drug can be withdrawn, the problem can be solved effectively. However, in some cases operations are contraindicated by the hematologic disorder unless they are lifesaving. Such is the case in patients with thrombocytopenia or marked leukopenia. In others, the administration of blood or blood products may provide a temporary improvement during which a necessary operation can be performed. In all instances careful evaluation of the individual patient and the risks involved is necessary.

INFECTIONS

It is important to find out if an acute infection is present before an operation or procedure because untreated infection may jeopardize the operation and because it may make the diagnosis of postoperative complications more difficult. Important clues may be obtained from a thorough history and physical examination, in which the presence of fever is the most important sign. Other signs may indicate a local infection, for example, of the upper respiratory tract or the bladder, or fail to point to a specific site. Results of laboratory studies may corroborate evidence of general infection, e.g., leukocytosis with an increase in immature cells, or specific problems such as white blood cells and bacteria in the urine.

Current concern about sexually transmitted diseases (STD) requires that a history of these problems be thoroughly investigated. In particular, patients at risk for acquired immune deficiency syndrome (AIDS) should be identified by questions such as (1) Have you had sex with a bisexual man? (2) Have you had sex with a man who is an IV drug user? and (3) Are you an IV drug user?

Specific infections are covered under the separate organ systems discussed later. Further diagnostic steps required to identify the type of general infection include chest x-ray, blood cultures (for unexplained temperature over

102°F), serologic tests and virologic tests. For detailed descriptions of general infections a textbook of infectious diseases should be consulted. The presence of an unexplained fever or infection is generally cause for delaying an operation unless the operation is urgent. If a specific infection has been diagnosed, it should preferably be cured prior to the operation. However, immediate control and/or adequate antibiotic levels are usually sufficient, particularly if the operation is designed to treat the infection, e.g., drainage of a tubo-ovarian abscess.

Apart from active infection, certain factors increase the possibility of postoperative infection (Table 2–4). In patients who have one or more of the first six factors listed in Table 2–4, tests of immunocompetence should be considered, since the function of the immune system may affect response to infection. Tests are similar to those used to evaluate nutritional status and include the less precise studies (serum albumin and transferrin levels, arm muscle circumference and creatinine concentration), height index and the more specific but as yet not definitive tests for cellular and humoral immunity such as skin testing with delayed hypersensitivity antigens, total lymphocyte counts and serum levels of immunoglobulins and complement.

Prophylactic antibiotics appropriately used reduce the incidence of postoperative infection. While these antibiotics are covered in relation to specific organ systems and operations, a few general principles are important:

1. In clean operations in which the intestinal tract, urinary tract and vagina are not entered, the risk of complications from the antibiotics usually exceeds the possible reduction of incidence of infection.

2. In potentially contaminated operations such as hysterectomy or cesarean section, prophylactic antibiotics are often indicated.

3. The first dose of a prophylactic antibiotic should be given just before (one hour) operation, and one to three doses should be given thereafter.

4. Cephalosporins, for example, a first or second generation agent, are the most useful and generally effective agents to use prior to obstetric and gynecologic procedures (Cartwright et al, 1984).

CARDIOVASCULAR SYSTEM

Hypertension

Evaluation of blood pressure is an important part of the preoperative workup since about 20% of women may have hypertension and be asymptomatic. Upper limits of normal are generally considered to be 140/90, with the diastolic component being the most important. Since blood pressure varies with anxiety, physical activity, discomfort or stress, a single determination is inadequate. If the blood pressure is found to be elevated, it should be taken again one or more times in different positions. A fall to normal indicates labile hypertension; little change indicates stable hypertension.

Since blood pressure is usually measured early in the course of a physical examination, there is ample opportunity to determine other relevant physical signs and whether the hypertension is labile or sustained. These include careful examination of the heart, palpation of the arteries in the arms and legs and fundoscopic examination for retinopathy. If the hypertension appears to be labile, routine diagnostic laboratory tests, including electrocardiogram and chest x-ray, usually suffice. If the hypertension is mild (systolic pressure less than 160 mm Hg, diastolic pressure less than 100 mm Hg), most elective procedures can be undertaken, although the patient should later be encouraged to attempt control of her blood pressure by weight reduction, moderate salt restriction and exercise under the supervision of her family physician or internist. Moderate or severe hypertension (sustained systolic pressure of 160 mm Hg or over or diastolic pressure of 100 mm Hg or over) requires medical con-

Table 2–4. *Factors Predisposing to Postoperative Infection**

Malnutrition
Age over 65
Type and severity of underlying disease
Prolonged hospitalization
Recurrent or remote infection
Recent antibiotic therapy
Immunosuppressive drugs
Anergy to skin tests
Poor tissue perfusion (shock, vasoconstriction)
Obesity
Indwelling catheter

*Adapted and reprinted with permission from Alexander JW: Infection, host-resistance and antimicrobial agents. In American College of Surgeons: *Manual of Preoperative and Postoperative Care.* Philadelphia, WB Saunders Company, 1983.

sultation and possibly further studies to identify any specific cause. Moreover, in elective operations, it is generally best for the blood pressure to be under reasonable control prior to operation because of the risk of coronary infarction or significant arrhythmias.

If a patient is already known to be hypertensive and is receiving medications, it is usually best to continue these up to the time of operation and immediately postoperatively so that the blood pressure will remain under control. However, it is important to be sure that no electrolyte imbalance exists, as, for example, in hypokalemia associated with some diuretics. Also the anesthesiologist should be alerted to the patient's possible increased risk.

Heart Disease

Preoperative screening for heart disease consists initially of a detailed history. Specific inquiries should be made about (1) heart disease in the family, (2) heart murmurs in childhood (congenital heart disease?), (3) rheumatic fever or rheumatic heart disease, (4) chest pain, (5) exercise tolerance, (6) palpitation or irregular heart beat, (7) evidence of heart failure (e.g., shortness of breath, especially at night, or persistent swelling of the ankles) and (8) heart medications. Physical examination of the heart for murmurs, arrhythmias and signs of heart failure is also important. An electrocardiogram is essential. These measures should identify the presence or likelihood of heart disease. Significant types of heart disease include:

Valvular Disease

This may be due to rheumatic fever or another cause and includes mitral valve prolapse. Although the significance of mitral valve prolapse (especially when diagnosed primarily by echocardiography) is not entirely clear, the possibility of such patients developing endocarditis when bacteremia occurs has to be considered. Therefore, antimicrobial prophylaxis is usually important prior to any surgical procedure, including minor ones such as D & C, which may cause bacteremia. Although modifications of the regimen may be necessary in individual cases, recommended prophylaxis for gastrointestinal and genitourinary procedures (American Heart Association Guidelines) is as follows:

Ampicillin (2.0 gm intramuscularly or intravenously) plus gentamicin (1.5 mg/kg but not over 80 mg intravenously or intramuscularly) or

streptomycin (1.0 gm intramuscularly) should be given. Initial doses are given 30 to 60 minutes prior to the procedure and may be repeated eight hours later. If the patient is sensitive to penicillin, vancomycin (1.0 gm intravenously) and gentamicin (as described earlier) should be given 30 to 60 minutes prior to the procedure and may be repeated in eight to 12 hours (Yurt, 1985).

It should be remembered that obstetric and gynecologic patients with valvular heart disease are at the same risk of endocarditis from common dental and upper respiratory tract procedures. They need prophylaxis with penicillin or, if they are sensitive to penicillin, with erythromycin.

Heart Failure

Patients whose heart failure is well controlled by medication such as digitalis are at slightly increased risk of recurrent failure during and immediately after an operation. This risk is greater in obstetrics immediately after delivery when the placental shunt is suddenly closed. Monitoring levels of digoxin or other cardiac glucosides is useful. Patients who are found to be in heart failure when evaluated preoperatively should be treated and be in as stable a condition as possible before the operation. In emergency situations rapid stabilization of the patient's condition with digoxin is indicated. As an example, digoxin may be given orally or intravenously in doses of 0.5 mg immediately and 0.25 mg every eight hours for three doses. Therapeutic levels of digoxin are 0.8 to 2.0 ng/ml.

Coronary Artery Disease

Patients who have a history of recent myocardial infarction have a 30% chance of repeat infarction intraoperatively or postoperatively. This falls to 15% at six months but is still 5% one year or more after the initial event. Therefore, elective procedures are best postponed, if possible, for at least six months in these patients. Patients who have angina are also at risk of infarction. The necessity of deferring the operation has to depend upon the degree of organic heart disease and the importance of the procedure. In both cases medication given prior to operation should be continued.

Arrhythmias

Bradycardia (heart rate 60 BPM or less) and tachycardia (heart rate 120 BPM or more) usually require preoperative investigation as does atrial fibrillation. Ventricular premature beats may be of significance, particularly if they are associated with organic heart disease, since they may in some instances presage ventricular tachycardia. Atrial premature beats are common and usually of little significance.

Cerebrovascular Disease

The hemodynamic changes and stress of anesthesia and operation increase the risk of cerebrovascular accidents (CVAs), whether from thrombosis, embolism, hemorrhage or ischemia, especially in women over 50 years of age.

PREDISPOSING FACTORS

These should be ascertained during the preoperative history and physical examination. They include:

History of Prior CVA. This means that another CVA is more likely, particularly if additional predisposing factors are present (see subsequent section). Residual cranial or spinal nerve defects more certainly identify a previous cerebral event.

History of Transient Ischemic Attacks. These are important because the risk of stroke occurring in the first year following such an attack is 6 to 7%. This rises to over 30% in five years. An ischemic attack is often difficult to identify. It is usually brief, lasting from a few seconds up to 30 minutes, occasionally longer, and consists of a transient "strange" feeling accompanied by symptoms localized to any part of the brain or spinal cord, e.g., transient monocular blindness, dizziness or muscle weakness.

Hypertension. Sixty per cent of cerebrovascular thromboses are associated with hypertension, especially if the blood pressure is greatly elevated, i.e., over 200/110. Therefore, control of blood pressure to a lower or even normotensive level is desirable before elective operations.

Diabetes. Twenty-five per cent of cerebrovascular thromboses are associated with diabetes. The effect of strict control of blood sugar upon the risk of stroke is not known clearly. However, it would seem prudent as a preventive measure to maintain reasonable control of the diabetes (blood sugar levels consistently under 250 mg/dl).

Other Factors. Heart disease, especially arrhythmias such as atrial fibrillation, and infec-

tion such as subacute bacterial endocarditis carry the risk of emboli being detached perioperatively. Oral contraceptives increase the risk of cerebrovascular disease by a factor of 4. How much this is affected by operations is not known. However, these medications should preferably be discontinued for at least one month in young women who are to undergo elective major operations.

MANAGEMENT

For an elective operation the risk of CVA must be balanced against the benefit of the proposed procedure. In any case and certainly in emergency situations, blood pressure and oxygenation must be maintained as well as possible, sudden falls in blood pressure, oversedation and rapid diuresis avoided, and hypotension and anemia promptly corrected.

Arterial Disease

Arterial disease is usually the result of atherosclerosis—a generalized and long-standing process. Discovery of arterial insufficiency in one part of the body, for example, the legs, implies the presence of vaso-occlusion in other areas such as the heart or brain, in which acute vascular occlusion may be a grave or even fatal event. Therefore, a history of pain in the legs on walking with recovery on resting or the absence of arterial pulsations in the feet or in the popliteal artery are important findings. Vasospastic disorders, such as cold sensitivities of various sorts, although of importance in themselves, are not so significant as far as complications of operations are concerned.

Venous Disease

Venous thrombosis and the subsequent silent detachment of a clot with the development of pulmonary embolism are among the most important complications of gynecologic procedures. The presence of clots in veins and the possibility of embolism must be evaluated preoperatively. It should be noted that many reports on thromboembolism (TE) are derived from the study of general or mixed surgical patients, and relatively few from the study of gynecologic patients alone.

PREDISPOSING FACTORS

Thromboses in the pelvic and leg veins are important in respect to local consequences and the possibility of emboli. Thromboses in the veins of the arm are common results of venipuncture to obtain blood samples or to give intravenous medication; they are rarely associated with pulmonary embolism. Their management is discussed in Chapters 4 and 12.

Both general and local factors predispose to pelvic and leg vein thromboses (deep vein thromboses or DVT). General preoperative risk factors include age, obesity, history of thrombotic (embolic) episodes and varicose veins. The presence of malignant disease is also important, particularly if migratory thromboses have occurred. Local risk factors include injury to the vessel wall, increased blood viscosity and stasis of blood. Injury to the large veins in the pelvis or to their tributaries can easily occur during radical procedures or even during a hysterectomy or minor operation for benign disease. Increased blood viscosity may result from hypercoagulability, for example in women taking oral contraceptives or in those with polycythemia. Changes in blood viscosity may also explain older findings of a higher incidence of pulmonary emboli in the spring and fall and of phlebothrombosis in the same seasons and with passage of a cold weather front, i.e., a rise in barometric pressure and a fall in temperature and humidity (Newton, 1951).

EVALUATION

It is possible to predict preoperatively the patient who may be at risk for postoperative thrombosis or embolism. An accurate history is most important. Clayton and co-workers (1976), in a study of 124 patients about to undergo major gynecologic procedures, developed a prognostic index based on obesity, weight and the presence of varicose veins. Preoperative stay in the hospital and presence of malignant disease were also important, but did not add further precision to the prognosis.

Venous thrombosis in the leg, especially in the calf, is often silent. Sometimes it may be detected on physical examination. In the thigh, tenderness may be noted over the course of the femoral vein. In the calf tenderness may be elicited on side-to-side or anteroposterior compression of the muscles. Pain in the calf may also be noted on sharp dorsiflexion of the foot with the knee relaxed (Homan's sign) (Fig. 2–2). Laboratory studies found by Clayton and co-workers (1976) to be useful were the euglobulin lysis time and the serum fibrin-related antigen level. Neither of these, however, is generally available. Doppler flow and impedance plethysmography may be helpful (Schroeder and Dunn, 1982). The ^{125}I fibrinogen test, described by Kakkar (1972), is reliable and has the advantage that repeated scans can be obtained postoperatively both as a routine precaution and if deep venous thrombosis is suspected. Venography is a definitive diagnostic procedure, but it is invasive and difficult to perform in the very obese patient. It should be used only when a diagnosis is urgently needed. The value of these tests as routine preoperative examinations has not been fully studied or established. Rather, the trend has been to take prophylactic measures in all patients who may be at risk.

PROPHYLAXIS

Prophylactic measures against thromboembolism may be taken preoperatively, intraoperatively and postoperatively. Preoperative and

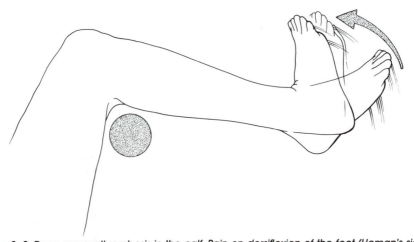

Figure 2–2. Deep venous thrombosis in the calf. Pain on dorsiflexion of the foot (Homan's sign).

intraoperative prophylaxis are closely related and will be considered together in the following discussion. Postoperative prophylaxis is covered in Chapter 4. Various preoperative measures have been used, indicating that no single one is completely successful. Older methods, now no longer used, included bilateral superficial femoral vein ligation and the use of warfarin products. The former is a major operative procedure and the latter is not easily reversible. Current methods include:

Adequate Physical Activity. Ambulation and leg movement are important, especially in the chronically ill or elderly patient. Increasing activity in these women before operation is essential.

Mechanical Stimulation of the Calf Muscles. Lindstrom and co-workers (1982) noted a decrease in both pulmonary embolism (PE) and DVT when the calf muscles were stimulated during operation by electrodes that had been placed preoperatively.

Compression of Calf Muscles. Calf muscles can be compressed passively by the use of fitted elastic stockings or actively by intermittent pneumatic compression. Short elastic stockings up to the knee are probably ineffective. On the other hand, full length hose, worn prior to, during and after operation, were found to be effective by Caprini and associates (1983). The disadvantages of long elastic hose are that some obese patients cannot be properly fitted, that postoperative movement by the patient is hampered and that avoidance of creases in and maintaining proper position of the stockings require constant attention.

Intermittent compression of the legs has been found to provide good prophylaxis against PE and DVT. Using pneumatic calf compression (Venodyne) during and for five days after operation Clarke-Pearson and co-workers (1984) found a significant decrease in PE and DVT in 55 patients undergoing major operations for gynecologic cancer as compared with 52 similar control patients not so treated. A compression device that sequentially compresses the lower calf, upper calf and thigh may be more effective in emptying blood out of the leg veins.

Antithrombotic Agents. Drugs with antiplatelet properties such as aspirin or persantin (dipyridamole) may be of value in patients with transient ischemic attacks or coronary insufficiency. However, the side effect of bleeding makes them unsuitable for use before, during or after operation.

Dextran. The use of Dextran 70 (molecular weight about 70,000 daltons) as prophylaxis

against postoperative PE and DVT was first described in the late 1960s. Subsequently Dextran 40 (molecular weight about 40,000 daltons) has also been used. The action of both is thought to decrease platelet adhesiveness and increase perfusion of smaller vessels. Although several methods of administration have been described, a common one has been to infuse 500 ml of 6% Dextran 70 at the beginning of the operation and then again at the end and/or during the first 24 hours postoperatively. Dextran 70 has been found to be effective prophylaxis. McCarthy and co-workers (1974) compared, in a prospective randomized study, the use of Dextran 70 with low-dose heparin and noted no significant difference in the incidence of DVT. Other studies, for example, that of Gruber and co-workers (1980), have confirmed the effectiveness of Dextran 70. Problems with the use of Dextran have been allergic reactions, 1.1% according to Gruber and co-workers (1980), and fluid volume overload and hemorrhage. The last occurs with similar frequency as when prophylactic heparin is used (see next section).

Heparin. Heparin has been widely used in recent years to prevent PE and DVT. Its action results from its ability to bind and activate antithrombin III, a heparin cofactor. Antithrombin III inhibits several activated coagulation factors in addition to thrombin, including factors IXa, Xa, XIa and XIIa. Clinically a near normal blood flow, as determined by Doppler flow studies, is maintained in the legs (Barsoum et al, 1982). Prophylactic heparin has generally been given in doses of 5000 units one to two hours before operation and every eight to 12 hours postoperatively for five to seven days. There is probably less risk of hemorrhagic complications if heparin is given every 12 hours rather than every eight hours. Regimens of this type have commonly been found to reduce thromboembolism. However, precise data and comparisons are difficult to obtain because different types of patients and operations are often included in the same series and because the diagnosis of both PE and DVT may be inexact. Moreover, there have been relatively few studies covering gynecologic patients alone. In patients with gynecologic cancer the effectiveness of prophylactic heparin has been summarized by Kotz and Geelhoed (1981). However, in a small randomized study of similar patients, Clarke-Pearson and associates (1983) found that low-dose heparin was of no prophylactic benefit. Low–molecular weight heparin (6000 daltons) has been shown by Kakkar and co-workers (1982), when given once a day, to have a prophylactic effect similar to unfractionated heparin (mean molecular weight 16,000 daltons).

Heparin and Dihydroergotamine. Dihydroergotamine appears to act synergistically with heparin. It has no effect on the coagulation system but increases the tone and capacitance of vessels and the velocity of blood flow within them. Clinically, in a multicenter randomized trial of 880 patients undergoing major surgical procedures (64 gynecologic operations) dihydroergotamine 0.5 mg with heparin sodium 5000 units two hours preoperatively and every 12 hours for five to seven days postoperatively proved significantly more effective in reducing deep venous thrombosis, detected by ^{125}I fibrinogen scan, than either drug alone, dihydroergotamine 0.5 mg with 2500 units heparin or placebo (Sasahara, 1984).

Complications of Prophylactic Anticoagulants. Bleeding in various forms is the most common complication of heparin prophylaxis. Even with prophylactic measures, postoperative thromboembolism still occurs in some patients. Moreover, in the Multicenter Study reported by Sasahara (1984) excessive bleeding at operation occurred in 2.6% of cases, hematoma at the injection site in 10.6%, hematoma in the wound in 2.3% and microscopic hematuria in 23.1% on postoperative day three and in 17.3% on day five. There were only minor variations with the different prophylactic regimens. Among gynecologic patients undergoing vaginal and abdominal hysterectomy and major gynecologic oncology procedures, increased blood loss has been noted. However, the loss has not been reported to be life-threatening. Minor bleeding at injection sites leading to bruising also troubles the patient although, again, it is not serious. Following radical vulvectomy and inguinal lymphadenectomy Piver and co-workers (1983) noted an increased incidence of lymphocysts in women receiving prophylactic heparin or Dextran. The reason for the hemorrhage is probably the higher heparin levels in the blood, but thrombocythemia and subtle effects may occur in a variety of coagulation factors. For further complications of anticoagulant therapy see Chapter 4.

PRACTICAL CONSIDERATIONS

Since TE is a serious and often silent complication of major and even minor procedures, preoperative evaluation of risk is essential. History and physical examination are most useful.

Diagnostic tests such as Doppler flow studies, ^{125}I fibrinogen scans or venography should probably not be performed routinely but only if current thromboembolic disease is suspected.

As prophylactic measures, discontinuation of potentially thrombotic medications such as oral contraceptives and adequate preoperative activity are essential for all patients. In obese, high-risk patients over 50 years of age who are undergoing major operations, additional measures are advisable. Compression of calf and/or thigh muscles by continuous or intermittent pressure is associated with few complications, but is more difficult for the anesthesiologist and the nursing staff to implement; it also makes movement and postoperative ambulation more cumbersome. Anticoagulants such as 5000 units of heparin with or without dihydroergotamine (0.5 mg) given one to two hours before and every 12 hours for five to seven days after the operation are easy to administer and apparently effective. However, they cannot be used in patients with abnormal coagulation factors and carry a small but definite risk of hemorrhagic complications.

EYES, EARS AND RESPIRATORY SYSTEM

Eye, ear, nose and throat symptoms, although important in themselves, may also be manifestations of other intracranial or systemic diseases such as brain tumors or other disorders or hypertension. These possibilities must always be kept in mind when a patient complains of EENT problems.

Eyes

Acute eye disorders are rarely coincidental with emergency obstetric or gynecologic procedures but may influence the timing and management of elective operations. Chronic eye disorders must be taken into account when planning or scheduling elective or emergency obstetric or gynecologic procedures.

Examination of the eyes is often omitted or performed perfunctorily by obstetrician-gynecologists. A screening history should, however, include inquiries about deficiencies in vision (especially recent changes), use of glasses or contact lenses, pain in the eye, swelling or itching, discharge from the eye or eyelids, unusual light flashes, black spots or incomplete vision. Screening examination includes inspection of the eye, rough determination of visual acuity and ophthalmoscopic examination. The latter is particularly important in evaluating such general diseases as hypertension or diabetes or, in pregnant women, preeclampsia.

The following ophthalmologic diseases require attention either because continued care is needed or because consultation with an ophthalmologist is indicated.

Acute, recent changes in vision require investigation before elective or semi-elective procedures. Patients who are blind need special care and instruction and sympathetic understanding of their problems. Patients who use glasses or wear contact lenses should only be deprived of their sources of vision when they are unconscious or unable to handle their own equipment; myopic individuals are particularly sensitive to this deprivation. Glasses and contact lenses should be returned to the patient promptly after operative procedures.

Tearing, spots in front of the eyes or photophobia usually require no treatment except reassurance. Conjunctivitis (redness of the conjunctiva) may be caused by bacteria, viruses or allergies. Antibiotic drops (10% sulfonamide) or ointment (0.5% erythromycin) may be helpful, especially if pus is present.

Pain in the eye unexplained by a local condition is usually of importance and requires consultation. Gross changes in visual fields should be investigated, since they may be associated with brain disorders.

Ear, Nose, Mouth and Throat

EAR

Routine preoperative examination of the ears is usually confined to a brief review of symptoms, an estimate of hearing acuity and examination of the external ear and external auditory canal. Significant complaints referable to the ear include hearing loss, dizziness, tinnitus, earache and discharge from the ear.

Hearing loss is usually not acute, is worse with increasing age, and is frequently partial and worse on one side than the other. Two points are important. First, the deaf person may not understand instructions and explanations unless one fully engages her attention and speaks slowly and distinctly into her good ear. Second, the deaf person who wears a hearing aid is like a person who cannot see well. Her hearing aid should not be removed unless she

is unconscious and should be restored to her promptly after the operation. Occasionally wax in the ear canal may cause some degree of deafness. The wax can usually be removed by easing it out with a blunt curette or loop. Audiometry does not usually need to be done preoperatively, although it may be helpful for the future management of the patient's deafness.

Dizziness may be a symptom of local disease, e.g., eustachian tube blockage, or of eighth cranial nerve malfunction; it should usually be carefully investigated. Tinnitus is often a symptom of drug use such as aspirin—an important piece of information, especially in regard to possible platelet malfunction and excessive operative bleeding. Pain in the ear may be associated with external or middle ear infection and also with other infections in the head and neck; it usually requires investigation and consultation. Discharge from the ear is a sign of external or middle ear infection and usually requires investigation, consultation and possibly preoperative treatment with antibiotics.

NOSE

Detailed preoperative examination of the nose is not usually necessary, being confined to a brief history and external examination. Significant symptoms are as follows:

Nasal Obstruction and Discharge. These may be due to an acute upper respiratory tract infection or to an allergic response. The former is usually accompanied by malaise and sore throat. The latter is more chronic and related to seasonal or other allergens. Acute upper respiratory tract infections should lead to postponement of an elective operation; allergic rhinitis can usually be treated with appropriate antihistamines before and after the procedure.

Pain. Pain in the area of the face or forehead may be due to sinusitis. This requires investigation and consultation.

Epistaxis. Epistaxis is a common nasal symptom. It should raise the question of hypertension or vicarious menstruation, but it is generally due to localized erosion of vessels in the nasal vestibule and can be treated locally by compression and instruction of the patient to avoid traumatizing the area.

MOUTH AND THROAT

Examination of the mouth is important for the identification of loose or absent teeth or evidence of ulceration. Loose teeth may be further damaged or knocked out during induction or maintenance of anesthesia unless special care is taken. The absence of teeth may be important in chronically ill patients pre- or postoperatively, since nutritious pureed or liquid food will be necessary to maintain or improve nutritional status. Patients who have false teeth will have to have them removed for anesthesia, but, as with other appliances, teeth should be restored as soon as possible since without them patients are unable to eat properly and feel embarrassed.

Inspection of the throat for redness or enlarged tonsils is important in identifying upper respiratory tract infection. Symptomatic pharyngitis may require bacterial culture while very large and/or infected tonsils may even obstruct the patient's airway.

Examination of the larynx is not normally a part of the preoperative evaluation. Hoarseness, the most significant symptom, unless it is related to an acute respiratory tract infection, is an indication for consultation.

Lower Respiratory Tract

ASSESSMENT

A history of previous lung disease, recurrent pneumonia, bronchiectasis, smoking, shortness of breath on exertion and current symptoms of cough, pain in the chest or hemoptysis should warn of a potential problem. Physical findings may confirm the impression of lung disease; of particular importance is the presence of emphysema with an enlarged thoracic cage and limited expansion on deep breathing. A chest x-ray (PA and lateral views) is essential because abnormalities can be found that were not discovered during the history or physical examination.

Respiratory function can be screened by simple tests requiring no special equipment.

1. Breath-holding. If the patient is unable to hold her breath for more than 10 seconds, she probably has considerably reduced respiratory reserve.

2. Expiration. Inability to exhale completely within four seconds indicates expiratory obstruction.

3. Match test. If the patient cannot blow out a match held three inches from her widely open mouth, her forced expiratory volume (FEV) is likely to be less than 1.6 liters (see following section).

Standardized pulmonary function tests (spi-

Table 2–5. Pulmonary Function Tests

Test	Normal	Restrictive Lung Disease	Obstructive Lung Disease
FVC	3L	Decreased	Normal
FEV_1	2L	Normal	Decreased
FEV_1/FVC	70%	Normal or High	Decreased
FEF_{25-75}	1.6L/sec	Normal	Decreased

rometry) are readily available and non-invasive. They should be performed prior to any major operative procedure or before one requiring general anesthesia in women with suspected lung disease, in heavy smokers (one pack or more per day) and in those over 65 years of age. Such tests can determine whether a patient has significant restrictive or obstructive lung disease. The former may be due to pain, atelectasis, pneumothorax, pleural effusion or obesity; the latter may be due to smoking, asthma or emphysema.

The simplest and most informative pulmonary function test is the measurement of the amount of air that can be forced out after a maximum inspiration (forced vital capacity or FVC). The amount of air that can be expelled in the first second of such expiration (FEV_1) and in the first three seconds (FEV_3) is also important. The maximum midexpiratory flow is a measure of the mean flow rate in the middle half of the forced expiration (FEF_{25-75}). The results of spirometry are usually expressed as a percentage of expected function. Table 2–5 shows expected figures for a "normal" woman together with the changes indicative of lung disease. In addition the results of FEV_3 may be indicative of small airway disease.

Severe lung disease is indicated by an FVC of less than 1200 cc or an FEV_1 of less than 800 cc. When moderately or severely decreased function is found, arterial blood gas determinations should be obtained. The normal range for pH is 7.38 to 7.41, for $PaCO_2$ is 38 to 43 mm Hg and for PaO_2 is 70 mm Hg or greater.

MANAGEMENT

Patients with No Pulmonary Disease. Preoperative instruction in deep breathing is most important for all patients over 50 years of age and for those about to undergo major or prolonged procedures. This can be done by personal teaching by the nursing staff or respiratory therapist or by the use of an incentive spirometer. Since smokers are prone to postoperative pulmonary complications they should, in addition, be encouraged to stop smoking for a minimum of 24 hours prior to operation, or, if that is impossible, to reduce the number of cigarettes smoked during that time.

Patients with Lung Disease. The precise nature of a lung disorder should be determined as well as possible before operation and appropriate treatment given. In emergencies such treatment may have to be abbreviated or even omitted, but the additional risks of postoperative pulmonary complications must be recognized by the anesthesiologist and by the obstetrician-gynecologist during the postoperative course.

ASTHMA. About 3% of the population have asthma; it is more common in young women. Typically it is an episodic disorder triggered by a variety of allergic and other factors that cause bronchial constriction; it may be persistent as in status asthmaticus. It is characterized clinically by cough, dyspnea and expiratory wheezes. The patient will usually give a history of asthmatic attacks and be aware of the medication (bronchodilators) used to control them. Expiratory wheezes and emphysema may be demonstrable on physical examination of the lungs. Chest x-ray is seldom diagnostic. Alterations in the results of respiratory function tests depend on the severity and duration of the disease. It is important to be aware of the possibility of an asthmatic attack, so that the use of drugs causing histamine release, such as narcotics and curare, can be minimized and treatment for asthma can be readily available. Treatment consists of (1) epinephrine, 0.5 ml of 1:1000 solution, (2) aminophylline (6 mg/kg initially in 20 min and 0.45 mg/kg/hr thereafter) or (3) aerosolized bronchodilators such as isoproterenol. In severe cases consultation with an internist specializing in respiratory diseases is advisable; in these situations the risk of any major operative procedure is greatly increased.

INFECTIONS. When the patient has a history of repeated lower respiratory tract infections due to viruses or bacteria such as bronchitis or bronchiectasis, it is desirable to obtain a sputum culture and give prophylactic antibiotics, preferably a cephalosporin (see Chapter 4), before and after the operation. Current infections should be treated adequately, when possible, prior to operation.

PLEURAL EFFUSION. Significant amounts of fluid in the pleural cavity should be removed preoperatively by thoracentesis both for diagnosis and to improve lung function.

PRIMARY OR METASTATIC LUNG CANCER. This may be related to the gynecologic disorder being treated, e.g., cancer of the corpus uteri or ovary. The abnormal findings should be further elucidated by CT scan of the lung, sputum cytology, bronchoscopy or guided needle biopsy.

CHRONIC OBSTRUCTIVE PULMONARY DISEASE (COPD). This may be due to chronic bronchitis, emphysema or abnormalities in the smaller airways. Although history, physical examination and x-ray changes may be helpful for diagnosis, the important question is how much lung function is impaired. Pulmonary function tests show that FEV_1 is reduced and the FEV_1/VC (vital capacity) and FEV_1/FVC ratios are usually reduced to less than 60% with significant COPD. Supporting evidence is obtained from the finding of a low (less than 60%) PaO_2. The danger of COPD is the possibility of postoperative development of acute respiratory failure or adult respiratory distress syndrome. Unfortunately, there is no good treatment for established COPD. When sputum is present, respiratory physical therapy such as postural drainage with clapping and vibration may assist in expectoration of sputum. Deep breathing exercises with emphasis on expiration are particularly valuable in preparing to counteract the usual postoperative respiratory depression. Intermittent positive pressure breathing (IPPB) is of uncertain value, but high humidity helps prevent inspissation of sputum in the bronchioles, which may lead to further obstruction.

GASTROINTESTINAL TRACT

Preoperative management of the gastrointestinal (GI) tract involves two principles, the detection and treatment of prior or current gastrointestinal disease and the preparation of the intestine so as to minimize postoperative complications.

Diagnosis

Prior GI disease may or may not be relevant to the success of a gynecologic operation, but it is important for the surgeon to know about it. A screening history of previous operations or treatments and a review of current GI symptoms is of first importance. Common conditions and their chief symptoms include:

Hiatus hernia—regurgitation of bile, upper abdominal distress, melena.

Gastric or duodenal ulcer and carcinoma of

the stomach—epigastric pain relieved by food, possible nausea and vomiting, weight loss, melena.

Cholecystitis or cholelithiasis—attacks of right subcostal, back or shoulder pain; intolerance of fatty food.

Small bowel obstruction—history of abdominal operation(s), intermittent crampy abdominal pain, distention, nausea and vomiting, constipation and failure to pass gas.

Inflammatory small bowel disease (Crohn's disease)—crampy and steady abdominal pain, blood in stool (usually occult).

Inflammatory large bowel disease (ulcerative colitis)—intermittent diarrhea, often severe; mucus and blood in stool.

Large bowel obstruction and carcinoma of the colon—increasing constipation, occasionally alternating with diarrhea; late nausea and vomiting; blood in stool.

Diverticulitis—intermittent lower abdominal pain, perhaps with fever; constipation; blood in stool.

Hemorrhoids—bright red blood in stool, especially associated with constipation; pain on defecation.

If any of the listed conditions are suspected prior to elective or semi-elective operations, further investigation is indicated. Physical examination of the abdomen may suggest intestinal obstruction—distention, hyperactive peristalsis with rushes, pelvic or abdominal mass—but is not very helpful in revealing the other conditions listed. Routine laboratory studies will disclose major abnormalities in blood count or electrolyte concentrations. Further studies may include ultrasound (gallstones), upper GI contrast x-ray films (gastric or duodenal ulcer or high intestinal obstruction), flat plate x-ray films of the abdomen (obstruction with excess air and fluid levels in small or large intestine), small intestinal contrast x-ray films (inflammatory disease, obstruction), large intestinal contrast x-ray films (colonic obstruction, diverticulitis) or proctoscopy, sigmoidoscopy or colonoscopy (disease of colon, rectum or anus). More elaborate studies include ultrasonography, CT scans or MRI (abdominal or pelvic masses).

With so many tests available it is essential to prioritize them and arrange them in a way that is most convenient and least disturbing to the patient. For example, if colonic obstruction is suspected, endoscopy should be performed first and then a barium enema x-ray. To give barium by mouth runs the risk of increasing the ob-

struction with inspissated barium. Ultrasound examination of the gallbladder can most easily be performed prior to x-ray contrast studies. If urinary tract contrast studies are to be obtained, they should precede GI studies, because residual barium in the intestine may obscure renal and ureteral details. For all tests it is important that the physician and the nurses or other personnel be fully aware of the preparation required and the possible discomforts of the tests, and that these be explained fully (and in writing) to the patient in advance.

Management

When a diagnosis of gastrointestinal disease has been established a decision must be made by the obstetrician-gynecologist, usually with consultation from an internist, whether or not to treat it prior to operation. In elective or even semi-elective cases treatment is necessary for acute gallbladder disease, complications of peptic ulcers such as hemorrhage or obstruction or for very active inflammatory bowel disease. However, in the case of intestinal obstruction (small or large bowel) or diverticulitis, the exact diagnosis may depend on surgical exploration. In this case either the operation should be performed by a gynecologist experienced in major pelvic operations and intestinal surgery or a consultant general surgeon should be readily available.

Preoperative Preparation of the Intestine

When no GI disease is present or suspected and major anesthesia and/or laparotomy is planned, the bowel should be as empty as possible before operation to minimize the possibility of aspiration of gastric contents and of postoperative ileus. This is most conveniently done by withholding oral intake for at least eight hours before operation and by emptying the lower colon and rectum with an enema or suppository, usually given the night before operation. When oral medication *must* be given immediately before operation, this may be done with a very small amount of water. In an emergency it may be necessary to empty the stomach by means of a nasogastric tube just before the operation or after induction of anesthesia.

When there is a possibility that the intestines

Table 2–6. Preoperative Bowel Preparation*

Day 1:	Low-residue diet.
	Bisacodyl, 1 tablet at 6 p.m.
Day 2:	Continue low-residue diet.
	Magnesium sulfate, 30 ml of 50% solution (15 gm) at 10 a.m., 2 p.m., and 6 p.m.
	Saline enemas in evening until return clear.
Day 3:	Neomycin, 1 gm, and erythromycin base, 1 gm, orally at 1 p.m., 2 p.m., and 11 p.m.
	Clear liquid diet.
	Magnesium sulfate, 30 ml of 50% solution at 10 a.m. and 2 p.m.
	No enemas.
	IV maintenance fluids started in afternoon.
Day 4:	Operation in a.m.

*Reprinted with permission from Condon RE, Nyhus LM: *Manual of Surgical Therapeutics*, Ed. 6. Boston, Little, Brown and Co., 1985.

may be entered with consequent intraperitoneal bacterial contamination or that intestinal anastomoses or construction of stomas may be necessary, additional preparation is indicated. The essential steps are: (1) a low-residue diet, (2) laxatives or cathartics and (3) intestinal antibiotics. Although various protocols are available, a useful one is shown in Table 2–6. Modifications may be made for individual patients. For example, fewer laxatives may be given to elderly patients (who tolerate diarrhea poorly) or the regimen may be shortened when the chance of intestinal involvement is less, as for an ovarian cyst in a relatively young woman that has little likelihood of being malignant. Intestinal intubation is seldom necessary prior to the usual gynecologic procedures, although with primary and recurrent ovarian cancer or severe pelvic inflammatory disease it may be indicated. The technique and complications of intubation are covered in Chapter 4.

Diseases of the Liver, Pancreas and Spleen

A history of hepatitis, jaundice or gallbladder disease (infection or stone) requires further investigation. Hepatitis may be exacerbated or prolonged by anesthesia and a major operation, and it may lead to deteriorating liver function as well as being an infection hazard to other patients and medical personnel. Jaundice may be related to many local and generalized diseases such as obstruction of the common bile duct, metastatic lesions or other liver diseases or a hemolytic process. Gallbladder problems

such as cholecystitis or common duct obstruction may appear first postoperatively.

Screening liver function tests are of help. They are usually part of screening blood chemistry tests and, as such, should be obtained routinely before major operations and before other procedures and treatments if liver disease is suspected. Liver function tests may be affected by many factors within and outside the liver. However, determination of concentrations of bilirubin, alkaline phosphatase and enzymes such as aspartate transferase (AST, formerly SGOT) and alanine transferase (ALT, formerly SGPT) are most useful. Bilirubin is indicative of the extent of jaundice, but is not diagnostic of its origin. A high alkaline phosphatase level suggests an obstructive process, whereas a high AST (SGOT) or ALT (SGPT) concentration suggests hepato-cellular disease.

If the history is positive for hepatitis with or without abnormal screening tests, antigen-antibody studies for hepatitis are appropriate (Table 2–7). If a specific diagnosis of liver disease can be made, consultation with an internist is advisable. More refined chemical tests can be performed. Further investigation of the liver parenchyma by CT scan, radioisotope studies, needle biopsy or angiography or of the gallbladder and bile duct by ultrasonography or endoscopic procedures may be indicated.

Diseases of the pancreas may be suspected because of a history of repeated attacks of upper abdominal pain, biliary tract disease or alcoholism. Serum amylase levels, ultrasound and a CT scan are the most helpful steps in a difficult diagnostic process.

Diseases of the spleen are usually traumatic or secondary to other disorders. Acute or subacute rupture of the spleen with peritoneal signs, shoulder pain and evidence of blood loss may be confused with rupture of an ectopic pregnancy or other gynecologic source of intraabdominal bleeding. The most common sign

Table 2–7. Tests for Hepatitis

Stage of Disease	Hepatitis A	Hepatitis B
Early, acute	Hepatitis A antigen (HAAg) IgG antibody	Hepatitis B surface antigen (HBsAg) (Australia antigen)
Chronic		Hepatitis B core antigen (HBcAg)

Hepatitis non-A, non-B is diagnosed by exclusion on the basis of the clinical picture.

of disease of the spleen is enlargement of the organ. This indicates the need for detailed hematologic and other studies to ascertain the primary disease. Treatment of diseases of the pancreas and spleen is beyond the scope of this book but is likely to take precedence over any but the most acute gynecologic condition.

URINARY TRACT

Evaluation

Preoperative evaluation of the urinary tract is important because (1) urinary symptoms are often related to or associated with gynecologic disease; (2) information about prior or present infection or other disorders of the lower genital tract provides a baseline for postoperative findings since injury to the ureter, bladder or urethra may occur during operation and infection may result from the frequently used invasive procedure of catheterization; and (3) abnormalities of the upper urinary tract may be relevant to operative procedures in the pelvis, e.g., displacement of the ureter, pelvic kidney or absence of one kidney.

The screening history includes the incidence and frequency of urethral or bladder infections, incontinence, upper urinary tract infection, symptoms of pressure on the bladder or a past history of diseases or operations involving the urinary tract. Physical examination of the bladder and urethra is an intrinsic part of the gynecologic examination; it is usually conducted while the patient is in the lithotomy position. Important factors to determine are prolapse or tenderness of the urethra and bladder, including protrusion of a diverticulum, especially on straining. If the patient has complained of incontinence, she can be asked to cough, gently at first and then more vigorously to see if urine leaks from the urethra; repeating this test while the patient is standing is informative. Theoretically, if the urethrovesical angle is restored by the examining finger or an instrument and urine does not then leak on coughing, operative cure may be possible; the value of this test is limited because it really does not simulate the effect of sutures or a sling repair. Evaluation of the laxity of the tissues in the area of the urethrovesical angle and the movement of the angle on coughing can, however, be a guide to the need for and extent of repair.

Urinalysis is the simplest and most important laboratory test for the urinary tract. Ideally, a midstream specimen should be obtained in the morning when the patient has not urinated for at least three hours. The introitus should be washed with a cotton ball soaked in sterile saline. Antiseptic solutions should not be used. If vaginal bleeding is present, a tampon should be placed in the vagina. The first part of the urinary stream is permitted to flow into the toilet, and the second is collected in a sterile container. Catheterization is to be avoided when possible because bacteria may be carried into the bladder. Suprapubic bladder puncture with the bladder full is a good way of obtaining an uncontaminated specimen but is unnecessarily invasive. Microscopic examination of the urine is performed first. If there are a large number of white blood cells or bacteria per high power field, the urine is cultured. Screening dipstick tests for pus and nitrites may be helpful.

Further studies include intravenous pyelography, renal ultrasonography, cysto-urethroscopy and cystometry. A preoperative intravenous pyelogram is indicated when a pelvic mass is present that may obstruct or distort the ureters or as a baseline before radical hysterectomy or similar procedures. Cystoscopy is indicated when there is a history of repeated lower urinary tract infections or of hematuria or prior to radiation therapy for gynecologic cancer. Cystometry is a valuable adjunct to the preoperative diagnosis of urinary incontinence, particularly in identifying a neurogenic bladder; it can conveniently be combined with cystoscopy. Details of the technique of cystoscopy and cystometry are covered in gynecologic urology textbooks. It is advantageous for the gynecologist to learn these techniques, particularly air cysto-urethroscopy, so that he can then undertake routine screening examinations, if necessary, and refer the patient to a urologist if the findings are not clear or more expertise is needed.

Management

LOWER URINARY TRACT

The discovery of a tumor of the urethra or bladder and its treatment takes precedence over the management of a concomitant benign gynecologic disorder. Some lower urinary tract problems such as urethral diverticulum, incontinence or cystocele can be managed at the same time as the gynecologic disorder. However, the presence of a neurogenic bladder with incontinence or overflow incontinence must be recognized and the patient made aware that it will not be cured by the proposed gynecologic procedure. Lower urinary tract infections are best treated with appropriate antibiotics (see Chapter 4) prior to operations or procedures; they are likely to be exacerbated or perpetuated by operative catheterization.

UPPER URINARY TRACT

If it seems likely that the gynecologic disorder is responsible for deviation or obstruction of the ureter(s), no preoperative management is necessary unless renal function is impaired. Preoperative insertion of ureteral catheters to facilitate dissection of the ureters is very rarely necessary. If upper urinary tract obstruction or abnormalities are due to other causes such as retroperitoneal or renal tumors, further preoperative investigation and consultation are indicated.

The most important part of upper urinary tract investigation is to determine renal function. An elevated BUN may be due to prerenal causes such as dehydration or to renal disease. The presence of the latter is confirmed by an elevated plasma creatinine level. If poor renal function appears to be due to obstruction, preoperative decompression by passing a ureteral catheter or by percutaneous nephrostomy (see Chapter 4) may be indicated. If intrinsic renal function is reduced, the risk of further operative impairment must be weighed against the benefits of the proposed operation.

SKIN

Most gynecologic procedures involve incising the skin or the vagina, which for the purpose of this section is regarded as an intact epithelial lining similar to skin. Usually skin incisions heal by first intention without undue scarring. However, the process may be complicated by bleeding, delayed healing, infection or keloid formation. Preoperative, intraoperative and postoperative factors are involved. The latter two will be considered in Chapters 3 and 4.

Preoperative factors that predispose to complications of skin incisions include (1) the patient's general condition, (2) previous scars and local therapies and (3) actual or potential skin infections.

Long-term malnutrition adversely affects cutaneous wound healing. This may be of concern in patients with recurrent ovarian or cervical cancer. Long-term hyperalimentation may be valuable, but short-term hyperalimentation does not increase the tensile strength of wounds. Severe deficiencies of vitamin C and zinc may interfere with wound healing, but temporary perioperative decreases of these or other vitamins or minerals are of uncertain importance. General disease states such as diabetes or cirrhosis of the liver may affect incisions. Therefore, reasonable control of diabetes is important. Hemorrhage with reduced blood volume decreases healing and should be treated, but anemia does not necessarily affect healing unless hypoxemia is present.

Preoperative administration of corticosteroids inhibits the development of new blood vessels and fibrous tissue and alters the normal inflammatory response; vitamin A may reverse this effect. Other agents that may affect wound healing include cytotoxic drugs, such as antifolates (methotrexate), alkylating agents (cyclophosphamide), or antibacterials (actinomycin D, doxorubicin), in therapeutic doses. Therefore, when postoperative chemotherapy is to be given, the possible effects on the incision must be weighed against the need for prompt adjuvant therapy. In general, the latter is more important, for example, in Stage III carcinoma of the ovary.

Much attention has been paid to the prevention of infections in incisions by preoperative treatment of the skin. Although the inclusion of hair in the incision is undesirable, shaving causes trauma to the skin and allows bacterial growth within a few hours. Therefore, shaving should be done immediately before the operation and not the previous night. Moreover, clipping the hair results in significantly fewer infections than shaving (Alexander et al, 1983). Use of depilatories the night before the operation, followed by a hexachlorophene shower, has also been found to be more effective than razor shaving (Shannon et al, 1985). This procedure may carry some risk of an allergic or irritative response.

The skin contains resident and transient bacteria, both of which may contribute to postoperative infection. The former are difficult to eradicate by the ordinary methods of scrubbing and antiseptics. However, the latter can and probably should be reduced as much as possible by adequate washing, i.e., by a shower or tub bath using hexachlorophene on the evening before the operation, re-enforced by scrubbing the (abdominal) wall just prior to operation and using a skin antiseptic (see Chapter 3). If an infection is already present in the area to be incised, preoperative preparation should be intensified, and the use of prophylactic antibiotics such as a cephalosporin should be considered.

No good measures are available to prevent keloids. It is important to know if the patient has a prior tendency to keloid formation so that she may be warned that they may recur.

The vagina is a more likely potential source of infection than the skin of the abdominal wall because of the variety of resident bacteria, its proximity to the intestinal bacteria at the anus and the difficulty of eradicating its bacteria prior to operation. Preoperative douches with water, povidone-iodine or other solutions have been widely used, as have antibacterial vaginal suppositories such as those containing various sulfa drugs. There is no evidence that any of these measures decreases postoperative infection. Prophylactic antibiotics and cleansing the vagina immediately before operation with an antiseptic such as povidone-iodine is probably sufficient.

NEUROLOGIC FACTORS

General

Neurologic disorders may affect a patient's ability to understand operative procedures and their necessity, to tolerate anesthesia or to make a smooth postoperative recovery. Neurologic diseases are often established and well known by the patient and her family so that they can be easily ascertained by a careful screening history. Established neurologic diseases are covered in standard textbooks of internal medicine or neurology and will not be discussed here. The possibility of acute perioperative deterioration must be remembered in such conditions as multiple sclerosis, metastatic brain disease or spinal cord degenerative processes such as syringomyelia. Also, appropriate medications for diseases such as epilepsy or parkinsonism must be continued in the perioperative period.

Whether or not there is a history of neurologic disease, a brief screening neurologic examination should be included in the pretreatment physical examination for all but the smallest procedures. This should include assessment of state of consciousness, mental and behavioral problems, visual and auditory acuity, peripheral movements, muscle tone, motor and sensory function and reflexes.

When a patient is comatose, operation is only feasible in an emergency. The cause of the coma must be determined rapidly and its progression or improvement carefully monitored. Peripheral nerve and muscle disorders usually do not contraindicate operative procedures, although they may modify the use of positions such as the lithotomy position for vaginal procedures, and they must be accurately identified for comparison with the patient's postoperative status. Specific tests, such as lumbar puncture, CT scan of the brain, electroencephalogram or myelogram are best conducted only after advice from a consultant neurologist.

Specific Neurologic Problems

MENTAL RETARDATION

Severe forms of mental retardation are well known from childhood to the patient's family. In the rare event that such a patient presents with obstetric or gynecologic problems, any decision to operate or treat must be made within the context of the individual's (usually) institutional life, for life-threatening conditions only and with the permission and understanding of the individual's guardians. Slight mental retardation may not be fully appreciated during the initial interview and physical examination, particularly if the individual is being protected by a caring relative. An IQ test, obtained through a consultant psychiatrist, neurologist or psychologist, may be necessary to determine the patient's mental status more precisely. Such patients with IQs in the 70 to 90 range require simpler preoperative and postoperative instructions than those of normal mental ability. It is sometimes difficult to be sure that the patient clearly understands the proposed procedure and its possible outcomes.

DRUG DEPENDENCE

Substances with the potential for dependence include (1) CNS depressants such as opiates, barbituates and alcohol; (2) minor tranquilizers such as meprobamate and benzodiazepines; (3) stimulants such as amphetamines and cocaine and (4) hallucinogens such as marijuana and LSD. In the first two categories drug dependence is important because postoperative withdrawal may precipitate acute symptoms, seriously affect the patient's ability to cooperate with necessary procedures and instructions and throw medical and nursing personnel into confusion because of the patient's attempts to obtain the needed medication. Gross drug dependence may be suspected at the initial interview from the patient's bizarre behavior or strange responses to questions. However, dependence may be occult and difficult to identify. This is particularly true of alcoholism. In a screening interview questions about the amount of alcohol (or other "social" drugs) should be included; however, the amounts drunk or taken will usually be minimized by the patient. Close family members may vouchsafe more information. Detailed questions about alcohol and other drug intake are likely to meet a hostile response, even if asked in the context of helping the patient through the planned procedure. However, problem drinking can be identified when a person responds affirmatively to three or four of the following questions: (1) Have you ever thought that you should cut down on your drinking? (2) Have you ever been annoyed at others' complaints about your drinking? (3) Have you ever felt guilty about your drinking? (4) Do you ever take morning eye-openers? Investigation of the possible effects of alcoholism is initially confined to general physical examination, including the liver for possible cirrhotic enlargement, and to liver function tests. In the event that severe drug dependence is identified, the help of a drug dependency unit should be sought prior to operation. In general, it is not wise to attempt to wean a dependent patient from a drug during the perioperative period. However, if she needs pain relief, higher than normal doses are likely to be necessary; all supporting personnel should be made aware of this. If the patient is a social drinker, there is usually no harm in permitting her to continue her alcohol intake preoperatively and postoperatively when she can take oral feedings. Perioperatively illegal drugs such as marijuana cannot be continued, and the possible effects of withdrawal have to be accepted.

PAIN

Pelvic pain is a prominent symptom in many gynecologic conditions. Often, however, either it is difficult to relate the described pain to the abnormalities found on examination or no obvious cause can be found for it. When possible, it is important to identify the reason for the pain before performing an operative procedure such as a hysterectomy, ovarian cystectomy or vaginal repair, since if another cause is present

the patient may continue to have pain postoperatively.

Three points should be considered when a patient complains of pain that is disproportionate to the physical findings. First, neurologic mechanisms may be important. Slocumb (1984) describes the identification of trigger points in the abdominal wall, vagina and sacral areas in patients with chronic pelvic pain. Eighty-nine per cent of 122 patients with demonstrable trigger points showed relief or improvement after injection of the specific areas with a local anesthetic. Application of the trigger point technique may therefore be useful in some instances. Second, psychologic factors probably play an important part, both with trigger point pain and especially with pain experienced over a general area. This should prompt preliminary discussion of possible life stresses and marital conflict (see following section). Third, pain may be conditioned by and related to the use of analgesic medications, particularly those with dependency potential. Thus, a more detailed appraisal of the possible use of these drugs should be made.

PSYCHOSOCIAL AND PSYCHOSEXUAL FACTORS

Social and sexual data can often be gathered together as part of the screening history, since they are closely related. The former include an evaluation of the enviromental stresses faced by the patient and her response to them, and the possible effect of the operative procedure on both. Past and present sexual behavior and attitudes are important, since obstetric and gynecologic procedures frequently alter reproductive capacity and thus affect the woman's view of herself and her family's and partner's view of her. In turn, these opinions may contribute to the success of the procedure. Important questions include:

1. Present job (within or outside the home); satisfaction with it; job history.

2. Stresses related to work; economic status.

3. Stresses related to family responsibilities, especially older parents, problem children.

4. Relationship with husband or partner—length, stability, crises.

5. Previous obstetric experiences, including pregnancy, labor, delivery and breast feeding and the patient's attitude toward them.

6. Feelings about menstruation—premenstrual tension, pain.

7. Current sexual activity—frequency, variety and contraceptive methods used.

8. Satisfaction with current sexual activity, i.e., orgasm, pain, dyspareunia. In this regard Plouffe (1985) found the following three simple questions to be useful: (1) Are you sexually active? (2) Are there any problems? (3) Do you have any pain with intercourse? If further details were needed, questions were asked in the following areas: (1) difficulty with lubrication, (2) pain at penetration, (3) deep dyspareunia, (4) difficulties in achieving orgasm, (5) degree of satisfaction with sexual activity, (6) number of partners and (7) any other concerns.

Brief analysis of data obtained from the above questions should enable one to reach one of several conclusions:

1. There is no major psychosocial or psychosexual problem, and the patient will be able to go through the planned operation, procedure or treatment with minimal disturbance of her equilibrium.

2. There are some psychosocial or psychosexual problems that will not be altered by the procedure. In this case, it must be recognized by patient and physician that the same stresses will continue.

3. There are major psychosocial or psychosexual stresses and tensions, and they are likely to be made worse by the proposed operation. In this case, the benefit of the operation must clearly exceed the possible emotional cost. This is most likely to be true in operations performed for acute or life-threatening conditions, i.e., ruptured ectopic pregnancy, severe bleeding or cancer. When benefit and emotional cost are approximately equal, the indications for the procedure may need to be reevaluated.

4. The psychosocial or psychosexual disability is so great that it must be solved before the procedure is performed. At this point consultation from a social worker, marriage counselor or psychiatrist may be necessary.

MISCELLANEOUS FACTORS

Allergy

Determination of specific allergies is important preoperative information. These include, among others, iodine (skin or vaginal preparation, radiologic contrast studies), analgesics such as demerol or codeine (postoperative pain relief), antibiotics and adhesive tape. For details of reactions to drugs, see Chapter 13. It is often difficult to determine when a patient really has an allergy to a particular substance because the term "allergic" can mean different things to different people. A history of acute onset of breathing difficulty, swelling of the face or throat, severe hives or an acute skin rash following the use of a particular substance is pathognomonic. If the history is not clear, it is better to avoid the possible allergen. If use of the allergen is really indicated, desensitization or protection with corticosteroids may be necessary. The allergic history should be clearly noted on the patient's chart.

Medications

An accurate record should be made of all medications that the patient is taking, since they may need to be continued and may affect her perioperative care. Gaps in the use of essential drugs, for example, medications for hypertension, diabetes or epilepsy, should be minimal.

The patient's use of bronchodilators and other respiratory drugs may alert one to the special need for postoperative respiratory toilet. The chronic use of laxatives may make postoperative bowel function sluggish. Urinary tract antiseptics and antibiotics will usually have to be continued, particularly if catheterization is needed. Recent use of oral contraceptives may increase the danger of postoperative thromboembolism. If these drugs cannot be discontinued for at least four weeks prior to a major operation, special attention must be paid to the prophylaxis of thromboembolism, even in the younger patient. If corticosteroids have been used in the past month, additional doses need to be given perioperatively. Psychoactive drugs of all sorts may lead to postoperative difficulties in diagnosis because of the underlying disease or because their side effects may include confusion, drowsiness or extrapyramidal symptoms.

An administrative problem may arise when the hospitalized patient brings her own medications and wishes to take them herself. There is no reason why the conscious patient of average intelligence who has been doing this without nursing supervision for some time should not continue to do so. However, it is important for the obstetrician-gynecologist and the nursing staff to know what the patient is taking, to determine that it will not adversely affect her current therapy and to oversee her use, particularly if she undergoes a major surgical procedure and/or is unable to take anything by mouth.

Appliances and Devices

Knowledge and care of appliances worn or commonly used by patients in the perioperative period is essential. These include glasses, contact lenses, hearing devices, dentures, artificial limbs, canes and walkers. When possible, patients should bring their own appliances to the hospital and should be encouraged to use them as they do at home. Hospital authorities are rightly concerned about appliances being lost or broken, particularly because many people see and handle them, especially if the patient is anesthetized, recovering from an operation or medicated for pain. Proper care requires special attention by the patient's primary nurse and, if possible, shared responsibility on the part of a close family member. If an appliance cannot be brought to the hospital and is necessary for the patient's daily existence, it is the hospital's responsibility to see that an appropriate substitute is provided without delay.

PRETREATMENT AND PREOPERATIVE DISCUSSION

Preparation of the patient for an operation or procedure can be divided into four phases—the medical decision, the initial discussion with the patient, secondary discussion and re-enforcement and instruction.

The medical decision that an operation or procedure is necessary is usually made in the course of an office visit. In spite of the pressure of time, the decision has to be a firm one, with adequate reasons. Sometimes, a decision may have to be delayed pending the results of laboratory tests, further evaluation of the patient's symptoms or feelings or changes in physical signs.

Initial discussion with the patient means explaining to her the reasons for the proposed treatment, the alternative therapies, the precise nature of the procedure, the expected results and the possible complications. It is essential to use simple language that she can understand. In spite of the dissemination of medical knowledge through the media, the terms "biopsy," "laparoscopy," and "D & C," to give a few examples, may mean very little to the individual patient. Simple explanatory drawings are useful. Explanations obviously need to be less detailed for procedures such as colposcopy or cervical biopsy than for hysterectomy or vaginal repair. This preliminary discussion will often result in the patient giving her informed consent to the procedure. A note of explanation about this should be entered on her chart. This is particularly important for office procedures, such as cervical biopsy, which are frequently performed as an extension of a regular examination. When the operation is to be scheduled for a later date, the signing of a consent form by the patient should be delayed until just before the procedure. It is best explained and witnessed by the patient's physician, although this can be delegated to a resident physician who is a member of the team and who understands the nature of the procedure to be performed.

Secondary discussion with the patient may be necessary if she wishes further information or more time to reach a decision. Additional data may be provided by educational literature; it is important that the physician be familiar with any material given to the patient to read. She may also wish or be required by her insurance company to obtain a second opinion about the necessity of operation. This practice is now so common that it should be handled in routine manner and the patient assisted to make the necessary arrangements. The most important data for a second opinion consultant are copies of operative reports, pathologic reports and results of *relevant* laboratory and x-ray studies. Many consultants also wish to review or to have reviewed pathologic slides from biopsies or operative specimens. The office secretary and nurse should have a clear understanding of the necessity of providing this information at the patient's request and without argument.

Once the patient has decided to proceed, further education and instruction regarding the process of hospitalization (if that is planned), the operation itself and the recovery period are necessary. It may be given in several ways, by the physician himself, by his office nurse, by audiovisual aids such as pamphlets, films or TV tapes, by group discussions or by nurses or resident physicians in the hospital. The patient's physician is responsible for overseeing this program. It is essential to remember that:

1. Repeated instruction is necessary because the patient is unfamiliar with the procedure and

its accompanying routine and cannot assimilate all the details at once.

2. The physician or the nurse who works closely with him is the most effective instructor.

3. Audiovisual aids may be helpful, but they deal with average cases and may be unsuitable for certain individuals. The physician must be thoroughly familiar with their contents.

4. Group instruction is very hard to arrange except in a large institution where it may be possible to bring together a number of patients about to have the same or a similar operation. Under such specific circumstances group instruction may be helpful.

5. Differences in instruction, advice and prognosis are most likely to come from preoperative teaching by nurses and resident physicians who may not understand the patient's particular problem and may have their own preconceived notion of what should be done. It is essential that the responsible physician give the members of his team adequate preadmission information about each patient and that he be aware of and approve any routine preoperative teaching given by hospital nurses.

Discussion with the patient's family is an essential part of the preoperative preparation. Most important is her husband or partner; other relatives who play a significant part in her life must often be included. Sometimes the discussion can be accomplished at the initial visit; sometimes it must wait until a later visit or hospitalization. The explanations given to close family members should be the same as those given to the patient herself. Their special fears and concerns should be addressed. The same degree of technical education about the procedure and hospital routines is not so necessary for them as for the patient herself. However, they will wish to know about hospital visits, opportunities for discussion with the physician in the hospital, what may be expected in the recovery period and how they may best arrange the patient's convalescence. Care should be taken not to discuss the patient's condition, operation or prognosis with distant and unknown relatives or friends except with the patient's express permission.

When the patient is a minor child or an adolescent or is mentally incapable of understanding what is to be done, the parent, guardian or caretaking relative must receive the same information as would be given to an adult patient. It is equally important, however, that the dependent person hear the same information, even if simple language must be used, because the patient's cooperation is essential at all ages.

References

Adkins RB, Scott HW Jr.: Surgical procedures in patients aged 90 years and older. *South. Med. J.* 77:1357, 1984.

Alexander JW, Fischer JE et al.: The influence of hair-removal methods on wound infections. *Arch. Surg.* 118:347, 1983.

Barsoum MS, Boulos FI et al.: The effect of prophylactic heparinization on the venous blood flow using the Doppler ultrasonic flowmeter. *Br. J. Surg.* 69:207, 1982.

Blackburn GL, Bistrian BR et al.: Nutritional and metabolic assessment of the hospitalized patient. *JPEN* 1:11, 1977.

Bonnar J: Venous thromboembolism and gynecologic surgery. *Clin. Obstet. Gynecol.* 28:432, 1985.

Caprini JA, Chucker JL et al.: Thrombosis prophylaxis using external compression. *Surg. Gynecol. Obstet.* 156:599, 1983.

Cartwright PS, Pittaway DE et al.: The use of prophylactic antibiotics in obstetrics and gynecology. A review. *Obstet. Gynecol. Surv.* 39:537, 1984.

Clarke-Pearson DL, Coleman RE et al.: Venous thromboembolism prophylaxis in gynecologic oncology: a prospective, controlled trial of low-dose heparin. *Am. J. Obstet. Gynecol.* 145:606, 1983.

Clarke-Pearson DL, Synan IS et al.: Prevention of postoperative venous thromboembolism by external pneumatic calf compression in patients with gynecologic malignancy. *Obstet. Gynecol.* 63:92, 1984.

Clayton JK, Anderson JA, McNicol GP: Preoperative prediction of postoperative deep vein thrombosis. *Br. Med. J.* 2:910, 1976.

Ferraris VA, Swanson E: Aspirin usage and perioperative blood loss in patients undergoing unexpected operations. *Surg. Obstet. Gynecol.* 156:439, 1983.

Girtanner RE: Preoperative and postoperative nutritional support. *Contemp. Obstet. Gynecol.* 25:155, 1985.

Gruber UF, Saldeen T et al.: Incidences of fatal postoperative pulmonary embolism after prophylaxis with dextran 70 and low-dose heparin: an international multicentre study. *Br. Med. J.* 1:69, 1980.

Huffman JW: Examination of the premenarchial child. In Huffmann JW, Dewhurst CJ, Capraro VJ (Eds.): *The Gynecology of Childhood and Adolescence*, Ed. 2. Philadelphia, WB Saunders Company, 1981.

Jain MG, Harrison L et al.: Evaluation of a self-administered dietary questionnaire for use in a cohort study. *Am. J. Clin. Nutr.* 36:931, 1982.

Kakkar VV: The diagnosis of deep vein thrombosis using the ^{125}I fibrinogen test. *Arch. Surg.* 104:152, 1972.

Kakkar VV, Djazaeri B et al.: Low-molecular-weight heparin and prevention of postoperative deep vein thrombosis. *Br. Med. J.* 1:375, 1982.

Kotz HL, Geelhoed GW: Lethal thromboembolism and its prevention in pelvic surgery: a review. *Gynecol. Oncol.* 12:271, 1981.

Lindstrom B, Holmdahl C et al.: Prediction and prophylaxis of postoperative thromboembolism—a comparison between preoperative calf muscle stimulation with groups of impulses and dextran 40. *Br. J. Surg.* 69:633, 1982.

McCarthy TG, McQueen J et al.: A comparison of low-dose

subcutaneous heparin and intravenous dextran 70 in the prophylaxis of deep venous thrombosis after gynecological surgery. *J. Obstet. Gynecol. Br. Comm.* 81:486, 1974.

Newton M: Relationship of weather to postoperative phlebothrombosis. *Am. J. Surg.* 81:607, 1951.

Orr JW, Shingleton HM: Importance of nutritional assessment and support in surgical and cancer patients. *J. Reprod. Med.* 29:635, 1984.

Peters JL (Ed.): *Central Venous Catheterization and Parenteral Nutrition.* Bristol, John Wright and Sons Ltd., 1983.

Piver M, Malfetano JH et al.: Prophylactic anticoagulation as a possible cause of inguinal lymphocyst after radical vulvectomy and inguinal lymphadenectomy. *Obstet. Gynecol.* 62:17, 1983.

Plouffe L Jr.: Screening for sexual problems through a simple questionnaire. *Am. J. Obstet. Gynecol.* 151:166, 1985.

Rayburn W, Wolk W et al.: Parenteral nutrition in obstetrics and gynecology. *Obstet. Gynecol. Surv.* 41:200, 1986.

Salzman EW: In American College of Surgeons: *Manual of Preoperative and Postoperative Care.* Philadelphia, WB Saunders Company, 1983.

Sasahara AA: Dihydroergotamine-heparin prophylaxis of postoperative deep vein thrombosis, a multicenter trial. *J. Am. Med. Assoc.* 251:2960, 1984.

Schroeder PJ, Dunn E: Mechanical plethysmography and Doppler ultrasound. Diagnosis of deep-venous thrombosis. *Arch. Surg.* 117:300, 1982.

Shannon J Jr., McComas B, de Koos PT: Preoperative skin preparation and wound infection. *Infect. Surg.* 4:451, 1985.

Sharnoff JG, Rosenberg M, Mistica BA: Seasonal variation in fatal thromboembolism and its high incidence in the surgical patient. *Surg. Gynecol. Obstet.* 116:11, 1963.

Slocumb JC: Neurological factors in chronic pelvic pain: trigger points and the abdominal pelvic pain syndrome. *Am. J. Obstet. Gynecol.* 149:536, 1984.

Yurt RW: Preventing bacterial endocarditis—The American Heart Association guidelines for prophylaxis. *Infect. Surg.* 4:221, 1985.

INTRAOPERATIVE COMPLICATIONS

3

MICHAEL NEWTON

This chapter covers intraoperative complications that are common to a variety of operations. Those that are related to specific operations are covered in later chapters. Although many of the intraoperative problems discussed occur with abdominal operations, some are associated with the vaginal approach; in these cases differences in management are indicated.

INCISION

Any skin or vaginal incision has potential complications. These may be related to the incision itself, e.g., bleeding, difficulty of closure, hematoma, breakdown or infection, or to the appropriateness of the incision for the operative procedure. As the operation is begun, the initial considerations are maintenance of asepsis and precautions against infection. Preoperative prophylactic measures are outlined in Chapter 2, and wound infections are covered in Chapter 4. At operation, attention to attire and proper handwashing techniques are still important. Many different techniques of skin cleansing have been described. The traditional and effective one is to scrub the skin with hexachlorophene soap and paint it with an iodine compound, provided the patient is not allergic to iodine; 70% alcohol may be used as an alternative. Adhesive antimicrobial incise-drapes are of possible value, although they take slightly longer to apply than cloth or edge-adhesive paper drapes. Also, separation of these drapes from the skin during the operation may result in an increased infection rate (Alexander et al, 1985). As the incision is made a second knife is often used for the deeper tissues. This does not appear to reduce wound infections (Hasselgren et al, 1984).

Many factors affect the choice of incision for abdominal procedures. They include the type of operation, the presence of previous scars, the patient's habitus and the likelihood of satisfactory healing without complications. If the operation is likely to involve only the removal of a small or moderate-sized mass (less than 10 cm) from the pelvis, a transverse lower abdominal incision may be made, with transverse division of the rectus sheaths and vertical entry into the peritoneal cavity (Pfannenstiel's incision) or transverse entry with division of one or both rectus muscles. If large pelvic tumors have to be removed or the upper abdomen requires exploration, a vertical midline incision is usually best; this may curve around the umbilicus. A transverse incision below the umbilicus will serve the same purpose. This incision takes longer but may be somewhat stronger if other factors are equal. In a very obese woman, a low transverse incision in the fold of skin may not heal well because the skin becomes macerated and does not receive air; a long vertical incision above the skinfold is better. When there is a previous midline scar it should be excised, but if there is a paramedian scar located well laterally, a separate midline incision should be made. An incision made at right angles to a previous incision is unsightly but may be necessary. The type and direction of the incision probably contribute little to incisional complications. More important are the patient's underlying disease or current problems, asepsis and avoidance of infection and the type of closure (see page 54 and Chapter 4).

The complications encountered as the abdominal wall is incised include excessive bleeding, failure to identify the fascial, muscular and peritoneal layers because of previous scars and entering bowel or bladder that is unexpectedly adherent to the anterior peritoneum. In vertical incisions excessive bleeding is unusual. It can be controlled by pressure on the skin edges as the incision is deepened and by electrocoagulation or fine ligature of specific bleeding vessels. Electrocoagulation is faster but results in more tissue necrosis and may predispose to infection. In transverse incisions bleeding may be encountered from vessels in the bellies of the rectus muscles as they are cut or from the inferior epigastric artery or vein, which lie beneath the lateral edge of the rectus muscle. In a Pfannenstiel's incision, when the rectus muscles are dissected upward and downward from their overlying sheaths, bleeding may occur because of perforation of vessels between the muscle and the sheath. Unless these vessels are carefully ligated or coagulated, a postoperative hematoma may result. Persistent generalized bleeding as the incision is made should

raise the suspicion of coagulopathy (see following section).

The intestine may be opened unexpectedly if a rapid incision that traverses all layers at once is made or if the intestine is adherent to the anterior abdominal wall and the presumed peritoneal cavity is entered incautiously. This complication can usually be avoided by opening the peritoneum away from any anticipated adhesions. Sharp dissection with knife or scissors is better than blunt sponge dissection, which is liable to cause larger tears. An opening into the intestine can be recognized by the appearance of intestinal contents; when the colon has been entered the fecal smell is usually obvious. Repair should be performed immediately (see page 44).

The bladder may be opened as the peritoneal incision is extended downward, particularly if the bladder has not been emptied prior to operation or if it has been attached high on the front of the uterus at a previous operation such as a cesarean section. It is most important to recognize the opening if it occurs. Urine is not as obvious as intestinal contents, but the color and appearance of the bladder mucosa are diagnostic. The bulb of the Foley catheter may be felt or seen. Enlargement of a small opening may be necessary. This should be of little concern at this point, since the opening is usually in the dome of the bladder and a slightly larger opening is no more difficult to repair; in fact, it may be easier since the layers are more clearly definable. Repair of the bladder should be performed promptly; details of closure are given in a subsequent section (page 49).

During vaginal incisions the bladder and rectum are also in danger of being opened; management is described in Chapter 5.

HEMORRHAGE

Control of Bleeding

Essentials for handling intraoperative bleeding are a knowledge of anatomic structures and their variations, adequate exposure of bleeding points and use of the appropriate instruments and suture material to ligate bleeding vessels.

The main arteries and veins supplying the female pelvic organs are shown in Figure 3–1. Anatomic variations commonly encountered in the arteries include (1) high bifurcation of the aorta and/or common iliac arteries (Fig. 3–1), (2) origin of the superior vesical and uterine

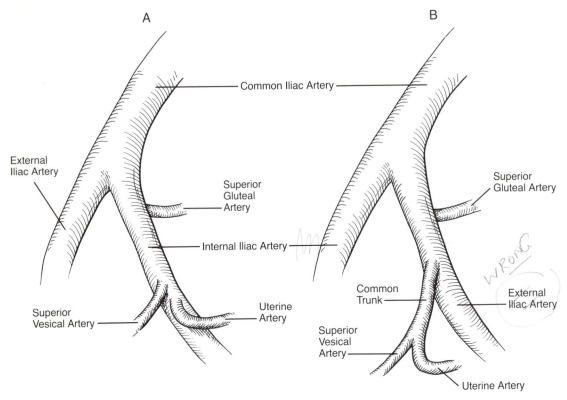

Figure 3–1. *Main arteries of the pelvis (right side).* A, *Separate origins of the superior vesical and uterine arteries.* B, *Superior vesical and uterine arteries arising from a common trunk.*

arteries from a common branch of the internal iliac artery (Fig. 3–1) and (3) anomalous vessels developing as a result of collateral circulation or the growth of a large tumor. Examples of these are omental blood supply to a parasitic myoma or enlarged descending branches of the uterine artery supplying a hypertrophied cervix. Although major veins tend to accompany arteries, the number and location of such veins, e.g., the various tributaries of the internal iliac vein deep in the pelvis, are unpredictable.

Adequate exposure and good light are essential. An important part of surgical training in an obstetric-gynecologic residency is to learn how to retract effectively and how to instruct others to do so. The Deaver retractor (narrow or wide blade) is best for general use, although large or heart-shaped retractors may occasionally be helpful and narrow or wide malleable retractors are invaluable in certain situations. Once the bleeding area has been exposed, the specific bleeding vessel(s) is gradually exposed by sponging or suction. Thin tape sponges are most useful. Suction must be used cautiously. Continuous or indiscriminate use of suction may

increase blood loss very rapidly. The most important aspect of good overhead lighting is the experience and skill of the circulating nurse. A headlight is valuable for dissection in a deep, small pelvis.

Instruments suitable for clamping a variety of blood vessels should be available on every gynecologic operating tray. Of these the most useful are small curved hemostats, right-angled clamps of two sizes, such as Mixter's clamps, and long fine curved clamps such as Boettcher's clamps. Rubber-shod vascular clamps for occluding large vessels should be readily available. Since they are seldom needed and only in an emergency, all operating room personnel should know where they are stored.

The ideal ligature is one that can be tied easily with a secure first knot, causes minimal tissue reaction and is absorbed, but only after the healing process is well established. The synthetic sutures such as Dexon or vicryl, available in the last 15 years, satisfy the last two criteria reasonably well. Catgut, the oldest absorbable suture, is easier to tie, especially deep in the pelvis and has a more secure knot, but it causes more tissue reaction and loses its strength more rapidly than the synthetic materials.

The effectiveness of a ligature depends not only on the size and strength of a suture but also on the number of knots and the likelihood of the knot slipping. The more knots, the weaker the suture. A square knot (conventionally identified as 1 = 1) slips less than a sliding knot (1 × 1). For most suture material three square knots (1 = 1 = 1) are least likely to slip, except that coated sutures (for example, vicryl) need four square knots (1 = 1 = 1 = 1) (Trimbos, 1984). A surgeon's knot (2 = 1 or 2 = 2) gives the greatest security but adds to the stress on the suture material.

The choice of sutures actually used is a peculiar amalgam of the surgeon's training, the materials available, i.e., the hospital's purchasing policy, and the persuasiveness of the suture company's salesperson. This attitude was well illustrated by a survey of suture material used in residency training programs in the United States by Hartko and associates (1982).

Similarly, knot tying is conditioned by training and experience, and it is not easy to change one's habits. However, for the young surgeon, several important points should be made. First, when exposure is good, the use of three square knots with synthetic material such as Dexon or four square knots with vicryl is appropriate. For greater security an added surgeon's knot (2 = 1 = 1 or 2 = 1 = 1 = 1) is helpful. Second, when exposure is poor and first knot security is important, catgut suture material may be more effective. Third, it is essential to be alert to possible improvements in suture materials and, prior to making a change, to become as familiar as possible with the data on the subject.

The use of metal clips has improved control of bleeding. At present, individual clips in a clip-holder are easiest to use in the pelvis or beside large vessels. The smallest effective clip is best, usually the "medium" size. Holders containing several clips obviate clips falling out of the holder, but need to be of appropriate length and shape so that they can be placed on vessels that are difficult to reach and expose. The least possible number of clips should be used. Even though they are inert, the long-term effect of one or many is unknown, nor is it certain whether they remain in one place or possibly migrate. Large numbers of clips may obscure subsequent x-ray findings and, indeed, may prevent the use of CT scans or be hazardous with MRI. Absorbable clips may be the answer to these problems, but they must be easy to apply and must provide secure hemostasis.

Intraoperative Hemorrhage

Any sudden unexpected and temporarily uncontrolled bleeding of more than 50 to 75 ml should be regarded as hemorrhage because of its potential for increasing severity.

Bleeding may arise from incision or division of a small or medium-sized artery or vein, from a major artery or vein in the pelvis or from many small vessels. The three principles of initial management are (1) control by pressure, (2) adequate exposure and (3) rapid, precise clamping and ligature or suture. Once the immediate bleeding is controlled by finger or sponge-stick pressure, ample time should be taken to obtain good exposure by retraction and to assemble the necessary clamps or sutures. The finger (or sponge-stick) is then slowly removed and, with judicious use of suction, the actual bleeding point is exposed. A small or medium-sized artery or vein can usually be clamped and ligated or clipped. A vessel of this size that is half divided should be completely divided; otherwise part of the vessel may escape the clamp.

Damage to a major artery or vein is usually recognized by the large amount of blood loss. If an artery is involved, pressure must be exerted by a sponge-stick or by securing the whole vessel in an arterial clamp above and below the laceration. The artery may then be sutured using a continuous non-absorbable monofilament suture. Pressure is then maintained over the suture line for two to three minutes to control oozing. If an artery has been completely divided, it can be anastomosed with fine silk. However, a graft may be necessary, and consultation with a vascular surgeon is advisable. When a large vein is injured, the same principles of management apply, except that attempts should be made to isolate the vein above and below the laceration only with great caution; pressure is safer and usually equally effective. The major venous problem in gynecologic surgery is injury to the internal iliac vein or its tributaries deep in the pelvis.

Failure to control bleeding in the pelvis may indicate the need for proximal arterial ligation. The vessel that needs to be ligated depends on the type of operation being performed. Usually the uterus has been removed, so the logical vessel to ligate is the internal iliac. If the uterus is to be preserved, ligation of the uterine artery alone may be appropriate. However, this requires more dissection closer to the ureter in a pelvis that is often filled with blood. Thus, internal iliac artery ligation may be best. In either case the surgical approach is the same. The retroperitoneal space is entered lateral to the external iliac artery; the bifurcation of the common iliac artery and the ureter, which is usually attached to the medial leaf of the peritoneum, are identified. The ureter is drawn medially and a Mixter's clamp is passed under the artery from the lateral to the medial side about 2 cm below the bifurcation. During this maneuver, care should be taken to avoid the internal iliac vein. A doubled silk suture is drawn back under the artery and divided, and both sutures are tied a short distance apart. There is no need to expose the superior gluteal artery nor to ligate the internal iliac artery below it; the danger of loss of blood supply to the buttocks is minimal. The artery should not be divided between the ligatures. It is generally wise to tie both hypogastric arteries because of the collateral circulation in the pelvis. As Burchell (1964) pointed out, occlusion of the internal iliac arteries does not completely stop bleeding from the distal branches of the arteries in the pelvis but reduces blood flow (48%) and pulse pressure (85%) so that ordinary hemostasis by pressure becomes effective. If the uterine

artery alone is to be ligated, it is best done as the artery leaves the internal iliac artery (either as a single branch or after it leaves the combined trunk with the superior vesical artery). If the uterus is left in place, ligation of the uterine branches of the ovarian arteries is useful because they are an important source of blood supply to the uterus. This may be done in the region of the utero-ovarian ligament where the utero-ovarian anastomosis is located (Fig. 3–2) (Cruikshank and Stoelk, 1983). The effect of ligation of the internal iliac artery on the pelvic organs appears to be slight. Collateral blood supply comes from the ovarian artery, the inferior mesenteric artery, the external iliac and femoral arteries, the middle sacral artery and the lumbar arteries. Ligation of the ovarian artery in the infundibulopelvic ligament rather than the uterine branch results in more complete loss of blood supply to the ovary and therefore a decrease in function is possible. However, normal ovarian function, pregnancy and term delivery have been reported following ligation of both internal iliac and ovarian arteries (Mengert et al, 1969).

When bleeding is generalized and no major bleeding vessels can be identified, it is important to check hemostasis (see following section) and replace blood or blood constituents. At the same time prolonged pressure and hemostatic agents can be used locally. The latter include oxidized cellulose (Oxcel), topical thrombin, absorbable gelatin sponge (Gelfoam) or micro-

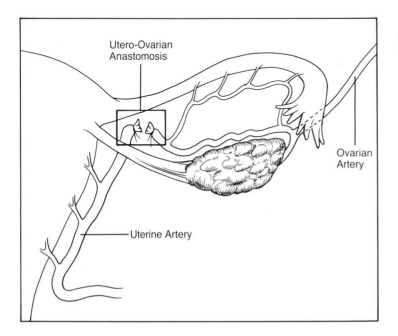

Figure 3–2. Ligation of the utero-ovarian arterial anastomosis in the utero-ovarian ligament.

Utero-Ovarian Anastomosis

Ovarian Artery

Uterine Artery

fibrillar collagen (Avitene). Each one or combinations of them have proponents. Part of the expressed satisfaction in their use is due to the surgeon's feeling of having taken definitive action; often it is likely that the bleeding would have stopped spontaneously. The author's preference is for the use of Gelfoam soaked in topical thrombin.

If massive bleeding continues despite all attempts at hemostasis and adequate replacement of blood, it may be necessary to pack the bleeding area in the pelvis and conclude the operation. One or more five-yard rolls of gauze can be used and brought out through the lower end of the abdominal incision or through a separate lateral incision. The pack is removed when the patient's condition is stable and bleeding appears to have ceased, usually in two to four days. Removal usually requires general anesthesia or intravenous analgesia.

Replacement of Fluids, Blood and Blood Constituents

PREPARATION

When blood loss of more than 500 ml is anticipated, two to four units of blood should be prepared in advance. Gynecologic operations with such blood loss include most major operations for cancer and any hysterectomy or exploratory laparotomy in which there is already blood in the peritoneal cavity or which is likely to be difficult or lengthy. When this blood loss is possible but unlikely, the patient's blood should be typed and held, but blood is not crossmatched until need arises, thus considerably decreasing expense and wastage of fresh blood.

MEASUREMENT OF BLOOD LOSS

Estimates of blood loss are somewhat unreliable even when made by experienced surgeons or anesthesiologists. One's natural tendency is to estimate too high for small losses and too low for large ones. Actual methods of measurement are not necessarily accurate but should be attempted in any major procedure. They include measurement of blood in suction bottles and by weighing sponges before and after use. Suctioned blood may be mixed with other body fluids such as ascites or may be diluted by clearing the suction system with fluid. Blood in sponges may be measured by weighing dry sponges before and after use. Alternatively, a standard weight for a dry or wrung-out wet sponge should be established for the operating room or the particular case and should be subtracted from the used weight. Devices for collecting blood loss at vaginal hysterectomy include plastic adhesive drapes that funnel blood into a receptacle. These devices are helpful, but their use still requires that blood on sponges or drapes be measured or estimated. Whatever method of determining blood loss is used, the loss should be repeatedly evaluated during any surgical procedure, particularly if it is long.

REPLACEMENT

Initial therapy for operative blood loss consists of crystalloids, normal saline or preferably lactated Ringer's solution. The use of colloids such as 5% albumin, Dextran 70 or Hetastarch is not necessary under ordinary circumstances, but may be important in severe acute bleeding when blood is not immediately available (see following section). The effect of crystalloids on intravascular volume is limited because the majority (70 to 80%) end up in an overexpanded interstitial space. The decision to administer whole blood or other blood products is not clear-cut, but depends on the clinical judgment of the surgeon and the anesthesiologist. In general, if the preoperative hematocrit is over 35% and the estimated blood loss is less than 500 ml, transfusion is not necessary. Whatever the preoperative hematocrit, an estimated blood loss of over 1000 ml is an indication for transfusion. Whole blood is generally appropriate since whole blood has been lost, but the lesser volume of packed red cells reconstituted with normal saline offers less chance of cardiac failure in patients with limited cardiac reserve. Many authors have decried the use of the single unit blood transfusion because the benefit is not sufficient to justify the risk of complications. However, during operations, future blood loss often cannot be determined, and a single unit of blood may be necessary and useful.

The drawing, handling and dispensation of blood and blood products is to a large extent standardized in the United States. Details are contained in the "Circular for Information for the Use of Human Blood and Blood Components" prepared by the American Association of Blood Banks and the American Red Cross Blood Services (1984). At the time of administration the responsible physician must check the specific data on the blood container, including the dates and identification of the correct recipient. When possible blood should be warmed to about 37° C and filtered before being administered.

Rapid or massive blood loss, over 1000 ml, occurring within minutes, makes the need for blood replacement urgent. Type O-negative blood may be necessary as a lifesaving measure, but group and Rh specific blood is preferable and can be obtained within a few minutes, exclusive of transportation time. When possible, it is best to wait until a rapid (30 minutes) or complete (1 hour) crossmatch can be done. In such an emergency the use of colloids such as 5% albumin or plasma, if readily available, can be used while waiting for crossmatched blood.

When more than four units of blood are given, there is danger of abnormal coagulation. Platelets, Factor V and Factor VIII, at least, deteriorate in stored blood. Therefore, patients who receive four units of blood should have coagulation studies at regular intervals during a long operation. Sometimes it is difficult to get these done quickly. One unit of fresh frozen plasma can be given empirically for every four units of whole blood, with the use of cryoprecipitate (for fibrinogen, Factor VIII and Factor XIII) or platelets if a demonstrated deficiency and clinical evidence of coagulation failure are evident. Prophylactic calcium does not appear to be necessary. Warming the rapidly given blood and monitoring the patient's temperature are important to prevent cardiac arrhythmias.

Blood and blood products have significant side effects and risks that emphasize the need for caution in administering them. They include:

1. Immediate hemolysis. Severe reactions consist of shock, chills, fever, dyspnea, chest or back pain, headache or abnormal bleeding. Hemoglobinemia, hemoglobinuria, bilirubinuria and possible renal failure may ensue. Treatment is to discontinue the transfusion and give 1000 ml of lactated Ringer's solution, 100 ml of 20% mannitol for diuresis and 44 mEq of bicarbonate to alkalinize the urine. The blood must be returned to the issuing blood bank so that the crossmatching can be rechecked.

2. Delayed hemolysis. This may occur one to several days later and is usually less serious than immediate hemolysis. The same principles of management apply.

3. Transmission of infection. Transfused blood or blood products may cause bacterial or viral infection. Bacterial infection is usually the result of a break in aseptic technique during collection, storage or administration. The patient experiences high fever and prostration characteristic of septicemia. Cultures confirm the diagnosis, and treatment is by appropriate antibiotics (see Chapter 4).

Hepatitis may be transmitted by blood products. Routine testing of donor blood for Hepatitis B surface antigen (HBsAg) is mandatory. However, non-A–non-B hepatitis cannot yet be detected in donor blood and is probably the cause of most transfusion-related cases of hepatitis.

Parenthetically, it should be noted that medical personnel (especially surgeons and obstetrician-gynecologists) who are in frequent contact with blood or blood products are 50 times more likely to acquire HBV (Hepatitis B virus) infection than the general U.S. population. The FDA and other authorities recommend that such persons, among others, be screened for anti-HBs or anti-Hbc, since either antibody is evidence of prior infection. If they are antibody-negative, they should receive HBV vaccine. The vaccine appears to be safe and very rarely associated with side effects. In particular, the inactivation process used in making the vaccine appears to eliminate the chances of its transmitting AIDS. Vaccination of patients at high risk should also be considered.

The possible transmission of AIDS (acquired immune deficiency syndrome) is the most serious current problem. Enzyme-linked immunoabsorbent assays (ELISAs) are now available to test blood for antibodies to the virus presumed to be responsible for AIDS (human T cell lymphocytotrophic virus, HTLV-III/HIV [human immunodeficiency virus]). However, the possibility of a false positive test means that all positive tests should be confirmed by a second assay (Western Blot test). Even so, a large proportion (perhaps 2/3 or more) of persistently positive tests represent false positives. Also, as many as 10 to 15% of patients with AIDS may have negative assays (false negative). The development of more precise screening tests is an urgent necessity. Guidelines for handling AIDS problems are listed by Lotze (1985).

4. Immunization of the recipient. This may be a danger in the future, and subsequent crossmatching may be very difficult.

5. Fever. This occurs in 0.5 to 1% of patients transfused and frequently appears to be due to the action of donor antigens on the recipient's leukocytes or platelets.

6. Allergy. Urticaria occurs in about 3% of

recipients. It is usually less marked when washed red cells are used and may be ameliorated in patients with a positive history of allergy by premedication with an antihistaminic agent such as diphenhydramine.

Alternative methods of replacing blood include use of the patient's own stored blood (autologous transfusion) or autotransfusion. The former consists of removing 500 ml of blood from the patient at least three weeks prior to operation, freezing it and having it available for transfusion at operation, if needed. Autotransfusion has been used primarily in cardiovascular surgery but may also be useful in severe intraabdominal bleeding from such conditions as ruptured ectopic pregnancy. However, it is less applicable when severe blood loss is not anticipated but occurs unexpectedly as is the case in most gynecologic operations. The principles of autotransfusion are described by Jacobs and Hsieh (1984). A variety of devices have been developed with or without cell-washing capacity. In essence, blood is sucked into a container under strictly aseptic conditions, anticoagulant is added and the blood is retransfused through a filter. Autotransfusion results in a decrease in platelets, fibrinogen and Factors V, VIII and X. For these reasons these blood components need to be added in the same manner as after large transfusions of stored blood. The risks of autotransfusion include hemolysis, sepsis, microemboli and the remote possibility of air embolism.

Some patients, for religious reasons, refuse to accept blood or blood products under any circumstances. Often a difficult clinical and ethical (see Chapter 16) decision is involved. Assuming that this ethical question has been settled preoperatively, and that the surgeon and the patient have agreed to proceed without blood transfusion, then if major blood loss occurs and replacement would normally be required, colloids such as Hetastarch or Dextran must be used. Fluosol DA, an acellular oxygen carrier, is of uncertain value (Gould et al, 1986).

INTESTINAL TRACT

Local damage to the intestinal wall or injury to a whole segment of the intestine may occur during any gynecologic procedure, especially during the removal of a pelvic mass due to endometriosis, inflammatory disease or cancer. About one-third of such injuries occur during entrance into the peritoneal cavity, one-third during the dissection or removal of a pelvic mass and one-third during laparoscopy, vaginal operations or dilatation and curettage or evacuation (Wheelock and Krebs, 1984).

Prevention

Careful surgical technique can prevent some but not all intestinal injuries. First, the peritoneal cavity should be entered away from any previous scar whenever possible, for example, at the upper end of an old incision. The peritoneum and its outer coverings should be picked up and incised layer by layer, the surgeon attempting to see if the intestine slides back and forth beneath the presumed peritoneum. Second, lysis of adhesions from the abdominal wall and between loops of bowel should be done with a knife or fine (Metzenbaum) scissors, separating the adhesions at the "white" peritoneal line and using traction with a Kocher clamp on the peritoneum and fascia or a Deaver retractor and countertraction with a sponge and/ or fingers (Fig. 3–3). Third, when the intestines are to be packed away from the pelvis, adhesions to the pelvic structures must first be divided so that neither the bowel nor its mesentery is torn when packs are inserted. Fourth, when a pelvic mass is being dissected off intestine, particularly the sigmoid colon, maximum exposure should be maintained. Also it is better, if there is no suspicion of cancer, to leave some of the inflammatory or endometriotic tissue on the colon rather than vice versa. When cancer is present, complete removal is advisable, even at the expense of intestinal injury. Fifth, when the pelvic or parietal peritoneum is being closed, the intestinal wall must be protected from inclusion in a suture by appropriate retraction and maintenance of adequate depth of anesthesia. This is a special risk when through-and-through sutures of the Smead-Jones type are used. These should be inserted under direct vision, left untied and all or several of them held up as each one is tied down.

Diagnosis

Whatever the cause of intestinal injury, prompt recognition is essential. Injuries to the serosa may be difficult to identify among many adhesions. All the involved intestine should be carefully inspected after the adhesions have been divided. If the lumen of the small intestine is entered, the yellow intestinal content can be easily identified, especially if it is profuse or

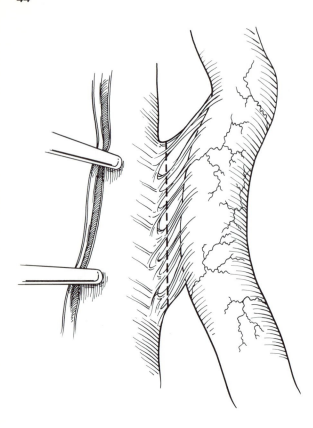

Figure 3–3. Division of adhesions between the intestine and the anterior abdominal wall. Clamps enable traction to be placed on the peritoneum, permitting adhesions to be cut close to the peritoneum and away from the intestine.

the intestine is distended. If the colon is opened, the fecal smell is diagnostic. Injury to the mesentery may lead to loss of blood supply to the affected segment of intestine. This turns dark blue or even black and is quite distinct from the neighboring healthy, pink intestine. If there is doubt about its viability, all tension should be relieved, hot packs should be placed on the intestine and it should be observed for five to ten minutes. If the color returns to normal, it should be checked again later in the operation. When the intestine remains dark, it is best treated as non-viable and the appropriate segment resected.

Treatment

The gynecologic surgeon who has had experience in bowel surgery and/or gynecologic oncology should handle all injuries to the intestine. The inexperienced gynecologist should be able to repair simple tears of the serosa, even if the mucosa has been entered. If the situation is complicated or there is doubt in the gynecologist's mind as to the best management, he should obtain consultation from a general surgeon.

Intestinal injury should generally be repaired promptly so that it is not forgotten and continued contamination of the peritoneal cavity is prevented. The only exception may be when further dissection is needed to expose the damaged intestine properly. The types of intestinal injury include (1) a serosal or seromuscular tear, (2) a single incision into the intestinal lumen, (3) multiple incisions in the intestine, (4) lacerations of the mesentery and (5) necrosis of intestine due to injury to the mesentery or involvement of the intestine with tumor.

Small serosal or seromuscular tears should usually be repaired with one or more inverting silk sutures (Fig. 3–4) so as to minimize subsequent adhesions. When many adhesions have to be divided, only the major serosal injuries should be closed.

When the small intestine has been entered, the remaining peritoneal cavity should be packed off. Rubber-shod clamps, closed at the first notch only, should be applied to the intestine above and below the laceration to prevent peritoneal contamination. The intestine should be repaired in two layers, a first layer of continuous 30 chromic catgut, including all layers of the intestinal wall, and a second layer of interrupted 30 silk sutures inverting the serosa; 30

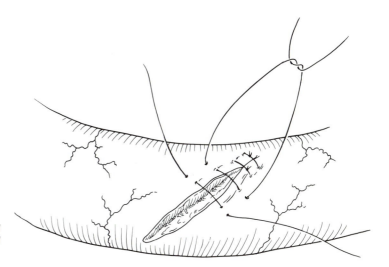

Figure 3–4. Closure of a superficial tear of the intestine with interrupted inverting sutures.

vicryl may be used for both layers. Some authors prefer interrupted sutures. The suture line should usually be placed transversely so as not to narrow the lumen (Fig. 3–5). If an incision has been made in the colon, infection is a more serious problem, and the degree of contamination is important. If contamination is minimal, the incision may be closed like one in the small intestine, except that, because of the distensibility of the colon, it is not usually necessary to place the suture line transversely.

Tears in the mesentery, particularly of the small intestine, result from ill-advised traction or packing. They are more likely to occur in obese women. Bleeding vessels must be ligated, and the intestine supplied by them should be observed for color and viability. Usually collateral circulation is sufficient to prevent necrosis, unless a major vessel at the root of the mesentery has been tied. The mesentery should be approximated with fine synthetic sutures such as 30 vicryl.

Long or multiple incisions in a segment of intestine, radiation damage or involvement of a segment in a pelvic tumor requires resection of a portion of intestine and end-to-end anastomosis. Stapling devices have made this a quicker and easier task. Details of the use of the GIA and TA instruments for anastomoses and the LDS instrument for dividing the mesentery are given by Wheeless (1982). In principle, the loop to be removed is identified and the mesentery divided for a short distance at each end, starting close to the intestine. The intestine is then divided with the GIA instrument and the two limbs approximated. The antimesenteric edges and their staples are cut off, and the GIA instrument is inserted into the

two lumina so formed and fired. The approximated open ends are then closed with the TA instrument, thus producing, in effect, a side-to-side but functional end-to-end anastomosis. The mesentery is then closed with 30 vicryl. The same stapling instruments can be used for anastomoses in the colon or for end-to-side or side-to-side bypass procedures (Fig. 3–6). When a low colonic anastomosis is necessary the EEA instrument can be used (for details see Wheeless, 1982).

The immediate complications of stapled anastomoses appear to be no different from those of the conventional ones in which sutures are used. Blood supply is usually excellent at the edges, and breakdown of the anastomosis with leakage is most likely to be due to the underlying disease, i.e., cancer, radiation damage or poor nutritional status. The long-term complications of stapling are unknown. The presence of the metal may be an impediment to the future use of CT scans or NMR. Also the staples may migrate, but the effect of this is uncertain.

For many years intestinal anastomoses have been performed by a variety of suture techniques. These are still preferred by some surgeons and may be applicable to specific situations, such as anastomosis of the colon low in the pelvis where the staplers cannot be maneuvered or when the EEA is not available or cannot be used. The author's preference is for a two layer anastomosis using an inner continuous layer of 30 chromic catgut and an outer layer of interrupted inverted 30 silk sutures (see Fig. 3–5). Several points of technique are important. First, excess intestinal content should be milked away from the loop and the proximal and distal bowel occluded by rubber-shod

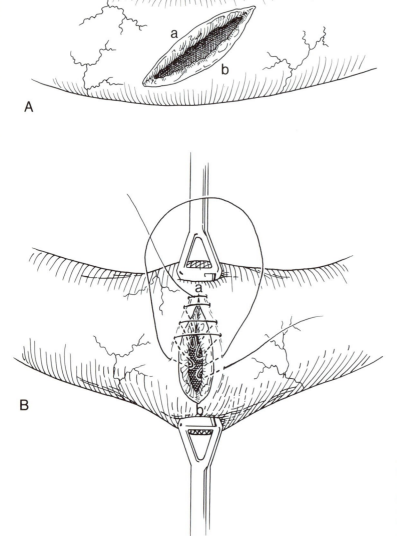

Figure 3–5. Closure of an oblique tear through all layers of the intestine. A, Oblique tear. B, The tear is closed transversely. The first continuous inverting suture is shown. A second layer of interrupted serosal sutures will then be placed.

clamps, secured at the first notch only so as not to injure the intestinal wall. Second, after division of the appropriate amount of mesentery, straight clamps should be placed across the intestine at an angle so as to give a larger lumen, and then the intestine is divided. Third, fat and mesentery should be removed from the ends of the bowel that are to be anastomosed. Fourth, sutures should not be placed far away from the lumen so as to avoid inverting a large wad of tissue. Fifth, particular care should be taken with the sutures at the angles of the anastomosis. Sixth, the resulting lumen should be checked with the finger and thumb for

adequate patency. Seventh, the mesentery should be closed with 30 vicryl sutures.

Whenever the intestine has been opened, there is a possibility of infection, which is more likely if the colon is involved. Intestinal content should be removed as completely as possible after the anastomosis by sponging, suction and irrigation with normal saline. Broad spectrum antibiotics such as a second generation cephalosporin should be started as soon as possible (during the operation); intraperitoneal or intraintestinal antibiotics are of limited value. Intestinal decompression should be started by inserting a nasogastric tube (not a long tube)

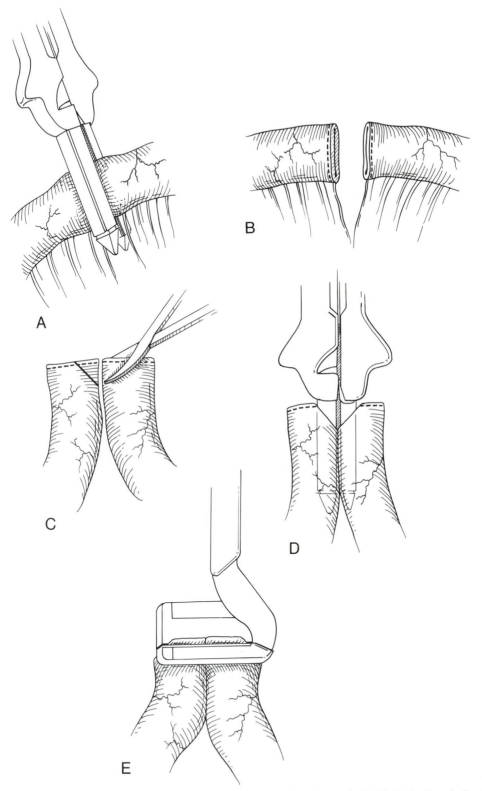

Figure 3–6. Intestinal resection using staplers. A, Application of GIA Stapler. B, Divided intestine. C, Excision of approximated anti-mesenteric corners. D, Insertion and firing of GIA Stapler to join the two lumina. E, Closure of open corners with TA Stapler.

while the patient is still under anesthesia; its presence in the stomach can be confirmed by palpation. If a long tube is already in the stomach, it can usually be manipulated, if necessary, into the duodenum.

The postoperative care of patients whose intestinal serosa alone has required closure does not differ from the normal postoperative care following laparotomy. If the intestinal lumen has been opened and closed or an anastomosis has been performed, oral intake should be prohibited until the patient has passed gas by rectum and there are no signs of intraperitoneal infection, ileus or obstruction. Appropriate intravenous fluids are required during this time. If a nasogastric tube has been inserted, it should be left in place on suction for two to five days (primarily to remove swallowed air), depending on the extent of the operation and the patient's progress. If a long intestinal tube is in place, it is important before pulling it out to be sure that it will no longer be needed, because of the time and difficulty required in inserting it. Thus, it should first be clamped for several hours. Then, liquids should be given with the tube in place. If no ileus or obstruction occurs, the tube may then be pulled out. For complications of intestinal tubes see Chapter 4.

Intestinal Stomas

The commonest stoma required for intraoperative complications in gynecology is a transverse colostomy. Very rarely, an end colostomy (see Chapter 6) or ileostomy is necessary in recurrent ovarian cancer. Gastrostomy or jejunostomy may occasionally be chosen to provide a portal for alimentation (see Chapter 4).

A transverse colostomy is most often indicated as a temporary diversion of the fecal stream when the colon has been opened during a pelvic operation and there has been considerable contamination. A transverse incision is made on the left side of the abdomen, preferably below the belt line. The rectus fascia is divided vertically, the rectus muscle split and the peritoneal cavity entered. A loop of transverse colon, on the left, is identified and brought through the abdominal wall with the distal loop to the left and the proximal loop to the right. The mesentery is opened close to the bowel and a retaining rod, usually fitted to a bag, is passed underneath it. The fascia and skin are closed loosely around the intestine. The unopened intestine is covered with petroleum jelly (Vaseline), gauze and dressings.

Twenty-four hours later the antimesenteric wall of the intestine is opened transversely ($\frac{1}{3}$ to $\frac{1}{2}$ of its width) with a knife or cautery. Postoperative care and closure are described in Chapter 4.

URINARY TRACT

Bladder

The incidence of injury to the bladder will vary with the difficulty of the operation and the skill of the surgeon. Precise data are difficult to obtain. Wheelock and associates (1984) report bladder injuries to have occurred in at least 1.8% of abdominal hysterectomies and 0.4% of vaginal hysterectomies. Management of bladder injuries should be within the capability of every well trained gynecologist. However, consultation with a urologist may be advisable.

The bladder is susceptible to damage at several different points during gynecologic procedures. When the abdomen is opened, the bladder may be entered if the peritoneal incision is extended downward too far or if the bladder has been pulled up as the result of scarring from a previous operation such as a cesarean section. During abdominal hysterectomy the bladder may be entered in the midline as it is being dissected or pushed downward off the cervix. The lateral angle of the bladder may be injured if it is adherent to a pelvic mass. When the vagina is being closed at its lateral angle or in the midline, the bladder may be included in a stitch. Finally, in suprapubic vesico-urethral suspension the bladder may be torn as exposure is maintained and sutures are being placed in the periurethral tissues. All of the above problems are more likely if the normal structures are distorted by tumors, inflammatory disease or endometriosis or if a radical hysterectomy is being performed.

The likelihood of injury to the bladder in an abdominal procedure may be lessened by several techniques. First, the bladder should be emptied before operation and kept empty by use of an indwelling Foley catheter. Caution should be used in opening the peritoneum after a previous lower abdominal operation. Often the bladder can be recognized by holding the thin peritoneum above it to the light. When the bladder is dissected off the cervix, the proper plane should be established by sharp dissection in the midline with the points of the scissors directed toward the cervix rather than the bladder. Blunt dissection with finger or sponge should be used only after a good plane has been established. Laterally, dissection should remain close to the tumor or pelvic mass, pushing the bladder carefully downward. Finally, as the vagina is closed, the bladder edge should be identified below the sutures as they are placed.

During vaginal hysterectomy or repair of the anterior vaginal wall the bladder may be entered as it is being dissected or pushed upward off the cervix. This can be avoided by dissecting close to the cervix in the midline, thus also avoiding bleeding that may be encountered from the bladder pillars laterally and that may obliterate the usual landmarks. Again, the relationship between the bladder and cervix may be distorted by large tumors, adhesions or inflammation. In such cases it may be better to perform the operation abdominally rather than vaginally.

It is most important that bladder injuries be recognized promptly. The appearance of urine, not always easy to identify, its smell or the sight of the bulb of the indwelling catheter are diagnostic. The appearance of blood in the urine, a common occurrence during pelvic procedures, is simply a sign that the bladder wall is being traumatized, but its presence should caution the surgeon to look carefully for any injury. On occasion injection of methylene blue or sterile milk (the former is usually easier to obtain in the operating room) through the indwelling catheter can identify a small leak. If necessary, the incision in the bladder may be extended so that the inside of the bladder can be seen more clearly. Repairing a somewhat larger laceration does not increase the difficulty or decrease the success rate.

If the bladder wall has merely been included in the suture, it is best removed; nothing else need be done. If there is a laceration into the bladder, it should be repaired promptly before continuing with the definitive procedure. This is to prevent continued leakage of urine, possible contamination of the peritoneal cavity or increase in size of the laceration with retraction. Also, the laceration may conceivably be forgotten if it is not repaired promptly.

Various methods have been described for closing the bladder. The author's preference is first to identify the ends of the laceration with Allis or Babcock clamps and be sure that it does not come close to the ureteric orifices. This may mean opening the bladder further. The bladder wall is then closed with two layers of continuous 30 chromic catgut. The first layer includes the mucosa (there is no need to avoid it) and the deep part of the muscularis. The second layer closes the superficial part of the muscle. Non-absorbable sutures may form a nidus for stone formation, and the delayed absorption of polyglycolic sutures may impede healing. Interrupted sutures do not provide a watertight closure and take longer to insert. A continuous locking suture may compromise the blood supply and cause breakdown of the repair.

When the bladder has been entered and repaired there is always the possibility of postoperative urinary leakage. If this occurs and the urine cannot escape, a urinoma or collection of urine develops with resultant pain, fever, infection and possibly development of a vesicoperitoneal, vesicocutaneous or vesicovaginal fistula. The chance of this occurring can be lessened by keeping the bladder empty and by inserting an extraperitoneal drain. Either a suprapubic catheter (inserted away from the repair) or an indwelling urethral catheter may be used (see Chapter 5). Extraperitoneal drainage is indicated when there has been considerable bleeding or chance of contamination or when the space of Retzius has been opened. The drain (Penrose or suction) is brought out through a separate stab incision. The catheter should be left in place for at least five days. The drain should be left in a day longer than the catheter and longer still if urine continues to drain. When bladder laceration occurs during vaginal hysterectomy, a retropubic drain is not necessary because leaking urine can escape through the vagina. However, urethral or suprapubic bladder drainage for at least five days is essential. If only the superficial part of the bladder wall has been injured and can be repaired by a single continuous suture, bladder drainage is not usually necessary for more than 24 hours, and extraperitoneal drainage is not needed.

Urethra

Injuries to the urethra are most likely to occur with anterior vaginal repair or suprapubic vesico-urethral suspension. They are covered in Chapter 4.

Ureter

Injuries to the ureter, either real or suspected, usually require consultation with a urologist, unless the gynecologist is experienced in handling these problems. However, it is essential that the gynecologist understand the principles of diagnosis and management that follow, in the event that he is unable to obtain the necessary consultation.

The course of the ureter in the pelvis and its proximity to the ovary, cervix and upper vagina make it liable to injury in almost every major gynecologic procedure. The exact incidence of ureteral damage in gynecologic procedures is not known, because many injuries may never be recognized during or after operation and because data are difficult to collect. Symmonds (1981) gave the incidence as 0.5 to 2.5%. These data were, however, obtained in the 1950's and 1960's, and current data are not available except for radical hysterectomy where the incidence has fallen from 5 to 10% to 1% or less in the past 20 years.

The sites at which ureteral injury is most likely are (1) anterior and lateral to the cervix and vagina, (2) medial to the uterine artery and (3) posterior to the infundibulopelvic ligament (Fig. 3–7). Distortion of the ureter in its course by a pelvic tumor increases the chance of injury.

Because of the grave consequences of ureteral injury all possible preventive measures should be taken. A preoperative intravenous pyelo-

gram, ultrasonogram or CT scan is important in demonstrating ureteral displacement or obstruction. The preoperative insertion of a urethral catheter when dissection of the ureter is likely to be difficult is of little or no value. First, it takes considerable time and coordination of effort. Second, it may give a sense of false security and, in fact, permit the ureter to be stripped bare of adventitial tissue, thus denuding its blood supply and causing later necrosis. Third, the situation intraoperatively may not be nearly as difficult as was anticipated, thus, post hoc, making the insertion of catheters unnecessary. The most important factor in preventing ureteral injury is adequate exposure and avoiding blind clamping of bleeding points, especially near the uterine artery and vein and at the corner of the vagina and bladder.

The ureter should be identified in every abdominal hysterectomy. This procedure is usually simple and takes little time. The posterior peritoneum is divided from the round ligament upward and lateral to the infundibulopelvic ligament, including division of the round ligament if that is part of the operation. The retroperitoneal space is entered by blunt and sharp dissection of the areolar tissue until the external iliac artery is felt and then exposed.

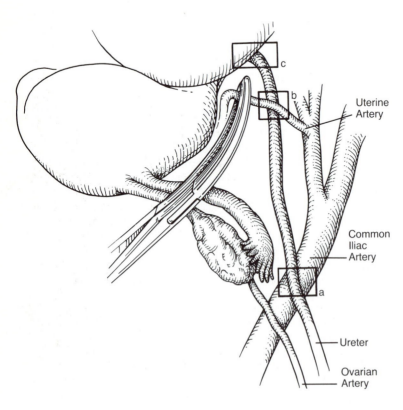

Figure 3–7. Sites of possible injury to the right ureter. A, Where the ureter crosses the common iliac artery and is close to the infundibulo-pelvic ligament. B, Where the ureter passes medial to the uterine artery. C, Where the ureter turns medially, close to the cervix, to enter the bladder.

Uterine Artery

Common Iliac Artery

Ureter

Ovarian Artery

The medial leaf of the peritoneum is retracted medially. The ureter may be felt by compressing this medial peritoneal flap between finger and thumb starting at the bony pelvis and moving anteriorly. The ureter is a firm structure that can be snapped between the finger and thumb. In addition, it should be exposed at about the point where the infundibulopelvic ligament is to be divided so that the ligament can be isolated and divided without damage to the ureter. The ureter can then be followed down, if necessary, to the point where it passes medial to the uterine artery and even to where it enters the bladder. In dissecting out the ureter, as much adventitia as possible should be left on it. A long Babcock clamp is very useful for holding the ureter and supplying gentle traction. Lower down, medial and upward traction on the uterus is helpful. When the ureter has been partially freed, it must be carefully avoided and not kinked during closure of the pelvic peritoneum.

Ureteral injuries include crushing in a clamp, ligation, incision and division. The diagnosis is important but sometimes difficult to make, since the injury occurs when exposure is poor and is complicated by heavy bleeding. Failure to recognize the problem is likely to result in ureteral obstruction or leakage of urine into the peritoneal cavity, retroperitoneal space or vagina. If a ureteral injury is suspected, the ureter must be exposed above the point of concern and carefully traced downward past that point. Sometimes it is helpful to inject methylene blue into the ureter above the area in question with a 22-gauge needle to determine if there is obstruction to the injection or leakage at the site of possible incision or division.

Once it has been determined that a ureter has been clamped or ligated, the clamp should be released or the ligature cut. The viability of the constricted segment must then be determined. If occlusion has been partial or momentary, the wall of the ureter may appear entirely normal in color and peristaltic waves may pass through it. If the inclusion has been complete or maintained for more than a minute or two, the wall will appear dusky in comparison with the ureter above and below it. If the ureter appears entirely normal, an extraperitoneal drain (Penrose or suction) should be placed at the site of injury and brought out through a lateral stab incision. If there is any doubt about viability, the ureter should be splinted and an extraperitoneal drain placed. Various techniques of splinting have been described. The

author's preference is to open the dome of the bladder vertically, identify the ureteric orifices using, if necessary, a retractor in the bladder, and insert a No. 5 or No. 6 French silastic catheter up the ureter to the renal pelvis. The distal end is then passed through the urethra and secured to the indwelling Foley catheter. It may also be attached to a suprapubic drainage catheter. The bladder is then closed as described previously. Another method involves placing a catheter or T-tube through the damaged area by making a separate incision in the ureter above the injury. This increases the danger of urinary leakage and possible later stricture. If a large area of ureter appears nonviable, it must be resected and either reanastomosis or reimplantation performed.

If it is determined that the ureter has been incised or partly divided, it should be repaired with fine (40) vicryl sutures and splinted, and an extraperitoneal drain placed.

If the ureter has been completely divided or a necrotic segment has to be excised, reestablishment of continuity is necessary. If the injury is within 8 to 10 cm of the bladder, it is best to reimplant the ureter into the bladder (ureteroneocystostomy). The distal ureter should first be ligated. Then, the simplest technique is to spatulate the end of the ureter (Fig. 3–8). A 30 chromic catgut suture is inserted into each spatulated end. A small incision is made in the most convenient part of the bladder. The sutures are placed through the incision and each end is brought out of the bladder wall and tied so that the spatulated ends are spread inside the bladder. The periureteral tissue is then sutured to the outside of the bladder with several 30 chromic catgut sutures to relieve tension. A second method is to sew the ureteric mucosa directly to the bladder wall with several interrupted sutures. In this technique the ureter may be tunnelled within the bladder wall, reproducing its normal course, in the hope of preventing reflux. The submucosal tunnel is made with a curved instrument for about 3 cm, and the ureter is then drawn through it before making the anastomosis. If there is tension on the ureter in making the anastomosis, the bladder may be drawn up and fixed with two or three 0 vicryl sutures to the psoas muscle on the same side. This is best done prior to the anastomosis; the surgeon should keep a finger inside the bladder as he performs this procedure. After the ureteroneocystostomy has been performed, splinting is indicated if there is concern about the security of the anastomosis.

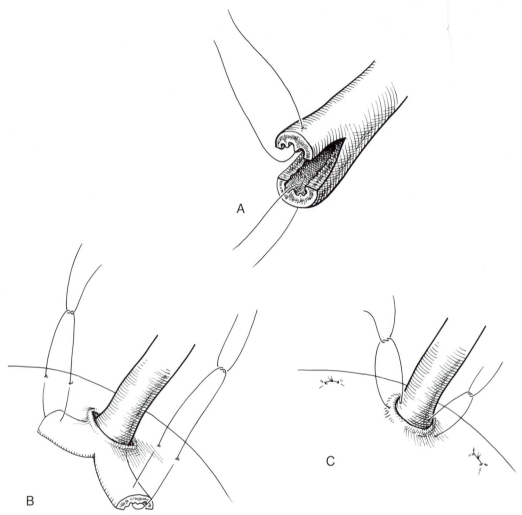

Figure 3–8. Reimplantation of ureter into bladder. A, Spatulation of end of ureter. B, Insertion of ureter into bladder and fixation of spatulated ends. C, Suture of periureteral tissue to superficial bladder wall.

The splint can be attached to the indwelling Foley catheter or to a suprapubic catheter inserted into the bladder through a separate stab incision. In all cases an extraperitoneal drain should be placed.

If the ureter is divided at or above the pelvic brim and cannot be brought down to the bladder, an end-to-end anastomosis is necessary. The ureter must be freed so that there is no tension on it. Holding sutures are placed 2 to 3 cm away from each end through the ureteral muscle but not into the lumen. A splint is inserted as described before. The upper and lower ends of the divided ureter are spatulated to increase the lumen at the site of anastomosis and the ends are sutured with four to six 40 vicryl sutures. The holding sutures are then tied to the psoas muscle to relieve tension on the anastomosis. An extraperitoneal (suction) drain is placed near but not touching the anastomosis.

Occasionally the section of damaged ureter is so long that repair by either of the above methods will not be possible. Alternatives then consist of joining one ureter to the other (transureteroureterostomy), interposing a segment of intestine as a substitute ureter, bringing the upper end of the ureter to the skin (cutaneous ureterostomy), creating a nephrostomy or in extreme circumstances ligating the ureter, effecting a nephrectomy.

The postoperative care of patients who have had ureteral injuries repaired by any of the methods just discussed is similar. Urinary antibiotics (see Chapter 4) should be used. Ureteral splints should be removed about seven days postoperatively and extraperitoneal drains one to two days later if there is no urinary leakage. If leakage continues around the drain, it should be left in place until the drainage ceases, which may be up to 14 days after operation. Postoperative follow-up intravenous pyelograms are necessary (see Chapter 4).

NEUROLOGIC COMPLICATIONS

Intraoperative injury to the nerves of the pelvis is rare. The nerves most likely to be involved in gynecologic procedures are the femoral, genitofemoral, obturator, ilioinguinal and lateral cutaneous nerve of the thigh. In obstetrics, fibers of the lumbosacral cord (and particularly the common peroneal nerve) and the pudendal nerve are most susceptible to injury. Most injuries are not recognized at operation, and therefore intraoperative management is largely preventive.

The femoral nerve (L2, 3, 4) descends through the psoas muscle, emerges between the psoas and iliacus muscles and enters the thigh underneath the inguinal ligament lateral to the femoral artery. It gives off the intermediate and medial cutaneous nerves of the thigh, supplying the skin of the medial and anterior aspects of the thigh down to the knee and muscular branches to the sartorius. The posterior branch gives off the saphenous nerve, supplying the skin of the medial part of the leg and foot. Muscle branches go to the quadriceps femoris. Injuries occur from the use of deep retraction, especially with a transverse incision, or from hyperflexion of the thigh in vaginal hysterectomy. The symptoms are recognized at various times postoperatively. They consist of sensory loss, usually numbness, over the area covered by the nerve and motor loss of the quadriceps, resulting in inability to extend the leg and walk properly. Management is discussed in Chapter 4.

The genitofemoral nerve (L1, 2) lies in front of the psoas muscle and lateral to the external iliac artery. The genital branch accompanies the round ligament and supplies the skin of the mons pubis and the labium majus. The femoral branch supplies the skin over the femoral triangle. Injury results in sensory loss (numbness) over the areas supplied. Injury is likely to occur when a large pelvic mass is adherent to the sidewall or when biopsy or removal of the external iliac lymph nodes is done. When possible, the nerve should be isolated and preserved. If, however, it has to be removed, the consequences do not seriously affect function.

The obturator nerve (L2, 3, 4) lies in the obturator fossa posterior to the external iliac vein (Fig. 3–9). Its anterior branch supplies the hip joint, the adductor longus muscle, the gracilis, the adductor brevis and rarely the pectineus. Its posterior branch supplies the adductor magnus. The nerve is susceptible to injury when an adherent pelvic mass is being removed or when biopsy or removal of the obturator nodes is done. Injury results in inability to adduct the thigh and some instability of motion, particularly when running. Therefore, exposure and preservation of the nerve is important. The external iliac vein must be carefully held back with a vein retractor. Dissection should be performed parallel to the nerve, and the space lateral and posterior to it should be avoided because of the danger of bleeding that may be heavy and difficult to control, thereby increasing the problem of exposure of the nerve.

The iliohypogastric (L1) and ilioinguinal (L1) nerves usually lie outside the gynecologic field. They are closely related and perforate the transversus muscle near the anterior part of the iliac crest and then pass through the internal oblique muscle and the inguinal ring to supply the skin of the upper medial part of the thigh, the mons pubis and the labium majus. They may be susceptible to injury if a lower transverse incision extends far laterally or if the external oblique muscle is divided during extraperitoneal pelvic lymphadenectomy. Loss of function of these nerves produces no serious deficit.

The lateral cutaneous nerve of the thigh (L2, 3) passes laterally into the thigh behind the inguinal ligament and supplies the skin of the anterior and posterior aspects of the lateral thigh. It may be divided into two parts by a portion of the inguinal ligament. Branches of this nerve are inevitably divided when inguinal lymphadenectomy is performed for carcinoma of the vulva. Injury gives rise to paresthesia and pain in the lateral aspect of the thigh, a condition sometimes known as meralgia paresthetica.

Obstetric injuries to the lumbosacral plexus are usually not recognizable at delivery. Involvement of the common peroneal nerve leads to loss of function of the peroneal muscles and the skin of the lateral and dorsal parts of the foot and toes. This results in foot-drop and also

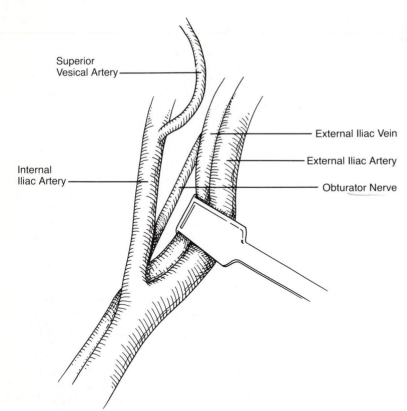

Superior
Vesical Artery

External Iliac Vein

External Iliac Artery

Obturator Nerve

Internal
Iliac Artery

Figure 3–9. *Exposure of the right obturator nerve.*

an alteration in or absence of sensation in the area supplied. Contusion or damage to the pudendal nerve may occur as it passes medial to the ischial spine, and this may lead to altered perineal sensation. It is difficult to distinguish pain due to nerve injury from that due to other disorders in the same area. The only prophylaxis against obstetric nerve injuries is to avoid prolonging the use of the lithotomy position for delivery and to minimize difficult vaginal operative procedures.

Changes in the spinal cord and peripheral nerves due to anesthesia are discussed in Chapter 15.

Operative management of nerve injuries is limited. Repair of small nerves, the loss of which has no serious functional sequelae, is not indicated. If a larger nerve such as the obturator nerve is bruised, no treatment is indicated. Recovery is likely in weeks or months (see Chapter 4). If such a nerve is completely divided, immediate repair is unlikely to be successful, but should be attempted with neurosurgical consultation. Nerve repair ideally requires the operating microscope and the use of very fine sutures to approximate the nerve

bundles. Since this is hardly feasible in the case of the obturator nerve specifically, closure of the perineurium with the finest sutures available and release of tension on the joined nerve by approximating the surrounding tissue is the best that can be done.

Later management and prognosis of nerve injury are discussed in Chapter 4.

CLOSURE OF INCISION

Intraoperative complications of closing incisions are relatively few. However, later problems arise from difficulties with closure. Therefore, several important prophylactic steps should be taken during closure.

The first structure to be closed is usually the pelvic peritoneum. Continued adequate exposure is necessary so that ureter, bladder and colon may be avoided. It is important not to let the ureter kink, especially if it has been freed from its surrounding attachments. If there is a large denuded area in the pelvis, it is better not to reperitonealize it.

Before the parietal (anterior) peritoneum is closed, a careful sponge and instrument count is mandatory. The prevention of postoperative intraperitoneal adhesions is also a matter of concern. The number of raw areas encountered or caused during operation should be minimized. In operations such as tubal plastic procedures in which postoperative adhesions can cause tubal obstruction, the instillation of 250 ml of 32% Dextran 70 (Hyskon) decreased adhesions significantly on second-look laparoscopy performed eight to 12 weeks later (Adhesion Study Group, 1983), although a randomized study by Jansen (1985) showed no beneficial effect from intraperitoneal 32% Dextran 70 or 0.5% hydrocortisone sodium succinate. Allergic reactions and impaired hemostasis occasionally result from the intravenous use of Dextran, but do not appear to occur when it is used intraperitoneally. However, Magyar and co-workers (1985) reported that 4% of 234 women had spontaneous leakage of fluid from the incision; 8% had painless swelling of the labia, and bloating and weight gain were also noted. The last symptom may have been related to the concomitant use of dexamethasone, while the amount of Dextran used (200 ml) may have contributed to the first two. Postoperative shoulder pain has been reported after the use of intraperitoneal Dextran; it may be greatly lessened by inserting the Dextran with the patient in the semi-sitting position (45 degree elevation) and maintaining her in that position for 48 hours (Fanning and Awad, 1985).

The type of fascial closure can contribute to the prevention of postoperative wound dehiscence. Most studies report the incidence of wound disruption after major abdominal operations to be 1 to 3%, and the median mortality rate is 18.1%. Local mechanical factors are important causes, along with general nutritional status, increased intraabdominal pressure postoperatively, the nature of the operation and infection. Traditionally transverse incisions have been thought to be stronger than vertical ones, but this does not seem to be true. Of the vertical incisions, a midline is stronger than a paramedian or more lateral rectus incision. In closing fascia, the use of chromic catgut should be abandoned, but most other sutures, absorbable and non-absorbable, are equivalent to one another, with monofilament sutures probably preferable. Interrupted fascial sutures should be placed as far away from the wound edges as they are from each other. Internal retention sutures of the Smead-Jones type or through-and-through (mass closure) sutures are thought to have advantages, especially in patients with cancer or infection. However, a continuous suture with each stitch placed well laterally is quicker and probably as effective. Subcutaneous stitches are needed only if there is likely to be much dead space. Careful skin closure (unless the wound must be left open because of infection) with clips or subcuticular sutures is important for cosmetic reasons (Poole, 1985).

During peritoneal closure the chief danger is that of placing a suture through intestine or omentum. Adequate depth of anesthesia is important. When retention sutures, such as those of the Smead-Jones type, are placed, care should be taken to see that a loop of intestine or a piece of omentum is not caught as each suture is pulled up and tied.

The complications of closure of the fascia and skin occur postoperatively in the form of wound hematoma, wound breakdown, infection, dehiscence and later hernia. Their management will be considered in Chapter 4. The performance of abdominoplasty, removing excess fat, at the time of laparotomy for gynecologic disease, is often desired by obese patients. However, both intraoperative and postoperative complications, e.g., operating time, blood loss, fever and pulmonary emboli, are significantly increased in such patients (Voss et al, 1986). Thus careful patient selection is necessary, and the combined procedure should certainly be avoided in high-risk patients.

In some gynecologic procedures the peritoneum, retroperitoneal space, retropubic space or subcutaneous tissues require drainage because of infection or possible leakage of lymph or urine. Suction drains (Jackson-Pratt, Hemovac) are useful prophylactically when considerable accumulations of fluid are anticipated. They should be placed extraperitoneally rather than transperitoneally. Sump drains are best used for infection and to prevent closure of an abscess cavity. Penrose drains (¼, ½ or 1 inch) can be used when small amounts of drainage are expected. Whenever possible, drains should be brought out through a separate incision, lateral to a midline incision, below a transverse one. Drains must be fixed to the skin to prevent their being pulled out or retracted below the skin (Fig. 3–10). The use of drains for specific operations is covered in other chapters. Drains should be removed as soon as possible, usually when drainage has ceased.

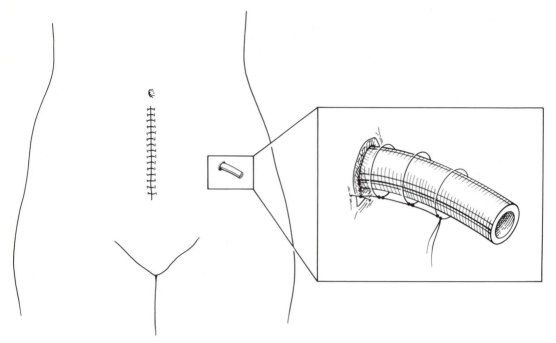

Figure 3–10. Site of exit and method of securing drain to skin.

IMMEDIATE POSTOPERATIVE DISCUSSION

How the patient and her family react to the news of a complication, both immediately and later, depends upon appropriate intraoperative behavior by the surgeon and his team and upon the immediate postoperative discussions with the patient's family and with her. Careful handling of these situations will help to ensure their help in the management of the complication and may prevent a later lawsuit or legal complication.

Discussion about the patient's disease, the findings or the prognosis should be minimal during induction of and recovery from anesthesia, since the patient's auditory sense lingers longer and begins earlier than one would expect. Also, special care must be observed if the patient is receiving local or regional anesthesia. Even casual conversation is susceptible to misinterpretation by the patient, who tends to feel that any comments on another interesting case apply to her. During the operation the surgeon or designated operating room personnel should keep in touch with the patient's waiting family, particularly if there is a delay in starting the operation, if an unexpected or major complication occurs or if the procedure takes longer than expected.

The patient and her family should be informed of the results of the operation as soon as possible afterwards. Several considerations are important. First, the operating team—surgeon and assistants—should decide what information should be given to the patient and her family, so that their messages can be consistent. In most gynecologic or obstetric operations this message can be straightforward and factual, but preliminary discussion is important when cancer has been found, when pelvic organs have had to be removed unexpectedly or when there has been an intraoperative complication. When possible the recovery room nurse and the patient's nurse on the gynecologic floor should receive the same information.

Second, since the patient is usually recovering from anesthesia, the family is the first to know the results of the operation. It is best to talk to the nearest relative first, such as husband, mother, daughter, son or brother rather than addressing a large group at once and to conduct the discussion sitting and in a relaxed manner. At this time families are concerned about future treatment, how long the patient will be in the recovery room and in the hospital and how she will feel and what she may do when she goes home. Explanations should be simple and understandable and should avoid medical jargon. When plans are uncertain, discussion about them should be deferred.

Third, the patient herself must be informed about the operation as soon as possible and from her surgeon rather than from a nurse or by overhearing a conversation between medical personnel. This means that a brief word of reassurance should be given in the recovery room, and a slightly more detailed explanation should be given later in the same day if feasible. The patient may not remember these discussions. Therefore, full details should be given after she recovers from anesthesia, often the next morning.

The report given to the family and the patient should almost always be the same. Requests not to tell the patient certain facts should be resisted. Although some patients may appear to prefer not to know about what was found, few are totally without curiosity about their bodies. A simple statement of the facts, together with repeated opportunities to ask questions, is appropriate.

A few special circumstances arise. If the news is bad, e.g., the discovery of advanced ovarian cancer, the gravity of the situation must be mentioned but the possibilities of help from further treatment emphasized. If a decision about such treatment cannot be reached until further information is obtained (e.g., from the pathology laboratory), it is well not to outline the possible modes of treatment in detail but rather to be encouraging about the possible ameliorative effects of therapy and not to be drawn at this point into an unprofitable discussion of longevity or disability.

The exact method of handling the news of a complication will vary with its severity. Generally, the complication should be mentioned in a matter-of-fact manner, plans for management discussed and the effect on the patient's recovery assessed. Questions must be answered frankly without self-reproach and without putting the blame on any member of the team. The same attitude toward the complication must be shown by all other members of the team who come in contact with the patient and the family. It is important that the complication be mentioned in the chart or operative note in a similarly matter-of-fact manner. Plans for further specific treatment should be included as soon as they are known. Finally, if the patient or her family has trouble speaking or understanding English, it is doubly important to use simple language and/or to obtain a good interpreter.

References

Adhesion Study Group: Reduction of postoperative pelvic adhesions with intraperitoneal 32% dextran 70: a prospective, randomized clinical trial. *Fertil. Steril.* 40:612, 1983.

Alexander JW, Aerni S, Plettner JP: Development of a safe and effective one-minute preoperative skin preparation. *Arch. Surg.* 120:1357, 1985.

American Association of Blood Banks, American Red Cross, Council of Community Blood Centers: Circular of information for the use of human blood and blood components, 1984.

Burchell RC: Internal iliac artery ligation: hemodynamics. *Obstet. Gynecol.* 24:737, 1964.

Cruikshank SH, Stoelk EM: Surgical control of pelvic hemorrhage: method of bilateral ovarian artery ligation. *Am. J. Obstet. Gynecol.* 147:724, 1983.

Fanning J, Awad L: Sitting position to reduce postoperative shoulder pain associated with intraperitoneal dextran. *Fertil. Steril.* 44:136, 1985.

Gould SA, Rosellen AL et al: Fluosol DA as a red cell substitute in acute anemia. *N. Engl. J. Med.* 314:1653, 1986.

Hartko WJ, Ghanekar G, Kemmann E: Suture materials currently used in obstetric-gynecologic surgery in the United States: a questionnaire survey. *Obstet. Gynecol.* 59:241, 1982.

Hasselgren P, Hagberg E et al: One instead of two knives for surgical incision. *Arch. Surg.* 119:917, 1984.

Jacobs LM, Hsieh JW: A clinical review of autotransfusion and its role in trauma. *JAMA* 251:3283, 1984.

Jansen RPS: Failure of intraperitoneal adjuncts to improve the outcome of pelvic operations in young women. *Am. J. Obstet. Gynecol.* 153:363, 1985.

Lotze MT: AIDS: a surgeon's responsibility. *Bull. Am. Coll. Surg.* 70(9):6, 1985.

Magyar DM, Hayes MF et al: Is intraperitoneal Dextran 70 safe for routine gynecologic use? *Am. J. Obstet. Gynecol.* 152:198, 1985.

Mengert WF, Burchell RC et al: Pregnancy after bilateral ligation of the internal iliac and ovarian arteries. *Obstet. Gynecol.* 34:664, 1969.

Poole GV: Mechanical factors in abdominal and wound closure: the prevention of fascial dehiscence. *Surgery* 97:631, 1985.

Symmonds RE: Urologic injuries. In Schaefer G, Graber EA (Eds.): *Complications in Obstetric and Gynecologic Surgery.* Hagerstown, MD, Harper & Row, 1981.

Trimbos JB: Security of various knots commonly used in surgical practice. *Obstet. Gynecol.* 64:274, 1984.

Voss SC, Sharp HC, Scott JR: Abdominoplasty combined with gynecologic surgical procedures. *Obstet. Gynecol.* 67:181, 1986.

Wheeless CR Jr.: Use of staples in pelvic surgery. *Internat. Advances Surg. Oncol.* 5:173, 1982.

Wheelock JB, Krebs HB: How to repair bowel injuries during gynecologic surgery. *Contemp. Obstet. Gynecol.* 24:135, 1984.

Wheelock JB, Krebs HB, Hurt WG: Sparing and repairing the bladder during gynecologic surgery. *Contemp. Obstet. Gynecol.* 24:163, 1984.

GENERAL POSTOPERATIVE COMPLICATIONS

4

MICHAEL NEWTON

PRINCIPLES OF EARLY POSTOPERATIVE CARE

Recovery Period

Complications occurring after the operation are best classified according to the organ system involved. This format is followed in the later sections of this chapter. However, during the first few hours (recovery period), when the patient is in the recovery room or the intensive care unit, her condition is often unstable and may be critical. Thus, complications arising during this period require separate consideration.

The recovery period varies from an hour or less for a minor procedure to several hours for a major abdominal operation and one or more days for a radical operation for cancer in a high-risk patient.

Immediately after operation the patient is usually transferred to a recovery room close to the operating room, staffed by trained recovery room personnel under the direction of the anesthesiologist and/or the surgeon. The chief parameters that require monitoring are her respiratory system, cardiovascular system, cerebral function, and urinary function.

RESPIRATORY SYSTEM

Monitoring initially consists of determining the adequacy of the patient's ventilatory effort. Anesthetic agents, muscle relaxants and analgesics given during the operation may delay return to effective spontaneous respiration. Ventilatory failure may result in death within a few minutes or in several days. Sudden failure may be due to aspiration of vomitus, development of a large mucus plug or sudden misplacement of an endotracheal tube. Constant surveillance and prompt suction are essential. Prolonged inadequate ventilatory failure is more insidious but can be suspected and managed by well trained personnel. Serial arterial blood gas determinations may be very helpful. The types of respiratory assistance are described in a later section (page 82).

CARDIOVASCULAR SYSTEM

The primary functions to be monitored are heart changes and blood pressure. Heart rate, rhythm and wave-form changes can be detected by a continuous electrocardiogram recorded on a screen with an alarm system to call attention to abnormalities. Blood pressure is initially measured by the standard sphygmomanometer. If an arterial catheter is in place, mean, systolic and diastolic pressures can be continually recorded.

Cardiac changes of concern include alterations in rate, rhythm and/or the appearance of the electrocardiogram. Some rise in heart rate is likely after any major operation, especially if the patient has been given an atropine-like drug before or during the operation. Bradycardia may be due to preexisting disease, a conduction defect or medication (digitalis). Arrhythmias are of more concern, particularly ventricular premature beats. The possibility of myocardial infarction must always be kept in mind. The usual symptom of pain cannot be elicited, so the initial diagnosis must come from changes in the electrocardiogram when compared with that obtained before or during operation. Classically, these include changes in the T waves (ischemia), S-T segments (injury) and QRS complexes (infarction). The extent and site of the infarction require more detailed analysis and consultation with an internist or cardiologist is necessary.

Alterations in blood pressure occur commonly in the recovery phase. Hypotension (systolic pressure less than 90 mm Hg or more than 40 mm Hg below the preoperative level) may be due to (1) cardiovascular acccidents such as myocardial infarction or pulmonary embolism, (2) cardiorespiratory factors such as residual anesthetic effects, (3) pharmacologic factors such as the postoperative administration of opiates, (4) neurogenic factors such as pain and (5) blood loss. In addition to respiratory and cardiac monitoring, venous pressure, hemoglobin-hematocrit determinations, urinary output and evaluation of possible sites of bleeding may be helpful in establishing the diagnosis. Cardiovascular accidents or ventilatory inadequacy may be detected by monitoring as described previously. If hypotension is due to medication, there is usually a noticeable change from the blood pressure observed prior to the medication being given. On the other hand, if the hypotensive patient is restless and sufficiently alert to complain of pain, the use of a small amount of opiates, i.e., 1 to 2 mg of morphine, given intravenously may restore the blood pressure to normal. Blood loss from the vagina or from an incision is usually obvious, although the amount may be difficult to measure. For vaginal loss, the pads underneath the patient should be carefully observed and saved and the amount of blood in them estimated. Internal bleeding (intra- or extraperitoneal) is less easy to evaluate. In addition to hypotension, venous pressure and urinary output are low. The hemoglobin concentration may not change unless blood loss is excessive, since dilution takes several hours or days. If the bleeding is intraperitoneal, distention and shifting dullness may eventually appear. Abdominal paracentesis in one or both lower quadrants with a No. 20 needle may be diagnostic. Culdocentesis might be better but is difficult to perform in the immediate postoperative period. If the bleeding is extraperitoneal, bulging in the flanks and discoloration of the skin may be noted. If other causes of hypotension have been excluded, one or two units of blood should be given rapidly. Recurrent hypotension may now be associated with other signs that point more clearly to bleeding.

The decision to reoperate within the first 24 hours is not an easy one. But it must be made if the signs of continuing bleeding are clear. The previous incision is reopened and the procedures described in Chapter 3 for control of hemorrhage should be followed. The incision can be closed again with the layer technique, although some authors prefer through and through sutures that include all layers.

Hypertension is less common. It may be due to pain, emergence from anesthesia with excitement, hypothermia with shivering, hypercapnia, hypoxia or poorly controlled preoperative hypertension. Medication is given when hypertension is serious (greater than 180/110) and persists. Analgesics (morphine 1 to 2 mg) or antihypertensive agents such as hydralazine (5 to 10 mg), diazoxide (1 to 3 mg) or sodium nitroprusside (1 to 3 mcg/kg/min) (all given intravenously) are among the primary agents used.

CENTRAL NERVOUS SYSTEM

The patient recovering from general anesthesia normally shows gradually increasing alertness and experiences some pain. Delay in recovering consciousness may simply mean prolonged depression by anesthesia. Rarely it may be due to a cerebrovascular accident (CVA). Complete neurologic examination is not usually possible, but at least motor activity and sensation (response to painful stimuli) can be tested. The management of the patient with a CVA presents major difficulties in the postoperative period; it should be under the direction of a neurological consultant. Immediate postoperative pain is usually managed by small single or repeated intravenous doses of analgesics (morphine 1 to 2 mg or Demerol 25 mg). Excessive pain is an indication for further investigation. It may be due to bleeding or some complication with the incision (see later section).

URINARY SYSTEM

After any major operation urinary output should usually be monitored by an indwelling urethral or suprapubic catheter. An output of at least 30 and preferably 50 ml/hr is desirable. Reductions may be due to antidiuresis following operative stress and anesthesia, inadequate replacement of operative fluid and blood loss, segregation of fluid into the extravascular or third space, urinary tract obstruction or renal failure. If enough urine can be obtained, specific gravity determination and microscopy should be performed. With antidiuresis and inadequate fluid replacement, specific gravity is high. Hypotension and low venous pressure may also be present if the low output is due to continued bleeding. When fluid is lost into the extracellular space, specific gravity is also high, but edema may be apparent. Urinary tract obstruction is likely to be mechanical, i.e., due to catheter blockage, since bilateral ureteral obstruction is very rare. In renal failure both the urinary output and specific gravity are low. Initial management of low urinary output consists of rapid administration of 200 to 300 ml of intravenous fluid (5% dextrose in water). This may have to be repeated, but must be done with caution for fear of overloading the heart. For later management see the section on the urinary tract. An intravenous diuretic (furosemide 10 to 20 mg) may be given, if mobilization of fluid is desired.

Intensive Care Unit

If a patient has made a satisfactory recovery from anesthesia without any of the complications described above and her vital signs are stable, she may be sent to her room. If her recovery is very slow and/or complications have occurred, consideration must be given to transferring her to an intensive care unit, since most recovery rooms are usually not organized for prolonged care. The primary need for intensive care is inadequate ventilation, requiring continued endotracheal intubation and repeated arterial sampling. Other indications are possible myocardial infarction, pulmonary embolism or cerebrovascular accident, all of which require continued careful monitoring. The decision to transfer a patient to an intensive care unit and the reasons for it must be communicated to the patient, if possible, and certainly to her family.

General Postoperative Care and Postoperative Orders

Care after operations, procedures or treatments is crucial to the prevention and early detection of complications. When the procedure has been minor or performed on an outpatient basis, this consists of detailed oral and written instructions and a specific telephone or return visit follow-up. When the patient is in the hospital and the procedure has been a major one,* the number and type of postoperative hospital visits and the format of postoperative orders are important. There is no substitute for regular, thorough postoperative care by the surgeon who performed the operation or by a qualified associate. Patients should be seen at least twice daily until they are ready to go home. Each visit should include a discussion with the patient's nurse and should consist of a review of the chart, vital signs, intake and output, any recently recorded laboratory data and nurses' notes. The patient herself should be given an opportunity to mention any complaints, particularly in relation to the gastrointestinal or genitourinary tracts. Examination will depend on the kind of operation performed. If it has been major, the lungs, heart, abdomen and perineal drainage should be examined at each visit, at least until the patient is well recovered. Orders should be changed appropriately. The use of routine printed postoperative orders is acceptable for minor cases. Fol-

---

*A major procedure in gynecology is one in which the peritoneal cavity has been opened (either abdominally or vaginally) or such extraperitoneal procedures as suprapubic urethral suspension, extensive vaginal repairs, radical vulvectomy or inguinal or pelvic lymphadenectomy have been performed.

lowing major operations, however, it is not possible to predict the patient's course from day to day and printed orders may be constrictive, making it difficult to adjust the patient's care to the circumstances and easy to overlook necessary changes. Finally, the visit should end with any necessary discussion about diagnosis and future plans for treatment or discharge from the hospital. In this connection it is wise to decide on recommendations about treatment plans before discussing them with the patient or with her family.

Documentation in the chart of postoperative findings is essential. If complications occur, they should be noted in a factual manner. There should be no written speculation about their possible causes. Treatment given should be described. Members of the medical team (except consultants) should not write recommendations for treatment in the chart; if they are not followed for any reason, later reviews may raise questions as to the correctness of the actual management.

METABOLISM

Fluid and Electrolytes

NORMAL REQUIREMENTS

After any operative procedure it is desirable that the patient resume oral feedings as soon as possible. Oral feeding within a few hours of the operation is usually feasible when the anesthesia has been of short duration and the procedure minor. Most extraperitoneal operations and some brief intraperitoneal ones such as laparoscopy or tubal ligation fall into this category. However, when the peritoneal cavity has been open for some time and the intestines handled, intravenous fluids are needed and should be ordered for at least the first 24 hours.

Elaborate calculation of fluid balance is not usually necessary. Replacement can be planned simply from a knowledge of the usual loss of fluids and electrolytes (see Table 2–1). A range of amounts is shown because they will depend on age, weight, body surface and ambient temperature. In general, slightly more than the minimum loss, i.e., 2000 to 2500 ml of water, should be given because the healthy kidney can excrete any excess. It is usually unnecessary to give potassium during the first 24 hours postoperatively since operative stress, tissue break-

down and blood transfusion, if given, provide sufficient amounts. Also, sodium chloride and water may be retained postoperatively as a result of the release of aldosterone and antidiuretic hormone; thus in the older patient and in those with poor renal or cardiac reserve, the amount of fluid should be reduced. For the average patient a useful rule for the first 24 hours is to give 1500 to 2000 ml 5% dextrose in water and 500 ml normal saline (78 mEq Na).

MODIFICATIONS OF NORMAL REQUIREMENTS

The above guidelines have to be modified if (1) there was an uncorrected preoperative blood volume deficit; (2) operative losses of blood or fluid (ascites, intestinal fluid) were inadequately replaced or were overreplaced; (3) there is evidence that a large amount of interstitial fluid or plasma has been sequestered during or immediately after operation; on the average this may amount to 500 to 750 ml but may be increased in such procedures as pelvic or inguinal lymphadenectomy; (4) unusual losses continue, for example, from the gastrointestinal tract; or (5) the patient is elderly or has limited cardiac or renal reserve.

After the first 24 hours the administration of 5% dextrose in water and normal saline is insufficient to meet the patient's electrolyte needs. Potassium (40 mEq) should be added to the daily fluids, usually in amounts of 20 mEq/liter. For the short term (less than seven days) calcium and magnesium and the other constituents of plasma are not necessary. The addition of a multivitamin ampule may help wound healing. Fluid loss from other sites such as drains or the gastrointestinal tract should be replaced milliliter for milliliter, with attention to the electrolytes especially likely to be lost (Table 4–1).

Table 4–1. Electrolyte Content of Intestinal Fluids (mEq/l)*

Fluid	Na	Cl	K
Gastric juice (pH < 4.0)	60	100	10
Succus entericus (mixed small bowel fluid)	100	100	20
Diarrhea	60	45	30

*Adapted from Condon RE, Nyhus LM (eds.): *Manual of Surgical Therapeutics*, Ed 6. Boston, Little, Brown & Co., 1985, p. 203.

COMPLICATIONS OF FLUID AND ELECTROLYTE THERAPY

Too little, too much or the wrong kind of fluid results in complications. Often the problem is failure to reevaluate the orders for fluid at regular intervals or to appreciate the amount lost through various portals. Orders for fluid should be written once a day and not continued from day to day without review. This is especially true when a complicated major operation has been performed, but it is important for the young obstetrician-gynecologist to get into this habit with uncomplicated cases so that it will persist if complications occur.

Clinically, inadequate fluid replacement results in dehydration—thirst, dry tongue, dry skin and urine of inadequate amount with a high specific gravity. Laboratory studies may show hemoconcentration and unduly high serum electrolyte levels. Increase in fluids is appropriate, but it is important to be sure that other factors are not producing the same symptoms, e.g., segregation of fluids in the third space. Electrolyte loss from unexpected sites must also be covered. Details of this replacement have been given in Chapter 2.

Overreplacement of fluid may result in shortness of breath, edema and normal or diminished urinary output. Evidence of cardiac failure may appear, consisting of distended neck veins, tachycardia and appearance of S_3 or gallop rhythm. Fluids must be restricted and diuretics given. Treatment for cardiac failure may be needed (see later section).

Diabetes

REGULAR MANAGEMENT

Diabetics are at high risk for a variety of complications because they often have associated arteriosclerosis and cardiac disorders including silent myocardial infarction. Postoperatively specific problems include the possibility of ketoacidosis with its attendant electrolyte disturbance, poor wound healing and inadequate response to infection. However, control of blood sugar levels during and after the operation may decrease these complications.

Using the blood sugar levels described in Chapter 2, the diabetic patient should be brought to operation with a blood sugar between 100 and 250 mg/100 ml. In this case, no special treatment is needed for the patient who takes no or only oral hypoglycemic agents, except that the oral medication is withheld on the day of operation. Patients taking either intermediate insulin or a combination of regular and long-acting insulin should be given half their usual dose before the operation. This is because they will receive fewer calories than usual on the day of operation. In addition, an infusion of 5% dextrose in water should be started early on the morning of operation to prevent hypoglycemia. Management is made easier by operating early in the day.

The effect of operative stress on diabetes is unpredictable. Additional insulin may be needed. Blood sugar determination is the best method of monitoring the situation. Measurement of glucose and ketones in the urine is not accurate because of the elevated renal threshold for glucose in the diabetic and the possible effect of operative stress and medications. Blood sugar levels can now be obtained with reasonable accuracy by instruments that require only a drop of blood from the finger, obtained by a spring-triggered device. A reagent strip such as Chemstrip gives a rough approximation of glucose levels by allowing the examiner to visually compare colors with a standard. However, on a surgical floor one of the available machines such as Glucoscan, which gives a more precise level, should be available and used by the nursing staff.

The schedule of obtaining blood sugar levels postoperatively varies with the severity of the diabetes and the progress of the individual patient. As a minimum, determinations should be made during and immediately after the operation and then once during each eight-hour nursing shift. Stable values in the first 24 hours after operation make it unnecessary to continue this schedule. An early morning (7:00 AM) and if necessary a mid-afternoon (3:00 PM) blood sugar determination is sufficient.

Elevated blood sugar levels may be satisfactorily managed on a "sliding scale." If the blood sugar level is over 400 mg/100 ml, 15 units of regular insulin are given. If it is between 300 and 400 mg/100 ml, 10 units are given, and if it is between 250 and 300 mg/100 ml, five units are given. Once the immediate postoperative period is over and the patient is able to resume normal eating and activity her daily dose of insulin can be raised gradually to what she was taking before the operation.

UNCONTROLLED DIABETES

Diabetes may become out of control in the postoperative period because it was uncontrolled prior to the (emergency) operation, because of the stress of operation or because a complication such as infection develops. Uncontrolled diabetes may lead to ketoacidosis or hyperosmolar coma. Ketoacidosis occurs in insulin-dependent diabetes. It is identified clinically by altered consciousness, deep (Kussmaul) breathing and dehydration. Shock may occur, especially when infection is present. The blood sugar level is high, often over 500 mg/100 ml. Serum ketone levels are elevated and ketonuria is present (detected by Ketostix). Acidosis and electrolyte disturbance may be marked, with a CO_2 of 10 mEq/L or less and a pH of 7.2 or less in severe cases. Hypokalemia and elevated BUN are often present. Treatment consists of giving insulin and correcting the dehydration. An initial bolus of regular insulin, 25 or more units, is given intravenously, and 5 to 10 units are added every hour until the plasma glucose level falls to less than 300 mg/100 ml. A rapid bolus of 1000 ml of intravenous fluid (normal saline) is given to which bicarbonate, 2 ampules of 44 mEq each, may be added if the pH is below 7.2. Potassium may also be necessary during therapy, and potassium levels need to be checked frequently. A central venous line and repeated electrocardiograms are useful in monitoring patients with diabetic ketoacidosis. After initial management, diabetes is then treated as described previously.

Hyperosmolar coma occurs in older patients. It is like diabetic ketoacidosis except that ketosis is not prominent. Management is similar to that for ketoacidosis. Less insulin may be needed. The danger of fluid overload must be kept in mind.

Endocrine Problems

Adrenal Cortex

The body's ability to withstand the stress of anesthesia and operation depends upon the capability of the adrenal cortex to produce cortisone in larger amounts than normal. Exogenous cortisone results in failure of the pituitary to release ACTH (adrenocorticotrophic hormone) as needed and in suppression of the adrenal gland so that the normal response to stress is reduced or absent. Symptoms of adrenal deficiency include weakness, nausea and vomiting and hypotension. Hyponatremia and hyperkalemia may also be present.

Patients who are receiving corticosteroids currently or who have received them for more than one week during the six month period prior to operation should be considered to be at risk for postoperative adrenal insufficiency. The extent of adrenal suppression is difficult to determine, although it probably depends on the dose given and the duration of treatment. In any case, the patient undergoing any major operation should be covered during the operative and postoperative periods by excess cortisone. One method is to give 50 to 100 mg hydrocortisone succinate or phosphate intramuscularly two hours before and four and eight hours after the operation. For patients undergoing radical procedures hydrocortisone succinate or phosphate is given as follows: 100 mg IM one to two hours before operation, 100 mg intravenously during operation and every eight hours for the first 24 hours postoperatively and then decreasing doses for three to five days. If the patient is able to take at least liquids by mouth hydrocortisone acetate may be substituted in the same dose. It is well, also, to maintain an adequate potassium intake. Changes should be made in the above regimen according to the needs of individual patients.

Acute Thyrotoxic Crisis (Thyroid Storm)

Thyroid storm is an acute postoperative complication that occurs rarely in patients with thyrotoxicosis and even more rarely in those with nodular goiter or others. It is characterized by (1) high fever (106° F or higher), (2) tachycardia (180 BPM or more), (3) nervousness, irritability and even psychotic symptoms, (4) vomiting and diarrhea and (5) cardiac failure. The diagnosis is made clinically since tests for thyroid function, although elevated, cannot be obtained immediately. Administration of adequate doses of propylthiouracil preoperatively may prevent crisis. Immediate treatment consists of cooling (mattress, blanket, ice packs), hydration (10% dextrose intravenously), oxygen, sedation and digitalis or other treatment for cardiac failure. More specifically, propylthiouracil, 150 to 250 mg every six hours, is given orally. One hour after propylthiouracil has been started iodide should be given orally or intravenously in a dose of 50 mg twice daily. Propranolol should be given to control restlessness and tachycardia in doses of 20 to 80 mg orally every six hours or 0.5 to 2 mg intravenously every four hours. Since there may be an element of adrenal failure, cortisone may be helpful.

Nutritional Support

For most gynecologic and obstetric patients the gastrointestinal tract remains intact during and after abdominal and vaginal operations. Oral intake of liquids and solids can be resumed one to four days postoperatively, and even a patient with borderline nutritional status can be supported with high protein and calorie supplements early in the postoperative period. Intraoperative complications such as closure of the the intestine following incision, resection of intestine or a colostomy do not usually prevent oral intake for more than seven days.

Patients who were severely deficient nutritionally before the operation and were receiving total parenteral nutritional support and who undergo major abdominal procedures are likely to continue to need hyperalimentation. Also, patients whose nutritional status is borderline and who undergo major intestinal resection, for example, in ovarian cancer or after radiation damage to the intestine or fistula, may require nutritional support postoperatively.

The techniques of postperative nutritional support include enteral feeding, gastrostomy or jejunostomy tube feeding, or total parenteral nutrition (TPN) (Meguid et al, 1985). Enteral feeding has been covered previously (Chapter 2). There is relatively little occasion for its use postoperatively except in the elderly or incompetent patient who is unable to eat.

When the intestinal tract is found to be intact at operation and remains so, nutritional support may be supplied through a gastrostomy or through a needle-catheter jejunostomy performed either as a separate procedure or as part of the main operation. The Stamm gastrostomy (or jejunostomy) is probably the best of the techniques described. It is performed by inserting a Malecot or similar catheter into the fundus of the stomach, securing it with three concentric purse-string sutures of 20 chromic catgut and then fixing the stomach to the anterior abdominal wall. A needle-jejunostomy offers less possibility of leakage and is more easily removed. A loop of proximal jejunum is selected and a purse-string suture of 20 chromic catgut placed on the anti-mesenteric surface. A 14-gauge needle is inserted within the purse-string, tunnelled distally for 3 to 4 cm submucosally and then passed into the lumen. A polyvinyl catheter is threaded through the needle down the jejunum for about 10 cm, and the needle is withdrawn. The purse-string suture is tied. A similar 14 gauge needle is inserted through the anterior abdominal wall to the left of the umbilicus, and the catheter is threaded out through it. The jejunum is fixed to the anterior abdominal wall with two 20 chromic catgut sutures (Fig. 4–1). In the recovery room radiopaque dye is injected into the catheter, and an x-ray is taken to insure patency. Feeding through the catheter may be begun promptly with a variety of elemental dietary formulas. These should be dilute at first, reaching full strength only after several days.

Catheter jejunostomy feeding is reported to be safe and relatively free of complications (Ballon, 1982). In three of 40 insertions the catheter did not work well because of kinking. Six patients experienced intolerance to the formula with abdominal cramps, bloating, nausea and diarrhea. Leakage of formula into the peritoneal cavity did not occur. Paregoric added to the formula may help to avoid some of the intestinal symptoms. The catheter may be left in place for a long time, although 10 to 14 days would seem to be sufficient unless the patient continues to be unable to eat. Catheter jejunostomy feeding can be continued on an outpatient basis. Removal of the catheter usually presents no difficulty since the jejunum should be adherent to the anterior abdominal wall. A malfunctioning catheter can be replaced using a guide wire (Stogdill et al, 1984).

The principles of intravenous hyperalimentation have been described in Chapter 2. If intravenous hyperalimentation is being used preoperatively, it is tapered off slowly over a 12-hour period and then discontinued for 12 hours immediately prior to the operation, only 5% dextrose in water being given. After operation, resumption of hyperalimentation should be delayed for 24 hours because of the metabolic changes occurring during recovery. It is then begun slowly as was done when it was first started.

The duration of hyperalimentation depends on the individual patient's problem. In the most frequent instance, an intestinal anastomosis should be healed in 10 to 14 days and, theoretically, the patient should then be taking most of her calories by mouth. However, appetite is usually decreased during hyperalimentation. Therefore, if the patient's condition is satisfactory and her weight is rising progressively, the hyperalimentation is stopped empirically at 12 to 14 days after operation. If the intestine has been radiated or if a large portion has been removed, hyperalimentation may need to be prolonged. If at operation intestinal function is found to be compromised by extensive cancer, hyperalimentation should be continued only if

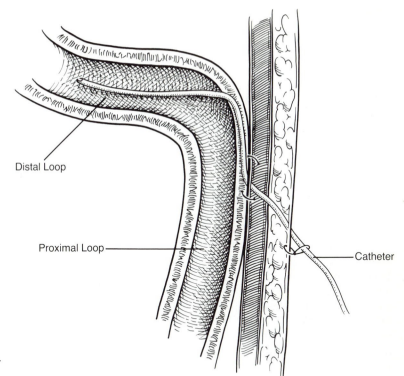

Figure 4–1. Catheter jejunostomy.

multiple courses of chemotherapy are to be given with hope of cure. Although hyperalimentation will prolong life in patients with advanced cancer who cannot take food by mouth, the possible complications and expense (whether given in hospital or at home) make this therapy of uncertain value for both ethical and practical reasons. Hyperalimentation is often discontinued gradually, but there appears to be no serious risk to doing this rapidly.

HEMATOPOIETIC SYSTEM

Bleeding

Bleeding in the immediate postoperative period has been discussed before. Subsequently, bleeding may become apparent because (1) it occurred immediately after operation but did not appear externally or affect the patient's vital signs; (2) it continued to occur slowly in the immediate postoperative period and subsequently; (3) it started later when clots in one or more blood vessels were lysed or broken off or (4) there was a persistent or new coagulation defect.

EARLY POSTOPERATIVE BLEEDING

Early postoperative bleeding may be defined as that which occurs after the immediate recovery period, i.e., after the patient has left the recovery room. The patient's vital signs may be stable and normal. Often the only evidence is a sharp fall in hemoglobin or hematocrit, greater than would be expected from the blood loss estimated to have occurred at operation. Immediate management involves:

1. Repeating the hemoglobin to check for laboratory error.

2. Identifying the site of bleeding. Signs are more reliable than in the immediate postoperative period. It is obvious if it is vaginal. Intraperitoneal bleeding may give peritoneal signs of tenderness, rebound tenderness, diminished or absent peristalsis and intestinal distension. An intraabdominal fluid wave may be present, and paracentesis may yield blood. Extraperitoneal hemorrhage may cause bulging, tenderness and discoloration in the flank. If there is a hematoma in the pelvis, vaginal or rectal examination may indicate a fluctuant mass.

3. Deciding whether the bleeding has stopped or is continuing. Continued slight fall in hemoglobin or hematocrit is to be expected as hemodilution occurs for 72 to 96 hours.

Greater fall than might be expected, deterioration in vital signs (i.e., rise in pulse) or postural hypotension may point to continued blood loss.

4. Replacing blood lost. Two units of packed red cells can be given initially; more can be given later, depending upon the evidence of continued bleeding and the hemoglobin level.

5. Reaching a decision about active operative or conservative treatment. In general, if bleeding appears to have ceased and it is more than 24 hours since the original procedure, reoperation is not advisable because of the difficulty of identifying structures, the danger of causing new bleeding and the real likelihood of infection.

The extravasated blood may be absorbed without forming a definite mass. More likely a hematoma will become palpable abdominally or on pelvic examination. It may eventually be absorbed or it may drain vaginally. The temptation to incise it should be resisted since infection may occur and represents a serious complication. An attempt to prevent infection by prophylactic antibiotics is of little value. When infection occurs, fever and tenderness over the hematoma are noted. Broad spectrum antibiotics (see following section) should be given intravenously because anaerobic organisms are common.

LATE BLEEDING

Late bleeding may occur five to 10 days or more after the operation. After hysterectomy, a small amount of bloody discharge is very common at this time as the sutures at the top of the vagina loosen. Similar bleeding may occur after conization of the cervix. No treatment is needed initially; the patient should be advised to rest for 24 hours and observe the amount of bleeding. If bleeding continues or becomes more severe, the patient should be examined promptly with a good light and adequate instruments. If one or two bleeding points are seen at the vaginal cuff, it may be possible to clamp them with a long curved hemostat and ligate them. More likely there will be generalized oozing from the vaginal cuff or bleeding from above the cuff. In the former case, Monsel's solution or hemostatic substances such as Gelfoam, Oxycel or Avitene may be placed at the top of the vagina against the bleeding point and the vagina packed. An indwelling Foley catheter is usually necessary, and antibiotics should be given. Twenty-four to 36 hours later the packing is cautiously removed. Usually bleeding

will have ceased and will not recur. If it does, repacking once may be advisable. Persistent bleeding from the vaginal cuff is handled in the same way as intractable bleeding (described later).

If the bleeding occurs from above the vaginal cuff and is profuse, intraperitoneal or extraperitoneal exploration may be needed as for immediate postoperative hemorrhage. Transfusions should be given as necessary to replace blood lost. Intraperitoneal hemorrhage occurring five to 10 days postoperatively without intervening signs is rare, but is handled as if it had occurred in the immediate postoperative period.

INTRACTABLE BLEEDING

During operation ligation of the hypogastric arteries may control persistent severe bleeding (Chapter 3). This may also be a valuable measure when hemorrhage occurs in the immediate postoperative or postpartum period. It is best performed transperitoneally by the technique described previously (Chapter 3). A possible and less invasive alternative is embolization of the appropriate artery in the pelvis. The Seldinger technique is used to puncture the femoral or axillary artery. A No. 5 or No. 6 French catheter with a curved tip is passed into the internal iliac artery with the use of fluoroscopy. An angiogram is performed to determine the exact site of the bleeding vessel (for this reason the procedure is best done during active bleeding). Emboli of Gelfoam or metallic coils are then injected to occlude the involved vessels. The procedure may be brief or may take two or more hours. Small series of successful cases have been reported (Mann et al, 1980; Rosenthal and Colapinto, 1985). In experienced hands the complications of embolization are few. There is a possible danger of the emboli migrating to the external iliac artery and occluding it. Pelvic pain and fever occur quite commonly. The use of prophylactic antibiotics is recommended by some.

As a last resort, a gravity suit (MAST [Military Anti-Shock Trousers]), if available, may be used. In principle this consists of circumferential pressure on the legs and abdomen by an inflatable garment with three chambers, one for each leg and one for the abdomen. The patient is placed in a supine position in the suit (with a Foley catheter in place) and the leg and then the abdominal chambers successively inflated to pressures of 10 to 20 mm Hg (but not more than 30 mm Hg). The effect of the compression suit is to shunt blood (750 to 1000 ml) to the vital structures in the chest and head and specifically to lessen bleeding by decreasing the caliber of the vessels. Compression should be discontinued as soon as possible, 12 to 24 hours after bleeding has ceased. Pressure should be decreased slowly, the abdominal compartment first, followed by the leg compartments. Isolated cases of successful use of the gravity suit in obstetrics (especially) and gynecology have been reported (Sandberg and Pelligra, 1983).

COAGULATION DEFECTS

Continued bleeding from operative sites—incision or vagina—may be an indication of a coagulation defect. This should usually have been detected and managed earlier. If not, detailed coagulation studies should be performed as described above in Chapter 2.

Anemia

Following major operations the patient's hemoglobin level is frequently lower than it was preoperatively even in the absence of detectable bleeding. This is usually due to unreplaced operative blood loss and subsequent hemodilution. If the hemoglobin is between 10 and 13 gm (borderline anemia), treatment should be with iron and foods containing iron. The simplest iron compound ($FeSO_4$) is appropriate. If this causes constipation, diarrhea or upper abdominal distress, ferrous gluconate or another iron compound may be substituted. Foods containing iron are shown in Table 4–2. If the hemoglobin is below 8 gm, transfusion of at least two units of packed red cells is indicated to improve wound healing and speed recovery. Transfusion should be followed by oral iron and iron containing foods. A hemoglobin of between

Table 4–2. Some Good Dietary Sources of Iron (over 2 mg/average portion)*

Beans—lima, soya, white, lentils
Brewers yeast, wheat bran, wheat germ
Dried fruit—apricots, dates, prunes, prune juice
Eggs
Enriched bread and cereals
Giblets—chicken, beef heart, kidney
Liver—beef, calf, chicken
Meats—beef, chicken, pork
Vegetables—mustard and other "greens," spinach

*Recommended Daily Allowance (RDA) is 10 to 18 mg. Amount of iron varies with the size of the portion and the particular food or enrichment.

8 and 10 gm may be treated as frank anemia with transfusion or as borderline anemia, depending on the circumstances. For example, a patient with a hemoglobin of 9 gm who urgently needs a major operation or who is about to receive chemotherapy for ovarian cancer or radiation therapy to the abdomen or pelvis should usually be transfused. In addition, if there is reason to suspect that vitamins A, D, E or K may not be normally absorbed from the small intestine these substances should be added to the diet. Operations bypassing or excising the distal ileum, such as an ileo-ascending colostomy, remove that part of the intestine from which vitamin B_{12} is absorbed. In these circumstances vitamin B_{12} (cyanocobalamine) is given intramuscularly in doses of at least 100 micrograms/month. All patients who have had anemia postoperatively should have their blood counts checked two to four weeks postoperatively, and anti-anemia measures should be continued as necessary.

INFECTIONS

Definitions and Diagnosis

Infection is a serious complication of major and even minor operations in women. Since the results of infections may have far-reaching effects on the success of operations and upon subsequent function, it is important that they be recognized and treated promptly.

The primary clinical finding in postoperative infection is fever with or without other symptoms or signs. Thus, identification of a specific infection and its site begins with the detection and work-up of fever. The classic definition of febrile morbidity, used primarily in obstetrics, is the presence of a "temperature of 100.4°F (38° C) on any two of the first 10 days postpartum, exclusive of the first 24 hours." This definition served an important purpose in calling attention to puerperal infections. It has also been used to define postoperative morbidity. However, it is not specific enough; nor does it help to determine the cause of the fever. Nevertheless, some standard is necessary in order to decide when laboratory and other studies are appropriate and cost effective. A useful critical temperature level is 101° F (38.3° C) on two occasions at least four hours apart and at least four hours after operation or a temperature of 102° F (39° C) on one occasion at least four hours after operation. When fever occurs, the

Table 4–3. Postoperative Fever

Hours After Operation	Most Likely Causes
0–48	Atelectasis
48–96	Urinary tract, lung infection
Over 96	Intraperitoneal or pelvic abscess, wound infection, urinary tract infection

usual postoperative history and examination should first be repeated. The most likely causes of the fever should then be considered; they vary according to the length of time after operation (Table 4–3). Physical examination should be directed chiefly to those organ systems. Miminum laboratory studies for all patients with fever include complete blood count with differential count, clean-catch or catheterized urinalysis and culture and chest x-ray. Respiratory tract, urinary tract and wound infections are considered later in this chapter.

Intraperitoneal Infection

Peritonitis

Abdominal pain is an important symptom of intraperitoneal infection if the peritoneal cavity or intestine has not knowingly been entered, for example, after D & C, hysteroscopy, conization of the cervix or application of radioactive sources. When the peritoneal cavity has been opened, postoperative pain is usually present. Pain varies greatly, and it is difficult to distinguish that due to infection. On examination, tenderness and rebound tenderness, distension and diminished peristalsis may be more marked than one would normally expect. Repeated observations are particularly important. Persistence of fever and leukocytosis with failure of peritoneal signs to improve support the diagnosis of infection.

Treatment is primarily by antibiotics (see later section). Oral intake is stopped and intravenous fluids given. Suction with a nasogastric tube is used if vomiting occurs. Laxatives and enemas are not given, since the intestine needs temporary rest.

Abscess

Diagnosis. A postoperative abdominal abscess may develop from (1) loculation of pus after peritonitis, (2) an infected hematoma, (3) prior infection in the reproductive tract, e.g., gonorrhea or other tubo-ovarian disease, (4) dissem-

ination from a septic focus elsewhere in the body, (5) perforation of the intestine that was not appreciated at operation and developed silently into a collection of pus or (6) rupture of a colonic diverticulum, appendix, Meckel's diverticulum or gastric or duodenal ulcer.

An abscess usually takes several days to develop. Symptoms may be few except for the effects of fever. Pain may be noted when a pelvic abscess develops. Pain may become localized after previously being generalized. In the case of a subphrenic or high retroperitoneal abscess, pain may be absent. Fever is almost invariable and may be spiking in type, with a low near normal in the morning and a high of 101° to 103° F in the evening. Chills may be present. Leukocytosis with increased numbers of band forms is characteristic. Physical examination may be inconclusive except that a pelvic abscess may be felt on vaginal or rectal examination (which should not be omitted).

Newer radiologic methods have made the diagnosis of abdominal abscess easier. Because of the different techniques available, personal consultation with the radiologist is important. Initially, plain flat and upright x-rays of the abdomen may show displacement and distortion of the intestine or a soft tissue density. A chest x-ray is helpful in showing pleural reaction or fluid above the diaphragm when a subphrenic abscess is present. Contrast material in the gastrointestinal tract or injected into a fistulous tract can further localize an abscess. If the diagnosis is not clear, ultrasonography or a CT scan is helpful. The advantages of real-time ultrasonography are that (1) it can be done at the bedside, (2) it does not take a long time, (3) it is particularly useful in the upper abdomen or pelvis where there are few other gas-filled structures, (4) no ionizing radiation is used and (5) it is less expensive than, for example, a CT scan or MRI. On the other hand, its use is limited by confusion of an abscess with intraabdominal gas and contrast material, and the results depend considerably on operator skill. CT scanning is valuable because it has high resolution, can be used in the mid and upper abdomen and may be the best way to guide percutaneous drainage (see later section) (Fig. 4–2). However, it is expensive, lengthy, requires pretreatment with oral contrast material and necessitates the patient being moved to the radiologic facility. Arranging adequate nursing care for a sick patient under these circumstances is very important. Contrast studies such as Gallium scans have limited value because they are non-specific and take time to perform.

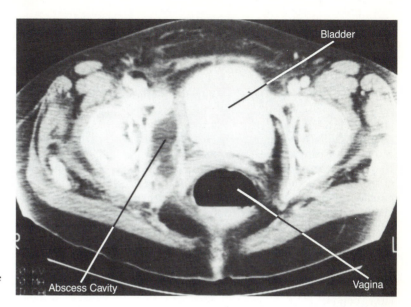

Bladder

Abscess Cavity

Vagina

Figure 4–2. *CT scan of pelvic abscess.*

Management. When an abscess has been diagnosed clinically it should first be identified by aspiration with a fine (22-gauge) needle and then drained. If the abscess is in the pelvis, is fluctuant and points at the apex of the vagina or in the cul-de-sac, aspiration is followed by a small incision, which is made with the patient under anesthesia. The opening is enlarged and loculations broken up, preferably with the finger. If the opening is not large enough, a T-tube or Foley catheter drain is inserted or a straight tube, sewn to the vaginal wall, is used. Drains are left in three to five days. This is usually successful unless the abscess extends upwards and contains pockets that cannot be reached vaginally (Hevron and Llorens, 1976).

Other intra- or extraperitoneal abscesses may present difficulties in drainage. If the abscess points superficially, surgical drainage is performed by incision, removal of pus and insertion of Penrose or suction drains. Drains are removed when the patient is afebrile and no further purulent drainage is present. Percutaneous drainage using CT scan is useful when the abscess is deep. Aeder and associates (1983) point out that percutaneous drainage should usually not be attempted if (1) more than two abscess cavities are present, (2) the drainage route traverses bowel or uncontaminated organs or (3) the viscosity of the abscess material does not permit complete initial aspiration. One technique of percutaneous drainage is to aspirate the cavity and outline its dimensions with contrast material. A No. 7 or No. 8 French pigtail catheter is then inserted over a guide wire, the pus removed and the cavity irrigated. A larger catheter or a double-lumen sump catheter may also be used for more superficial abscesses. The catheter is fixed to the skin and leads to a drainage bag or low suction. Irrigation may be continued one to three times daily. The decrease in size of the cavity is monitored by CT scan, and the catheter is removed when drainage has been minimal for two or three days.

Treatment of an abscess is successful if drainage ceases, the patient remains afebrile and no further abscesses or loculations are found. Glass and Cohn (1984) noted a failure rate (patients requiring reexploration) in 51 out of 252 collected cases (20%) when CT-guided drainage was used. In their own series of 71 cases, 51 received surgical drainage with a success rate of 88% and a major complication rate of 23% (wound infection, hemorrhage, wound dehiscence or intestinal perforation); 17 underwent CT-guided catheter drainage with a success rate of 47% and a major complication rate of 6%. It should be noted that most series of procedures performed for drainage of abdominal abscesses contain both non-gynecologic and gynecologic cases, the former usually predominating.

RUPTURED ABSCESS

A postoperative abscess may rupture spontaneously. Rupture most commonly occurs into the vagina and may be curative, although the opening may need to be enlarged as described before. When rupture of an intraabdominal abscess occurs within the peritoneal cavity, the patient experiences sudden generalized abdominal pain. On examination she usually appears acutely ill with a rapid pulse, hypotension and evidence of shock. Excision of the abscess or external drainage is needed promptly. In the case of a tubo-ovarian abscess, excision may involve a total abdominal hysterectomy and bilateral salpingo-oophorectomy, a difficult procedure in a patient already in poor condition. If only extraperitoneal drainage can be provided, drains should be placed in the lowest possible dependent position. Suction with a Hemovac or sump drain is useful. Drains are left in place until drainage has almost completely ceased, fever has disappeared and the patient's general condition is satisfactory. Rupture of an intraabdominal abscess may lead to an enterocutaneous or enterovaginal fistula (see later section).

Septic Shock

PATHOPHYSIOLOGY

Any patient with infection may develop septic shock. It occurs more often in hospitalized patients and in those who are debilitated by underlying disease such as diabetes or cancer (particularly in those receiving chemotherapy), by major surgical procedures or postoperative complications or by urinary tract or uterine instrumentation. Although septic shock is popularly attributed to gram-negative organisms (gram-negative shock), it can be caused by many organisms, both gram-negative and gram-positive ones and fungi.

The underlying pathophysiologic mechanism in septic shock, from whatever cause, is the presence of bacteria in the bloodstream accompanied or followed by bacterial toxins. Among the important early effects are enhanced coagulation and fibrinolysis, which may lead eventually to disseminated intravascular coagulation. Release of histamine may cause transient vasodilatation, increased capillary permeability and decreased peripheral resistance, leading to a rise in heart rate and cardiac output. The patient appears warm, flushed and maximally vasodilated, a condition termed early or warm shock. Continued sepsis results in activation of the sympathetic nervous system with increased release of corticotropin releasing hormone and ACTH from the hypothalamus and anterior pituitary gland respectively and generalized catecholamine release (late or cold hypotensive shock). Intense widespread vasoconstriction occurs, and this affects many organs, particularly those of the cardiovascular and respiratory systems. Continuation of the syndrome leads to secondary or irreversible shock (Duff, 1982).

DIAGNOSIS

The diagnosis of septic shock must be suspected in any patient with fever accompanied by shaking chills, restlessness, confusion and disorientation. If there is evidence of hypotension and generalized vasoconstriction, supportive treatment is of first importance and often lifesaving.

Initial studies essential for any patient with suspected septic shock include:

1. Aerobic and anaerobic blood cultures.
2. Cultures of any draining incision or abscess.
3. Urinalysis and culture of urine.
4. Chest x-ray and electrocardiogram.
5. Complete blood and platelet count and determination of coagulation factors.
6. Blood chemistry survey.

Additional studies may be needed to identify the source of the infection, e.g., abdominal flat and erect x-rays, CT scans of the abdomen or an intravenous pyelogram. All studies may have to await stabilization of the critically ill patient.

MANAGEMENT

Septic shock is life-threatening. Management of the patient with fully developed shock, i.e., with hypotension, vasoconstriction and oliguria, requires careful monitoring, treatment of the infection and attention to the function of several organ systems. This condition is best handled with the resources of an adequately staffed and equipped intensive care unit. Even in the early stages of "warm shock" when the blood pressure is relatively normal but the threat of hypotension and progression of the shock syndrome is present, modified monitoring together with adequate antibiotic therapy is essential.

Monitoring. Basic monitoring includes:

1. Evaluation of central venous pressure (CVP) or pulmonary artery wedge pressure (PWP) by central venous or Swan-Ganz catheter. A double- or triple-lumen catheter may be useful.

2. Determination of arterial blood pressure and repeated measurements of arterial pO_2 and pCO_2 by means of an indwelling arterial (radial) catheter.

3. Measurement of cardiac function by continous electrocardiograms.

4. Continuous measurement of urinary output by means of an indwelling Foley catheter.

5. Frequent determinations of white blood count and hemoglobin, hematocrit, platelet, coagulation factor and serum electrolyte levels.

6. Chest x-rays on a daily basis, at least initially.

Antibiotics. The infecting organism is not known at first and may not be identified for 24 to 48 hours. *Escherichia coli*, group B *streptococci*, anaerobic *Streptococci*, *Aerobacter*, *Pseudomonas*, *Klebsiella* and *Bacteroides* may all be responsible as well as *Staphylococci* and on occasion *Candida albicans*. A combination of antibiotics with as broad a spectrum as possible should be given intravenously on an empiric basis and changed as necessary when the reports of cultures are available. One such combination is penicillin (5 mil units every six hours), gentamicin (or tobramycin) (3 to 5 mg/kg/day in three divided doses) and clindamycin (600 mg every six hours). Treatment for a possible fungal infection should be deferred until later. For further discussion of antibiotics and their use and complications see later section.

Restoration of Effective Blood Volume. Central venous pressure, blood pressure and urinary output are the best guides to the amount of fluid to be given. Lactated Ringer's solution is most useful initially. Because of the metabolic acidosis (determined by arterial blood gases) that commonly occurs, the addition or substitution of bicarbonate may be necessary. The dose is calculated as mEq $NaHCO_3$ needed = $0.3 \times$ body weight in kg $\times$ (25 − measured serum bicarbonate). One half of the deficit is given at once. In addition, colloids are often necessary. Albumin may be most useful if the colloid osmotic pressure is less than 24 cm H_2O (Grundmann and Heistermann, 1985). Blood transfusions are indicated if there has been demonstrated blood loss, a low hemoglobin level or unexplained anemia.

Various drugs have been suggested to support the circulation. Peripheral vasoconstrictors are of limited value when peripheral vasoconstriction is already great, unless the drug used has selective regional vasodilation in central organs. Dopamine serves well in this capacity. In a dose of 2 to 5 micrograms/kg/min, increasing to as much as 15 to 20 micrograms/kg/min it helps to preserve essential renal, splanchnic, coronary and cerebral blood flow, although it also causes alpha adrenergic vasoconstriction. The use of corticosteroids is advised by many authors. They may be given by continuous intravenous infusion, for example, dexamethasone (6 mg/kg/day) or methylprednisone sodium succinate (30 mg/kg/day) after loading doses of 20 mg dexamethasone or 125 mg methylprednisolone. Cavanagh (1981) reports lower mortality among patients with septic shock treated with glucocorticoids (7%) compared with those not so treated (50%).

Pulmonary Insufficiency. In septic shock the lungs are at risk from fluid overload as attempts are made to restore blood volume and also from specific intrinsic damage due to interstitial edema, perhaps related initially to microemboli and the effect of sepsis on capillary permeability. The later stages of this disorder are known as shock lung or adult respiratory distress syndrome (ARDS) and are characterized by increasing pulmonary insufficiency. The best guide to management is the arterial pO_2. Persistent levels of less than 60 mm Hg in spite of added oxygen are an indication for assisted respiration through an endotracheal tube (see later section).

Cardiac Function. The management of the heart in septic shock is closely allied to fluid management. The primary risk is circulatory overload. Changes in heart rate and rhythm and abnormalities of coronary circulation may be specifically related to intrinsic cardiac function and are determined by continuous electrocardiograms. Circulatory overload may be suspected when the CVP is 15 cm H_2O or greater or if the response to a small 200 ml fluid challenge is a rise in CVP of more than 2 cm H_2O. A more sensitive measure of fluid overload is the pulmonary wedge pressure (PWP). A PWP of more than 15 mm Hg shows an abnormal elevation of ventricular filling pressure. When it measures less than 10 mm Hg there is low to normal filling. Administration of digoxin is indicated if there is suspicion of congestive heart failure. A loading dose of 0.5 mg digoxin is followed by three divided doses of 0.25 mg four to six hours apart and daily maintenance doses of 0.125 to 0.25 mg. Digoxin levels should be obtained regularly and maintained between 0.8 and 2.0 ng/ml. Further management of cardiac abnormality is discussed in a later section.

Urinary Tract. Measurement of urinary output is a good index of circulatory status. A volume of less than 30 ml/hr is of concern. The simplest test of renal function is urine specific gravity. If specific gravity is high (over 1.010), more fluid is usually needed. If it is low (less than 1.010) and urine volume is also low, renal failure should be considered. Although more sensitive tests of glomerular and tubular function can be performed (see later section), a loop diuretic such as furosemide (10 to 20 mg intravenously) can be given empirically and repeated with or without an osmotic agent such as mannitol. Lack of response confirms the presence of renal failure and requires fluid restriction and further management as outlined later in this chapter.

OUTCOME

Improvement in the condition of the patient with septic shock is shown by (1) maintenance of normal blood pressure, CVP and PWP without support, (2) increased urine output, (3) improvement in respiratory status, (4) fall in temperature, (5) maintenance of hemoglobin levels and (6) return of platelets and coagulation factors to normal. Fluid and electrolyte management remain crucial during the subsequent diuretic phase, which lasts three to five days, and antibiotic coverage should be maintained for an adequate time. Failure of the patient to improve and the approach of an irreversible state is accompanied by multiple organ failure and deterioration of the monitored signs. Such patients show increasing sensory confusion. Blood pressure and urinary output are difficult to maintain and cardiac arrhythmias may develop. Most important is progressive respiratory failure, which requires intubation and/or tracheostomy and control of respiration from which the deteriorating patient cannot be weaned.

Toxic Shock

Toxic Shock Syndrome (TSS) has received considerable attention because of its association with use of highly absorbant vaginal tampons during menstruation. However, the syndrome has also been found in non-surgical focal infections, surgical wound infections and following obstetric conditions such as vaginal delivery, cesarean section or abortion. In many respects it is similar to septic shock. The difference lies in the pathophysiology, since it appears that the primary cause of TSS is staphylococcal infection and the release of one or more toxins by the staphylococci. Thus, bacteremia is not commonly found. The typical clinical manifestation as described by Wager (1983) are:
1. Fever.
2. Diffuse, generalized macular rash appear-

ing in the first 48 hours, similar to an eruption caused by allergy to a drug, and resulting in desquamation at the fifth to twelfth day of the illness.
3. Hypotension, characteristic of shock of any sort.
4. Involvement of three or more organ systems—gastrointestinal (nausea and vomiting at onset in up to 100% of patients); muscular (severe myalgia with creatine phosphate levels twice normal); mucous membranes (hyperemia of vagina, oropharynx or conjunctiva); renal (rise in BUN and/or creatinine); hepatic (total bilirubin, AST or ALT twice normal); hematologic (platelets less than 100,000/mm^3); or nervous (disorientation and loss of consciousness).

The management of TSS is essentially the same as that for septic shock and requires intensive monitoring and supportive care as well as appropriate antibiotics. Toxic shock syndrome is largely preventable. Patients should be advised not to wear tampons for prolonged periods, four to six hours at the most, and not to use them at night. Recurrence is an important feature of TSS. Approximately 30% of patients have more than one episode, and as many as five have been recorded in one patient.

Antibiotics

Antibiotics are indicated for the treatment of postoperative infection. The problems are to decide when to start using them, which antibiotic(s) to use, how much to give and by what route, when to change them and how long to continue them.

Antibiotics should be started when the patient has fever, as defined on page 67, and infection is the most likely cause for it. No antibiotics should be given until minimum laboratory studies have been set in motion. If prophylactic antibiotics have been given before the operation, they should generally be continued therapeutically if the patient has significant postoperative fever, pending appropriate studies.

The choice of antibiotic(s) is not easy, since neither the offending organism nor its sensitivity to various drugs is known. When the patient is desperately ill, i.e., in septic shock, the primary use of multiple antibiotics is appropriate in order to combat as many as possible of the microorganisms likely to be responsible. However, such a shotgun approach is not justifiable when the patient's condition is less serious, since combinations of drugs increase the possibility of toxicity, antagonism between drugs and superinfection and add expense. The problem is complicated by the limitations of the particular hospital pharmacy and the dazzling claims for the newest drugs. Nevertheless, some help can be obtained from the likely site of the infection (Table 4–4) and from the results of a Gram stain of pus or other material (Table 4–5).

During the early postoperative period the parenteral route of administration (intravenously, rather than intramuscularly), as a rule, is the most effective and often the only one available. Later in the postoperative course and for less serious infections, antibiotics may be given by mouth. Representative doses are shown in Table 4–6. Antibiotics differ greatly in cost. Table 4–6 also includes an estimate of the cost of one day's treatment with various drugs.

Once a culture report, including the sensitivity of the organism(s) to the various antibiotics, has been received a change of therapy is often necessary. If relatively few colonies are cultured, usually less than 100,000/ml (or less than this in urinary tract infections), and the patient's condition is improving, antibiotics should be stopped. If the organisms are not sensitive to the drugs used, it is necessary to change the antibiotic or add another agent. Because of the large number of organisms and agents, it is not possible to detail here all the specific actions of each drug. However, Table 4–7 shows a number of organisms commonly encountered in obstetrics and gynecology and the first and second choices of antibiotics to cover them. Doses will vary according to the weight of the patient and the severity of her illness. Possible side effects must also be considered; these are covered in Chapter 12.

Under normal circumstances, antibiotics may be expected to control infection within 72 hours. By that time fever and symptoms and signs of infection should have disappeared. If

this does not happen, there may be several possible reasons.

1. The blood level(s) of the antibiotic(s) is too low. Expected effective levels may be found in the manufacturer's product information, supplemented by data from the local (hospital) laboratory.

2. There may be other (additional) microorganisms which were not cultured originally and which are not sensitive to the antibiotics used. Repeat cultures should be taken from any available site. Antibiotics can then be changed according to the new information or a second choice antibiotic can be substituted.

3. Superinfection may have occurred. This possibility should spur a thorough examination and perhaps further cultures. In poorly nourished patients with prolonged illnesses, e.g., cancer, fungal infections are a real possibility.

Table 4–4. Initial Antibiotic Therapy

Suspected Site of Infection	Drug(s) of Choice
Lung	Cephalosporin (1)*
Urinary tract	Ampicillin
Incision	Clindamycin + Aminoglycoside or Cephalosporin (3)
Peritoneal cavity	Cephalosporin (2)
Pelvis	Cephalosporin (2)

*Cephalosporin (1), (2), and (3) indicate 1st, 2nd and 3rd generation cephalosporins.

Table 4–5. Initial Use of Antibiotics Based on Gram Stain

Suspected Organism	1st Choice	2nd Choice
Gram-positive cocci	Penicillin G	Cephalosporin
Gram-negative bacilli	Gentamicin	Piperacillin
Anerobic Gram-negative bacilli	Clindamycin	Chloramphenicol or Metronidazole
Gram-negative cocci	Penicillin G	Erythromycin
Undetermined	Gentamicin + Cephalosporin	Gentamicin + Piperacillin

Table 4–6. Typical Intravenous Doses of Selected Antibiotics

Drug	Dose	Cost Category*
Ampicillin	0.5–2.0 gm q 6 hrs	1
Penicillin G	1–5 mil units q 4–6 hrs	1
Ticarcillin	250–300 mg/kg/day (q 4 hrs)	3
Piperacillin	200–300 mg/kg/day (q 4 hrs)	3
Nafcillin	1.0–2.0 gm q 4 hrs	2
Cephalothin (1)†	0.5–2.0 gm q 4 hrs	1
Cefoxitin (2)†	2.0 g q 4 hrs	2
Moxalactam (3)†	50 mg/kg/day (1 gm q 8 hrs)	2
Gentamicin	3–5 mg/kg/day (q 8 hrs)	1
Amikacin	15 mg/kg/day (q 8 or q 12 hrs)	2
Clindamycin	150–900 mg q 8 hrs	2
Vancomycin	1.0 gm q 12 hr	3

*Costs vary greatly by hospital and by brand name of drugs. Those marked 1 are less expensive, 2 moderately expensive and 3 expensive.

†The markings (1), (2) and (3) refer to 1st, 2nd and 3rd generation cephalosporins.

Table 4–7. Antibiotics of Choice for Commonly Encountered Organisms in Gynecology and Obstetrics

Organism	1st Choice	2nd Choice
Actinomyces	Penicillin G	Tetracycline
Bacteroides	Clindamycin	Choramphenicol or Metronidazole
Chlamydia	Tetracycline	Erythromycin
Enterobacter sp.	Gentamicin	Piperacillin
Enterococci	Penicillin G + Gentamicin	Vancomycin + Gentamicin
Escherichia coli	Ampicillin	Gentamicin
Hemophilus influenzae	Ampicillin	Tetracycline
Mycoplasma pneumoniae	Erythromycin	Tetracycline
Neisseria gonorrhoeae	Penicillin G	Tetracycline
Proteus, Indole (−)	Ampicillin	Cephalosporin or Gentamicin
Proteus, Indole (+)	Gentamicin	Piperacillin
Pseudomonas	Trimethoprim/ Sulfamethox- azole	Chloramphenicol
Serratia marcescens	Amikacin	Cephalosporin (2nd generation)
Staphylococcus aureus (Methicillin- sensitive)	Penicillase- resistant Penicillin	Vancomycin or Erythromycin
Staphylococcus aureus (Methicillin- resistant)	Vancomycin	
Streptococci	Penicillin G	Cephalosporin or Erythromycin
Streptococci, anaerobic	Penicillin G	Cephalosporin
Treponema pallidum	Penicillin G	Erythromycin or Tetracycline

4. An abscess has formed, which cannot be penetrated by the antibiotics and may, indeed, be sterile. Surgical drainage is indicated (see previous section).

5. The antibiotics themselves may be causing fever. If none of the four causes listed seem likely, all antibiotics can be discontinued for 24 to 48 hours and the effects noted.

During antibiotic therapy the patient should be evaluated regularly for signs of toxicity. Peak and trough levels of drugs may be useful, for example, with aminoglycosides which may have renal toxicity especially in patients with reduced renal function. Automatic Stop Orders on antibiotics are a useful method of avoiding side effects.

Antibiotics should usually be continued for 24 to 72 hours after the signs of postoperative infection have disappeared. In some instances, such as urinary tract infection, it may be necessary to continue therapy for a week or even much longer.

Systemic fungal infections present a special problem. They are usually due to *Candida* species of which the commonest is *C. albicans.* They rarely occur in gynecologic or obstetric patients, and specific cases are usually included in larger series of patients who have had a variety of primary diseases. Candidiasis appears to be an infection usually acquired in a debilitated patient after a long hospital stay. Risk factors include antibiotic therapy (usually prolonged), bacterial sepsis, hyperalimentation, cancer, steroid therapy and diabetes. When fungemia is present, mortality is high, with death in these very ill patients often being caused by other factors besides candidiasis.

Vaginal and urinary candidiasis are relatively common findings in obstetric and gynecologic patients. The problem is to decide when the infection is disseminated and of serious prognostic importance. Two positive blood cultures 24 hours apart, of specimens that are not from a central venous catheter, are evidence of generalized infection. Culture of the organism from tissues such as kidney or lung, endophthalmitis or a positive culture from peritoneal fluid are also evidence of dissemination. In addition, isolation of fungi from at least three colonized sites, e.g., urine, sputum, wound or incisional drain, is presumptive evidence of dissemination (Burchard et al, 1983).

Vaginal, oral and cutaneous candidiasis are usually treated with nystatin. Since a primary site of *Candida* growth is the gastrointestinal tract, treatment with oral nystatin would appear to be useful, but this has not so far been proved. The only currently effective systemic fungicidal drug is amphotericin B. This is given in a daily dose of 0.25 mg/kg, increasing to 1.0 mg/kg per day. A total dose of at least 3 mg/kg is apparently necessary for effective treatment (Solomkin et al, 1982). Amphotericin B is difficult for the patient to tolerate because it causes many adverse reactions, e.g., nausea and vomiting, thrombophlebitis at the site of injection, hyperkalemia and renal damage (see Chapter 12). Intravenous miconazole has recently been suggested as therapy for candidiasis, but its efficacy has not been clearly demonstrated.

Prophylaxis

The use of antibiotics prior to a procedure depends on the nature of the procedure and the susceptibility of the patient to infection. Their use in potentially infected operations is described previously (Chapter 2), and their value has been shown in several studies, for example, that done by Ferrari and co-workers (1984). In clearly contaminated operations such as tubo-ovarian abscess or infected pelvic hematoma, antibiotics in therapeutic doses should be given before and after the operation.

Patient susceptibility to infection varies. Compared with young healthy women, women with known heart disease, including mitral valve prolapse, and women who are debilitated and suffering prolonged serious illnesses such as ovarian cancer require prophylactic antibiotics. More specific prophylaxis is needed when resection of the intestine and especially the colon is anticipated; under these circumstances the intestine should be as empty as possible and its bacterial contents reduced. Details of the use of prophylactic antibiotics in relation to specific preoperative conditions and operations are given in Chapter 2.

CARDIOVASCULAR COMPLICATIONS

Cardiac Complications

Cardiorespiratory Arrest

Failure of either heart or respiration may occur first, but the other rapidly follows. Cardiac causes include (1) mechanical asystole, occurring in the operating room, which is usually due to inadequate ventilation, (2) ventricular fibrillation, occurring in intensive care units and following myocardial infarction and (3) ineffective ventricular contraction due to depression of contractility by drugs associated with cardiac abnormalities. Respiratory arrest may be due to obstruction (foreign body) or ineffective gas exchange from such causes as atelectasis, pulmonary embolism, pneumonia, adult respiratory distress syndrome or cardiac failure.

The clinical signs of cardiorespiratory arrest occur in rapid sequence. First is evidence of anoxemia—restlessness, anxiety, disorientation and combativeness. Respiratory signs include dyspnea, tachypnea and inability to get enough air. Cardiovascular signs include cyanosis, weak or irregular pulse, hypotension and profuse sweating. Very soon the pulse disappears, breathing stops, visible blood becomes dark, the pupils dilate, the body becomes flaccid and convulsions may occur.

Cardiopulmonary resuscitation (CPR) involves the rapid application of a series of measures to restore function. Training (and certification) in CPR has become generally available (and required) in the past few years for health care personnel of all kinds. Although seldom needed, it can be life-saving in many situations, and the needed skills should be maintained by annual recertification. The essentials of CPR (1986) are as follows:

1. Establishing an airway. With the patient on her back, the shoulders are lifted up so that the head is hyperextended. Foreign bodies such as food in the mouth and throat can be removed with the finger. If the patient is upright or can be raised up, the Heimlich maneuver may dislodge a foreign body from the throat or larynx. This consists of grasping the patient's body from behind with the arms at the lowest part of the chest wall and jerking the arms sharply inward and upward.

2. Artificial respiration. If the above maneuvers do not clear the airway, mouth-to-mouth ventilation should be started. The patient's nose is pinched and the resuscitator takes a deep breath in and blows it into the patient's mouth so that her chest rises. Expiration is allowed to occur naturally and the insufflation is repeated 12 times a minute.

3. Cardiac resuscitation. If no carotid pulse is felt after four or five effective lung inflations, striking the sternum sharply with the fist may start the heart. If not, pressure is applied with the heel of one hand covered with the other hand over the lower part of the sternum. The sternum is compressed one to two inches and then suddenly released. Compression should be maintained at a rate of about 80/minute. Sets of 15 compressions should be interspersed with two breaths.

These measures are temporary. In most hospitals a CPR team is available for these emergencies. Its functions are to monitor vital functions, continue resuscitation and restore metabolic abnormalities. Immediate monitoring consists of continuous recording of the electrocardiogram and repeated blood pressure determinations. Intravenous and intraarterial lines are inserted. Blood gases are obtained. Sodium bicarbonate (2 mEq/kg) is given to combat acidosis. If necessary, a permanent airway is established with an endotracheal tube. If the electrocardiogram shows ventricular fibrillation, defibrillation is attempted with a direct current stimulus of 200 watt-sec to the chest wall, increasing to 400 watt-sec if necessary. Cardiotonic drugs that may be useful include epinephrine (1 to 2 ml 1:1000 in 10 cc) or calcium chloride (100 to 200 mg). Both are injected into the ventricle. Additional cardiac drugs (lidocaine, atropine, isoprotorenol) may be necessary for persistent arrythmias.

The outcome of cardiorespiratory resuscitation depends on the underlying cause of cardiorespiratory arrest and the speed with which CPR is started. Recurrences are common unless the basic pathophysiology can be corrected. Resuscitation started more than five minutes after the arrest is likely to fail. If resuscitation succeeds, at least temporarily, the patient should be promptly transported to an intensive care unit for adequate monitoring. It is important to check thoroughly for pneumothorax or possible damage to ribs, liver or spleen that may result from vigorous resuscitative efforts. If resuscitation was started too late or appears to be failing, the length of time it should be continued has to be decided in each case individually. The longer it is pursued the less likely is the patient to recover adequate function.

The results of resuscitation, particularly in the postoperative period, are difficult to ascertain but are worse for patients with underlying cardiorespiratory disease. Reported series usually contain few gynecologic or obstetric patients. Bedell and co-workers (1983) studied 294 consecutive resuscitated patients. Fourteen per cent were discharged from the hospital and 50% of these were alive six months later. Ninety-three per cent of those discharged were mentally intact then and six months later. There were no survivors when resuscitative efforts took more than 30 minutes, but 42% of those who survived for 24 hours left the hospital.

Myocardial Infarction

Myocardial infarction may occur at any time postoperatively. In the recovery phase it is an important consideration in the differential diagnosis of hypotension and shock (see earlier discussion). Later, although the postoperative state, particularly with regard to pain, may confuse the diagnosis, at least two of the following findings are necessary: (1) chest pain; (2) electrocardiographic changes, consisting of the presence of abnormal Q waves and changes in the ST-T segment; (3) elevation of cardiac enzymes, CK (creatine phosphokinase), GOT (glutamic oxaloacetic transaminase) and LDH (lactic dehydrogenase) or the isoenzymes MBCK and LDH (serial studies are important) and (4) pyrophosphate scans. The immediate management of a patient with presumptive myocardial infarction includes transfer to a coronary or intensive care unit, cardiac monitoring particularly with regard to arrhythmias, pain control, sedation and administration of oxygen. Further therapy should be directed by an internist or cardiologist.

Cardiac Arrythmias

Abnormalities of cardiac rhythm occur most commonly in the immediate postoperative recovery period, but may occur as a postoperative complication at any time. The precise diagnosis can only be made from an electrocardiogram either obtained routinely or as a result of a patient's complaint of irregular heartbeat or from observation of rhythm changes by the physician or nurse. Changes of minimal consequence include atrial premature contractions or first degree heart block. Changes of future concern that present no immediate danger include multiple ventricular extrasystoles or atrial fibrillation. Severe conditions that may cause immediate circulatory problems include marked bradycardia (less than 50 BPM), marked tachycardia (more than 160 BPM) or chaotic rhythms.

The minimal changes require only repeated observations. Atrial fibrillation generally requires the administration of digoxin (0.75 to 1.5 mg digoxin in 24 hours) and may need further measures. Frequent ventricular extrasystoles (more than 6 per minute) can be managed with lidocaine. A 100 mg bolus is given intravenously, followed by a continuous infusion of 4 mg/min with an additional bolus as needed. Failure of these measures or the presence of any of the severe conditions requires transfer to an intensive care unit for continuous monitoring and cardiology consultation.

Cardiac Failure

Heart failure may arise de novo or in a patient with known heart disease. The most likely cause, apart from intrinsic cardiac disorders (such as myocardial infarction or severe arrhythmias), is fluid overload either from crystalloids or colloids. The primary symptom is acute shortness of breath. Diminished urinary output and edema of the feet and sacrum may be noted. The pulse is rapid (110 or greater) and the neck veins may be distended. A hepatojugular reflex may be elicited—pressure over the liver with the patient in the sitting or semireclining position causes distention of the neck veins. Rales are heard in the lungs usually at the right base or at both bases, extending a varying distance up the lung fields. Treatment consists of (1) restricting intravenous fluids and particularly sodium, (2) diuretics (furosemide 20 to 40 mg intravenously, repeated every two hours as needed), (3) morphine in small doses, e.g., 4 to 8 mg hypodermically, (4) nasal oxygen and (5) digitalis (digoxin 0.5 mg immediately and 0.25 mg every 8 hours for three doses). If these measures fail or other cardiac problems arise, the patient should be transferred to an intensive care unit for more elaborate monitoring.

Vascular Complications

BLOOD PRESSURE CHANGES

Hypotension may be a sign of many postoperative complications. It is particularly important in the recovery period. When it occurs later in the postoperative period, it is evidence of a serious problem such as rapid blood loss, septic shock, acute cardiac problems such as a myocardial infarction or a pulmonary embolus. Management of these conditions is covered in other sections.

Hypertension occurring postoperatively is most commonly a continuation of the preoperative condition. Some patients with preexisting hypertension are normotensive during the first few postoperative days and revert to their previously higher levels only after they become ambulatory and more active. Regular monitoring is essential, with blood pressures taken and recorded on each nursing shift. Under these circumstances antihypertensive medication should be temporarily discontinued and then resumed as the need arises. A prompt postoperative rise in blood pressure to hypertensive levels indicates the need for use of antihypertensive drugs as soon as possible. In some patients hypertension develops acutely, usually in the immediate recovery period, but sometimes later. Initial treatment is outlined in an earlier section, i.e., the use of intravenous medications such as hydralazine, diazoxide or sodium nitroprusside. For the early postoperative period diuretics, hydralazine, methyldopa or propranolol are useful. Once blood pressure is under control and the patient can take fluids by mouth, oral antihypertensive agents should be used.

VENOUS COMPLICATIONS

Superficial Thrombophlebitis. Superficial thrombophlebitis is an almost invariable complication of administering intravenous fluids or repetitive blood drawing. While it does not usually result in the detachment of clots and embolization, it is painful and very obvious to the patient. The affected vein and the surrounding area are red and tender, particularly if there has been some extravasation of fluid or an irritating medication has been given through the intravenous line. The incidence and severity of superficial thrombophlebitis can be lessened by using a small catheter for no more than 48 to 72 hours; a change is easy to defer because of the nuisance and discomfort to the patient of inserting another catheter. Once the signs of superficial thrombophlebitis are obvious, the intravenous line should be removed and the area treated with moist heat and elevation. In most instances the condition will have subsided or improved within 48 to 72 hours. However, the patient may notice redness and induration of the vein for many weeks and should be warned about this. Superficial thrombophlebitis also occurs in the leg if a foot vein has been used for intravenous therapy. Because of the incapacity that results and the possible but still rare chance of embolism, foot veins should only be used in an emergency.

Deep Venous Thrombosis. Preoperative diagnosis of and prophylactic measures for deep venous thrombosis are discussed in Chapter 2. The true incidence of postoperative deep venous thrombosis (DVT) is not known. Crandon and Koutts (1983) using ^{125}I-labelled fibrinogen, found DVT to be present postoperatively in 37.9% of patients undergoing operations for gynecologic malignancy, as compared with an expected rate of 10 to 15% in the general gynecologic population. DVT occurred significantly more frequently in nonsmokers than in smokers. It is often silent (up to 50%) and may involve both legs. The small veins of the leg, extending to the popliteal vein, are probably first involved. Subsequently thrombosis may extend upwards to involve the femoral and then the iliac veins. In the early stages symptoms may be absent or consist of pain in the calf on walking or even at rest. Slight swelling of the foot and ankle may be noted and superifical veins may be prominent in the lower leg. Tenderness on lateral compression of the calf may be noted and sudden dorsiflexion of the relaxed foot (with the knee bent) may produce sharp pain in the calf (Homan's sign) (see Figure 2–2). Femoral vein involvement usually results in leg pain, swelling extending into the thigh and tenderness over the femoral and popliteal veins. When the iliac veins or inferior vena cava are occluded the leg is cool, swollen and very painful. Generalized signs such as tachycardia and fever may be present. Thrombosis may also occur in the pelvic and/or ovarian veins, either as a result of clots starting at operation or from an infectious process, giving rise to septic pelvic thrombophlebitis (Duff and Gibbs, 1983).

DIAGNOSIS. The diagnosis of femoral or iliac thrombosis is usually clear upon clinical examination of the leg. The only confusion may be with lymphatic obstruction, occurring after radical hysterectomy or similar procedures. The diagnosis of beginning thrombosis in the foot or leg may not be easy. Muscular pain may result from early ambulation, and patients may have had leg cramps prior to operation. Daily history and clinical examination of the leg are important, including repeated measurements of the circumference of the leg and thigh at the same point each day, if indicated. Laboratory studies are described above in Chapter 2. Postoperatively the least invasive procedures, Doppler ultrasound and impedance plethysmography, should be used first. Measurement of ^{125}I-labelled fibrinogen uptake is of limited value postoperatively because of the necessary delay of 24 to 48 hours between the injection of the isotope and scintillation counting. The definitive study is an x-ray venogram, but this presents problems because of the time taken, the invasive nature of the procedure, the difficulty of performing it in the obese postoperative patient and the fallibility of interpretation (Sandler et al, 1984).

MANAGEMENT WITH ANTICOAGULANTS. The primary treatment of postoperative venous thrombosis is currently by the use of anticoagulants. While this has complications, chiefly hemorrhagic, the risk of pulmonary embolism is sufficiently serious so that treatment is advisable if there is a reasonable suspicion of deep venous thrombosis. Anticoagulation is started with heparin after baseline prothrombin time (PT) and partial thromboplastin time (PTT) have been obtained. Although regimens vary, a common protocol is to give a bolus of 8000 to 12,000 units of heparin, and follow this with a continuous intravenous infusion of about 1000 units per hour. The dose is regulated so as to keep the PTT at 1½ to 2 times the normal level (Bjornesson and Greenberg, 1985). Heparin is continued for five to seven days. After two to four days oral warfarin (Coumadin) is started at a dose of 10 mg/day for three days. The PT is checked daily and the warfarin dose is adjusted

to keep it at two to three times normal. The duration of heparin therapy does not appear to be critical to its effectiveness. If it is shorter, the duration of hospitalization and, therefore, the cost is less (Rooke and Osmundson, 1986). How long warfarin anticoagulation should be continued is uncertain. Three months appears to be a reasonable time.

The chief danger of both heparin and warfarin given in therapeutic doses is bleeding. Therefore contraindications to anticoagulation include any bleeding tendency or any condition in which a small amount of bleeding is likely to have serious consequences, e.g., peptic ulcer. It is important to watch for bleeding from operative sites, the gastrointestinal tract or mucous membranes. Heparin is rapidly excreted, disappearing from the plasma less than four hours after discontinuation. If earlier neutralization is needed, protamine sulfate is effective but it must be given intravenously and slowly at a rate of no more than 10 mg/min or a maximum of 100 mg. The total amount needed is based on the amount of heparin presumed to be circulating and should be guided by PTT determinations. Initially, 1.0 mg should be given for each 100 units of presumed circulating heparin.

The action of warfarin is much longer than that of heparin, its half life being 2½ days. Thus the PT only gradually returns to normal. This return can be accelerated by the administration of phytonadione (vitamin K_1) in doses of 2.5 to 10 mg by mouth or 5 to 25 mg intramuscularly or intravenously (the latter given slowly at a rate of 5 mg/min).

MANAGEMENT WITH OTHER MEASURES. Initially bed rest with the legs elevated promotes venous drainage. As anticoagulation proceeds (in 24 to 48 hours) the patient should be allowed to use a bedside commode and her activity gradually increased. Sitting with the legs bent should be avoided; a small stool should be used to support the feet. Warm, wet compresses may sometimes decrease pain. Broad spectrum antibiotics, for example, a second generation cephalosporin, are given if fever and leukocytosis are present, especially if septic pelvic thrombophlebitis is suspected. As a last resort with progressive thrombosis, thrombectomy may be performed under local anesthesia using suction to remove thrombi above the inguinal ligament and tight bandaging of the leg to express distal clots.

SEQUELAE OF DEEP VENOUS THROMBOSIS. A small proportion of patients who have had deep venous thrombosis develop the postphlebitic syndrome. It is more common in patients who have had iliofemoral thrombosis than in those with thrombi in the calf veins. About half the patients (49%) had pain in the leg(s), while edema was noted to be present in 21%, pigmentation in 26% and ulceration in 2% (Killewich et al, 1985). Treatment is conservative, difficult and prolonged.

MANAGEMENT DURING PREGNANCY. Heparin has a molecular weight of 10,000 to 40,000 daltons and does not appear to cross the placenta. On the other hand, warfarin has a molecular weight of about 1000 daltons and readily crosses the placenta. It may cause fetal anomalies if given in the first trimester of pregnancy. Heparin, therefore, is the safest drug to use, at least during the first 16 weeks of pregnancy while organogenesis is proceeding and after 36 weeks when the danger of prolonged anticoagulation poses the risk of bleeding during and after delivery. Intravenous heparin cannot usually be given for prolonged periods. However, small, self-administered subcutaneous doses (5000 units twice daily) may be an effective way of providing therapy as well as prophylaxis and may be continued over many weeks (Bonnar, 1979). If necessary, warfarin can be given from the 16th to the 36th week of pregnancy and heparin before and after this. Heparin is stopped when labor starts and this usually permits the PTT to return to normal before delivery. The mangement of DVT in pregnancy is difficult and represents a major psychosocial as well as a medical stress to the patient (and her family).

PULMONARY EMBOLISM

Pulmonary embolism is one of the most serious postoperative complications because it is usually unsuspected and may be fatal. Symptoms depend on the size and number of the emboli in the pulmonary arterial tree and whether or not pulmonary infarction occurs. Small emboli may be asyptomatic. Emboli of minor or moderate severity that are in the periphery of the lung may produce the classic symptoms of dyspnea, pleuritic pain on deep breathing and hemoptysis. Major emboli may result in acute dilatation and failure of the right ventricle (cor pulmonale), resulting in acute anxiety, tachypnea, tachycardia, cyanosis and hypotension. Sudden cardiorespiratory failure and death may occur.

Diagnosis. Clinical findings are often non-specific and may be due to other lung diseases.

The following laboratory and radiographic studies are useful, but their results may be difficult to interpret.

1. Arterial pO_2. This is particularly valuable if a prior study is available. However, the results are non-specific.

2. Chest x-ray. Classically a wedge-shaped density is present, and the diaphragm may be elevated. These changes are usually not present immediately and may be non-specific.

3. Electrocardiogram. Many findings are reported. The S_1–Q_3–T_3 pattern of cor pulmonale is somewhat specific. An important function of the electrocardiogram is to rule out other disorders such as myocardial infarction.

4. Lung Scan. A ventilation-perfusion lung scan is a useful noninvasive test (Rosenow et al, 1981). The probability of a correct diagnosis of pulmonary embolism is usually rated as low, intermediate or high. A high probability (90%) exists when there are two or more segmental or larger perfusion defects with normal ventilation, a V/Q (ventilation/perfusion) mismatch.

5. Angiography. A pulmonary angiogram is the definitive study if done within 24 to 72 hours of the suspected embolism. Later, resolution of the clots makes interpretation difficult. It is invasive and results in a mortality of 0.2% and a morbidity of 4% (Rosenow et al, 1981).

If pulmonary embolism is suspected from the history, thorough physical examination should be performed and an electrocardiogram, chest x-ray and ventilation-perfusion lung scan performed. An angiogram is indicated only if the scan indicates a low or intermediate probability of embolism and it is essential to obtain a diagnosis.

Treatment. Initial treatment for a pulmonary embolus that is not immediately life-threatening is by the use of anticoagulants as described above for deep venous thrombosis. Anticoagulants (warfarin) are continued for at least three months. Thrombolytic therapy with streptokinase or urokinase has been shown to be superior to heparin alone in major cooperative trials. It may be of special value in patients with massive pulmonary emboli, but must be used with caution because of febrile and allergic reactions (Sasahara et al, 1983).

Surgical management may take two forms, embolectomy or occlusion of the inferior vena cava to prevent recurrent emboli. Embolectomy is indicated when the degree of acute pulmonary occlusion is sufficient to produce transient or sustained hypotension, requiring vasopressor support, provided that angiography confirms the clinical diagnosis (Greenfield et al, 1982). These authors reported catheter embolectomy in 19 patients; in 16 (84%) definite emboli were removed and in three fragments only were obtained. The mortality was six or 32%. Open embolectomy was performed in four patients with success in three and death in one (25%).

The inferior vena cava can be occluded when anticoagulants are contraindicated or recurrent emboli occur in spite of the use of anticoagulants, especially from septic thrombophlebitis (Keller et al, 1985). Occlusion is performed by open operation and ligation or application of a multichannel serrated teflon vena cava clip or more recently by insertion of a filter or umbrella through the internal jugular or femoral vein. Open operation carries considerable risk in a sick patient, but enables the ovarian veins, an important source of emboli, to be ligated at the same time. Filter or umbrella placement is somewhat easier in experienced hands. However, problems with positioning and migration of the filter have been encountered. With either method of occlusion recurrent emboli are rare. Approximately 50% of patients have persistent swelling of the legs, necessitating the use of elastic stockings and other measures. The incidence of stasis may be related to venous occlusion prior to interruption of the vena cava and/or to the completeness of caval closure.

ARTERIAL OCCLUSION

The most common sites of arterial embolism are the vessels of the leg. This occurs rarely in the postoperative period. An important predisposing factor is atrial fibrillation. Sudden occlusion presents a dramatic clinical picture. The patient notices pain followed by paresthesias and paralysis. The leg is cold and pale. No arterial pulsations can be felt below the occluded vessels, although this is sometimes difficult to determine. There is usually no swelling of the leg, in contrast to deep venous thrombosis. If no treatment is given, gangrene of the leg will occur. Non-invasive Doppler ultrasound is helpful in locating the site of occlusion. The diagnosis is confirmed by arteriography. Treatment is by anticoagulation and immediate embolectomy.

RESPIRATORY COMPLICATIONS

Atelectasis (collapse of a lung or part of a lung) is the commonest postoperative compli-

cation. It is usually treatable but if treatment is not successful and predisposing factors are present, pneumonitis or pneumonia may follow. Preoperative respiratory diseases such as emphysema, asthma and bronchitis may become worse postoperatively. Pneumothorax and pleural effusion may follow special procedures, more commonly performed in surgical than in gynecologic patients. Respiratory insufficiency, adult respiratory distress syndrome (ARDS) and respiratory failure represent the end, life-threatening stages of pulmonary complications.

Atelectasis

Atelectasis is due to obstruction of the bronchial tree by increased thickness or amount of bronchial secretions plugging small (or large) bronchi, defective expiration mechanism and reduction of bronchial caliber. It most commonly occurs in the early postoperative period (12 to 72 hours). The early signs are moist rales heard posteriorly over the lung bases with diminished and bronchial breath sounds over a localized segment of the lung. Later, fever and tachycardia develop. If the atelectasis is massive with collapse of a large part or all of one lobe, the trachea, mediastinum and heart may shift to the involved side. If the atelectasis is patchy or segmental, this shift will not usually occur. Physical findings may be confirmed by x-ray. However, specific radiologic changes may not be present in patchy atelectasis. Moreover, since the patient is in the early postoperative state, it is often necessary to obtain x-ray films with portable radiology equipment; the quality of such films may be such as to show only gross changes.

The management of atelectasis consists primarily of adequate preoperative assessment and treatment (where possible) of preexisting lung disorders and early postoperative encouragement of respiratory effort. This includes analgesics to relieve pain (best given in small doses frequently, every two to three hours), stimulation of deep breathing with an incentive spirometer and frequent coughing, encouragement to breathe deeply and changes of position. Older, debilitated patients, smokers and those with prior chronic obstructive pulmonary disease (COPD) require extra attention to these measures. Additionally, intermittent positive pressure breathing (IPPB) to inflate the lungs and nebulize mucolytic agents such as acetylcysteine may be helpful. Endotracheal suction with a soft tube (transnasally) may be necessary. Antibiotics are not indicated initially. In rare instances, usually in patients with poor preoperative lung function, respiratory insufficiency may develop as a result of atelectasis (see later section).

Pneumonia, Bronchitis, Bronchopneumonia

Pneumonia inevitably develops after atelectasis has persisted for 72 hours or more. Unless it is lobar in type, there are few changes in physical or x-ray signs. Fine patchy rales and bronchial breath sounds continue. Lobar pneumonia presents a well-demarcated area of dullness with bronchial breath sounds and egophony. It is important to obtain a sputum culture if possible. Antibiotics should be started at this point. Initially penicillin G (2 mil units every 4 hours intravenously) or a first generation cephalosporin, for example, cephalothin 1.0 gm every 6 hours intravenously, are appropriate.

Patients with bronchopneumonia or exacerbation of bronchitis, in contrast to those with lobar or lobular pneumonia, are more likely to be older, debilitated and to have hospital-acquired infections. A wide variety of organisms may be responsible. Initial empirical antibiotic therapy should include an antipseudomonal aminoglycoside such as gentamicin or tobramycin together with a second generation cephalosporin such as cefoxitin or a betalactamase-insensitive penicillin such as piperacillin.

Once the report of the sputum culture and sensitivity of the organisms cultured has been received, a change in antibiotics may be necessary. Chest physical therapy should be continued and nasal oxygen is indicated if dyspnea, cyanosis or low arterial pO_2 occurs.

Asthma

Acute attacks or exacerbations of asthma may occur postoperatively. Precipitating causes include anesthetic agents, stress or allergic response to medications. Narrowing of the airway (bronchospasm) and increased bronchial secretions cause shortness of breath with, in some instances, respiratory insufficiency. Expiratory wheezes are characteristically heard.

Recognition of a history of asthma enables one to be forewarned. Treatment is directed to bronchodilation, hydration, oxygenation and in extreme cases ventilatory support. Immediate bronchodilation can be obtained by the subcutaneous injection of aqueous epinephrine 0.3 to 0.5 ml of a 1:1000 solution. This dose can be repeated every 20 minutes. As continuing therapy intravenous aminophyllin is useful. A loading dose of 6 mg/kg is given over 15 to 30 minutes and this is followed by continuous intravenous infusion of 0.5 to 1.0 mg/kg/hr. Therapeutic levels of theophylline (if available) should be maintained at 10 to 20 micrograms/ml. Oral aminophyllin (200 to 400 mg four times daily) should be started as soon as possible. A variety of aerosol solutions, used three to four times daily, may also promote bronchodilation. Corticosteroids may also be given.

Pneumothorax

Pneumothorax may occur in the postoperative period either spontaneously, from perforation by a central catheter (with hemothorax) or as a result of thoracentesis. If more than 15% of the lung is collapsed, thoracostomy is indicated with insertion of a No. 32 to No. 35 French tube leading to underwater drainage. Within three to four days the tube is clamped, and if pneumothorax does not recur, the tube may be removed. The chance of pneumothorax may be lessened by care in performing a thoracentesis, i.e., not penetrating the lung and not letting air in through the system (see Chapter 12).

Pleural Effusion

Postoperative pleural effusion may be due to infectious lung disease, pulmonary embolism, cardiac failure, metastatic disease in the pleural cavity, migration of ascitic fluid across the diaphragm or subdiaphragmatic abscess. Its amount can be roughly determined by the upward extent of percussion dullness and by chest x-ray. Indications for removal of fluid by thoracentesis are to obtain a diagnosis or therapeutically if the amount of fluid is large enough to compromise lung function. Thoracentesis is usually performed with the patient sitting and leaning forward. Local anesthetic is injected in the posterior axillary line above the 8th or 9th rib, since the intercostal nerve, artery and vein run below each rib. A needle is attached to a three-way stopcock and syringe (with an airtight connection), inserted into the pleural cavity through the anesthetized area and its position maintained constantly. Only a small amount of fluid needs to be withdrawn for diagnosis. For therapeutic purposes caution should be exercised in removing more than 1000 ml because of possible mediastinal shift and respiratory distress. The thoracentesis site should be covered with an occlusive dressing for 24 hours. Following the procedure, the patient may require analgesics for pleural pain. If the fluid reaccumulates rapidly, as in postoperative ovarian carcinoma, thoracentesis may be repeated. However, if this has to be done more than two or three times, thoracostomy should be performed. If drainage through the tube then continues to be profuse pleurodesis with tetracycline or other sclerosing substance is indicated.

Respiratory Insufficiency and Failure

Postoperative respiratory insufficiency and/or failure may result from (1) obstruction by a foreign body, (2) aspiration of gastric contents, (3) progressive decrease in respiratory function from underlying lung disease, exaggerated by atelectasis or infection and (4) adult respiratory distress syndrome (ARDS) (shock lung) due to septicemia, amniotic fluid or trophoblastic embolism or overinfusion of crystalloids or colloids.

A clinical diagnosis of obstruction or aspiration is dramatic and obvious. With a progressive decrease in functions or ARDS respiratory problems often appear to develop suddenly, but there is always a prodromal stage in which the patient shows restlessness, anxiety and later air hunger, labored respiration with the use of accessory muscles of the nose and throat, circumoral pallor and cyanosis.

The management of the respiratory difficulty is linked to the management of the associated cardiovascular system problems and to the treatment of the underlying disorder. The first question is whether or not the patient requires mechanical ventilatory support, as opposed to oxygen and chest physical therapy. Criteria for making this decision are given in Table 4–8. Ventilatory support can be given through a tightly fitting face mask or preferably through an endotracheal tube. The patient must be in an intensive care unit with comprehensive monitoring, round-the-clock nursing (on a 1:1 or a 1:2 basis) and medical care immediately available. The face mask with continuous positive airway pressure (CPAP) avoids possible damage to the larynx and trachea. However, it is difficult to avoid leaks and the mask is very uncomfortable for the patient. In a critically ill patient insertion of an endotracheal tube and attachment to a ventilator provides a better method of controlling respiration and oxygenation. Modern ventilators permit control of tidal volume (V_t) (12 to 15 ml/kg), respiratory rate (10

Table 4–8. Indications for Respiratory Support*

	Oxygen Therapy Chest Physiotherapy	Intubation Ventilation
Respiration rate	25–35/min	>35
Vital capacity	30–15 ml/kg	<15
pO_2	70 (40% O_2)	<70
pCO_2	45–60	>60

*From Webb WR, Moulder PV: Postoperative pulmonary complications. In Hardy JD (ed.): *Complications in Surgery and Their Management.* Philadelphia, W. B. Saunders, 1981, p. 107. Reprinted with permission.

to 12/min) and inspired oxygen concentration (F_iO_2) (50%). It is essential to be familiar with the settings and working of the available machine. The addition of positive end expiratory pressure (PEEP) of 5 to 15 cm appears to be helpful in preventing small areas of atelectasis, which cause arteriovenous shunting in the lung (Weisman et al, 1982). The objective of ventilation is to maintain the arterial pO_2 at 60 mm Hg or greater and the pCO_2 at about 40 mm Hg. An experienced respiratory therapist is essential for good management. In addition to ventilator orders and cardiac monitoring (Swan-Ganz catheter) patients on respiratory support may need narcotics, sedation or a neuromuscular relaxant such as pancuronium bromide (Pavulon). All other organ systems (e.g., gastrointestinal tract and urinary tract) and nutritional status need constant monitoring.

Weaning from ventilatory support should be carried out as soon as the patient's underlying disease is stable. Intermittent mandatory ventilation (IMV) is a useful step in weaning. This allows the patient to breathe at her own rate and tidal volume, but, in addition, the respirator delivers a preset volume usually at a rate less than the patient's existing respiratory rate. When weaning does not appear practical in 72 to 96 hours a tracheostomy should generally be performed. This reduces the chance of permanent damage to the larynx, decreases the dead space and permits easier tracheal toilet (Grillo, 1983). The moribund patient who cannot be weaned from the respirator after a prolonged period of ventilation presents a complex medical and ethical problem. The latter is discussed in Chapter 16.

GASTROINTESTINAL TRACT

Gastrointestinal complications are likely to occur after any operation or procedure that involves entering the peritoneal cavity. Complications are related to (1) the preoperative condition of the patient (i.e., poor nutritional status, prior radiation therapy), (2) the patient's disease, (3) the extent and length of the operation, (4) intraoperative contamination of the peritoneal cavity by intestinal contents, (5) the amount of manipulation the bowel has received and (6) infection. Abdominal operations are more likely to be followed by gastrointestinal complications than vaginal procedures.

Postoperative Function

After the operation the motility of the stomach and colon is usually decreased for a varying time. Motility of the small intestine continues but may be diminished. In an exaggerated form this inactivity leads to acute gastric dilatation, paralytic ileus or constipation with, eventually, fecal impaction. These changes are compounded by the anti-peristaltic action of narcotics given to relieve postoperative pain.

Routine postoperative orders should take into account intestinal function. Although doubtless many patients can begin to drink and eat soon after operations that involve entering the peritoneal cavity, it is wisest to withhold oral intake of all sorts until 24 hours after operation (except laparoscopy) or, if any but a minor procedure has been performed, until the patient passes flatus, has a bowel movement or has very active peristalsis and is hungry. In this situation there is no substitute for palpation and auscultation of the patient's abdomen by the operating surgeon or his qualified delegate at regular (8 to 12 hour) intervals. Listening in the left upper quadrant of the abdomen just above the umbilicus with the dressings off is most productive when peristalsis is diminished.

When a decision has been reached to permit oral intake, the patient should be given small amounts of clear liquids at regular intervals. After the first few hours unlimited liquids may be given and in 24 hours the patient may eat what she wishes. The use of a so-called soft diet is an unnecessary intermediate step between liquids and a self-selected diet of the patient's choice.

The final evidence of a functioning gastrointestinal tract is regular bowel movements. This may take several days and is often of great concern to the patient who is used to having daily bowel movements or to the nursing staff who think that she should have a bowel movement as soon as possible. Gentle oral laxatives such as milk of magnesia (30 to 60 ml) given on the second or third postoperative evening, supplemented later, if necessary, by a glycerine or bisacodyl (Dulcolax) suppository is usually sufficient to initiate bowel action. Enemas should rarely be necessary.

Disorders of Motility

ACUTE GASTRIC DILATATION

This occurs so rarely in gynecology and obstetrics that the diagnosis can be missed. It is more common when the upper abdomen has been manipulated or when a long tube has been passed into the small intestine, and gas is swallowed above it. The patient may be nauseated. She looks distressed and may have an unusually rapid pulse. On examination the upper abdomen is distended and tympanitic. Treatment is by aspiration of the stomach contents through a nasogastric tube. The tube should be left in place only if there is a continuing contributory cause to the dilatation such as upper gastrointestinal obstruction.

PARALYTIC ILEUS

Paralytic ileus occurs when swallowed air passes into the small intestine but can go no further because of decreased motility, closure of the ileocecal valve or reduced colonic motility. It, therefore, depends on the amount of air swallowed as well as upon the type of operation, the amount of intestinal handling and the presence of intraperitoneal infection. The patient feels full, belches, and may become nauseated and vomit. On examination the abdomen is distended and peristalsis is usually diminished or absent. Signs of peritoneal irritation are not characteristic of uncomplicated ileus. Abdominal flat and upright x-rays show air in the small intestine and usually in the colon. The small intestinal loops are diffusely located throughout the abdomen. Intestinal obstruction is the chief differential diagnosis. Findings distinguishing between ileus and obstruction are shown in Table 4–9 and Figure 4–3.

The management of ileus consists of withholding oral fluids, replacing fluid and electrolytes with appropriate intravenous fluids and nasogastric suction. The use of a long intestinal tube is not usually necessary, at least initially. Conservative management is usually effective. Persistent signs of ileus suggest that there is an underlying intraperitoneal cause such as infec-

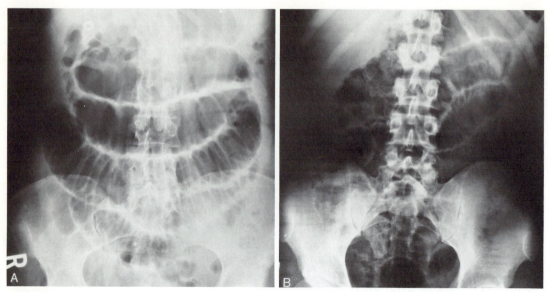

Figure 4–3. Differentiation of ileus and obstruction. A, Intestinal obstruction, showing step-ladder effect. B, Paralytic ileus, showing gas in both the small and large bowel.

tion or that small bowel obstruction is present, masquerading as ileus.

Impaired motility of the colon may occur postoperatively. This gives rise to pseudo-obstruction (Ogilvie's syndrome). Typically the abdomen becomes acutely distended with relatively few abnormal signs or laboratory findings unless perforation of the bowel is imminent or has occurred. Flat and upright abdominal x-rays are usually diagnostic, although distal colonic obstruction has to be differentiated. Vanek and Al-Salti (1986) advise conservative treatment with nasogastric suction, bowel stimulants and cautiously given enemas. If the diameter of the cecum exceeds 12 cm, there is danger of perforation, and decompression by colonoscopy

or operation is advisable. In a review of 400 cases these authors found that the problem was resolved in an average of 5.2 days.

Prolonged constipation can be very distressing to the patient and inspissated stool can lead to fecal impaction. When possible severe constipation should be prevented by the appropriate use of laxatives and suppositories. If prolonged use of narcotics has been required, regular administration of stool softener, e.g., docusate sodium, is important. A true fecal impaction can only be diagnosed by rectal examination. Abdominal x-rays may confirm a large amount of feces in the colon. Manual removal of at least some of the impaction is necessary, together with the use of mineral oil and laxatives by mouth. Enemas, including oil retention enemas, may be used after disimpaction.

Intestinal Obstruction

The incidence of obstructive complications after gynecologic operations is impossible to determine because the majority of cases occur months to years later and are not recognized nor recorded as complications by the primary surgeon. Also, such patients are likely to be seen by a general surgeon rather than a gynecologist.

Most postoperative bowel obstructions are due to adhesions. The prevention of adhesions

Table 4–9. Differential Diagnosis of Ileus and Intestinal Obstruction

Findings	Ileus	Obstruction
Time of appearance after operation	24–72 hours	Over 5 days
Abdominal pain	Slight, due to distension	Crampy (?)
Nausea and vomiting	Present	Present
Fever	Absent except with peritonitis	Absent except with strangulation
Abdominal distension	Marked	Present
Bowel sounds	Absent or hypoactive	Hyperactive (?)

is discussed in Chapter 3. The fact of the matter, however, is that some individuals are more prone to develop adhesions than others for reasons that are largely unknown. Soon after the operation, adhesions are usually thin. Later, they become fibrous and fixed. Adhesions cause kinking of the bowel, attachment of bowel loops to one another and even volvuli and intussusception. Postoperative obstruction may also be due to other factors not related to adhesions, including cecal or sigmoid volvulus or an incarcerated hernia not previously appreciated. Further, in closing the abdomen, intestine, mesentery or omentum may be caught in sutures, leading to kinks and subsequent obstruction. After gynecologic operations, obstruction occurs most commonly in the small bowel and rarely in the large, expect for inspissation of feces leading to de facto obstruction.

Various classifications have been applied to intestinal obstruction. It may be partial or complete, or it may be simple or strangulating; the latter occurs when bowel vascularity is compromised and necrosis takes place due to prolonged obstruction or mesenteric vascular change such as thrombosis. These distinctions are important in diagnosis and management. Special problems arise in gynecologic oncology after exenterations and when bowel obstruction is associated with widespread intraabdominal cancer.

DIAGNOSIS

The typical symptoms of bowel obstruction are crampy abdominal pain, failure to pass gas or feces, abdominal distension and nausea and vomiting. These apply to both partial and complete obstruction, although with the latter, symptoms may be more dramatic and acute. In early postoperative obstruction, crampy abdominal pain is confusing because it occurs commonly under normal circumstances. Its persistence beyond four to five days should make one suspicious of obstruction. Steady abdominal pain associated with the other symptoms suggests strangulated obstruction. Nausea and vomiting may be a late symptom if the obstruction is low in the ileum. A fecal appearance and odor of the vomitus is characteristic of long-standing, low obstruction.

On examination the patient with bowel obstruction characteristically has a distended, nontender abdomen with hyperactive high-pitched peristalsis, with peristaltic rushes that coincide with the crampy pain. These signs may be muted in the early postoperative period. In the early stages of simple obstruction, pulse and temperature may be relatively normal. Feces may or may not be present in the rectum as determined by rectal examination. Laboratory data will usually show a normal white blood count. Electrolytes are usually unchanged, although later shifts may be noted as fluid accumulates in the intestine. Strangulating obstruction presents a more acute picture with localized or generalized abdominal tenderness, rebound tenderness, tachycardia, fever and leukocytosis.

MANAGEMENT

The three principles of managing postoperative intestinal obstruction consist of correction and maintenance of fluid and electrolyte balance, intestinal intubation and reoperation. Management of fluid and electrolytes are covered in Chapter 2. Intubation serves the purposes of preventing further ingestion of air and removing air and fluid above the point of obstruction. This permits the bowel to return to a more normal diameter and reduces the swelling of its wall. The author's preference is for a single-lumen, long intestinal tube (Cantor), although a double-lumen tube is quite satisfactory. If the clinical picture is clear and early operation seems indicated, nasogastric suction alone may be sufficient. However, there is a reasonable chance that intubation with a long tube may be successful in simple, partial or possibly in complete obstruction—65% and 25% respectively—Peetz et al (1982).

The Cantor tube is a 16 or 18 French single-lumen tube with a balloon at the end. Two to four milliliters of mercury are injected into the balloon, and the well-lubricated tube is passed through the nose into the stomach. Transit into the duodenum is aided by having the patient lie on her right side and by having the head of the bed elevated. Low intermittent suction is begun. It is important not to advance the tube beyond the P (pylorus) mark. Otherwise it may coil in the stomach. Metaclopramide may be given intravenously (10 mg) to aid gastric relaxation. Clinically, passage of the tube into the duodenum is shown by a change in the suction drainage from the greenish, flecked stomach contents to the bile-colored and (in obstruction) more fecal small bowel contents. If the tube fails to pass into the duodenum in one to two hours, it should be withdrawn to above the P mark and positioning repeated. Sometimes having the patient walk will permit the tube to enter the duodenum by gravity. If doubt remains as to its passage in three to four hours, abdominal x-rays are indicated, with, if possible, fluoroscopy to position the tip of the tube at the pyloric end of the stomach. When the tube has entered the duodenum it should continue to progress spontaneously. Failure to progress is usually a sign that the tube is nearing the point of obstruction. This may be confirmed by x-ray examination after injection of Gastrografin through the tube. A free loop of tube should be left outside the nose to permit further passage. Intermittent low suction is continued.

Nasogastric and long tubes have some complications. These include:

1. Difficulty of insertion. Nasal obstruction may make the use of the nose impossible and oral insertion is not satisfactory. Bleeding from the nose may occasionally be troublesome. Passage through the pharynx may be aided by an anesthetic spray. The air should be removed from the balloon of the Cantor tube to reduce its bulk. In addition, to prevent diffusion of intestinal gas into the balloon, small punctures may be made in it with a 22-gauge needle.

2. Patient discomfort. Prolonged intubation is uncomfortable. At first, the tube may be tolerated because the abdominal pain and distension are relieved. Later, nasopharyngeal irritation may be somewhat relieved by having the patient suck hard candy. Lubrication of the tube with a very small amount of oil may help. Anesthetic lozenges or sprays should not be used for fear of ulceration if the tube remains in one place in the anesthetized pharynx.

3. Rupture of the balloon. This results in free mercury in the intestinal tract. It is not of serious consequence.

4. Passage of the balloon all the way through the intestinal tract. If the balloon emerges through the anus (a very rare event, which can usually be avoided by monitoring its passage) it is cut off and the tube withdrawn upwards in the usual manner.

5. Intussusception. This is a rare but serious complication (Redmond et al, 1982). It may be due to fixing the tube at the nose or to fixed plications in the bowel that permit the balloon to act as the leading point of an intussusception. Persistence of obstruction and x-ray findings assist in making the diagnosis. The tube may be pulled back gently or an operation may be required to reduce the intussusception.

6. Removal. Slow removal is advisable to prevent reverse intussusception or bowel laceration. About one foot should be removed at a time, every two to five minutes. When the balloon is in the stomach, it is brought up quickly. The very rare knot in the tube may require gastrotomy for removal.

The decision to operate depends on the type of obstruction and the success of conservative measures, i.e., intubation. When strangulating obstruction is believed to be present, prompt exploration is indicated, as soon as the patient's fluid and electrolyte balance have been stabilized and appropriate broad spectrum antibiotics given. Intubation is important since anastomoses are likely, but it is not necessary to wait for a long tube to enter the duodenum; a nasogastric tube will do as well.

When the obstruction is simple but complete, large amounts (over 500 ml/8 hrs) of fluid continue to drain from the Cantor tube, and the material drained often appears thick and particulate. Distension and x-ray signs may improve slightly but peristalsis remains hyperactive and no gas or stool is passed. As soon as these facts are ascertained and the patient is in fluid and electrolyte balance, operation is indicated (in 12 to 48 hours).

Relief of the obstruction by intubation is shown by the fact that the amount of suction drainage decreases to less than 300 ml/eight-hour nursing shift and becomes clearer and golden in color. The patient passes gas and feces. Peristalsis, abdominal distension and x-ray signs return toward normal, with more gas apparent in the rectum. Once improvement is clearly established, suction is continued for 24 hours. The tube is then clamped in the morning and remains clamped unless the patient has abdominal pain or nausea and vomiting. In the evening, it is opened for 30 minutes. If there is little drainage, it should remain unclamped overnight and oral liquids started the next morning. If these are tolerated and retained for 24 hours, the tube is removed. Failure of this progressive return to normal function is usually an indication for operation. It implies that the condition causing the obstruction is still present. Moreover, the patient's nutritional status is being steadily depleted. After seven to ten days of obstruction, suction and minimal oral intake, intravenous hyperalimentation must be considered.

In gynecology there are two situations in which conservative treatment of obstruction may be extended. The first is after exenteration, when reoperation presents a significant hazard and the second is in ovarian cancer with widespread intraperitoneal metastases. In the latter case reoperation is likely to be useless because little or no bowel may be free for bypass or anastomoses, and the operation may have to be concluded with nothing accomplished or with an unanticipated small bowel stoma. Moreover, in advanced ovarian cancer, the obstruction is most often partial and its degree may fluctuate from time to time. If the patient's condition is terminal or near-terminal, there is no reason to subject her to another operation unless something can be accomplished by it (Baines et al, 1985).

The principles of operation for intestinal obstruction are as follows:

1. The abdomen is opened through a vertical midline incision. In gynecology and obstetrics when a similar incision has been used previously it is usually best to extend it around and above the umbilicus and attempt to enter the peritoneal cavity at the upper end.

2. All adhesions are divided and the intestine followed from the ligament of Treitz until the point of obstruction is reached. This procedure can be very tedious. Appropriate countertraction and sharp dissection are essential.

3. When the obstruction is reached, it may be possible to free it by untwisting the intestine or dividing adhesive bands. If gangrenous bowel is present, it should be excised and the ends reanastomosed. The only exception is when abdominal radiation has been used or widespread carcinoma is present. Then a bypass procedure (from jejunum or ileum to ileum or ileum to ascending or transverse colon) is advisable with creation of a mucous fistula from the distal end of the divided bowel if there is likely to be obstruction of the excluded loop. A residual blind pouch without a mucous fistula may lead to continued gastrointestinal symptoms and anemia (Schlegel and Maglinte, 1982). The mucous fistula is brought out at the lower end of the incision or through a right lower quadrant stab incision. The use of automatic stapling devices has greatly simplified such intestinal anastomoses.

4. Broad spectrum antibiotics, such as second-generation cephalosporins, are advisable before and after operations for intestinal obstruction.

Perforation

Perforation of the intestine into the peritoneal cavity occurs rarely in gynecology and obstetrics. It may follow complicated procedures done for inflammatory disease, endometriosis or cancer. The clinical picture consists of the relatively sudden onset of generalized abdominal pain. Fever, tachycardia and possibly hypotension may be present. The abdomen is distended and rigid with diminished or absent peristalsis and generalized rebound tenderness. Leukocytosis is present. Flat and upright x-rays of the abdomen show free air outside loops of bowel. Aspiration of the cul-de-sac or lower abdominal quadrants may show nonspecific cloudy exudate, brownish intestinal fluid or frankly fecal material (with vegetable fibers). The differential diagnoses which must always be considered include ruptured appendix, colonic or Meckel's diverticula, gallbladder or peptic ulcer or pancreatitis. Prompt operation is indicated. The patient is prepared by appropriate fluids and broad spectrum antibiotics. At operation a thorough search is made for the perforation. When found, it is closed. The peritoneal cavity is irrigated thoroughly with saline. If the colon is involved, proximal colostomy is usually indicated even if primary resection and anastomosis is feasible. Resection or bypass of the intestine may be necessary. If contamination is considerable, it is advisable to drain the peritoneal cavity and/or to leave the skin and subcutaneous tissue open for later closure.

Fistula

Intestinal fistula is one of the most serious complications of gynecologic and obstetric operations. Fistulas can be classified as enterocutaneous (intestine to skin), enterovaginal (small intestine to vagina), colovaginal (colon to vagina) and rectovaginal (rectum to vagina) (Fig. 4–4).

ENTEROCUTANEOUS FISTULA

Communication between the small or large intestine and the skin is usually due to unrecognized operative injury to the intestine, often following prior abdominal radiation therapy, or to a leaking intestinal anastomosis. Such fistulas may be accompanied by active or recurrent cancer and may be multiple. An enterocutaneous fistula is usually manifested by the discharge of small or large intestinal contents through (the lower part of) the abdominal incision. Measurement of the amount of loss is important in order to maintain fluid intake. A karaya-sealed bag of the appropriate size is most effective for doing this. The site of the fistula in the intestine is identified by injecting radiopaque material into the fistula (sinogram or

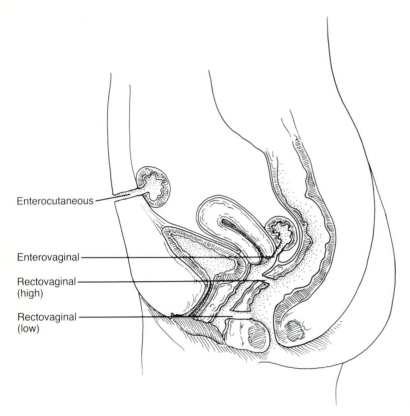

Enterocutaneous

Enterovaginal

Rectovaginal
(high)

Rectovaginal
(low)

Figure 4–4. Intestinal fistulas.

fistulogram) and/or by upper and lower gastrointestinal examinations, which also serve to exclude areas of obstruction in the remainder of the intestine.

The patient who develops an enterocutaneous fistula frequently has major intraabdominal disease. The primary treatment is restoration and maintenance of fluid and electrolyte balance. The intestine is put at rest by interdiction of oral food and fluids; intestinal intubation with a long tube may also be helpful, although not all authors agree with this. Hyperalimentation is usually advisable to restore nutritional status, to encourage closure of the fistula and to improve healing should operation be necessary. If the discharge decreases sharply during this regimen, conservative therapy may be continued for longer than the seven to ten days that are strictly necessary for improving nutritional status up to a maximum of three weeks. Such a regimen is expensive and difficult for both patient and physician. Usually, however, operation is needed for cure, after appropriate intestinal antibiotic prophylaxis; this is especially important if the colon is involved. At the time of operation the fistula and fistulous tract are excised, the involved segment of intestine excised and the intestine reanastomosed. The

fistula may also be bypassed. Few series of enterocutaneous fistulas are reported and many of them include patients with various primary diseases. In gynecologic cancer, Smith and coworkers (1984) described 23 cases with an 86% successful closure rate.

ENTEROVAGINAL FISTULA

The diagnosis of enterovaginal fistula is made from the vaginal discharge of intestinal contents. If this discharge is at all profuse, it is most irritating to the skin of the vulva and perineum. The fistula is identified by contrast x-ray of the small intestine and demonstration of the fistulous tract. In management, the perineum can be temporarily protected by zinc oxide ointment or Maalox. Although conservative treatment can be tried, as described before, operative treatment is necessary in most instances; successful closure was reported in 91% of 14 cases by Smith and co-workers (1984).

COLOVAGINAL FISTULA

Occasionally injury to the sigmoid colon results in a colovaginal fistula. Such fistulas may also be complex, involving the uterus and even the bladder. Radiation injury is the most likely cause, often related to the proximity of the sigmoid colon to the radioactive sources in the vaginal vault or top of the uterine fundus. Unanticipated penetration of the radioactive source through the fundus and adherence to the colon may also be responsible. The vaginal discharge is thicker, less profuse and more malodorous than with enterovaginal fistula. It usually occurs independently of bowel movements. Irritation of the vulvar and perineal skin is less marked than with an enterovaginal fistula. The diagnosis is made by the fact that although fecal discharge is present the fistula cannot be felt on vaginal or rectal examination. The diagnosis may be confirmed by a sinogram or a barium enema x-ray. Treatment is by a preliminary colostomy (transverse) followed later by resection and repair.

RECTOVAGINAL FISTULA

Rectovaginal fistulas occur (1) after hysterectomy (simple, radical or anterior exenteration), usually in the upper third of the vagina; (2) after radiation therapy for carcinoma of the cervix or corpus uteri or in recurrent cancer, usually in the upper or middle third of the vagina and (3) after delivery or obstetric operations, or gynecologic procedures on the perineum or posterior rectal wall, usually in the lower third of the vagina. In the last instance, injury to the rectal sphincter or mucosa may also be present (fourth degree laceration).

The diagnosis is usually obvious because of the fecal discharge from the vagina. Discharge may only occur with loose bowel movements and may be minimal when the stool is formed, especially when the fistula is in the lower third of the vagina. The opening can usually be felt on vaginal or rectovaginal examination or can be seen with a speculum in the vagina. Occasionally no fistula may be visible in spite of the patient's complaints. Injection of methylene blue into the rectum above the sphincter with a tampon in the vagina may demonstrate the presence and sometimes the location of the fistula. A probe may be used (with great caution) to demonstrate the fistula.

The management of a rectovaginal fistula depends upon its cause and location and the amount of surrounding inflammation (Rothenberger and Goldberg, 1983).

Upper Vagina—No Previous Radiation Therapy. If the fistula is large or if there is much surrounding inflammation, a diverting colostomy is indicated. This should usually be a loop transverse colostomy in the left upper quadrant of the abdomen (see Chapter 6). Repair is performed at least two months later when the inflammation has subsided. After preparation of the distal bowel segment by saline enemas and antibiotics, operation may be performed transabdominally by dissection of the rectosigmoid off the vagina and separate closure of the two organs or a partial colpocleisis may be performed vaginally. The latter consists of denuding the mucosa from the anterior and posterior walls of the upper vagina and then apposing them with three layers of interrupted 30 vicryl sutures, the last closing the vaginal mucosa. In this way the fistula is excluded (Fig. 4–5). The disadvantage of abdominal closure is the necessity of another transperitoneal procedure; while the colpocleisis is easier but results in some shortening of the vagina. The loop colostomy is closed six to eight weeks after repair of the fistula. This is most easily done by dissecting the colostomy stoma from the abdominal wall, freshening the edges and closing the bowel with two layers of sutures, one of continuous 20 chromic catgut and one of interrupted 30 silk.

Middle Vagina—No Prior Radiation Therapy. This type of fistula is best closed in layers after bowel preparation (see later section).

Middle or Upper Vagina—Prior Radiation Therapy. These fistulas are extremely difficult to close because of their size, the surrounding inflammation, the poor healing potential of irradiated tissue and the possibility of persistent or recurrent tumor. They usually occur six to 24 months after radiation therapy for carcinoma of the cervix or vagina (possibly complicated by operation) and are preceded by rectal bleeding, diarrhea, tenesmus and rectal ulceration. A diverting colostomy is necessary. Many authors feel that this should be an end (permanent) colostomy in the left lower quadrant with the distal end of the colon closed if there is no rectal obstruction or brought out as a mucous fistula in the midline if distal obstruction is present. After colostomy the fistula will usually become smaller and may, rarely, close spontaneously. Adequate biopsy specimens should be taken to exclude persistent or recurrent cancer, and repair should not be attempted until at least two years after the primary treatment. Layer closure or even colpocleisis is not likely to be successful. Two possible alternative techniques are to use a bulbocavernosus flap or a segment of colon to cover the gap. In the former technique, a pad of fat and bulbocavernosus muscle is swung under the vaginal mucosa to cover the rectal closure and give new blood

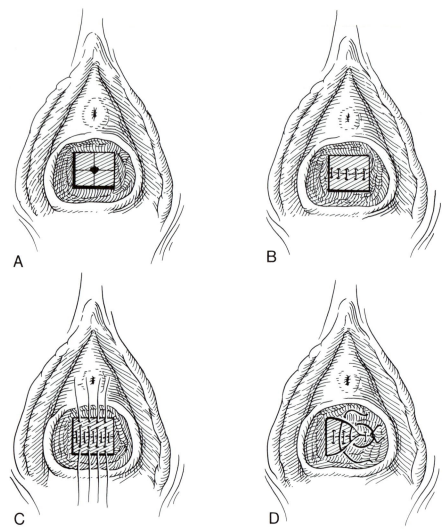

Figure 4–5. *Partial colpocleisis for high rectovaginal fistula. A, Denudation of the vaginal mucosa. B, Exclusion of fistula (first layer). C, Exclusion of fistula (closure of fascia). D, Closure of vaginal mucosa.*

supply to the area (Fig. 4–6). Boronow (1971) and others have reported successes in small series of cases. Bricker and associates (1984) fold the colon over, either in toto or using one half of the intestine, if a stricture is present, so as to interpose healthy bowel between vagina and rectum. These authors report success in 19 of 22 patients treated by one of these two methods.

Lower Vagina—With or Without Prior Radiation Therapy. Fistulas in the lower vagina most commonly follow obstetric trauma; they are seldom the result of radiation therapy, since this area is infrequently so treated. Gynecologic procedures on the posterior vaginal wall also may be responsible. Low fistulas are often as-

sociated with laceration of the external anal sphincter. Methods used for repair include (1) purse-string closure, (2) layer closure and (3) flap techniques. Before repair is undertaken the local inflammatory reaction should have subsided (three or more months). Delay also permits spontaneous healing, which may occur rarely. The only exception to this delay may be if the fistula is recognized at delivery or within 48 hours after delivery, when primary closure can be attempted. Bowel preparation and antibiotic coverage are advisable for repair of any rectovaginal fistula.

Purse-string sutures can be used for very small fistulas. The vaginal mucosa is dissected back around the fistula, and the fistula is in-

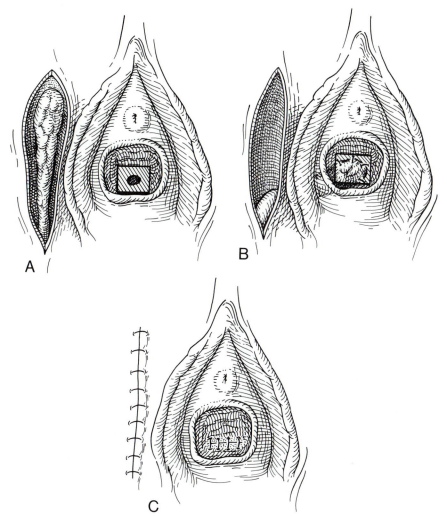

Figure 4–6. *Closure of a rectovaginal fistula, using the bulbocavernosus fat pad. A, Dissection around fistula and preparation of the right bulbocavernosus fat pad. B, Fistula closed and covered with fat pad. C, Labial incision and vagina closed.*

verted with two concentric purse-string sutures of 30 vicryl. The vaginal mucosa is then closed vertically with a continuous suture of the same material.

Layer closure is applicable to larger fistulas in the middle or lower vagina, except those close to the anal sphincter. The vaginal mucosa must be widely dissected laterally to permit closure of the bowel wall without tension by a continuous 30 vicryl suture inverting the lumen and by approximation of the outer rectal wall and fascia, such as is available, with a second layer of interrupted 30 vicryl sutures. Then the vaginal mucosa is closed vertically with a continuous 30 vicryl suture.

If the fistula is close to the anus and particularly if the external sphincter has been torn,

the fistula may be converted into a fourth degree laceration and sewn up in layers just as is done at the time of delivery. If a layer closure is not used, several other methods of repair have been described. Of these the Noble flap technique offers some advantages if the tissues can be adequately mobilized. In this procedure the vaginal wall is freed from the rectal wall and the fistula excised. The rectal wall is then pulled down to the anal opening and sutured to the skin. The external sphincter and perineal muscles are sutured in front of the new anterior rectal wall; the vaginal mucosa is freed, brought down and sewn to the skin at the new introitus (Inmon and Fish, 1977).

The number of different techniques for repair of low rectovaginal fistulas indicates that no single one is always successful. The primary problems are choosing the right procedure and the difficulty of dissecting the fibrotic tissues widely so that the layers can be closed without tension. Cure rates of about 80% may be expected (Rothenberger and Goldberg, 1983). Reoperation is much more difficult because of increased fibrosis and decreased tissue mobility.

URINARY TRACT

Anuria and Oliguria

After many major operations or in obstetric emergencies such as abruptio placentae or severe preeclampsia or eclampsia an indwelling urethral catheter is essential to determine urine output. Urine output can be obtained hourly by means of a graduated measuring device that can be emptied without disconnecting the catheter, thus minimizing contamination. When the patient's condition is stable, the catheter has been removed and she is ambulatory, it is sufficient to record total urinary output over an eight-hour nursing shift. If for any reason the patient's condition later becomes unstable, hourly measurement of output by means of a catheter is again advisable.

ANURIA

Complete absence of urine usually indicates urinary tract obstruction. Most commonly the catheter is blocked or a suture constricts the urethra, as after a vaginal repair. The patient's bladder becomes full and she has pain. The catheter should be checked and/or reinserted. Very rarely both ureters may have been occluded at operation; occlusion of one ureter causes no obvious decrease in urinary output unless the function of the remaining kidney is already badly compromised. If bilateral ureteral obstruction is suspected, ultrasonography or intravenous pyelogram may demonstrate it. Inability to pass ureteral catheters confirms the diagnosis. Bilateral nephrostomies (catheter) are indicated with later operative release of the constriction (see later section).

OLIGURIA

Postoperative urinary output should usually be more than 50 ml/hr. An output of 30 to 50 ml/hr is cause for concern, while one of less

than 30 ml/hr for two consecutive hours can be defined as oliguria. The causes of oliguria are prerenal and intrarenal. In prerenal oliguria perfusion of the kidneys is reduced because of hemorrhage or hypotension or sequestration of fluid into the extracellular space ("third space"). Intrarenal oliguria is caused by intrinsic kidney disease. The general term, acute renal failure (ARF), is widely used for this but the pathophysiologic changes are not yet completely clarified. A possible sequence of events is as follows. Ischemia or toxins produce injury to the proximal tubules. Then increased local production of renin and angiotensin results in renal afferent arteriolar vasoconstriction. Also of possible importance is tubular obstruction and backward diffusion of solutes across the necrotic tubular epithelium. The result of these changes is a decreased glomerular filtration rate and a reduced amount of filtrate. The term acute tubular necrosis (ATN) is often applied to acute renal failure, but it only describes one process, proximal tubular injury and its sequelae.

Management. When oliguria is evident, urinalysis should be performed. In the absence of obvious hematuria the gross appearance of the urine may be useful. Dark urine may be concentrated and/or contain casts. Light-colored urine is likely to be dilute. A specific gravity of 1.010 or over suggests a prerenal cause for the oliguria, whereas a specific gravity below 1.010 indicates intrarenal disease. The latter is confirmed by the presence of protein and casts in the urine. The presence of many white blood cells and bacteria indicates urinary tract infection; culture and determination of bacterial sensitivities to antibiotics should be obtained.

Although early postoperative oliguria is common, prompt treatment is necessary because intrarenal disease may follow even when it was not present initially, and this is a much more difficult problem. The first consideration is to establish and maintain adequate intravascular fluid volume. To do this properly may require monitoring by central venous pressure measurements, continuous blood pressure recording and/or measurement of pulmonary wedge pressure (PWP) by means of a Swan-Ganz catheter. Initially a fluid challenge of 200 ml 5% dextrose in water is helpful. An immediate rise in urine flow indicates intravascular volume deficiency. This may have to be remedied by blood transfusion if blood loss has been excessive or is continuing or simply by administering more crystalloids. The use of albumin may be of some value if colloid osmotic pressure is below 24 cm

H₂O. Fluid challenges may have to be repeated once or twice. If body fluids and injected solutions are being sequestered in the third space, i.e., in intestines, peritoneal cavity or subcutaneous tissues, oliguria may persist in spite of adequate replacement of intravascular volume. Excessive intravenous fluids may then cause cardiac failure. Thus, fluids should be carefully controlled and electrolyte balance maintained until the patient mobilizes her own fluids.

If intrarenal disease is suspected on the basis of low urinary specific gravity and the presence of casts and protein in the urine, further tests are indicated. These should include determinations of levels of plasma sodium, potassium, chloride and CO_2, blood urea nitrogen, creatinine and osmolality and urinary sodium, urea and osmolality. Table 4–10 shows the findings in intrarenal oliguria as compared with prerenal oliguria. While these laboratory data are being obtained, a therapeutic trial is advisable with mannitol (25 gm intravenous bolus), an osmotic diuretic, and furosemide (20 to 40 mg intravenously), which acts primarily on the ascending limb of the loop of Henle to inhibit chloride transport. If no increase in urinary output occurs, acute renal failure is likely, provided that plasma volume is adequate.

Acute renal failure has a significant mortality rate. However, unless it is already severely damaged, the kidney will recover in a varying length of time from days to weeks. The problem then is to maintain fluid and electrolyte balance and avoid infection or other complications until this happens. The principles of treatment are as follows:

1. Continued monitoring. A central venous catheter is essential. Plasma and urine studies mentioned previously should be repeated daily, together with serum calcium and magnesium determinations, complete blood counts and electrocardiograms. Transfer to or retention in an intensive care unit is advisable.

2. Fluid restriction to that required to match insensible loss (i.e., about 500 ml/day) plus urinary output and any other losses of body fluids.

3. Management of hyperkalemia. Unless treated this may lead to sudden cardiac arrest. A level above 6.5 mEq/l with no or equivocal electrocardiographic changes is an indication for sodium ion exchange resin (sodium polystyrene sulfate, Kayexalate) given as a retention enema (40 gm in 200 ml 25% sorbital-every six hours). A quicker (and temporary) effect is obtained by rapid intravenous administration of 44 mEq sodium bicarbonate, 50 gm hypertonic (10%) glucose and 10 units of regular insulin. A serum potassium level above 7.5 mEq/l or electrocardiographic changes, consisting of peaking of the T-waves, prolonged QT interval or widening of the QRS complexes, should be treated urgently with 5 to 10 ml of 10% calcium chloride given intravenously in two to five minutes.

4. Hyperalimentation. An effective solution contains essential amino acids plus glucose in the amount of 800 calories/gm of nitrogen (Nephramine). This is particularly important when dialysis is used.

5. Dialysis. Many authorities advise that dialysis be started early, especially to combat electrolyte imbalance, hyperkalemia and uremia. Either hemodialysis or peritoneal dialysis may be used; the latter is inappropriate after a recent abdominal operation. Consultation with a nephrologist is advisable.

6. Modification of drug dosage. Drugs that are excreted by the kidneys must be given in reduced doses or over longer intervals (see Chapter 12).

Rarely, renal failure may be associated with a high output of dilute urine but gradually rising blood urea nitrogen and creatinine. The same principles of management apply except that more fluid replacement will be needed.

When the kidneys recover from acute renal failure, a diuretic phase occurs in which large quantities of dilute urine are excreted. Monitoring must be continued and fluid balance carefully followed. Of particular importance are sudden decreases in electrolyte levels.

Hematuria

Hematuria (microscopic or visible red discoloration of urine) is common after radical hysterectomy, if the bladder has been traumatized by vigorous retraction or if the bladder has been entered or repaired. Hematuria usually decreases quickly in the first few hours after operation and disappears within 24 hours. Per-

Table 4–10. Prerenal vs Intrarenal Failure

Findings	Prerenal	Intrarenal
Urine Na	<20 mEq/L	>40 mEq/L
Urine urea/Plasma urea	<30:1	<10:1
Urine osmolality	>Serum	Isosmolar with serum
Urinalysis	–	Casts and epithelial cells

sistence suggests infection or unrecognized injury, such as inclusion of the bladder wall in a stitch. Conservative management is appropriate with antibiotics as indicated. Further urologic evaluation by intravenous pyelogram and cystoscopy can be delayed until after the first few postoperative days.

Severe bleeding from the bladder does not usually follow gynecologic or obstetric procedures. However, since it may occur after chemotherapy (especially with cyclophosphamide) or radiation therapy, it may complicate procedures performed in patients with cancer of the ovary or cervix. It may also be due to an unsuspected bladder or kidney tumor, to local invasion by tumor from neighboring organs or to hematologic disorders.

Severe or profuse urinary tract bleeding results in the passage of clots and, if the clots are large enough to fill the bladder, urethral and even ureteral obstruction. Pain and urgency are marked. Treatment is as follows:

1. Complete blood count and determination of coagulation factors, BUN and creatinine. Transfusions if indicated.

2. Insertion of a No. 22 (or larger) Foley catheter and irrigation with normal saline to remove as many clots as possible. A three-way catheter and continuous irrigation with saline may also be used.

3. If these methods fail, usually because clots are organized or adherent, cystoscopy under regional or general anesthesia is needed to break up the clots by irrigation or mechanical means. All clots must be removed. Bleeding points may be coagulated with a ball-tipped electrode.

4. The use of intravesical 1% formalin under general anesthesia. Postoperatively this is very painful. Vesicoureteral reflux is a danger (see Chapter 14).

5. Intravesical pressure balloon, which is rarely used.

6. Urinary antibiotics to reduce the risk of infection attendant upon repeated instrumentation.

7. A variety of secondary procedures such as arterial embolization or urinary diversion (Mitcheson and Sant, 1984).

Urinary Extravasation

Urine may leak into the vagina through a ureteral, vesical or urethral fistula (see later section). It may also leak into the subcutaneous tissues, retroperitoneal space or peritoneal cav-

ity as the first sign of a fistula. Extravasation may also result from drainage at the site of a ureteral anastomosis or bladder repair or around a suprapubic catheter.

Extravasated urine is extremely irritating. Pain is severe. Fever and tachycardia are also present. Intraperitoneal urine rapidly leads to peritonitis with diffuse tenderness, rigidity, rebound tenderness and diminished peristalsis. Given the history of the operative procedure, the site of extravasation can usually be deduced. If urine from the bladder is leaking into the peritoneal cavity no urine can be obtained from the urethral or suprapubic catheter. Paracentesis may produce urine-like fluid. If only one ureter is leaking into the peritoneal cavity, urine coming from the other ureter will be flowing into the bladder and draining from the catheter. In this case, contrast studies such as an intravenous pyelogram or cystogram are helpful. Urine in the peritoneal cavity is an indication for prompt laparotomy. The site of the leakage must be identified and the bladder or ureter closed. The ureter should be splinted. Intra- and extraperitoneal drains are necessary.

If the ureter is thought to be leaking extraperitoneally, an attempt should be made to pass a catheter up through a cystoscope or down through a percutaneous nephrostomy. If this cannot be done, a formal nephrostomy should be performed and extraperitoneal drains placed down to the site of leakage. Later repair will then be necessary.

Leakage from the bladder around a suprapubic tube is best handled by removing the tube and inserting a urethral catheter. Leakage from the bladder after repair of a laceration usually appears vaginally and is discussed later. In the rare event that such leakage after repair occurs suprapubically, it may be necessary to explore the space of Retzius, close the hole in the bladder, place drains on each side and insert a Foley catheter.

The success of these emergency measures in dealing with extravasation is difficult to ascertain since they are rare events, and the results depend on the general condition of the patient and associated infections. In general, however, both intraperitoneal and extraperitoneal extravasation require prompt urinary drainage and later surgical repair; if this is done, the results are usually satisfactory.

Urinary Retention

Retention of urine in women of reproductive age occurs in 4.8% of patients after abdominal hysterectomy and in 15% after vaginal hysterectomy (Dicker et al, 1982). It is more frequent in older women and when vaginal repair is added. A special problem arises after radical hysterectomy when the nerve supply to the bladder is necessarily damaged and may take several weeks to recover.

On the third day after simple abdominal hysterectomy the residual volume of urine in the bladder is increased and the voluntary capacity to void and the volume producing the first desire to urinate are decreased. By the seventh day the values are returning to but have not yet reached normal (Wake, 1980). These changes are most likely to be due to direct trauma to the bladder and consequent irritability, factors which vary with the individual operation. Vaginal hysterectomy results in similar changes, but suspension of the urethrovesical angle and repair of a cystocele may add an element of obstruction, depending on the tightness of the sutures.

Management is similar for all types of urinary retention, whatever their cause. Overdistension of the bladder should be avoided because it causes considerable pain, predisposes to infection and may be detrimental to a vaginal repair. Therefore, specific postoperative or postpartum orders should include single catheterization after a specific time (i.e., four to six hours), depending upon the patient's discomfort. If the patient is then again unable to void or if the catheter inserted at operation has been removed and the patient has required catheterization once, a second catheterization should be performed with a Foley catheter. If the residual urine is over 100 ml, the Foley catheter should be left in place for 24 to 48 hours. Repeated single catheterization increases the chance of infection significantly. Usually patients will be able to urinate after an indwelling catheter has thus rested the bladder. For those who cannot, a cholinergic agent such as bethanecol (Urecholine), 10 mg by mouth every one to two hours, is effective. A maintenance dose of 10 to 20 mg four times daily may be given. Once it has been demonstrated to the patient that she is able to urinate, the bethanecol is usually no longer necessary. An occasional patient will require repeated reinsertion of a Foley catheter. In these cases a cystometrogram may be necessary to rule out an unrecognized neurogenic bladder. If the cystometrogram is normal and the urethra easily permits passage of a 16 to 18 French catheter, i.e., there is no obstruction, the patient may have to be sent home with a Foley catheter in place. After an interval of one

to four weeks (the latter after radical hysterectomy), she is instructed to cut the catheter and remove it at home it. She then drinks several glasses of liquid and comes to the office within three hours. There she voids and her residual urine is determined, using a Foley catheter. Only if the residual urine is more than 100 ml is the Foley catheter left in place again. All patients who require catheterization more than once or who have a Foley catheter in place for more than 36 hours should receive urinary antibiotics. In very rare cases the obstruction of the urethra is so pronounced, as determined by the difficulty of catheterization, that reoperation must be performed to cut and replace the constricting sutures. Emotional factors are important in urination. Sometimes the patient who has been unable to void in the hospital surroundings can do so easily at home and may be discharged with what appears to be a rather large residual urine volume.

Urinary Tract Infection (UTI)

CAUSE

Urinary tract infection is the second most common postoperative complication in gynecology. This is due to the frequent presence of asymptomatic bacteriuria preoperatively (7% in women over 50, 4% in young women and 1% in schoolgirls) (Asmussen and Miller, 1983), frank preoperative infection, the manipulation of the bladder occurring during gynecologic procedures and the use of catheters before, during and after the operation. Preoperative evaluation or treatment should decrease the first cause. Intraoperative retraction of the bladder is inevitable, but should be minimized. Infection caused by catheterization remains the most serious problem. If the bladder is empty during pelvic operations, the chance of injury may be decreased and exposure improved. Thus, for major operations it has long been the custom to insert a urethral catheter before operation and leave it in place for at least 24 hours after operation and longer in cases of anterior colporrhaphy or radical hysterectomy. Repeated catheterization and additional insertions of indwelling catheters may be necessary in some of these patients. Urinary infection increases at a rate of 3% per day of catheterization (Thompson et al, 1984) and with the number of times a catheter is inserted. E. coli, derived from the neighboring lower gastrointestinal tract; is primarily responsible; other organisms frequently involved include *Pseudomonas*, *Proteus*, *Klebsiella*, *Enterobacter* and *Enterococci*. *Serratia marcescens* and *Candida* may also be found. Patients who have diabetes or are in a poor nutritional state are especially likely to develop urinary tract infections.

DIAGNOSIS

In many instances the presence of bacteria in the urine and the bladder causes no immediate postoperative symptoms. Spread to the upper urinary tract with development of pyelonephritis may cause flank pain and fever, often in the first 48 hours after operation, but also later, at any time that the urinary tract is invaded by a catheter. This fever has to be distinguished from that due to atalectasis or infection in other areas, e.g., the peritoneal cavity or retroperitoneal space. Urinary tract infection is demonstrated by examination and culture of the urine. In the patient without a catheter in place, a mid-stream urine specimen, after cleaning of the introitus with sterile normal saline, is satisfactory. In the early postoperative period urine can be obtained from the bladder or suprapubic catheter by aspirating from the tubing connecting the catheter to the drainage set (ideal) or after disconnecting the catheter and cleaning the outside with alcohol. The finding of pus cells and bacteria in an uncentrifuged drop of urine is prima facie evidence of infection, and treatment can be started empirically, although culture and bacterial sensitivities should always be obtained. A count of 100,000 (10^5) organisms/ml is generally regarded as evidence of active infection. However, 10^4 or possibly 10^3 organisms/ml may actually be significant.

TREATMENT

Acute postoperative urinary tract infection, most likely due to *E. coli*, can be treated satisfactorily with ampicillin or a first generation cephalosporin, usually given intravenously at first. Severe infections with bacteremia require combinations of antibiotics (see page 71). Since many hospital-acquired infections are caused by resistant bacteria, changes in antibiotics may have to be made when sensitivity reports are available. Therapy should be continued for seven days, changing to oral medication when possible. If the urinary tract infection occurs later in the postoperative course and is mild (i.e., minimal or no fever or flank pain), urinary acidification with ascorbic acid (500 mg four times daily) or cranberry juice (large amounts at frequent intervals) with suitable antimicrobial agents is appropriate (Table 4–11). These agents are continued for five to seven days or longer in the case of recurrent postoperative infection. Any anti-infective agent should be accompanied by adequate hydration, orally or intravenously.

PREVENTION

Many attempts have been made to reduce the danger of catheter-mediated urinary tract infection. The most important are suprapubic drainage, limitation of the number and length of catheterizations and sterile, closed-catheter drainage with avoidance of breaks in techniques. Other techniques are relatively ineffective. These include decreasing reflux from the drainage bag by inclusion of a valve, covering the catheter with antibacterial agents, occluding the external urinary meatus with a pad containing chlorhexidine or periodically instilling a disinfectant such as hydrogen peroxide. An interesting approach and one that has not received much attention is to empty the bladder by aspiration after the abdomen has been opened for laparotomy, rather than using an indwelling catheter (Sood, 1972). In many instances it might then be possible to avoid subsequent catheterization, although if the bladder is full or partly full at the beginning of the operation, there is danger of it being opened as the peritoneum is entered.

Recurrent infection may follow a postoperative UTI. On the first occasion a urine culture should be obtained. If the organism is the usual *E. coli*, and the symptoms mild (i.e., frequency, dysuria or suprapubic pain without fever), intermittent self-therapy with a single dose of trimethoprim/sulfamethoxazole (320 mg/1200 mg) appears to be as effective as long-term low-dose prophylaxis with small doses of the same drug (Wong et al, 1985). Persistence of symptoms or a more severe clinical picture requires further investigation and the use of different, appropriate antibiotics.

Table 4–11. Initial Treatment of Mild Postoperative Urinary Tract Infection

Drug	Dose
Trimethoprim/ Sulfamethoxazole	1 tablet bid (single or double strength)
Sulfisoxazole	1 Gm q6 hrs
Nitrofurantoin	100 mg q6 hrs
Nalidixic acid	1 Gm q6 hrs

Ureteral Complications

See Anuria

Bilateral Obstruction

Intraoperative ligation of both ureters is an unusual event. Early postoperative anuria is present, and bilateral nephrostomies are indicated (see later section for operative procedures). Later, bilateral ureteral obstruction may develop as a result of retroperitoneal fibrosis. Of 430 cases collected by Wagenknecht and Hardy (1981) 55 (8.7%) appeared to have been related to prior operations and 11 (1.7%) to urinary extravasation or retroperitoneal hematoma. The cause of the fibrosis is obscure and the symptoms are non-specific, consisting of back or abdominal pain, weight loss, nausea and vomiting, urinary tract infection and many others. The diagnosis is typically made by intravenous pyelogram, which shows ureteral obstruction and medial displacement of the ureters. Obstruction of the vena cava may also be demonstrated by venogram, and abnormalities of the abdominal aorta or its branches may be noted. Treatment is by freeing the ureters and transplanting them intraperitoneally. Recurrent stenosis occurred in 22% of the cases reported by Wagenknecht and Hardy, but this could be reduced by long-term corticosteroid therapy.

Unilateral Obstruction

During pelvic operations, particularly radical hysterectomy and procedures involving extensive pelvic dissection, the ureter may be ligated, part of its wall may be caught in a suture or it may be kinked by neighoring sutures or during reperitonealization of the pelvis. Ideally these problems should be avoided or recognized during operation. How often they occur without such recognition is difficult to determine. Over 25 years ago Solomons and associates (1960), in a classic study, performed intravenous pyelograms before and after abdominal hysterectomy in 204 patients and noted two instances of ureteral ligation (1%). One would like to think that improvement in surgical techniques has decreased this number, but it still seems reasonable to assume that unrecognized ureteral obstruction of some sort occurs in about 1% of hysterectomies or major pelvic procedures.

Complete unilateral ureteral obstruction may be silent and give no symptoms, or the patient may complain of slight pain and have some fever in the first few postoperative days. Tenderness may be noted in the costovertebral angle on sharply thumping the area with the side of the fist. Urinalysis may be negative, and if one kidney is functioning normally, there will be no change in the blood urea nitrogen or creatinine levels. The diagnosis is confirmed radiologically. An intravenous pyelogram will show that both kidneys are present and identify the degree and point of obstruction. Preparation of the bowel is not necessary, and the number of films should be limited since renal function and the degree of pelvo-ureteral dilatation and not minor calyceal abnormalities are being determined. Ultrasonography is almost as useful. Other non-invasive techniques such as MRI or CT scans are potentially helpful.

Management requires urologic expertise or consultation. If the obstruction is minor, no treatment is indicated but the intravenous pyelogram should be repeated in one week. If the obstruction is major or complete, an attempt should be made cystoscopically to pass a ureteral catheter up to the renal pelvis. If partial obstruction is found, the ureter should be splinted with a pigtail catheter. This is left in place for seven to ten days (or longer if constriction by a polyglycolic acid-type suture is suspected). It is removed cystoscopically. Complete obstruction indicates urinary diversion and subsequent repair (see later section).

Ureterovaginal Fistula

Unrecognized incisions into or division of a ureter lead to early postoperative intraperitoneal or extraperitoneal extravasation of urine (see previous section). When the incision is small or there has been necrosis of the wall of the ureter, leakage occurs later. The latter is more common when the ureter has been denuded and its blood supply compromised as in a radical hysterectomy (Fig. 4–7); in this case leakage usually occurs at 5 to 14 days but occasionally as late as 60 days after operation. The diagnosis is made by the discovery of thin fluid with a smell like that of urine coming from the vagina. It is important to distinguish a ureterovaginal from a vesicovaginal fistula. This is best done by inserting two or three cotton balls into the vagina and injecting methylene blue into the bladder through an indwelling catheter. After an interval of five to ten minutes, during which the patient should stand up, the upper cotton ball will be stained blue if a vesicovaginal fistula is present, but not if there is a ureterovaginal fistula, unless it is very close to the bladder and there is vesicoureteral reflux, a rare event. Leakage of the dye around the

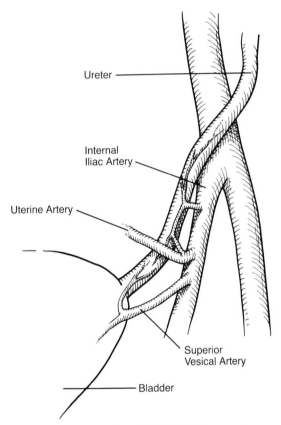

Ureter

Internal
Iliac Artery

Uterine Artery

Superior
Vesical Artery

Bladder

Figure 4–7. Blood supply to the left lower ureter.

urethral catheter will stain the lowest cotton ball, but the not the highest. Confirmation of the presence of the fistula is obtained by intravenous pyelogram; oblique views are usually necessary.

Initial management of ureterovaginal fistula is conservative, because inflammation and infection make immediate repair unlikely to be successful. First, an attempt should be made cystoscopically to pass a ureteral catheter through the area of the fistula into the renal pelvis. This is difficult because the recent operation will often have distorted or obscured the ureteral orifices, and there is a real danger of false passage of the catheter outside the ureter. If a ureteral catheter (preferably of the pigtail variety) can be so inserted, it should be left in place for 21 days, and there is a 50% chance of curing the fistula. If a ureteral catheter cannot be inserted, spontaneous healing may occur during the wait for the optimum time for repair, usually 60 to 90 days. However, since this may be associated with obstruction and loss of renal function on that side, follow-up intravenous pyelograms or ultrasonography

should be obtained at three- to four-week intervals.

The presence of a fistula is extremely uncomfortable and distressing to the patient. Urine is irritating to the perineum and vulva. Frequent washing with clean water and the use of large disposable pads (Depends) minimize such irritation. Urinary antibiotics should be given as long as the possiblity of bacterial contamination is present.

Urinary Diversion and Repair

Temporary Diversion. Drainage of the kidney is indicated if there is (1) acute and complete obstruction, (2) partial or severe obstruction and a catheter cannot be passed cystoscopically or (3) a ureterovaginal fistula with obstruction above it and deteriorating renal function, prior to the time when repair can safely be attempted.

The simplest method of temporary diversion is by percutaneous nephrostomy. This is best done under local anesthesia with fluoroscopic or ultrasound guidance. Complications include hemorrhage (4 to 42%), perinephric abscess (rare) or dislodgement of the catheter (4.3 to 29%) (Perinetti, 1982). The last can be avoided, if drainage must be maintained for a long time, by using catheters of gradually increasing size until a No. 18 Foley catheter can be inserted; this can usually be replaced easily. Open nephrostomy (through the substance of the kidney), either by catheter drainage from the renal pelvis or by a circle tube, has generally been discontinued in favor of the percutaneous route, although it may occasionally be necessary.

Reestablishment of Ureteral Continuity. The principles of operation are similar to those for repairing a clamped or divided ureter intraoperatively. Repair should usually be delayed for at least 60 days to permit the local inflammatory reaction to subside, temporary percutaneous nephrostomy being used if necessary. Knowledge of the site of the fistula from prior x-ray studies is helpful in deciding on the best procedure. If the fistula appears to be within 5 to 8 cm of the bladder, reimplantation into the bladder is best. Although the extraperitoneal approach can be used with success, a transperitoneal incision permits adequate exploration and exposure, which are important if the bladder and ureter must be widely mobilized. Wide mobilization is necessary when there is excessive fibrosis or the fistula is higher than anticipated. In these instances, the bladder may be fixed, after mobilization, to the psoas muscle. Kihl and co-workers (1982) reported success with ureteroneocystostomy in eight of nine ureterovaginal fistulas, six following malignant and three following benign disease, although kidney function was lost in one case. In the ninth case splinting with a ureteral catheter was successful. When the ureter cannot be brought down to the bladder, a tube of bladder can be used to shorten the distance between them. This can be done by the Boari or Demel technique (Symmonds, 1976). The kidney may also be mobilized downwards. It may be necessary to use a segment of ileum to replace a longer segment of damaged ureter (Fig. 4–8). Automatic stapling devices have greatly decreased the operating time for such procedures. For ureteral damage at the level of the pelvic brim or higher, secondary end-to-end anastomosis can be used in some instances, but, because of the lack of blood supply, failure to heal and breakdown are more likely to occur.

Permanent Urinary Tract Diversion. Although in most cases ureteral continuity can be restored after obstruction or fistula, a problem occurs when the lower part of one ureter has been lost and mobilization of the bladder is much decreased, for example, by radiation therapy. In this case the proximal end of the damaged ureter may be anastomosed to the other ureter (transureteroureterostomy). If both lower ureters are irretrievably damaged and/or the bladder is involved in extensive fibrosis resulting from radiation or infection, diversion of the ureters into a segment of ileum or colon or cutaneous nephrostomy is necessary.

Bilateral ureteroileostomy has been widely used since it was described by Bricker (1950). The technique and complications of the operation are discussed in detail in Chapter 7. Reported series of cases usually include operations performed for a variety of reasons, not only those addressed in this chapter. Early and late complications in 178 cases reported by Schmidt and associates (1973) were 34% and 68% respectively. The sigmoid and transverse colon have also been used as conduits, but long-term follow-up data are not available. More recently the creation of a continent reservoir, originally described by Kock (1971), although technically complex and lengthy to perform, has been found to be successful in 49 of 50 patients described by Skinner and co-workers (1984). Also, a variety of techniques using ileocecal conduits have been designed to prevent ureteral reflux and provide continence (Sagalowsky, 1986). Cutaneous ureterostomy is seldom indicated because it is not easy to bring

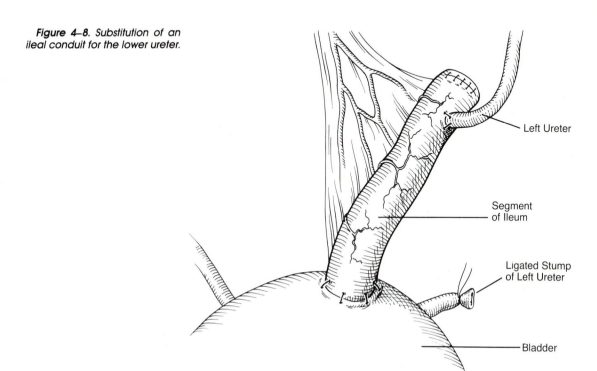

Figure 4–8. Substitution of an ileal conduit for the lower ureter.

Left Ureter

Segment of Ileum

Ligated Stump of Left Ureter

Bladder

the ureter to the skin if it is already shortened and because retraction, necrosis and stenosis of the stoma occur frequently.

Vesicovaginal Fistula

Vesicovaginal fistula has a special place in the history of gynecology because of the dramatic and eventually successful attempts at repair of such fistulas by J. Marion Sims in 1849. It still occurs in many parts of the world as a major physical and social problem following obstructed labor. Obstetric fistulas may involve the bladder alone, the bladder neck or both and may be associated with considerable loss of the urethra and extensive fibrosis. In developed countries obstetric causes are very rare, and most fistulas follow abdominal or vaginal hysterectomy, carcinoma of the cervix and vagina or treatment of those conditions with radiation therapy. Post-surgical fistulas are often very small and usually located at the top of the vagina. Fistulas following cancer of the cervix and radiation treatment may be of any size. Their walls are indurated by cancer or fibrosis and they may be associated with extensive loss of tissue in the pelvis and with rectovaginal fistulas. Primary consideration will be given to post-surgical fistulas.

Diagnosis

If injury to the bladder has not been recognized at operation, copious discharge of thin fluid, which smells like urine, is usually noted within 24 to 72 hours after operation. If the fistula is due to necrosis of the bladder wall or its inclusion in sutures, vaginal leakage may begin as long as several weeks after operation. If the diagnosis is in doubt, use of methylene blue in the bladder, as described previously, will usually be conclusive. A second method that is of use in small fistulas is to place the patient in the prone position, fill the vagina with saline and fill the bladder with CO_2. If bubbles rise to the top of the saline, there is a communication between the bladder and the vagina. Cystoscopy and urethroscopy are helpful in identifying the site of a fistula and its proximity to the ureters. An intravenous pyelogram is also important in excluding a concomitant ureterovaginal fistula or ureteral obstruction.

Immediate Management

An indwelling Foley catheter should be inserted; one with a large (30 ml) balloon should be used if a smaller one is ineffective. The catheter serves two purposes, to keep the patient dry and to permit healing, which occurred in 15 to 80% of cases collected by Hebert (1983). At the same time urinary antibiotics should be given to prevent ascending infection. If catheter drainage does not succeed, the problem of handling the leakage while awaiting the best time for repair is difficult. A vaginal occlusive device such as a contraceptive diaphragm or a menstrual cup (Tassette) with a catheter attached has been described, but it is of limited value, and reliance has to be placed on absorbent pads. Maintaining the transurethral catheter for a long period or placing a catheter through the fistula may keep the patient drier, although usually not completely so, but may cause persistent inflammation, thus further delaying repair.

Repair

The optimal time for repair has long been debated. Previously it was thought best to wait for at least six months to permit inflammation to subside. Collins and co-workers (1971) reported success in 72% of 29 patients who did not have cancer with the use of cortisone, 100 mg three times daily by mouth, in conjunction with an indwelling urethral catheter for 10 to 12 days after discovery of the fistula. If the fistula had not closed spontaneously, repair was performed immediately. Of the eight failures, five were cured at the second attempt and three at the third, using the same regimen. This work has not been followed up adequately, possibly because of the fear that cortisone will impede healing. Early repair has also been reported to be successful without the use of cortisone (Goodwin and Scardino, 1980). The condition of the fistula itself is probably the best guide to the time for repair. When it is clean, pliable, uninflammed and free of edema and granulation tissue, repair can be attempted with reasonable expectation of success. In postmenopausal women the use of oral estrogens (Premarin 1.25 mg daily), for two to four weeks, decreases the friability of the vaginal mucosa and increases vascularity so that healing is improved.

Techniques of Repair. Vesicovaginal fistulas can be repaired vaginally or abdominally. The vaginal route is traditional. It is often simpler for the gynecologist experienced in vaginal surgery and for the patient who has minimal postoperative discomfort. The abdominal (transvesical) route is indicated if the fistula is very close to one or both ureters or in some instances if previous repairs have failed.

VAGINAL REPAIR. The lithotomy position is preferable, although the prone knee-chest position has had its advocates. Partial colpocleisis or layer closure may be used (see previous section). The former is most useful when the fistula is small and located at the top of the vagina. In the classic layer closure the vaginal mucosa is opened in an anteroposterior direction. The vagina is dissected off the bladder laterally, then the edges of the fistula are excised and the bladder is inverted with a continuous suture of absorbable material, preferably 30 vicryl. The tissue between the bladder and the vagina and then the vagina itself are closed in a similar fashion.

Each vesicovaginal fistula is different and there are a number of maneuvers that can be used during the layer method of closure if they are needed in the individual case.

1. Ureteral catheters may be inserted if there is concern about the relationship of the fistula to the ureteral orifices; this is rarely necessary and if it is an abdominal approach should be considered.

2. Hypertrophied labia may be sewn to the skin of the thigh or to the drapes to improve exposure.

3. A small introitus may be enlarged by a deep mediolateral episiotomy (Schuchardt incision).

4. A local vasopressor (neosynephrine 1 mg in 20 ml saline) may be injected around the fistula to improve hemostasis.

5. The initial closure of the bladder may be tested by the injection of sterile milk into the bladder. Milk is better than methylene blue which makes subsequent exposure and suturing difficult.

6. Either continuous or interrupted sutures may be used. Continuous sutures are more watertight and therefore, in the author's view, preferable, although if tied too tightly they may strangle tissue. It should be noted that nonabsorbable sutures should be avoided in the deeper layers because they form a nidus for infection and stone formation.

7. The direction of the suture line may be varied. Vertical sutures are easier to orient, but the type of fistula may dictate a different direction. Some authors prefer to change the direction, i.e., place the first layer vertically and the second and third layers horizontally to prevent overlapping of suture lines. This is probably not necessary.

8. Bladder drainage is best obtained through a suprapubic catheter.

Special problems occur with large obstetric fistulas which may involve the base of the bladder and the urethra as well as the bladder itself and with postradiation fistulas. For the former Moir (1961) described the use of nonabsorbable nylon sutures to close the last layer. These sutures are removed in 21 days. A parallel relaxing vertical incision may also be made in the vaginal mucosa to relieve tension on the suture line; this is not closed and should heal spontaneously. In these large fistulas, also, the interposition of a bulbocavernosus muscle and fat pad between the bladder and the vaginal suture lines may provide necessary new blood supply (see Fig. 4–6).

Vesicovaginal fistulas following radiation therapy present the same difficulties as post-radiation rectovaginal fistulas. If persistent or recurrent carcinoma has been excluded and at least two years have elapsed since the original diagnosis of cancer, then there is good reason to attempt repair, since urinary diversion is more disabling for the patient than colostomy. However, the difficulties are similar. Again the use of a bulbocavernosus fat pad may be helpful.

ABDOMINAL REPAIR. Transvesical repair is performed through a vertical or preferably transverse lower abdominal incision. The peritoneal cavity is not entered. The bladder is opened widely and a self-retaining retractor inserted to expose the fistula and the ureteral orifices. The principles of repair are similar to those used in the vaginal approach, but they are applied in reverse. The edges of the fistula are excised and the bladder wall and vagina are dissected from each other. The vagina is first closed, then the tissue between the vagina and the bladder and finally the bladder itself. Absorbable sutures are used throughout. The ureters may be catheterized if the fistula is very close to them. Suprapubic drainage is obtained through a Foley or other indwelling catheter, placed as the bladder is closed. A drain is placed in the space of Retzius for three to five days. The results of abdominal repair are good in expert hands. O'Conor (1980) reports success in 37 of 42 selected patients (88%) with cure by reoperation in the remaining five. In large and difficult fistulas, especially those due to obstetric causes, successful use of an omental flap has been described by Orford and Theron (1985).

Urethrovaginal Fistula

A fistula between the urethra and the vagina may be the result of a difficult delivery, breakdown of an anterior vaginal wall repair, rupture or repair of a urethral diverticulum or miscellaneous causes such as trauma, carcinoma or granulomatous lesions. A high urethrovaginal fistula is often associated with damage to the internal urethral sphincter and a vesicovaginal fistula. It is usually accompanied by urinary incontinence. When the fistula is in the middle or lower third of the urethra, the patient may have no symptoms except spraying of the urinary stream.

Repair of a high fistula is similar to that used for a vesicovaginal fistula. When the fistula is in the middle or lower third of the urethra, and there has been little loss of the urethral wall, repair is performed by dissecting the paraurethral tissue from the vaginal wall, closing the

mucosa over a No. 22 catheter, covering the urethra with such paraurethral tissue as can be obtained and finally closing the vagina (Fig. 4–9). Because of the fibrosis, it is often difficult to cover the site of urethral closure. Non-absorbable sutures may be used and left in place for two to three weeks. A bulbocavernosus fat pad and/or relaxing vaginal incisions may be necessary. If a large part of the urethra has been destroyed, the paraurethral tissue is rolled over a catheter, and the tube so created will eventually epithelialize. The indwelling catheter should be left in place seven days for smaller fistulas and 14 days if the urethra has been reconstructed. Because of the importance of the catheter being retained, a silastic tube may be

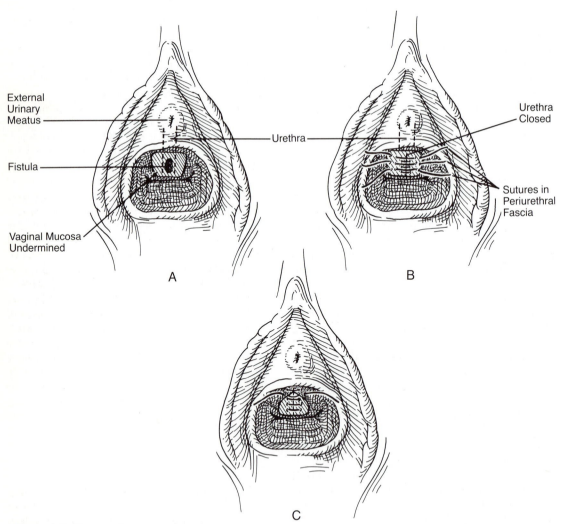

Figure 4–9. Closure of an urethrovaginal fistula. A, Dissection around fistula. B, Closure of urethra and fascia. C, Closure of vaginal mucosa.

used and sutured to the vaginal mucosa at the site of the future external urinary meatus. Urinary antibiotics are used while the catheter remains in place.

INCISIONS

In this section wound complications common to a variety of operations will be considered, primarily those of abdominal procedures. Those following vaginal operations tend to be specific for certain procedures, e.g., breakdown of the anterior vaginal wall, recurrence of a fistula, bleeding from conization of the cervix and so forth. These are covered in Chapter 5 in connection with the individual procedures. Wound complications are more common in obese, diabetic or nutritionally depleted patients. They are affected by the type of suture and the method of closure of the incision as well as by drugs such as chemotherapeutic agents, physical factors such as radiation therapy or previous scars. Even if appropriate prophylactic measures have been taken before and during the operation (see Chapters 2 and 3), some incisional complications do occur.

Hemorrhage and Hematoma

Slight oozing of blood between the skin staples or sutures is common. When oozing is discovered in the immediate postoperative period, local pressure for two to three minutes with or without the application of sterile adhesive strips is usually effective. Sometimes a specific bleeding point can be identified and resutured under local anesthesia. Continuous oozing of large amounts of blood suggests a coagulation disorder. Appropriate studies and management should be performed (see Chapter 2). After normal coagulation is restored it may be necessary and advisable to reopen the incision and resuture the skin; this can be done satisfactorily within 24 hours of operation but not later. When such bleeding occurs, hemorrhage deeper in the incision and within the peritoneal cavity must be suspected.

Bleeding in the layers of the abdominal wall with development of a hematoma is difficult to diagnose in the early stages. It is more common in Pfannenstiel incisions because of the necessary undermining. The pain it produces is confused with the usual postoperative pain. If the hematoma is of considerable size, however, the pain becomes localized and swelling and discoloration of the abdominal wall may be noted, even extending far laterally. Over a period of several hours hematocrit and hemoglobin levels may fall. If a hematoma is not increasing in size and the patient's condition is stable, it can be treated conservatively and watched. If a hematoma is increasing rapidly, the incision must be reopened under general anesthesia and the bleeding point sought. It is most likely to be in the rectus muscle or coming from the inferior epigastric artery (or vein) or one of its branches. The vessel is ligated and the skin closed again. If more than 48 hours have elapsed since the original operation or if there is evidence or suspicion of infection, the incision should be left open and secondary closure performed. If there is a large dead space, it may be drained for two to three days by a soft (Penrose) drain, brought out through a separate incision.

A hematoma of moderate or even large size that has been treated conservatively may eventually be absorbed and disappear or drain through the incision, or it may become infected (see following section). It should not be drained unless the last event occurs.

Infection

Risk factors for abdominal wound infections include the number (three or more) and severity of underlying diseases, the length of the operation (over two hours), and the classification of the wound (clean-contaminated or contaminated) (Haley et al, 1985). Obesity is also important. Pitkin (1976) noted infection in 29% of 300 women weighing over 200 pounds. Data on infections are usually obtained from general surgical patients or are collected from different services, rather than from gynecologic and/or obstetric patients alone. It is estimated that 2 to 4% of clean incisions become infected; this figure is probably lower for gynecologic and obstetric operations, but there are great variations from service to service and from time to time on the same service.

EPIDEMIOLOGY

Surveillance of wound (and other) infections is an important part of the quality control of medical care. The most effective way of doing this is to maintain accurate monthly statistics. Wound complications and especially infections

Table 4–12. Classification of Postoperative Wound Complications

Dehiscence
  First degree: skin, subcutaneous tissue
    with infection
    without infection
  Second degree: skin, subcutaneous tissue, fascia
    with infection
    without infection
  Third degree: skin, subcutaneous tissue, fascia,
    peritoneum (including evisceration)
    with infection
    without infection
Hemorrhage or Hematoma
  With external drainage
    with infection
    without infection
  Without external drainage
    with infection
    without infection
Coagulation defect

must be clearly defined, and the definitions must be understood by all physicians on the staff. A complication sheet with these definitions should be placed on each chart (Table 4–12). Attending staff members and/or residents should be required to complete these as part of their record-keeping obligations. Data should be recorded on a computer, ideally by record room personnel or, if not, by the department's secretarial or administrative staff. Monthly reports should be generated by the tenth of the following month and presented and discussed at the next monthly staff meeting.

Review of wound infection data will not only indicate the risk factors for individual patients or groups of patients, but also may show infection trends for individual physicians or groups of physicians and should stimulate investigation of possible causes. Among those to be considered are preparation of the patient's skin, aseptic precautions by the surgical team, ventilation and air quality in the operating room, cleaning and culture of the operating rooms, operative technique, wound care and the use of prophylactic antibiotics and antimicrobial products (Polk et al, 1983) (see Chapters 2 and 3).

DIAGNOSIS AND MANAGEMENT

Wound infections usually do not become apparent until at least three to five days after operation; the deeper the infection and the more obese the patient, the longer this takes. The incision appears red and there is tenderness and perhaps swelling beneath and lateral to it.

Temperature is not usually significantly elevated in superficial infections although it may be in deep ones.

Initial management is by the application of hot packs. Fluctuation may appear, but even before that the skin edges may separate. When this happens staples or stitches should be removed and the incision opened as far as can be done with minimal discomfort to the patient. Pus should be gently expressed. The depth of the abscess, i.e., down to or through the fascia or peritoneum (see later section on dehiscence), should be ascertained with a cotton-tipped applicator, Kelly clamp or uterine dressing forceps and a culture taken. The opened incision should be irrigated with hydrogen peroxide and packed lightly with gauze soaked in hydrogen peroxide. Irrigation and wet dressings should then be repeated every eight hours. The physician should do this once daily at first, and the nurses on the other two shifts should be carefully instructed and supervised in the technique. Dead tissue should be regularly and widely debrided; analgesics may be required either by mouth or intravenously. Antibiotics are not usually necessary except in very severe infections (see later section). When the incision appears clean and granulating, irrigations with saline and a dry dressing may suffice to promote further healing. Secondary closure is occasionally feasible. Skin stitches may be used under local anesthesia or partial approximation may be obtained with sterile adhesive strips. The time taken for an infected incision to heal varies with its size, but is usually longer than one hopes. Patients do not have to remain in the hospital after granulation tissue has begun to form, provided that family members or others have been instructed in wound care. At home a visiting nurse can supervise this.

Delayed primary closure may be advisable when gross infection of the incision is likely. The peritoneum and fascia are closed in the usual manner, preferably in these cases with Smead-Jones sutures. The subcutaneous tissue is irrigated with saline. Interrupted vertical mattress sutures are placed 1 to 2 cm apart in the skin and subcutaneous tissues and left untied. The subcutaneous tissue is packed with gauze, soaked in saline or povidone-iodine. The sutures may be tied loosely in a bow-knot over the pack. On the third or fourth postoperative day the gauze is removed and the sutures tied, gaps being closed with sterile adhesive strips. Delayed closure was found by Brown and co-workers (1977), in an excellent matched-pairs study of 292 patients, to result in significantly less wound infection. These authors also noted that the cosmetic results in the delayed suture group were at least as good as in the controls, where delayed closure had not been performed.

SEVERE INFECTIONS

Severe necrotizing soft tissue infections occasionally complicate incisions in gynecology and obstetrics. They may be due to *Clostridia* or to a variety of other organisms, particularly aerobic and anaerobic streptococci and staphylococci; usually several different organisms can be cultured. *Clostridia* may only be contaminants of other infections and confined to the superficial tissues or they may produce the classic anaerobic myonecrosis or gas gangrene. Clinical syndromes due to infection with organisms other than *Clostridia* have been given a variety of names such as necrotizing cellulitis, necrotizing fasciitis or Meleney's gangrene (Dellinger, 1981). The most descriptive term for these infections is necrotizing soft tissue infections (NSTI).

NSTI occurs most often in obese patients and in those at risk for infection because of systemic or nutritional factors or the type of operation performed. The onset is usually within three to four days after operation and may appear acute. Pain and swelling of the incision are present. Some thin exudate may be seen. Its odor is usually foul. A sweet odor is associated with clostridial myonecrosis. The patient appears to be in a toxic condition with fever and leukocytosis. Subcutaneous crepitation (gas) may be present. It is not necessarily diagnostic of clostridial infection. Toxic shock syndrome (see previous section) has been reported to occur in severe wound infections (Bartlett et al, 1982).

Primary management consists of antibiotic therapy and prompt and repeated surgical debridement of the incision. Penicillin (penicillin G) is the drug of choice for *Clostridia*, while clindamycin, chloramphenicol or metronidazole are effective against most of the other anaerobic organisms likely to be present (Serota and Finegold, 1982). Initial selection of multiple antibiotics should be on an empirical basis, to be modified by reports of bacterial sensitivities. Hyperbaric oxygen therapy has also been used. However, it is not easily available and oxygen toxicity in the form of seizures and pulmonary alveolar damage represent contraindications to its use.

The overall mortality for gynecologic or ob-stetric patients with NSTI is impossible to determine because of the rarity of the condition. It is probably not as high as the 29% reported by Kendrick and co-workers (1982), since many of these authors' cases followed severe trauma or major intestinal operations. An estimate of 10 to 20% mortality seems reasonable.

Severe infections of the abdominal wall or groin take many weeks to heal. Maintaining a clean granulating surface is important. Many techniques have been used. The application of commercial honey was used with success in 12 cases of groin infection after radical procedures on the vulva by Cavanagh and associates (1970). Knutson and co-workers (1981) reported successful use of a paste of 70 to 80% granulated sugar mixed with povidone-iodine ointment and povidone-iodine solution in 605 patients with a variety of skin ulcers and infections. Excision and secondary closure of the granulating incision or skin grafting can be considered, but simply waiting for eventual closure may be the wisest course after the grave initial illness.

Dehiscence

Wound dehiscence means separation of the layers of the abdominal incision. It may be partial, through skin, subcutaneous tissue, fascia and muscle but not peritoneum, or complete, through all layers. When intestine protrudes through the incision, the term evisceration is used. Common predisposing factors include obesity, old age, poor nutritional state and metabolic disturbances such as diabetes. Postoperatively, excessive coughing or abdominal distension are important immediate causes.

In partial dehiscence local factors that affect healing such as hematoma and infection are prominent. The management of these problems was discussed previously. The extent of the dehiscence must be determined early. If the fascia has not separated, healing, although lengthy, will usually not be complicated. If the fascia is no longer intact, the threat of complete dehiscence and evisceration is always present. Although the peritoneum rapidly thickens and provides a good barrier, healing is prolonged and an incisional hernia is very likely to develop. In view of this, immediate repair as for complete dehiscence should be strongly considered. This can be done with success if the wound is clean. Smead-Jones sutures are most effective for the fascia with secondary closure of the skin.

Complete dehiscence is often a traumatic and apparently sudden event. Its incidence is reported to be from 0.5 to 2.0% in gynecology and obstetrics, although this figure varies widely with the type of patient and the operations included in a given series. The type of incision and the sutures used have been greatly debated. In general, vertical incisions and layer closure with catgut have been accompanied by a higher incidence of dehiscence as compared with transverse incisions and closure with Smead-Jones sutures. It is probable that vertical incisions properly closed with this technique, even in elderly, obese, debilitated patients who have had major operative procedures, have a similar and irreducible incidence of dehiscence as compared with transverse incisions properly closed with polyglycolic sutures. There appears to be no difference in dehiscence whether the fascia is closed with continuous or with interrupted (polyglycolic) sutures. In a randomized prospective multicentric study Fagniez and co-workers (1985) found the overall dehiscence rate to be 1.6% in the continuous sutures group compared with 2.0% in the interrupted sutures group. The higher incidence in the latter was significant only in contaminated wounds. The authors also point out that the continuous suture technique is more economical and expeditious.

The classic premonitory sign of complete dehiscence is leakage of thin pink fluid from the incision four to seven days after the operation. Earlier discharge in a patient found to have ascites at operation may represent residual ascitic fluid; this usually ceases after two or three days. The patient may have slight persistent fever and leukocytosis. The incision should be inspected twice daily, and it may be helpful to use a tight binder of the Scultetus type to minimize possible intestinal extrusion. If the superficial part of the incision breaks down, probing it with a cotton-tipped applicator or hemostat may demonstrate the opening into the peritoneal cavity. In some instances intestine may be seen at the bottom of the incision or may indeed protrude through it.

When it is clear that the peritoneum is no longer intact, prompt repair is almost always indicated. Prior to operation, cultures of the wound should be obtained, and exposed bowel may be covered with sterile towels moistened with saline and pads and a binder applied. If delay is likely to elapse before repair, the bowel can be replaced using sterile gloves and gently packed in place with pads soaked in povidone-iodine (Morris, 1982). Broad spectrum antibiot-

ics should be started and baseline blood count and blood chemical studies obtained.

The eviscerated incision should be opened throughout its length and all necrotic tissue excised. The abdomen should not be explored except to determine that the protruding bowel or omentum is healthy. If the wound is relatively clean and the patient's condition is satisfactory, the incision can be closed with Smead-Jones sutures to the peritoneum and fascia, using a long-acting polyglycolic suture. The skin and subcutaneous tissues are left open for secondary closure (see page 104). If the wound edges are ragged and the patient's condition poor, it is quicker to place sutures of nonabsorbable material through all layers. Heavy silver wire has long been used because its tension can be adjusted by twisting or untwisting. However, No. 2 nylon or No. 5 silk is also satisfactory. Whatever material is used, the sutures are placed well away from the wound edges and 2 cm apart. To prevent inclusion of intestine in a suture, all are held up before the first one is twisted or tied. The skin edges are protected by passing the sutures through a short length of fine rubber tubing. It is important to tie the sutures with the right tension. If they are too loose, closure will be inadequate. If they are too tight, necrosis of the skin edges will occur. Later wound edema is inevitable, and this increases the tension. Unapposed skin between the through-and-through sutures is closed with interrupted non-absorbable mattress sutures. These are removed at the normal time, five to seven days later. The main sutures remain for 21 days. The author's preference is to use through-and-through single suture closure in most instances.

Patients who have had eviscerations are often critically ill, and they have an overall mortality of 10 to 20%. Death occurs from accompanying sepsis or other complications. Adequate monitoring and the use of appropriate antibiotics and nutritional support, including hyperalimentation, are essential. Nasogastric suction is necessary initially to help prevent intestinal distension.

Keloids

Keloids are raised hypertrophic scars that occur more frequently in women of dark-skinned rather than light-skinned races. They are more common and noticeable on exposed parts of the body, but are often of considerable concern to the patient when they occur in abdominal incisions. The exact cause of keloid formation is not known.

An individual's tendency to form keloids can usually be ascertained from her history or physical examination. Prevention of keloids in a new scar has limited success. The skin should be carefully closed with a subcuticular stitch and/or sterile adhesive strips. Local cortisone has been used for many years. Shell and Inmon (1959), in a well controlled study, used topical cortisone on half of 30 abdominal incisions and found no decrease in keloid formation in the treated area, but they also noted an increase in local wound infections. Later, the injection of a corticosteroid such as dexamethasone (4 mg/ml) with 1% lidocaine at the time of operation and at weekly or monthly intervals thereafter, depending upon the appearance and thickness of the scar, produced excellent or good results in 76% of patients reported by Wilson (1965). Excision and careful primary closure or excision with skin graft and the use of corticosteroids is recommended by Pollack and Goslen (1982). Other pharmacologic methods together with radiation are reviewed by Peacock (1981), but their effectiveness and safety are uncertain.

Other than keloid formation, some scars become much wider many months or years later because of stretching of the abdominal wall skin. There is little that can be done except excision and careful reclosure.

Miscellaneous

INCISIONAL HERNIA

The occurrence of incisional hernias following lower abdominal incisions is probably about 1%. This increases to about 10% after infection and 30% after dehiscence. The patient usually has minimal discomfort. She may notice a protrusion in or near the scar. On examination a defect surrounded by fascia can be felt, often in more than one place. If no treatment is given, incarceration and possible strangulation of intestine or omentum in the hernial sac, although rare, is always a possibility. Protrusion can be partly controlled by a tight girdle and/ or a specially fitted pad and belt. Repair is advisable for symptomatic, large or disfiguring hernias. Since many patients are obese, weight reduction prior to operation is essential, especially because it materially increases the chance of success. The principles of repair include (1) separation of the hernial sac from the skin, subcutaneous tissue and fascia; (2) identification

of secondary sacs; (3) excision of the hernial sac(s) with inspection of incarcerated bowel or omentum; (4) wide exposure of the fascia; and (5) primary closure with Smead-Jones polyglycolic sutures. When the defect is very large a Marlex mesh may be used to bridge the fascial gap after closure of the peritoneum.

SUTURE GRANULOMA

Intermittent breakdown of a small area of the incision with purulent and/or bloody discharge is a relatively common occurrence. It is associated with the use of subcutaneous sutures or slowly absorbable or non-absorbable fascial sutures. Occasionally a loose stitch will work its way to the surface spontaneously. If not, a small button hook should be inserted into the opening, using local anesthesia if necessary, and manipulated to try to pull up the offending suture so that it can be cut and removed. This manuever may have to be repeated, especially if there are several sutures in similar granulomas. Silver nitrate (on a stick) can be used to cauterize any granulation tissue. A suture granuloma may present only as a tender hard area deep in the incision, occasionally with redness of the skin and with low grade fever. Short of reopening the incision, usually an undesirable procedure, treatment should be conservative using heat and analgesics, since the inflammation is likely to subside or the suture will present near the surface.

ENDOMETRIOSIS

Endometriosis occasionally develops in abdominal or perineal incisions. It is most likely to occur when the uterus has been opened and closed. For example, Chatterjee (1980) reported an incidence of 1.08% in 1129 hysterotomies for second trimester abortion and 0.03% in 3729 patients who had had cesarean sections. Endometriosis is occasionally seen in episiotomy scars or at the site of a perineal repair. Characteristically, the scar becomes swollen and more painful during menstruation, and occasionally there is a little bleeding at that time. The diagnosis can be confirmed by fine needle aspiration and cytologic studies. The best treatment is wide surgical excision.

DESMOID

A desmoid tumor occasionally appears in a midline incision. This very rare proliferation of fibrous tissue seems sometimes physically connected with the scar, although its causation may be unrelated. The tumor behaves like a low-grade sarcoma. Wide surgical excision is the appropriate treatment (Reitamo et al, 1986).

RETAINED FOREIGN BODY

An unusual and distressing complication of an operation is the presence of a foreign body in the incision or particularly within the peritoneal cavity. This may be the result of an intrauterine device perforating the uterus or of a retained sponge, instrument or needle or of disappearance of a drain originally inserted through the primary or a separate incision. The former is an accepted though rare hazard of intrauterine conception. It is usually discovered on ultrasonography or x-ray when the tail of the IUD is no longer seen to protrude from the external os of the cervix (see Chapter 12). The latter situation, retention of a sponge or other object, should be prevented by using only sponges tagged with radiopaque material and by careful counting of sponges, instruments and needles before the end of the operation. The first count should be made before the peritoneal cavity is closed, so that if the count is incorrect, the cavity can be reexplored. If the discrepancy cannot be accounted for, or if the final count is incorrect, it is best to have an x-ray film of the abdomen taken immediately and, if necessary, to reopen the incision. However, in some cases the preoperative count (and so the final one) can be in error. Also, in major and complicated cases, the condition of the patient may be so desperate and the blood loss so great that insufficient attention is paid to the sponge and instrument count. Further, when drains are placed at operation, they may unexpectedly migrate into the incision or peritoneal cavity unless they are properly secured to the skin.

The clinical picture of a retained foreign body is protean. A small needle or portion of a needle may cause no symptoms and may not be detected until an x-ray is taken, perhaps many years later, for another purpose. An instrument or sponge is usually surrounded by inflammation and a (possibly sterile) abscess. It may cause fever and vague abdominal complaints or may result in intestinal obstruction or rarely perforation of the intestine at any time after operation. If the object is radiopaque, the first x-ray taken will permit the diagnosis. If the object is not radiopaque, its presence may be suggested by the appearance of an abscess on ultrasonography, CT scan or MRI. However,

the final diagnosis will have to await exploratory laparotomy.

A foreign body should be removed after division of adhesions, and any repair and/or resection of intestine is performed as necessary. Pathologic examination of the specimen and factual operative notes are essential. Clearly, the handling of discussion and communication with the patient and her family is a very delicate matter, since the presence of a sponge, legally speaking, is a classic instance of res ipsa loquitur. This means that a sponge (or other object) is not normally expected to be present within the peritoneal cavity. The fact that it is there is usually considered to be evidence of negligence on the part of the surgeon (see Chapter 16).

NEUROMUSCULAR

Postoperative Pain

MINOR PROCEDURES

For specific procedures and treatments such as venipuncture, biopsy of the vulva or cervix, endometrial sampling or fine needle aspiration, the preliminary apprehension and the discomfort of the procedure itself may be allayed by explanation, and, if indicated, by the use of local anesthesia. Post-treatment discomfort is not usually great and can be managed by common analgesics such as acetaminophen without or with codeine.

MAJOR PROCEDURES

Early Postoperative Pain (in the first 24 hours). Following operations that involve entering the peritoneal cavity, vaginal repairs or larger excisional procedures, pain is an expected complication and its management must be planned in advance. Writing postoperative orders for analgesia is often covered by a printed form or relegated to the most junior member of the surgical team. General guidelines are appropriate, but printed forms need careful preparation and regular review, while junior staff must be given clear instructions. In general, a narcotic analgesic such as meperidine, morphine or hydromorphine should be ordered initially on a regular basis every three hours (meperidine, morphine) or every four hours (hydromorphine). The practice of writing an order for medication to be given p.r.n. is unsatisfactory since the recovering postoperative patient cannot be expected to know how or when or why to ask for pain medicine and the nurse may be reluctant to administer a narcotic for pain that she does not yet consider severe. The danger of oversedation can be covered by writing an order for the nurse to withhold the full dose if the patient appears oversedated or her respiratory rate is below 12.

Modifications in dosage must be made in certain circumstances. Less should be given to older and debilitated women. More is needed in heavier women and in those whose pain threshold has been demonstrated to be low. Patients known to be dependent on narcotics should be given their usual amounts; the postoperative period is an inappropriate time to attempt to cure drug dependency.

Initially postoperative analgesics are commonly given subcutaneously or intramuscularly. This may result in irregular absorption, depending on the site of injection and the amount of fat. Alternatively they can be given intravenously, for example, morphine 1 to 3 mg/hr by infusion pump. This method is promising (Briggs et al, 1985) but requires more careful nursing surveillance.

Observation of the patient and individualization of analgesic doses are the most important aspects of postoperative pain management. These fall appropriately within nursing responsibility since nurses follow the patients most closely. Many patients do not request pain medication (when it is ordered p.r.n.) even when the are suffering from quite severe pain. Also, nurses tend to choose lower doses when ranges of doses are prescribed (Kampon et al, 1983). Many other factors affect narcotic administration such as (1) the patient's request for medications sooner than ordered; (2) possible side effects such as nausea, vomiting, or respiratory depression; or (3) the ability of nurses to respond quickly to patients' requests or to pass on relevant information from shift to shift. The upshot of these difficulties is that it is most important for the surgical team to monitor pain relief during the first 24 hours after the operation.

Methods of supplementing or even supplanting the early postoperative administration of narcotic analgesics include:

1. "Potentiating" drugs such as hydroxyzine or promethazine (25 to 50 mg) can be added when an analgesic is given. How much they increase analgesia is not certain. They may be useful in decreasing nausea and vomiting, but may cause hypotension or oversedation. Therefore, the use of a separate anti-emetic medication (e.g., prochlorperazine) is more appropriate.

2. Transcutaneous electrical nerve stimulation (TENS) may be used. This requires insertion of electrodes parallel to the skin incision and continuous electrical stimulation. It has been found to be effective in reducing the amount of narcotics needed (Rowlingson and Rogers, 1984). It is not clear whether the results are worth the trouble of inserting the electrodes.

3. Local anesthetic nerve block can be carried into the postoperative period by using long-acting agents or by repeating, for example, intercostal blocks. This is of limited value for the lower abdominal incisions commonly used in gynecology and obstetrics.

4. Epidural injections of 5 to 7.5 mg morphine in 5 to 10 ml of normal saline (both free of preservatives) can result in excellent anesthesia for 12 to 24 hours. Side effects of itching, nausea, vomiting and urinary retention as well as rare respiratory depression have been reported. The technique has not yet been fully evaluated (Rowlingson and Rogers, 1984).

Later Postoperative Pain (after 24 hours). Review of pain management is a most important aspect of the twice daily visits to the postoperative patient. Analgesics should be given by mouth as soon as the patient is able to take liquids orally. Commonly used drugs include acetaminophen with codeine (30 to 60 mg) or Percodan/Percocet. In major cases in which much handling of the bowel occurs, the parenteral route may have to be maintained for three to five days or even longer. Under these circumstances it is appropriate to reduce the dose gradually. If, in spite of being able to eat, the patient still appears to need injections or if she asks for them more frequently, it is clear that their effect is becoming less, but not necessarily that the patient is becoming dependent on them. In fact, dependence is most unlikely unless the patient has a history of previous dependence. Nevertheless, weaning patients from parenteral analgesics may be difficult. Combining decreasing amounts of narcotics with increasing amounts of promethazine may be useful. Often the firm substitution of equivalent oral medication is effective (Table 4–13). The diagnosis and management of chronic and persistent pain, especially that due to cancer, are covered in Chapter 7.

Table 4–13. Equivalent Doses of Commonly Used Analgesics

Drug	Dosage	
	Intra-muscular (mg)	Oral (mg)
Morphine	10	60
Codeine	130	200
Oxycodone	15	30
Pentazocine (Talwin)	60	180
Meperidine (Demerol)	75	300
Hydromorphone (Dilaudid)	1.5	7.5
Methadone (Dolophine)	10	20
Levorphanol (Levo-Dromeran)	2	4

Specific Neurologic Problems

Injuries to cutaneous nerves that may occur during gynecologic or obstetric procedures are described in Chapter 3. The resulting sensory losses are likely to improve, although some deficit may remain. Loss of muscle function from nerve injury to the obturator or femoral nerve in gynecology or to the lumbosacral plexus or pudendal nerve in obstetrics is more serious.

OBTURATOR NERVE

Injury to the obturator nerve is most likely to occur during biopsy or removal of the obturator lymph nodes. This results in inability properly to adduct the thigh. After contusion partial if not complete recovery may be anticipated, but this may take many weeks.

FEMORAL NERVE

Damage to the femoral nerve may follow abdominal hysterectomy (most common), vaginal hysterectomy or delivery. According to Kvist-Poulsen and Borel (1982), minor degrees of injury occur more frequently following abdominal hysterectomy than is realized. These authors noted it to be present to some degree in 17 of 147 patients (11.7%) undergoing elective total abdominal hysterectomy. They implicated retractors with large lateral blades and advised repeated intraoperative determination of the relationship of the retractor blades to the psoas muscle. Self-retaining retractors appear to be more likely to cause damage than hand-held retractors. The type of incision (transverse), the habitus of the patient (thin) and the length of the operation (prolonged) may also be of importance.

The symptoms of femoral nerve injury become apparent 24 to 48 hours after the operation. They consist of numbness of the antero-medial aspect of the thigh and leg, instability (buckling) of the knee when the patient attempts to walk, especially up steps, and pain localized to the area anterior to the hip joint. On examination the patient is unable to raise the straight leg off the bed, there is decreased or absent touch and pain sense over the anteromedial aspect of the thigh and leg and the patellar reflex is diminished or absent. Sometimes involvement is bilateral.

Spontaneous recovery of femoral nerve injury is to be expected. This occurs within a few days or may take up to six months. Conservative treatment is appropriate, using physical therapy such as gait training, passive exercises and the application of local heat and electrical muscle stimulation.

OTHER

Sciatic nerve injury with involvement of the common peroneal nerve and subsequent numbness of the foot and footdrop can occur after the use of the lithotomy position. The exact mechanism is unclear. In two cases Batres and Barclay noted spontaneous recovery within 60 days (1983).

Injury to the innervation of the pelvic floor may occur at childbirth more frequently than is recognized. Snooks and co-workers (1984) noted that fecal incontinence, attributable to damage to the innervation of the puborectalis and external and internal rectal sphincters, was more common in multiparas, with the use of forceps, after prolonged labor or in patients with a history of pelvic floor injury. Recovery within two months was the rule, although the effects appeared to be cumulative with repeated childbirth. Anesthesia may also contribute although Snooks and co-workers did not include data on this aspect in their series.

PSYCHOLOGIC, SOCIAL AND SEXUAL SEQUELAE

Psychologic, social and sexual complications are considered together because they are closely interrelated. There are certain common characteristics. First, although they may be related to operations and procedures in general, these complications are more likely to follow procedures or medications that have specific effects upon sexual function, such as hysterectomy, oophorectomy or sterilization. Second, foreknowledge of possible difficulties may help the patient to avoid them (see Chapter 2). Third, early postoperative signs, except for major psychiatric disorders, are few and often require careful observation for detection. Fourth, late development of these complications (particularly social and sexual) may be unexpected, and indeed, not known to the obstetrician-gynecologist who performed the original procedure because of the time elapsed and the length of follow-up necessary.

Early Postoperative Period

Emotional disturbances may occur after any major operation and occasionally after minor ones. They are not specific for gynecology and obstetrics. The characteristic symptom is inappropriate behavior. A patient may be out of touch with reality or in touch with reality but responding in an unusual manner to her surroundings. Both conditions require prompt attention.

The completely detached patient does not recognize where she is, the time of day, or familiar people. This disorientation may be accompanied by noisy or combative behavior, which is disturbing to personnel and other patients alike and detrimental to the patient's postoperative recovery. Organic causes must be exchanged, particularly the persistent effects of anesthesia and analgesic medication; this is an important consideration in older patients who sometimes react poorly even to small doses of narcotics, especially at night and in the unfamiliar hospital surroundings. If there is even a slight possibility that the disorientation is caused by medication, that medication should be stopped. Noisiness and hyperactivity are more difficult to handle. Tranquilizers such as thorazine (25 mg intramuscularly initially, repeated or increased as indicated) are useful. A patient in such condition should not be left alone. A knowledgeable and caring family member or a special nurse should be with her at all times until the acute episode ends or is treated appropriately. Restraint of the arms may be necessary to prevent the disoriented patient from pulling out essential intravenous lines, tearing off dressings or risking injury from getting out of bed and falling. However, restraints are very frightening. They should be used only as a last resort and not unless one-on-one nursing is ineffective. A patient placed in restraints should continue to have a personal companion or nurse to give her reassurance and explanation, since it is impossible to tell how much the apparently completely disoriented patient understands what is being done and said around her. If the patient's bizarre behavior continues, psychiatric consultation should be obtained promptly, especially if the patient has a history of previous psychiatric disorder and/or treatment.

More common behaviors are exaggerated responses to the operation and the hospital surroundings. Depression, denial and anger are normal components of the reactions to illness or operation. Patients who are completely unresponsive to attempts at communication, who firmly maintain that they are all right even when circumstances by no means justify such a statement, or complain constantly and are abusive to all their caregivers may be overreacting. A variation on the last theme is the patient, particularly the one with a serious problem such as cancer, who seeks answers to the same questions from all her caregivers and attempts to get favorable responses from someone. Caregivers tend to regard all these types of patients as "difficult." However, there is no such thing as a difficult patient, only an unhappy one. Appropriate methods of management are (1) to give courteous, consistent attention; (2) to spend time with the patient and allow her to express her feelings; (3) to talk with the family and see that they understand the situation; and (4) to communicate with other members of the health care team so that a consistent plan of care is followed.

Postoperative withdrawal from alcohol may present special behavioral problems. An accurate history of alcohol intake is important, but may not always be available because of the patient's tendency to minimize its use. Withdrawal may produce severe symptoms such as elevated pulse and temperature, sweating, confusion, tremor, restlessness and hallucinations (delirium tremens). Immediate management consists primarily of a benzodiazepine (diazepam 10 mg intravenously or intramuscularly followed by 5 to 10 mg every three hours or chlordiazepoxide 50 to 100 mg intramuscularly), hydration and vitamins B and C. If the patient is able to drink, continuation of a moderate amount of alcohol is temporarily useful. However, the occurrence of an episode of withdrawal should indicate the need for long-term follow-up and counseling.

Intensive Care Unit

The patient who is in an intensive care unit (ICU) is subject to special stresses because of the severity of her illness and the unusual nature of her environment. This means that behavioral symptoms are more likely to be present and/or exaggerated. In addition, the ICU produces (1) anxiety because of the patient's uncertainty about her condition and fear of failure of the mechanical devices to which she is attached; (2) exhaustion and lack of orientation, particularly related to noise, confusion between day and night and often reduced contact with the outside world especially if there are no windows; and (3) inability to communicate because of elaborate monitoring equipment and/or endotracheal intubation. These factors chiefly express themselves in overt anxiety and apparent lack of comprehension of what is being done. The difficulties increase the longer the patient remains in the ICU. It is essential that all medical personnel recognize the stress to which the patient is subjected and understand that her unusual behavior may be caused by this.

The management of psychologic problems in the intensive care unit has five aspects:

1. Appropriate medication to relieve pain and anxiety.

2. Emotional support from all ICU personnel.

3. Communication aids, such as visual devices for instruction, writing mechanisms or attachments to the endotracheal cannula that enable intubated patients to speak (Benzer et al, 1983).

4. Special encouragement of family members to provide support and/or the use of volunteer companions to provide continued emotional support throughout the patient's stay in an ICU.

5. Continuation of psychologic care after discharge from the ICU. Such patients tend to be more concerned about their own problems, more depressed, less affectionate and to rely more on others for decisions. In patients whose medical condition improves, these personality changes tend to decrease with time. However, recognition of their existence and continued provision of counseling are valuable.

Giving care to patients in the ICU has important complications as far as the caregivers are concerned. Depression, a sense of lack of accomplishment and guilt feelings are very common, leading to the "burn-out syndrome." The situation is similar to that occurring among those caring for cancer patients, especially the terminally ill. Established ICU policies and regular team meetings between all involved personnel (physicians, nurses, therapists) with discussion and participation in decisions can do much to mitigate the emotional issues.

Later Postoperative Period

Some emotional problems occur after the first postoperative week and extend for an indefinite period thereafter. After a laparotomy, for example, it is common for a woman to feel tired and depressed. This arises in large part from decreased muscle strength, persistent incisional pain and nutritional problems such as anemia or possible deficiencies of specific nutrients such as vitamins. Other psychophysiologic symptoms may have their origin in urinary or intestinal tract disorders.

Specific operations may result in specific emotional problems. For example, bilateral oophorectomy may lead not only to hot flashes but to accompanying emotional distress. Hysterectomy may result in feelings of worthlessness because of the inability to bear children. Operations on the external genitalia may result in a change in the woman's concept of her own body. These individual complications are discussed in detail in later chapters. However, many of them, as well as some of the general problems, have a psychosexual element.

The management of later postoperative psycho-sexual problems includes the following:

1. Detailed instructions before and at the time of discharge from hospital, particularly with regard to bathing, use of tampons and resumption of intercourse. In general, bathing is permitted, tampons should not be used until the initial bleeding has subsided and coitus can be resumed three to 14 days after minor vaginal procedures or laparoscopy and about four weeks after major abdominal or vaginal procedures in which the vagina is sutured. This postoperative advice should be given by the physician and not relegated to other personnel except for reinforcement. Opportunity must be provided for the patient and her partner to ask questions.

2. Psychosexual problems must be reviewed at the postoperative follow-up visits. Questions and sexual complaints such as dyspareunia, loss of libido and secondary orgasmic dysfunction deserve thorough and prompt investigation. They are usually psychologic rather than physical in origin.

3. When possible, the patient's partner should be included in any discussion about psychologic and psychosexual problems.

4. Long-term follow-up is important because difficulties may not appear for months or years after a procedure. It is important then to ascertain if new causes, other than the previous operation, are responsible for the symptoms.

5. Special problems occur with children and adolescents. A social worker or psychologist-counselor is most helpful.

6. Group therapy. Occasional patients may be helped by discussing their problems with others in similar situations. For example, self-help groups of hysterectomy or endometriosis patients, if available in the community, can be useful.

POSTOPERATIVE DISCUSSION

A routine should be established for talking to the patient and her family after an operation or procedure. The occurrence of a complication makes this even more important. The immediate postoperative discussion has been covered in Chapter 3. Additional guidelines for later discussion are as follows:

1. Do not, under any circumstances, omit mention of a significant complication. The patient must know that her physician is honest with her.

2. Write up or dictate a note on complications as they happen and what was done.

3. Do not suggest or imply fault at any time either in discussion or in written notes.

4. Give the patient and her family repeated opportunities at subsequent visits to ask questions about her progress and prognosis, but do not make off-the-cuff statements about percentages or plans of treatment until it has been decided what these are and what is to be done.

5. If a fee for the operation is charged, the occurrence of the complication should not change it. If a subsequent procedure is necessary, it should be charged at a reduced rate, possibly 50%.

6. Respect the patient's confidentiality. Do not discuss her disease or problems with her distant relatives or friends unless she has given her permission for this.

7. If the patient has a complication that is likely to prolong or affect her recovery, be sure that your insurance company, risk manager or lawyer is notified of the event in case a medicolegal complication arises (see Chapter 16).

REFERENCES

Aeder MI, Wellman JL et al: Role of surgical and percutaneous drainage in the treatment of abdominal abscesses. *Arch. Surg.* 118:273, 1983.

Asmussen M, Miller A: *Clinical Gynecological Urology.* Oxford, Blackwell, 1983, p. 186.

Baines M, Oliver DJ, Carter RL: Medical management of intestinal obstruction in patients with malignant disease. *Lancet* 2:990, 1985.

Ballon SC: Effective early postoperative nutrition by defined formula diet via needle-catheter jejunostomy. *Gynecol. Oncol.* 14:23, 1982.

Bartlett P, Reingold AL et al: Toxic shock syndrome associated with surgical wound infections. *J. Am. Med. Assoc.* 247:1448, 1982.

Batres F, Barclay DL: Sciatic nerve injury during gynecologic procedures using the lithotomy position. *Obstet. Gynecol.* 62:92S, 1983.

Bedell SE, Delbanco TL et al: Survival after cardiopulmonary resuscitation in the hospital. *N. Engl. J. Med.* 309:569, 1983.

Benzer H, Mutz N, Pauser G: Psychosocial sequelae of intensive care. *Int. Anesthesiol. Clin.* 21:169, 1983.

Bjornsson TD, Greenberg C: Heparinization in the surgical patient. *Infect. Surg.* 4:87, 1985.

Bonnar J: *Venous Thrombo-embolism and Pregnancy.* Vol. 9 in the series *Recent Advances in Obstetrics and Gynecology.* Edinburgh, Churchill Livingstone, 1979.

Boronow RC: Management of radiation-induced vaginal fistulas. *Am. J. Obstet. Gynecol.* 110:1, 1971.

Bricker EM: Bladder substitution after pelvic evisceration. *Surg. Clin. North Am.* 30:1511, 1950.

Bricker EM, Johnston WD et al: Reconstructive surgery for the complications of pelvic radiation. *Am. J. Clin. Oncol.* 7:81, 1984.

Briggs GD, Berman ML et al: Morphine: continuous intravenous infusion versus intramuscular injections for postoperative pain relief. *Gynecol. Oncol.* 22:288, 1985.

Brown SE, Allen HH, Robins RN: The use of delayed primary wound closure in preventing wound infections. *Am. J. Obstet. Gynecol.* 127:713, 1977.

Burchard KW, Minor LB et al: Fungal sepsis in surgical patients. *Arch. Surg.* 118:217, 1983.

Cardiopulmonary resuscitation (CPR) and emergency cardiac care (EC): Standards and Guidelines. *J. Am. Med. Assoc.* 225:2905, 1986.

Cavanagh D: Septic shock. In Schaefer G, Graber EA (eds): *Complications in Obstetric and Gynecologic Surgery.* Hagerstown, MD, Harper and Row, 1981, p. 166.

Cavanagh D, Beazley J, Ostapowicz F: Radical operation for carcinoma of the vulva: a new approach to wound healing. *J. Obstet. Gynaecol. Br. Comm.* 77:1037, 1970.

Chatterjee SK: Scar endometriosis: a clinicopathologic study of 17 cases. *Obstet. Gynecol.* 56:81, 1980.

Collins CG, Collins JH et al: Early repair of vesicovaginal fistula. *Am. J. Obstet. Gynecol.* 111:524, 1971.

Crandon AJ, Koutts J: Incidence of postoperative deep vein thrombosis in gynecologic oncology. *Aust. N.Z. Obstet. Gynecol.* 23:216, 1983.

Dellinger EP: Severe necrotizing soft-tissue infections. *J. Am. Med. Assoc.* 246:1717, 1981.

Dicker RC, Greenspan JR et al: Complications of abdominal and vaginal hysterectomy among women of reproductive age. *Am. J. Obstet. Gynecol.* 144:841, 1982.

Duff P: Recognizing and treating toxic shock. *Contemp. Obstet. Gynecol.* 22:43, 1982.

Duff P, Gibbs RS: Pelvic vein thrombophlebitis: diagnostic dilemma and therapeutic challenge. *Obstet. Gynecol. Surv.* 38:365, 1983.

Fagniez P-L, Hay JM et al: Abdominal midline incisions. *Arch. Surg.* 120:1351, 1985.

Ferrari A, Baccolo M et al: Randomized clinical trial of short-term antibiotic prophylaxis in 750 patients undergoing vaginal and abdominal hysterectomy. *Int. Surg.* 69:21, 1984.

Glass CA, Cohn I Jr.: Drainage of intraabdominal abscesses. A comparison of surgical and computerized tomography guided catheter drainage. *Am. J. Surg.* 147:315, 1984.

Goodwin WE, Scardino PT: Vesicovaginal and urethrovaginal fistulas. *J. Urol.* 127:370, 1980.

Greenfield LJ, Stewart J, Crute S: Results of surgical management of pulmonary thromboembolism. *J. Clin. Surg.* 1:194, 1982.

Grillo HC: When and how to do tracheostomy. *Contemp. Obstet. Gynecol., Update on General Surgery*: 83, 1983.

Grundmann R, Heistermann S: Postoperative albumin infusion therapy based on colloid osmotic pressure. *Arch. Surg.* 120:911, 1985.

Haley RW, Culver DH et al: Identifying patients at high-risk of surgical wound infection. *Am. J. Epidemiol.* 121:206, 1985.

Hebert DB: How to avoid or minimize urologic injuries in surgery. *Contemp. Obstet. Gynecol.* 22:213, 1983.

Hevron JE Jr., Llorens AS: Management of postoperative abscess following gynecologic surgery. *Obstet. Gynecol.* 47:553, 1976.

Inmon WB, Fish SA: Surgical repair of old fourth-degree lacerations. *South. Med. J.* 70:1080, 1977.

Kampon S, Weiss OF et al: Analysis of narcotic analgesic usage in the treatment of postoperative pain. *J. Am. Med. Assoc.* 250:926, 1983.

Keller SM, Papa M, Wilder JR: Inferior vena cava interruption. *Mt. Sinai J. Med.* 52:353, 1985.

Kendrick JH, Casali RE et al: The complicated septic abdominal wound. *Arch. Surg.* 117:464, 1982.

Kihl B, Nilson AE, Pettersson S: Uretero-neocystostomy in the treatment of postoperative uretero-vaginal fistula. *Acta Obstet. Gynecol. Scand.* 61:341, 1982.

Killewich LA, Martin R et al: An objective assessment of the physiologic changes in the post thrombotic syndrome. *Arch. Surg.* 120:424, 1985.

Knutson RA, Merbitz LA et al: Use of sugar and povidone-iodine to enhance wound healing. *South. Med. J.* 74:1329, 1981.

Kock NG: Ileostomy without external appliances: a survey of 25 patients provided with intra-abdominal intestinal reservoir. *Ann. Surg.* 173:545, 1971.

Kvist-Poulsen H, Borel J: Iatrogenic femoral neuropathy subsequent to abdominal hysterectomy: incidence and prevention. *Obstet. Gynecol.* 60:516, 1982.

Mann WJ Jr., Jander HP et al: Selective arterial embolization for control of bleeding in gynecologic malignancy. *Gynecol. Oncol.* 10:279, 1980.

Meguid MM, Elder S, Wahba A: The delivery of nutritional support. *Cancer* 55:279, 1985.

Mitcheson HD, Sant GR: Management of intractable bladder hemorrhage. *Infect. Surg.* 3:839, 1984.

Moir JC: *The Vesico-vaginal Fistula*. London, Bailliere, Tindall and Cox, 1961.

Morris DM: Preoperative management of patients with evisceration. *Dis. Colon Rectum* 25:249, 1982.

O'Conor VJ: Review of experience with vesico-vaginal fistula repair. *J. Urol.* 123:367, 1980.

Orford HJL, Theron JLL: The repair of vesico-vaginal fistulas with omentum. *S. Afr. Med. J.* 67:143, 1985.

Page CP, Carlton PK et al: Safe, cost-effective postoperative nutrition defined formula diet via needle-catheter jejunostomy. *Am. J. Surg.* 138:939, 1979.

Peacock EE: Control of wound healing and scar formation in surgical patients. *Arch. Surg.* 116:1325, 1981.

Peetz DJ, Gamelli RL, Filcher DB: Intestinal intubation in acute mechanical small-bowel obstruction. *Arch. Surg.* 117:334, 1982

Perinetti EP: Palliative urinary diversion. *Surg. Clin. North Am.* 62:1025, 1982.

Pitkin RM: Abdominal hysterectomy in obese women. *Surg. Gynecol. Obstet.* 142:532, 1976.

Polk HC, Simpson CJ et al: Guidelines for prevention of surgical wound infection. *Arch. Surg.* 118:1213, 1983.

Pollack SV, Goslen JB: The surgical treatment of keloids. *J. Dermatol. Surg. Oncol.* 8:1045, 1982.

Redmond P, Ambos M et al: Iatrogenic intussusception—a complication of long intestinal tubes. *Am. J. Gastroenterol.* 77:39, 1982.

Reitamo JJ, Scheinin TM, Hayry P: The desmoid syndrome. *Am. J. Surg.* 151:230, 1986.

Rooke TW, Osmundson PJ: Heparin and the in-patient management of deep venous thrombosis: cost considerations. *Mayo Clin. Proc.* 61:198, 1986.

Rosenow EC III, Osmundson PH, Brown ML: Pulmonary embolism. *Mayo Clin. Proc.* 56:161, 1981.

Rosenthal DM, Colapinto R: Angiographic arterial embolization in the management of postoperative vaginal hemorrhage. *Am. J. Obstet. Gynecol.* 151:227, 1985.

Rothenberger DA, Goldberg SM: The management of rectovaginal fistulae. *Surg. Clin. North Am.* 63:61, 1983.

Rowlingson JC, Rogers W: Current concepts of postoperative pain. *Infect. Surg.* 3:527, 1984.

Sagalowsky AI: Further experience with ileocecal conduit urinary diversion. *J. Urol.* 135:39, 1986.

Sandberg EC, Pelligra R: The medical antigravity suit for management of surgically uncontrollable bleeding associated with abdominal pregnancy. *Am. J. Obstet. Gynecol.* 146:519, 1983.

Sandler DA, Martin JF et al: Diagnosis of deep-vein thrombosis: comparison of clinical evaluation ultrasound, plethysmography, and venoscan with x-ray venogram. *Lancet* 2:716, 1984.

Sasahara AA, Sharma GVRK et al: Pulmonary thromboembolism. *J. Am. Med. Assoc.* 249:2945, 1983.

Schlegel DM, Maglinte DDT: The blind pouch syndrome *Surg. Gynecol. Obstet.* 155:541, 1982.

Schmidt JD, Hawtrey CE et al: Complications, results and problems of ileal conduit diversions. *J. Urol.* 109:210, 1973.

Serota AI, Finegold SM: Necrotizing soft tissue infections following abdominal surgery. *Infect. Surg.* 1:50, 1982.

Shell FM, Inmon WB: The effects of topical application of cortisone-antibiotic ointment on surgical incisions and keloid formation. *Miss. Doctor* 36:247, 1959.

Skinner DG, Boyd SD, Lieskovsky G: Clinical experience with Kock continent ileal reservoir for urinary diversion. *J. Urol.* 132:1101, 1984.

Smith DH, Pierce VK, Lewis JL: Enteric fistulas encountered on a gynecologic oncology service from 1969 through 1980. *Surg. Gynecol. Obstet.* 158:71, 1984.

Snooks SJ, Setchell M, et al: Injury to innervation of pelvic floor sphincter musculature in childbirth. *Lancet* 2:546, 1984.

Solomkin JS, Flohr AM, Simmons RL: Indications for

therapy for fungemia in postoperative patients. *Arch. Surg.* 117:1272, 1982.

Solomons E, Levin EJ et al: A pyelographic study of ureteric injuries sustained during hysterectomy for benign conditions. *Surg. Gynecol. Obstet.* 111:41, 1960.

Sood SV: Prevention of urinary tract infection after gynecological laparotomy. *J. Obstet. Gynaecol. Br. Comm.* 79:80, 1972.

Stogdill BJ, Page CP, Pestana C: Nonoperative replacement of a jejunostomy feeding catheter. *Am. J. Surg.* 147:280, 1984.

Symmonds RE: Ureteral injuries associated with gynecologic surgery: prevention and management. *Clin. Obstet. Gynecol.* 19:623, 1976.

Thompson RL, Haley CE et al: Catheter-associated bacteriuria *J. Am. Med. Assoc.* 251:747, 1984.

Vanek VW, Al-Salti M: Acute pseudo-obstruction of the colon (Ogilvie's syndrome.) *Dis. Colon Rectum* 79:203, 1986.

Wagenknecht LV, Hardy JC: Value of various treatments for retroperitoneal fibrosis. *Eur. Urol.* 7:193, 1981.

Wager G: Toxic shock syndrome: a review. *Am. J. Obstet. Gynecol.* 146:93, 1983.

Wake CR: The immediate effect of abdominal hysterectomy on intravesical pressure and detrusor activity. *Br. J. Obstet. Gynaecol.* 87:901, 1980.

Weisman IM, Rinaldo JE, Rogers, RM: Positive end-expiratory pressure in adult respiratory failure. *N. Engl. J. Med.* 307:1381, 1982.

Wilson WW: Prevention of postsurgical keloids. *South. Med. J.* 58:751, 1965.

Wong ES, McKevitt M et al: Management of recurrent urinary tract infections with patient-administered single dose therapy. *Ann. Int. Med.* 102:302, 1985.

COMPLICATIONS OF OPERATIONS ON THE VULVA, VAGINA AND CERVIX

5

MICHAEL NEWTON

OPERATIONS ON THE VULVA

Incision and Drainage

Vulvar infections and abscesses requiring incision, other than those involving Bartholin's glands, are rare. The chief complications include bleeding at the time of operation, failure to drain the abscess cavity properly and delayed closure of the incision.

Bleeding is usually minimal if the abscess is ready to be incised, i.e., if signs of local inflammation have progressed to fluctuation, and if the initial incision is small and is made at the most fluctuant area. Premature operation, failure to break up pockets of pus and an inadequate drainage opening may result in persistent infection and recurrent abscess. Delayed closure of the incision may be due to its direction. It should generally be placed in an anteroposterior line, and on the medial rather than the lateral aspect of the abscess.

Excision or Biopsy

DIAGNOSTIC BIOPSY

Biopsy specimens of vulvar lesions may be obtained by using the Keyes's punch (3, 4 or 5 mm diameter), by excision of a portion of a large tumor or by excision or biopsy of a small lesion. Complications include hemorrhage at the time of operation, postoperative infection and failure to heal. Bleeding from small incisions such as those made by the Keyes punch can usually be controlled by Monsel's solution (ferric subsulfate) and/or pressure. Sutures (catgut or vicryl) may be necessary. Non-absorbable sutures must be removed later and may become buried and difficult to find. More severe bleeding may be avoided by doing only small excision biopsies in the office (1.5 cm in diameter or less) or by ensuring adequate assistance, for example

116

in an ambulatory surgical unit, when larger incisions are made. Failure to heal and infection in the incision may be reduced by placing sutures in an anteroposterior direction, even if the excision is circular.

CONDYLOMATA

Condylomata acuminata are increasingly common growths of the vulva, perineum, vagina and cervix. They are caused by one of the many condyloma viruses. Various local treatments have been recommended, including the topical application of podophyllin (25% in tincture of benzoin) (not in pregnancy), cauterization, cryosurgery, excision and laser vaporization. For the last four procedures anesthesia is necessary. Local anesthesia suffices for small lesions, but with extensive disease general anesthesia is necessary. Complications include local reaction to the therapy, bleeding, scarring of the introitus and recurrence of condylomata.

Local reaction can occur after any type of therapy but is marked after the use of podophyllin, unless precautions are taken to treat only the condyloma(ta), avoiding the surrounding normal skin or using petroleum jelly on it, and having the patient take a warm soaking bath within three hours after the application. The most effective treatment of an established severe local reaction is the frequent application of cloths soaked in cold Burow's solution (1:40 or 1:20 solution of aluminum sulfate and calcium acetate).

Bleeding is most likely to occur after laser therapy. It is usually minor, but cauterization may be needed to control it.

Scarring may result from any type of therapy (less likely with laser therapy), particularly when the condylomata are large and extensive. It is likely to cause dyspareunia. Treatment requires dilatation and possibly plastic repair (see page 119). Counseling and support are essential, because of the emotional aspect of such scarring.

Recurrence (or persistence) of condylomata varies with the different therapies. It is highest after the use of podophyllin. After cauterization, cryosurgery, excision or laser therapy recurrence occurs in 10 to 20% of patients. In particular, when laser therapy was used in early pregnancy recurrence rates were reported to be 33% by Ferenczy (1984).

Uninformed handling of cautery, cryosurgery and particularly laser equipment may lead to complications in the form of damage to neighboring normal tissues.

VULVECTOMY

Partial or complete vulvectomy is performed for premalignant lesions such as hypertrophic vulvar dystrophy, intraepithelial carcinoma and Paget's disease of the vulva. The extent of the vulvectomy is determined by the extent of the the primary disease. Partial vulvectomy is a large excision-biopsy and is subject to the same complications as a simple biopsy (see page 116).

In complete (simple) vulvectomy (as contrasted to radical vulvectomy; see Chapter 7) the labia majora and minora, clitoris, some perineal skin and a small amount of vagina are removed but the dissection is not necessarily carried down to the deep fascia. Intraoperatively bleeding may occur from the pudendal artery, which enters the labia posterolaterally, and in the area of the clitoris. Damage to neighboring normal structures such as the urethra, bladder, rectum or anal sphincter should be avoided, since only the skin and skin appendages are removed. Wide removal of skin may result in some tension, which, during closure, can be overcome by more extensive undermining. In a woman who is or is likely to be sexually active there is danger of constricting the introitus. Upward dissection under the posterior vaginal wall enables the vaginal mucosa to be drawn down to the perineal skin and sutured from side to side thus laying the introitus more open (Woodruff et al, 1981) (Figure 5–1). If the excision of perineal skin is extensive, it may be necessary to construct skin flaps to cover the dead space (Figure 5–2).

Early postoperative complications include bleeding and pain. Severe bleeding may require that the incision be reopened. If specific bleeding vessels can be found, they are ligated. More often no specific bleeding point can be seen. Then, through and through large mattress sutures of vicryl as well as packing the vagina to give pressure is the best approach. Later, bruising of the skin due to subcutaneous bleeding is common but does not require specific treatment. Pain can best be controlled by ice packs and analgesics.

The main late complication is stricture of the introitus resulting in dyspareunia. This can be treated medically by dilatation (Rock and Jones, 1984). In the older woman the use of oral or intravaginal estrogens may be useful. Surgically, introital constriction may be managed by adequate undermining of the posterior vaginal wall and pulling it down to evert the introitus. As indicated earlier, this is the primary technique that is most likely to prevent this complication.

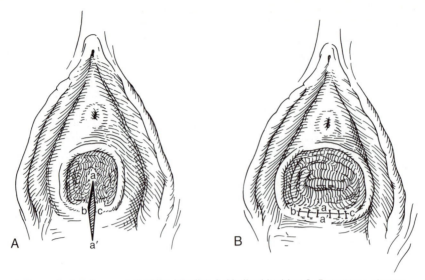

Figure 5–1. Enlargement of the introitus. A, Vertical incision. B, Transverse closure.

Specific Vulvar Organs

BARTHOLIN'S GLANDS

Bartholin's glands are located on either side of the introitus at 4 and 8 o'clock. They are particularly liable to infection with a variety of agents, especially *E. coli* and *N. gonorrhoeae*. Infection results in obstruction of the main duct and formation of a cyst or abscess. Other ab-

normalities of the gland are rare and include benign tumors and carcinoma (see Chapter 7).

Acute abscesses of Bartholin's glands require drainage. This is most easily done by incision under local (or general) anesthesia. The complications of the procedure include hemorrhage at the time of operation, and, later, recurrent abscess. The danger of the former is greater during pregnancy, and excision of Bartholin's

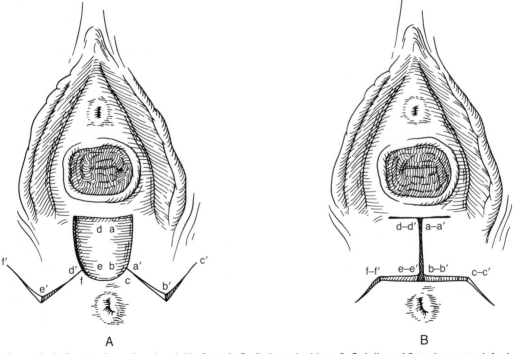

Figure 5–2. Construction of perineal skin flaps. A, Preliminary incisions. B, Rotation of flaps to cover defect.

glands should usually be avoided at this time. Hemorrhage necessitates finding the bleeding vessel and ligating it. If this is not possible packing may be used (see earlier discussion). Recurrent abscesses may be prevented by making a sufficiently large vertical incision through the vaginal mucosa, not the vulvar skin, and breaking up any loculations within the cavity with a finger or a curved instrument.

A more satisfactory way of dealing with an acute or subacute abscess or cyst of Bartholin's gland is by marsupialization. This involves making a vertical incision into the cyst over its medial or vaginal aspect and sewing the lining of the cyst to the vaginal mucosa and skin all around the opening with interrupted absorbable sutures. The complications of marsupialization include those common to other operations on the vulva, i.e., hemorrhage or injury to neighboring structures. Infection may recur, sometimes due to inadequate opening of the cyst or abscess. In this case complete surgical excision of the gland is necessary. Inevitably a cavity persists after marsupialization, often for a long time. This usually causes no symptoms since it has a wide mouth and squamous metaplasia occurs in the lining cells. The effect of marsupialization may also be achieved by inserting a balloon catheter into the cavity and allowing it to remain for four to six weeks (Word, 1964). There appear to be no complications to this technique except the continued presence of the slightly protruding catheter.

Perineal Scars

Repair of the vaginal outlet may be indicated for constriction of the introitus following previous vaginal operations, perineal procedures or extensive destruction of condylomata. This can be done by undermining the posterior wall and suturing it to the perineal skin so as to evert the introitus (see earlier discussion), or by the use of a Z-plasty (Figure 5–3).

Complications of such operations include rectovaginal fistula, fecal incontinence with loss of anal sphincter function, recurrence of scar tissue and dyspareunia. Most of these complications can be avoided by careful preoperative evaluation. Special precautions include investigation of infection by appropriate smears and cultures, determination of dysplasia by colposcopy and biopsy and attention to the emotional factors related to dyspareunia. Often medical and sometimes psychologic therapy is indicated prior to attempting surgical reconstruction of

the introitus. At operation the most important thing is to free the posterior wall of the vagina as far up as is necessary to lay open the introitus. Care must be taken to avoid injuring the anal sphincter, and if the perineal muscles are closed across the midline, closure should be done loosely so as to avoid a "bridge" of suture and tissue just inside the introitus. For repair of rectovaginal fistula or torn anal sphincter see page 89.

Circumcision

Female circumcision is not usually performed in developed countries, nor is there any therapeutic indication for it except as part of a vulvectomy performed for malignant or premalignant lesions. However, in developing countries and especially in Africa it is often performed in a ritualistic fashion in childhood or adolescence by medically untrained personnel. The procedure may consist of excision of the clitoris, the labia minora and the labia majora in part or in toto and the tissues may then be sewn together (infibulation). Subsequently the vulva heals leaving only a tiny opening for urine and menstrual fluid. Over 25% of women subjected to the more severe forms of circumcision suffer serious physical complications (Cutner, 1985). They include initial hemorrhage and/or shock, urinary retention, infection, injury to neighboring structures (urethra, rectum), scar and keloid formation, inclusion dermoid (usually in the region of the clitoris), difficulty with first coitus, dyspareunia, possible infertility and outlet obstruction at the time of delivery, requiring an extensive episiotomy. Treatment of these complications usually requires separation of the labia and reconstruction of the introitus as well as is possible in the individual case. Prevention involves discontinuation of the practice of female circumcision.

Urethra

The external urinary meatus may be considered part of the vulva since it is visible on inspection of the external genitalia. Operations on the external urinary meatus for acquired conditions are not common. They include those performed for urethral caruncle, prolapse of the urethra and cyst or abscess of the periurethral glands (Skene's glands) and consist of excision or, in the case of caruncle, destruction by fulguration, cryosurgery or laser. The main

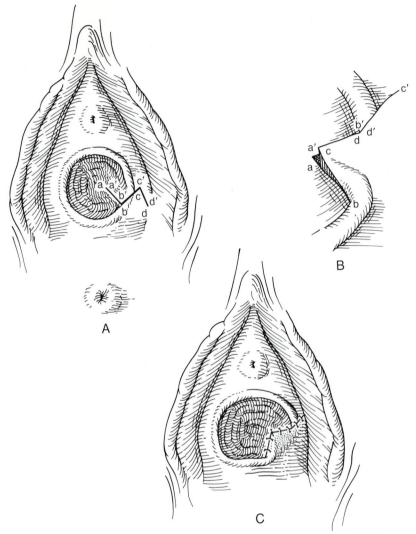

Figure 5–3. *Introital Z-plasty.* A, *Z-type incision.* B, *Transposition of flaps.* C, *Closure.*

complications include (1) removal of excess urethra (more than one half), with resulting incontinence, (2) stricture of the meatus and (3) urethrovaginal fistula.

The first may be very difficult to treat, although lengthening the urethra and/or a sling procedure may be tried (see Chapter 6). The second can be avoided by excision of no more than half of the circumference of the meatus. If it occurs, repeated dilatations are necessary, or the scar at the meatus may be excised and the urethra everted and sutured to the vaginal mucosa. The third complication, urethrovaginal fistula, can be avoided by including only the distal part of the urethra in the procedure. Its management is discussed in a later section and in Chapter 6.

Congenital Anomalies

IMPERFORATE HYMEN

Hymenotomy (or hymenectomy) may be performed when there is a congenital complete or nearly complete occlusion of the introitus by a hymeneal membrane. In infants, complete closure may lead, together with labial agglutination, to retention of fluid (hydrocolpos). In the adolescent girl menstrual fluid may be retained in the vagina and uterus (hematocolpos/hematometra).

In infants and young children (up to about 6 years of age) with hydrocolpos the local use of estrogen cream may permit the epithelium to mature and the labia to separate spontaneously. If this does not occur, simple surgical division followed by administration of estrogens is satisfactory. Gonorrhea or sexual abuse must be excluded.

In older girls with hematocolpos the hymen may be opened by cruciate incision or excision. Complications include infections of the upper genital tract and reocclusion. The former may be avoided by doing the minimal procedure, i.e., opening the hymen only, and by using prophylactic antibiotics such as a cephalosporin. The latter may be prevented by suturing the hymen open with fine absorbable sutures placed transversely. The retention of blood within the uterus and tubes may also lead later to endometriosis.

If the diagnosis of a thick hymen is made prior to first coitus in the adolescent or adult woman, the hymen may be excised or may be incised in a anteroposterior direction and the edges sewn together transversely with absorbable sutures. Complications include pain and the emotional trauma associated with operations in this area. Postoperative discomfort is inevitable for one to several weeks and, therefore, if possible, the procedure should only be performed when there is really a thick membrane and when there can be some delay before first coitus. The use of graduated dilators, beginning a week or so after operation, may accustom the patient to stretching of the introitus.

OPERATIONS FOR AMBIGUOUS EXTERNAL GENITALIA

A description of the types of ambiguous genitalia, their underlying causes, so far as they are known, and their management is given by Dewhurst (1981). Since most of these children should be reared as females, almost all the operations used in these rare cases are designed to reduce the size of the clitoris, separate the urethra, vagina and anal canal and provide a vaginal opening large enough for coitus and, if feasible, for childbearing.

Immediate postoperative complications are those inherent in performing surgical procedures on children and adolescents and injuries to neighboring structures such as urethra, bladder and rectum. The principles of their management are covered in Chapter 4. Long-term complications arise primarily from decisions about the time and appropriateness of the procedure. For example, a decision about the sex of rearing must be made, if possible, early in neonatal life. If the child is to be reared as a female, removal of a large clitoris is important to the parents' and later to the child's feelings about her sex. Also important early in life may

be procedures to separate urinary and fecal streams and prevent infection. However, enlargement of the vaginal opening can be deferred until the child is 2 or 3 years old or even until puberty if the repair is likely to be difficult.

MALE TRANSSEXUALISM

Operations for male transsexuals are designed to remove the male external genitalia, relocate the urethra and create a new vagina. The procedures that can be used and their complications are described by Turner and co-workers (1978). Immediate complications are frequent. For example, the same authors report that of their last 20 treated patients, eight (40%) required further operative procedures. The most serious complications are rectovaginal fistula, urethrovaginal fistula and introital and vaginal stenosis. Management of the first two is described on pages 89 and 101, whereas the latter may require the ingenious use of rhomboid (Barnhill et al, 1983) (see Fig. 5–2) or other local skin flaps or a skin graft. Long-term results are generally reported as satisfactory in terms of adjustment of patients to the new gender. However, all authors advise extremely careful selection of patients with extensive social and psychologic evaluations before operation.

EXCISION OF NUCK'S HYDROCELE

A cyst of the canal of Nuck presents as a sac containing serous fluid in the anterior part of the labium majus. It is a remnant of the processus vaginalis and may be confused with a gonad or a cyst of Bartholin's gland. During excision it is important to determine if the peritoneal sac extends upward and to repair any associated inguinal hernia.

Other Operations

OPERATIONS FOR CHRONIC PRURITUS OF THE VULVA

Intractible pruritus has been treated by (1) subcutaneous injection of 0.1 to 0.3 ml of absolute alcohol at 1-cm intervals over the whole vulva and perineum or (2) incising the skin and subcutaneous tissue around the vulva and perineum so as to divide the nerves to the area.

Subcutaneous injection of alcohol is followed by local swelling and loss of skin sensation for two to four months (Ward and Sutherst, 1975). Blistering and cellulitis may occur if the alcohol has been injected intradermally rather than subcutaneously. Surgical undermining of the skin may result in loss of sensation but there are usually no other significant complications.

Failure of both procedures to relieve itching may occur in 10 to 20% of patients. This can be obviated by restricting the procedures only to those women who have been thoroughly investigated for any possible cause of pruritus and to careful spacing of alcohol injections or complete division of the subcutaneous tissue.

OPERATIONS ON THE VAGINA

Vaginal Hysterectomy

INTRODUCTION

Historically the primary reason for removing the uterus vaginally has been prolapse of the organ when it projects outside the introitus and causes significant symptoms. As familiarity with the technique of operation grew in the United States, especially after 1950, the indications for the procedure were broadened to include cervical intraepithelial neoplasia, dysfunctional uterine bleeding not responsive to conservative measures, leiomyomata of the uterus of small or even moderate size and other pelvic conditions. Moreover, it has become clear that vaginal hysterectomy, with or without vaginal wall repair, can be performed successfully in women in their seventies and eighties (Ellenbogen et al, 1981), thus avoiding the continued use of a pessary.

Comparisons between vaginal and abdominal hysterectomy are frequently made. In fact, in the past 20 years there have been several major reports comparing these procedures in regard to complications. These reports are reviewed in Chapter 6. However, the two operations are only in part comparable, since they should be performed for different reasons. However, in general, vaginal hysterectomy is subject to less major complications than abdominal hysterectomy in the form of intraperitoneal infection or intestinal obstruction and thromboembolism. However, infections of the vaginal cuff and urinary tract, although usually not severe, are more frequent after the vaginal operation, and bleeding from the major vessels or the vaginal cuff is more visible and may also be more common after vaginal than after abdominal hysterectomy.

Although details of the procedure vary somewhat, according to different authors, the operation usually includes the following steps:

1. Circumcision of the vaginal mucosa 2 to 3 cm above the lowest point of the cervix and below the attachment of the bladder.

2. Exposure of the peritoneum of the posterior cul-de-sac and its incision, permitting entry into the peritoneal cavity.

3. Division and ligation of the uterosacral ligaments.

4. Division of the broad ligaments in one or several bites, including ligation of the uterine arteries.

5. Exposure of the peritoneum of the anterior cul-de-sac and its incision.

6. Delivery of the fundus of the uterus, either posteriorly or anteriorly.

7. Division of the round and utero-ovarian ligaments and removal of the uterus.

8. Inspection and possible removal of the ovaries and tubes.

9. Closure of any enterocele present with or without suspension of the vaginal vault.

10. Closure of the peritoneum.

11. Closure of the vaginal mucosa.

INTRAOPERATIVE COMPLICATIONS

Intraoperative complications are best considered in connection with the steps described previously.

Step 1. Prior to incising the mucosa, the cervix is grasped with a tenaculum. Since considerable traction will be exerted on the cervix throughout the operation, there is a tendency for the tenaculum to be pulled off, tearing the cervix and causing bleeding. If a single-toothed tenaculum has been used, it should be replaced by a double-toothed tenaculum on one or both lips.

As the cervix is circumcised, several problems may occur. First, the incision may not be at the right depth to enable the bladder (in front) or the rectum (behind) to be pushed off easily by the operator's finger covered with a single layer of gauze. Second, bleeding may be noted. Third, entry into the bladder may be suspected or may actually have occurred. Dissecting in the right plane is largely a matter of experience and trial and error. Bleeding may be avoided by pushing the bladder up in the midline so as not to injure the vascular pillars. The lower edge of the bladder may be identified and possible injury avoided by inserting a small metal catheter through the urethra. If only the bladder muscle is injured, nothing need be done provided that the right plane can then be found and the bladder properly pushed up. The muscle is closed with a continuous layer of 30 chromic catgut or vicryl. If the bladder has actually been entered it should be dissected off the cervix. The bladder mucosa is then closed with a continuous inverting suture of 30 catgut or vicryl and the muscle is closed by a similar continuous suture.

Step 2. During exposure of the cul-de-sac and entry into the peritoneal cavity, bleeding may occur from the vaginal edge and the prerectal tissue. It can be decreased by pressure and by sewing the peritoneum to the vaginal mucosa with a single or continuous stitch. This may also help to identify the posterior edge of the peritoneum later in the operation.

Difficulty in entering the posterior cul-de-sac may be due to its being obliterated by conditions such as endometriosis, inflammatory disease or adhesions; these can often be appreciated by careful preoperative examination under anesthesia. Persistent and unsuccessful efforts to enter the peritoneal cavity may result in injury to the rectum or small intestine. It is best to try to identify the peritoneal bulge again and to reassess the site of the incision, making it anteriorly near the back of the uterus rather than posteriorly near the rectum. If this does not succeed, an attempt should than be made to enter the anterior cul-de-sac after pushing off the bladder (see Step 5).

If rectal injury is suspected, it must be identified and repaired. Fecal odor and the appearance of feces are the most characteristic signs. Rectal examination with an extra glove on the rectal hand may help. A malleable uterine sound may be passed either from the vaginal incision and felt in the rectum or passed through the rectum and seen in the vaginal field. If entry into the rectum is demonstrated, the hole should be closed in two layers with continuous 30 chromic catgut or vicryl sutures, one inverting the mucosa and one closing the muscularis. Broad spectrum antibiotics, such as a second generation cephalosporin, if not already being given prophylactically, should be started during the operation. If the injury is small, a diverting colostomy is not necessary. If there is major fecal contamination, diversion may be necessary.

Injury to the small intestine can be identified by a bile-colored and often profuse discharge that has little odor. If the opening into the small intestine can be clearly exposed and identified, it can be closed from the vaginal approach, using an inverting 30 catgut or vicryl suture through all layers and interrupted 30 silk sutures through the serosa and muscularis. If there is the least doubt about the feasibility of vaginal repair, the vaginal approach should be discontinued and the abdomen opened by a midline incision without delay. The intestine should be completely examined and the perforation appropriately closed (see Chapter 3). The hysterectomy should be completed (from above, if necessary) and any contemplated vaginal repair should be carried out only if the patient's condition permits.

Step 3. If the uterosacral ligaments are not identified and adequately ligated, the pelvic floor repair may be jeopardized. They may be difficult to find, especially in the older woman with considerable prolapse. Exposure and identification may be improved by initially pushing the vaginal mucosa up on each side of the cervix with a gauze-covered finger.

Step 4. Two major complications may occur during the division of the broad ligament, bleeding and injury to the ureter. Bleeding usually comes from the uterine artery either because it has been completely or partially divided without being clamped or because it has slipped out of a clamp. The first problem can be avoided by recognizing that the cervix is often long and that more than one bite may be needed to reach the uterine artery and also by not cutting beyond the end of the clamps. The second can be obviated by using suture ligatures. Some authors recommend both a ligature and a suture ligature on the uterine artery but this requires a bigger pedicle with more lateral dissection and increased possibility of injury to the ureter. When bleeding occurs the artery must be identified and clamped. This is relatively easy if it has been partially divided but more difficult if it has retracted. Deliberate haste and adequate exposure are important. It is essential to avoid blind clamping, particularly laterally, because of the danger of clamping the ureter. Angled clamps, such as a Mixter or Boettcher, are useful. If the site of bleeding cannot be identified and blood loss is significant, it may be necessary to make a vertical lower abdominal incision and identify and ligate the uterine artery at its origin from the anterior branch of the internal iliac artery.

Ureteral injury, by clamping, cutting or incising, occurs very rarely during vaginal hysterectomy. It is usually due to failure to dissect the bladder fully off the anterior surface of the uterus and to placing clamps too far laterally across the paracervical tissue. Injury may be difficult to recognize since it is often associated with poor exposure and may only be appreciated postoperatively. If it is suspected during the procedure, an attempt should be made to expose the ureter. Principles of repair developed from the procedure of radical vaginal hysterectomy are useful. From the vaginal approach the ureter loops down medial to the uterine artery. Its identification is facilitated by opening the anterior cul-de-sac (Step 5) and retracting the bladder upward and to the opposite side. The ureter can be palpated in its retroperitoneal course and exposed by cautious dissection across the bladder pillar 2 to 3 cm from its base. It can then be pushed upward and injury avoided. Even if an injury to the ureter is discovered, repair or reimplantation into the bladder from the vaginal approach should usually not be considered. It is best performed through an abdominal incision (see Chapter 3).

Steps 5 and 6. Steps 5 and 6 in vaginal hysterectomy carry the risk of injury to the bladder or intestine. This should be handled as described previously. Good exposure and dissecting close to the uterus help to avoid these injuries.

At this point in the operation it may be recognized that the uterus cannot be pulled down satisfactorily either because of adhesions to the fundus or because the uterus (and accompanying leiomyomata) are considerably larger than was anticipated. Prolonged and unsuccessful attempts to remove such a uterus vaginally tend to lead to excessive bleeding and injury to neighboring structures. When adhesions seem to be the problem, better exposure and easier removal of the uterus can be achieved by promptly changing to an abdominal approach. Large leiomyomata can be reduced in size by removing them individually or by morcellation. This involves excising successive wedge-shaped pieces of the anterior uterine wall and fundus. However, bleeding can be considerable, and if there is doubt about the ease of removal, it is better to avoid heroic efforts and use the abdominal approach.

Step 7. During step 7 the major complication is bleeding from the utero-ovarian ligaments. It is important to check for this before closing the peritoneum by using a long sponge in the pelvis to push the intestine back. Since the vessels may retract and exposure is difficult, it may occasionally be necessary to secure the bleeding at its source through an abdominal incision.

Step 8. Removal of the ovaries at the time of vaginal hysterectomy is feasible in 60 to 70% of cases according to Capen and associates (1983). The difficulty of exposing the ovary and its blood supply predisposes to the risk of injuring

the ureter and to hemorrhage from the infundibulopelvic ligament.

Steps 9, 10 and 11. Steps 9, 10 and 11 do not present major complications other than those described for the earlier stages of the operation. If an enterocele is closed by plication of the uterosacral ligaments and pelvic peritoneum, there is danger of including the ureter in the stitches if bites are taken too far laterally. However, this complication is unlikely to be recognized at the time of operation and will appear later (see Chapter 4).

IMMEDIATE POSTOPERATIVE COMPLICATIONS

The chief immediate postoperative (in the first 24 hours) complication of vaginal hysterectomy, apart from the respiratory and cardiac sequelae of anesthesia and/or operative blood loss, is hemorrhage. In the first few hours shock resulting from bleeding must be differentiated from that due to myocardial infarction, pulmonary embolism, pain or excessive sedation. Bleeding after vaginal hysterectomy, although it may occur intraabdominally, is more likely to be visible externally, especially if the peritoneum has been closed so as to externalize the stumps of the ligaments below it. Packing the vagina tightly with 2-inch plain or iodoform gauze may be tried if the patient's condition is stable and the bleeding is not severe. However, once it has been determined that significant bleeding is occurring vaginally, the patient should be anesthetized, put in the lithotomy position and prepared and draped. The vaginal cuff is exposed and inspected. Sometimes the bleeding point can be identified and controlled by hemostatic sutures of catgut or vicryl. If no definite bleeding point can be seen, blind sutures at the lateral part of the cuff are inadvisable, because of the danger of injury to the ureter. In many cases, however, if the bleeding has been sufficient to bring the patient to the operating room, it is sufficient to indicate abdominal exploration and ligation of the uterine or even the hypogastric arteries for its control. Postoperative bleeding occurring intra- or retroperitoneally is covered in Chapters 4 and 6.

EARLY POSTOPERATIVE COMPLICATIONS

Bleeding. A small amount of bleeding or bloody discharge is common after an otherwise uncomplicated vaginal hysterectomy. It usually appears from 5 to 10 days after operation and is related to the loosening or partial absorption of sutures. Rarely it may be followed by more severe bleeding; this is less common than severe bleeding occurring in the first 24 hours after operation. If such bleeding occurs, the patient should promptly be examined in the office or emergency room in the lithotomy position and with a good light and adequate equipment. After removal of clots, the suture line at the vaginal cuff should be inspected. Sometimes a specific arterial bleeding point can be clamped and ligated, although exposure may be difficult. If the bleeding appears to be coming from above the cuff and to be profuse, laparotomy is indicated so as to ligate specific bleeding vessels. When the bleeding is in the form of a general ooze from the cuff, the vagina should be firmly packed with 2-inch plain or iodoform gauze. If sufficient pressure is used, the patient may not be able to void, so an indwelling catheter is necessary together with appropriate urinary antibiotics (see Chapter 4). Packing should be left in no more than 24 hours and should be removed in the morning (not at night). If the initial packing does not control the bleeding or if profuse bleeding recurs after removal of the pack, a second pack should generally not be inserted but laparotomy performed and the uterine, the ovarian or, if necessary, the hypogastric arteries should be ligated.

Urinary Tract. Urinary tract problems are covered in Chapter 4. They are particularly likely to occur after vaginal hysterectomy, especially if it is combined with anterior colporrhaphy. This is because (1) the bladder and urethra may be traumatized during the operation; (2) a catheter may be used, not only during operation but for a varying time afterwards; and (3) the position of the urethra and urethrovesical junction may be altered, especially when anterior colporrhaphy is performed.

Failure of the patient to void successfully after removal of a urethral catheter is common (see Chapter 4). If suprapubic drainage (Ingram, 1975) is instituted, the necessity for repeated catheterization is usually eliminated because bladder function can be tested by clamping the suprapubic tube. Moreover, in a comparison between suprapubic and vaginal drainage, Wiser and co-workers (1974) showed that the former was associated with decreased incidence of urinary tract infections, shorter hospitalization, increased ease of care by ward personnel and greater patient comfort. The various suprapubic catheters now available and the techniques of insertion and management are described by Montz and Stanton (1985). Sequelae include hematuria (usually not severe) for the first day or two or extravasation of urine outside the bladder, usually in the space of Retzius. The former usually responds to intermittent irrigation with 1% acetic acid. The latter is detected by the patient's complaints of suprapubic pain and extravasation of radiopaque dye injected through the catheter. If the suprapubic tube fails to drain the bladder adequately, transurethral drainage by Foley catheter should be instituted promptly. Problems with suprapubic drainage may be obviated by inserting the trochar and catheter prior to operation and with the bladder full.

Infection. Vaginal hysterectomy involves operating in a potentially infected area, the vagina, which cannot be rendered sterile by mechanical scrubbing or the use of antiseptic solutions. In addition, the operation results in a potential dead space and some necrotic tissue distal to the ligatures on the pedicles of the ligaments. The use of vasoconstrictors, specifically epinephrine, as the cuff is being circumcised (Step 1) may predispose to infection, according to a randomized prospective study reported by England and co-workers (1983). Postoperative infection may occur in as many as 50% of patients (see Chapter 6), depending upon the associated procedures, the blood loss, the length of the operation and the skill of the surgeon. Such infection is usually characterized by fever not attributable to other causes such as urinary tract infection. It may begin immediately after operation, is usually of low grade and is not accompanied by other symptoms except possibly some pelvic discomfort. Initial examination may show only induration at the suture line. This may resolve slowly with discharge of thin purulent material, may progress into an abscess in the cuff or may rarely develop into a major pelvic infection.

Initial management should be expectant. It consists of obtaining a culture of the vaginal cuff and administering a broad spectrum antibiotic such as a second generation cephalosporin. If the culture indicates bacteria that are not sensitive to cephalosporins and the patient's fever and cuff induration persist, the antibiotics should be changed appropriately. The temptation to explore the cuff with an instrument should be resisted at first, since spontaneous drainage usually occurs and injury or bleeding may be caused by blind probing. If a definite fluctuant abscess develops, it should be opened from below if possible and appropriate drains should be inserted and fixed to the vagina so as to remain in place for three to five days. If the infection appears to be spreading upward and a higher pelvic mass is palpable, an ovarian abscess may be suspected if the ovary(ies) have not been removed (see Chapter 4 for the diagnosis of an abscess). This may require a laparotomy, excision of the abscess and drainage of the peritoneal cavity.

Prophylactic antibiotics such as cephalosporins appear to reduce cuff infections. Various regimens have been reported, usually consisting of one dose of a second generation cephalosporin preoperatively and continuing doses for 12 to 24 hours postoperatively. Also, T-tube drainage through the cuff for 48 hours may be effective (Swartz and Tanaree, 1976), although the continued presence of a foreign body may lead to reinfection and possible delay in closure of the vaginal vault.

Fistulas. Vesicovaginal, rectovaginal, urethrovaginal or even enterovaginal fistulas may occur in the intermediate postoperative period. They are considered in Chapter 4.

LATE POSTOPERATIVE COMPLICATIONS

Vaginal Vault. Complications in the vaginal vault include granulation tissue, prolapsed Fallopian tube, endometriosis or ectopic pregnancy. These are covered in Chapter 6.

Pelvic Relaxation. Cystocele and rectocele may become more prominent or may develop after vaginal hysterectomy. Enterocele or prolapse of the vaginal vault occasionally follows vaginal hysterectomy, giving the patient the sensation of a protruding mass. The diagnosis is apparent on pelvic examination. Management is discussed in a later section.

The prolapsed vagina or enterocele may also contain intestine or very rarely may rupture. When this occurs, prompt reduction of the intestine by the abdominal approach is indicated, together with an attempt to repair the vaginal vault as well as possible.

Bladder and Rectum. Chronic urinary tract infection, obstruction or fistulae may result in the late postoperative period, but are more common when anterior or posterior repair accompanies the procedure. Their management is described in Chapter 4.

Sexual Sequelae. There is a dearth of information on the sexual effects of vaginal hysterectomy. On theoretical grounds there should be no change in sexual lubrication, since this occurs by transudation through the vaginal wall

and not from the cervical glands. On the other hand, the suture line at the apex of the vagina and the associated scarring may prevent the ballooning of the top of the vagina, which is reported to occur during coitus, and may result in some constriction of the vagina. Also, the mere fact of an operative procedure on the sexual organs and the fear of harming the repair may alter the patient's sexual response. Craig and Jackson (1975) found in a small series that intercourse was more satisfactory for 86% of 49 patients (out of 69 queried) who had had vaginal hysterectomy.

Vaginal Repairs

ANTERIOR COLPORRHAPHY

Anterior colporrhaphy is performed to correct cystocele and/or urethrocele and stress incontinence related to these conditions. Stress incontinence may occur without vaginal relaxation. In that case an abdominal or combined abdominal and vaginal approach is needed. These procedures are covered in Chapter 6. The principles of anterior colporrhaphy by the vaginal route include:

1. Dividing the vaginal mucosa in the midline from the free anterior edge of the vagina, which was circumcised as the first step in the vaginal hysterectomy or, if no hysterectomy was performed, from just above the cervix to about 1 cm below the external urethral meatus.

2. Dissecting the fascia off the vaginal mucosa.

3. Plicating the fascia below the bladder, including suspension of the urethro-vesical angle with the so-called Kelly stitch to correct or maintain that angle.

4. Excising the excess vaginal mucosa and closing it.

During operation the major complications are bleeding and injury to the bladder or urethra. Bleeding usually occurs because the plane between the mucosa and the fascia is not dissected properly or because dissection is carried too far laterally under the pubic bone. Bleeding can be controlled by ligature or cautery. Injury to the bladder is covered previously (page 122). Injury to the urethra should be repaired immediately. The hole is identified by inserting a Foley catheter through the urethra into the bladder. The cut edges of the urethra are identified and closed with interrupted 30 catgut or vicryl sutures. The fascial repair is then completed in the usual manner. The indwelling catheter should remain in place for seven days to splint the repaired urethra, and appropriate antibiotics should be given.

Important early postoperative complications of anterior colporrhaphy include bleeding, breakdown of the repair and urinary retention. Bleeding may occur soon after the operation or 5 to 10 days later. It is more likely to take the form of a hematoma under the suture line rather than a sudden external hemorrhage. It should be treated conservatively and antibiotics given. The hematoma will eventually drain. Breakdown of the suture line usually results in recurrence of the cystocele and/or urethrocele. Secondary repair is difficult but may be attempted at least six months postoperatively, after the local reaction has subsided. Urinary retention may be caused by the urethro-vesical angle suture being placed too tightly. If an indwelling urethral catheter is used, it may have to be left in place for some time, even after the patient goes home. If suprapubic drainage is used, sounding the urethra may help to determine the degree of constriction. Further urethral dilatation may then be necessary. Occasionally it may be necessary to cut the obstructive sutures (under anesthesia). Secondary repair will then have to await healing, usually at least three months.

Late complications of anterior colporrhaphy include stress incontinence and shortness of the anterior vaginal wall, the latter adversely affecting coitus. Stress incontinence may be due to obliteration of the posterior urethro-vesical angle. This requires appropriate work-up, as in patients who were not operated on, to distinguish between urethral sphincter incompetence, detrusor instability, neuropathy or other causes. Special diagnostic tests of value include urethrocystoscopy, uroflowmetry, cystometry, urethral pressure measurements and radiologic study (Stanton, 1980). Some improvement in stress incontinence can be expected from the use of perineal muscle exercises (Kegel exercises) with biofeedback (Burgio et al, 1986). In older women stress and urgency incontinence can be improved by bladder-sphincter biofeedback and toileting skills training (Burgio et al, 1985). Testing of the circumvaginal muscles may be helpful (Worth et al, 1986). However, management often requires suprapubic vesico-urethral suspension (see Chapter 6). Occasionally the vagina may be shortened and constricted by the repair, leading to dyspareunia. Some lengthening may be possible by application of the Z-plasty principle (see Fig. 5–3) within the vagina. In addition, the patients may need counselling in regard to coitus.

POSTERIOR COLPORRHAPHY, PERINEORRHAPHY AND ENTEROCELE REPAIR

Operations for relaxation of the posterior vaginal wall include repair of enterocele, rectocele or relaxed vaginal outlet. One or all of these may be performed, depending on the individual anatomic deformity and the patient's symptoms. They may accompany vaginal hysterectomy or be performed separately. The steps of the procedure, if all three parts are performed at once, are as follows:

1. Transverse incision of the mucocutaneous junction at the fourchette.

2. Separation of the vaginal mucosa from the anterior wall of the rectum, incising it vertically as high as is necessary for the type of repair needed.

3. Separation of the vaginal mucosa laterally from the rectum.

4. Isolation of the enterocele sac.

5. Excision and closure of the enterocele sac.

6. Provision of support for the enterocele repair by closing the remnants of the uterosacral ligaments beneath the sac or by plication of the cul-de-sac (McCall, 1957).

7. Plication of the fascia over the rectocele and possible fixation to the vaginal apex.

8. Closure of the fascia of the levator muscles across the midline.

9. Closure of the perineal muscles.

10. Excision of excess vaginal mucosa.

11. Closure of the vaginal mucosa and perineum.

During the operation the main complications are bleeding and injury to the rectum. The former usually occurs as a result of dissecting too far laterally and entering a paravaginal venous plexus (Step 3). Avoiding the latter involves considerable care in dissecting the vagina off the rectum (Step 2), since the septum is often thin and scarred. When rectal injury is suspected and confirmed by a finger in the rectum, the rectal mucosa should be repaired by a continuous inverting suture of 30 chromic catgut or vicryl and the posterior repair continued in the usual manner. Postoperative antibiotics and stool softeners should be given.

Early postoperative complications consist of pain, breakdown of the incision, rectovaginal fistula and adhesions at the vaginal apex. The perineal stitches often cause pain. This can be lessened by using a subcuticular stitch and applying ice to the perineum intermittently for the first 24 to 48 hours. Breakdown of the incision should be treated conservatively with Sitz baths; secondary repair should be delayed for at least three months. Rectovaginal fistula may develop when the incision breaks down or as a result of the rectal mucosa being included in a stitch; this can be avoided by rectal examination during or after the repair. Repair of a rectovaginal fistula is covered in Chapter 4. Adhesions at the vaginal apex can be avoided by not carrying the vaginal incision too high so that the stitches and tissue at the top of the posterior wall of the vagina do not adhere to the stitches involved in the vaginal hysterectomy or anterior repair. If such adhesions develop, they will need to be separated on one or more occasions, and dilatation of the top of the vagina may be required.

Late complications relate primarily to sexual dysfunction. Francis and Jeffcoate (1961) noted dyspareunia in 57 of 140 women (41%) who had had anterior and posterior colporrhaphy combined with a Manchester operation or vaginal hysterectomy. The cause was a tight introitus and narrow vagina in 30, a long perineum in two, stenosis of the upper vagina in three and shortening of the vagina in two. In 20 women emotional factors appeared to be important. These could be related to the initial discomfort of coitus and fear of damaging the repair, both leading later, especially in the older woman, to contracture of the vagina as a result of lack of coitus. These dismal results probably do not apply universally, particularly in younger women. However, they do point out the importance of performing colpoperineorrhaphy only when strict indications are present and of leaving an introitus of adequate width and a vagina of sufficient length without a bridge of skin or muscle at the introitus.

ENTEROCELE AND PROLAPSE OF THE VAGINA

A small enterocele may be present as part of the pelvic relaxation syndrome. It should be repaired at the time of the vaginal hysterectomy or other procedure. In this case, excision of the sac, plication of the uterosacral ligaments or fixation of the vaginal vault can be performed by the McCall technique (1957) or a modification thereof.

Larger enterocele and prolapse or eversion of the vaginal vault are important late complications of hysterectomy, both abdominal and vaginal. They present special problems in management. If sexual function is not desired, colpectomy or colpocleisis may be appropriate (see page 129). If sexual function is important, maintenance of adequate length and width of the vagina is necessary in addition to repair of the enterocele and suspension of the vaginal vault.

Much has been written about the repair of enterocele and vaginal vault prolapse. It is clear that no one technique is applicable to all cases, and that the type of procedure and the order in which procedures are performed have to be determined for the individual patient. Symmonds and associates (1981) believe that vaginal repair can be carried out satisfactorily in the great majority of cases. Of 160 patients so managed and followed over five years only 18 (11%) had failures or poor results, and in seven of these a second operation was successful. The essentials of the vaginal approach are to resect the enterocele sac, repair the cul-de-sac after the method of McCall (1957), excise a wedge of posterior vaginal wall and repair any associated cystocele and/or rectocele. An additional technique for vaginal support, which consists of fixing the vagina to the (right) sacrospinous ligament, can also be used. Nichols (1982) reported 97% success with this method in 163 patients. The abdominal approach is indicated primarily to suspend the vagina if there is a large prolapse, if the supporting structures are weak and attenuated and to maintain vaginal length and adequate sexual function. Several techniques have been described. First, the cul-de-sac can be closed with a series of purse-string sutures of non-absorbable material (Moschcowitz's technique). Second, the vagina may be fixed to the sacrum with a mersilene strip sewn from the back of the vagina to the front of the sacrum at the level of S2 to S3. Third, a strip of fascia lata may be used to attach the vaginal vault to the rectus muscle anteriorly (Beecham and Beecham, 1973). Fourth, the levator muscles may be sewn to the vagina, after exposure of the ureters, according to the method described by Zacharin and Hamilton (1980). When a combined vaginal and abdominal approach is indicated because of associated cystocele and/or rectocele, Addison and coworkers (1985) point out that vaginal repair should be performed first, since suspension of the vagina makes correction of cystocele and rectocele less accessible and more difficult. When the anterior or posterior wall relaxation is less marked, abdominal suspension of the vagina may reduce or even obliterate such weaknesses and should therefore be performed first. If stress incontinence is a problem, it may be advisable to combine the previously described procedures with a urethropexy.

Complications of the various procedures for repair of enterocele and the prolapsed vaginal vault, except for those associated with the greater age of many of these patients, are reported to be relatively minor. The chief dangers are injury to the rectum or bladder, primarily from the vaginal approach, and injury to the ureter from both approaches. A short vagina may result from the vaginal approach, whereas nerve damage was reported in two of 163 patients receiving transvaginal sacrospinous fixation (Nichols, 1982).

COLPOCLEISIS

Closure of the vagina is a useful and relatively simple solution to symptomatic pelvic relaxation in the older woman for whom intercourse is not a present or future possibility. This may involve colpectomy or partial colpocleisis. Colpectomy may be performed in conjunction with hysterectomy or as a separate procedure if the uterus has already been removed. If the uterus is still present a partial colpocleisis (Le Fort operation) is necessary.

In total colpectomy the vaginal mucosa is excised and the fascia of the anterior and posterior walls of the vagina is closed with a series of purse-string absorbable sutures or transverse interrupted sutures from above downward.

In partial colpocleisis rectangular pieces of vagina are removed from the anterior and posterior walls and the denuded area is closed with two layers of transverse interrupted sutures to the fascia and one to the mucosa, leaving lateral channels for the egress of fluid from the uterine cavity.

Less information is available about the complications of colpectomy than of partial colpocleisis. Since both procedures are performed rarely, they can be considered together in terms of their complications. Major intraoperative complications have not been reported. During the early postoperative period, the age of the patients and their general condition make them more prone to acute cardiovascular, thromboembolic and respiratory accidents. The addition of hysterectomy to colpectomy adds considerably to this risk. Goldman and co-workers (1981) reported that urinary retention occurred in 9%, urinary infection in 14% and complications of wound healing (usually superficial) in

5% of 118 Le Fort operations. These authors emphasized the use of postoperative estrogens to improve healing.

Late complications include (1) recurrence of prolapse, (2) urinary incontinence and (3) the difficulty of handling subsequent uterine disorders (after partial colpocleisis). Recurrence of prolapse after colpectomy may be very difficult to manage except by pessary and pad. After partial colpocleisis, hysterectomy and colpectomy may be performed if the patient's general condition is satisfactory. Urinary incontinence may have to be solved by use of absorbent pads or an indwelling catheter. It is caused by distortion of the urethro-vesical junction and may be minimized by adequate perineorrhaphy and by stopping the excision of the vaginal mucosa at least 2 cm above the external urethral meatus. Bleeding from the lateral vaginal channels after partial colpocleisis associated with uterine disorders presents a difficult problem in diagnosis and may require the colpocleisis to be taken down so that diagnostic studies and definitive procedures such as a hysterectomy may be performed.

Congenital Anomalies of the Vagina

Vaginal anomalies that require surgical correction include (1) transverse septa, partial agenesis or atresia, (2) complete agenesis and (3) mesonephric and paramesonephric duct cysts.

TRANSVERSE SEPTA AND PARTIAL AGENESIS

Transverse septa may occur at any level of the vagina and may be partial or complete. If the septum is partial and there is no obstruction to the flow of menstrual blood, the anomaly may not be noticed until coitus is experienced or a pelvic examination performed. When a portion of the vagina has failed to develop (complete septum) and the uterus and cervix are present, menstrual blood may be retained above the constriction. Regular cyclic pain and progressive dilatation of the upper vagina and upper genital tract may then occur.

Correction of a transverse vaginal septum is discussed by Rock and co-workers (1982). It is best performed at puberty or later. The septum is excised and the vaginal mucosa sewn transversely. A vaginal mold is then inserted and used continuously or intermittently for at least six weeks. When a considerable portion of the vagina is atretic, dissection through it to expose the cervix may be very difficult and entry into the bladder or rectum is a serious hazard. It is usually not possible to suture the upper and lower vaginal mucosa together without greatly shortening the vagina. Skin grafts do not take well in this area. However, growth of the epithelium across the deficit does occur if a mold is left in place continuously. Such a mold must have a canal in the center for the escape of menstrual blood.

Early and late complications of operation for transverse vaginal septum or atresia consist primarily of partial or complete closure of the newly created tract by fibrosis with resultant dyspareunia or obstruction to menstruation. Surgical treatment may be an extremely onerous task because of the difficulty, first, of establishing an adequate vaginal passage through the mass of scar tissue without injuring the bladder or rectum, especially if the interval since the primary operation has been long, and second, maintaining patency by skin graft or obturator. Failure of a secondary operation may make hysterectomy necessary. Pressure by the Ingram technique (1982) may be worth trying if the patient has partial closure and is willing to persist with the regimen.

COMPLETE AGENESIS

Complete absence of the vagina may be congenital or may result from exenterative procedures; the latter are covered in Chapter 7. Congenital agenesis is often associated with absence of the uterus and anomalies of the urinary tract, but with otherwise normal female development. A neovagina may be created by:

1. Pressure indentation by the classical Frank technique or by the Ingram modification (1982).

2. Surgical creation of a space between the bladder and rectum and insertion of a mold covered by a split-thickness skin graft (McIndoe, 1950). More recently amnion has been used to cover the mold (Morton and Dewhurst, 1986).

3. Vulvovaginoplasty after the method of Williams (1964).

4. Other methods, including the use of intestine and peritoneoplasty.

Ingram (1982) has reported an 83% success rate with his technique. No complications were noted except failure due to the patient's lack of sustained motivation.

Intraoperative complications of the McIndoe procedure include:

1. The difficulty in obtaining an appropriate skin graft, particularly if the patient expects to expose the skin of the buttock or thigh.

2. Injury to bladder or rectum.

3. Bleeding laterally and deep in the vaginal space. This must be controlled before the graft is inserted.

4. Use of an inappropriately heavy mold. Foam rubber covered by two condoms appears best.

Postoperative complications were reported by Rock and associates (1983) in 79 cases to have been minor and to have occurred in 21 patients (26%). They included granulation tissue resulting from variable graft loss in 19 patients and vaginal hematoma with infection in two. Evans and co-workers (1981), in a series of 160 operations, noted the occasional occurrence of rectovaginal, vesicovaginal and urethrovaginal fistulas; most of these followed premature resumption of sexual activity by the patients and occurred in the early part of the study. The same authors point out that fistula formation and other complications were more frequent in patients in whom a previous attempt to construct a neovagina had failed. Rarely carcinoma has been found to arise in the new vagina. Stenosis of the new vagina may occur unless dilatation is continued. Various forms and molds to maintain patency are described by Rock and Jonas (1984).

In the Williams vulvovaginoplasty the labia are used to form an external pouch. With the patient in the lithotomy position the long axis of this pouch initially lies in an anteroposterior direction, at a right angle to that of the normal vagina. It is a relatively simple procedure, and it is particularly useful when a vaginal dimple is already present (Fig. 5–4). Intraoperative complications include the difficulty of obtaining sufficient vaginal length when the perineal body is short; this may result in the urethral meatus being "hidden" by the external wall of the pouch. Also, when the labia are not well developed, it may be difficult to obtain enough tissue to create a sufficiently wide pouch. Early postoperative complications include the collection of secretions and/or urine within the pouch, infection and breakdown of the incision. It has been suggested that the first complication may be obviated by leaving a small opening at the base of the neovagina, but this may defeat the purpose of creating an adequate tube and predispose to breakdown of the incision. Irrigation with dilute hydrogen peroxide may be helpful. Data on the late results of vulvovaginoplasty are scanty. With dilatation and coitus the axis

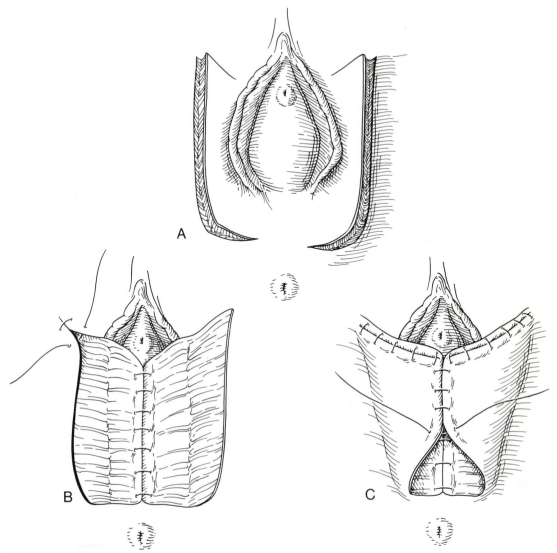

Figure 5–4. Construction of a neovagina from the labia. A, Labial incisions. B, Labial skin folded in to form a tube. C, External skin layer closed.

of the neovagina rapidly approaches normal. Adequate motivation on the part of the patient is needed for this. The presence of hair-producing skin on the inside of the neovagina may also present some problems; they are, however, largely unavoidable, since the skin used for the pouch is necessarily of this type. Stenosis does not seem to occur even if the neovagina is not used.

The use of isolated tubes of small or large intestine to create a neovagina has been reported in the past. These procedures minimize fibrosis of the neovagina, and the naturally occurring columnar epithelium changes into stratified squamous epithelium with dilatation and coitus. But the procedure itself is extensive, and the intestinal resection carries an unacceptable risk compared with operations performed from the perineal approach.

Peritoneoplasty, according to the method of Davydov and reported in one case by Rothman in the United States (1972), has been reported to be successful; the peritoneal lining of the neovagina is eventually converted to squamous epithelium and there is relatively little chance of stenosis. The problem, however, whether the perineal or a combined abdominoperineal approach is used, is to find and free sufficient peritoneum from the pelvic floor to obtain adequate length of the neovagina, and at the same time to avoid drawing tubes and ovaries into or close to the top of the neovagina.

CONGENITAL CYSTS

Mesonephric (Gartner's) duct cysts may become large, block the vagina and require removal. During excision it may be difficult to dissect the cyst from the vaginal wall. Vaginal constriction may occur if too much mucosa is removed. Transverse closure or vertical relaxing incisions may be useful.

Other

HISTORIC OPERATIONS FOR PELVIC RELAXATION

The Spalding-Richardson (composite) operation and the Watkins transposition operation are examples of procedures used in the early part of the 20th century to correct pelvic relaxation. The former, which required amputation of the cervix and part of the fundus and the middle part of the uterus after ablation of the endometrium, combined with anterior and posterior colporrhaphy, was used to support the apex of the vagina. The latter involved transposing the whole of the uterus anteriorly between the vaginal mucosa and the bladder. The most serious long-term complication of these operations was the later development of disease of the remaining uterine fundus. They are not performed nowadays and the end results are seldom seen. They have been superseded by vaginal hysterectomy.

The Manchester (Donald-Fothergill) operation has had a wide and more prolonged use, especially in England where it originated. In principle it involves amputating the lower part of the cervix (trachelectomy) and suturing the stumps of the divided cardinal ligaments to the front of the remaining cervix. The external os is reconstructed by inverting the vaginal mucosa with Sturmdorf's sutures (see later section), and repair is completed by anterior colporrhaphy with or without posterior colporrhaphy. This procedure, too, has been almost completely replaced by vaginal hysterectomy because (1) pregnancy and labor are complicated by the shortened and possibly incompetent cervix, (2) the support given by the attenuated cardinal ligaments is poor and (3) cervical stenosis and later intrauterine disease can be troublesome.

CULDOTOMY

Incision or puncture of the posterior fornix of the vagina has been used for:

1. Inspection of the peritoneal cavity (culdoscopy).
2. Operations on the tubes and neighboring organs (tubal ligation, division of uterosacral ligaments for dyspareunia, removal of ectopic pregnancy or appendectomy).
3. Aspiration of peritoneal fluid.
4. Aspiration or needle biopsy of pelvic masses.
5. Drainage of a pelvic abscess.

Culdoscopy provides a limited view of the peritoneal cavity and has been superseded by laparoscopy.

Tubal ligation is still performed through the vagina by some gynecologists (see Chapter 6). However, the difficulty of exposure has resulted in discontinuation of vaginal procedures to remove organs other than the uterus and, at the same operation, tubes and ovaries. Laparoscopy and, if necessary, laparotomy have taken their place.

Culdocentesis has an important place in the diagnosis of blood, fluid or pus in the peritoneal cavity. It is also used to aspirate pelvic masses for cytologic study or to obtain tissue for histologic examination. The complications of these procedures are covered in Chapter 12.

Culdotomy has been chiefly used for drainage of a pelvic abscess. It is properly performed when the abscess is in the midline, is fluctuant and is dissecting the rectovaginal septum. A transverse incision is made at the fluctuant area, the abscess is explored to break down adhesions and drainage is obtained through a self-retaining catheter or drains sutured to the vaginal mucosa. The intraoperative complication of failing to obtain pus can be avoided by selecting only appropriate patients for the procedure. Postoperatively, fever and evidence of continued abscess by physical examination and/or ultrasonography is an indication for exploratory laparotomy with an attempt at removal of the abscess and usually the pelvic organs together with appropriate drainage. Development of signs of peritoneal irritation following culdotomy suggests leakage of pus into the peritoneal cavity and requires prompt laparotomy. Late complications may include recrudescence of pelvic inflammatory disease, requiring reoperation, or inability to conceive. This topic has recently been reviewed by Rivlin (1983).

URETHRAL OPERATIONS

Diverticulectomy. Urethral diverticula vary in size and may be multiple. Larger ones may give symptoms of dysuria, the presence of a lump in the vagina, dyspareunia and discharge of urine or pus with pressure upward on the anterior vaginal wall or with coitus. Repeated bladder infections may occur. The principles of surgical treatment include dissection of the diverticulum from the surrounding tissue, excision at the neck, closure of the urethra with inverting sutures and approximation of the fascia and vaginal mucosa beneath the urethra. The bladder is drained for five to seven days by a suprapubic or indwelling urethral catheter.

Postoperative complications occurred in 16% of 414 cases collected from the literature by Ginsburg and Genadry (1984). These complications are discussed in the following paragraphs and are listed in Table 5–1.

Urethrovaginal fistula close to the urethrovesical junction may cause continuous leakage of urine. More distal fistulas result in little or no leakage and in the lower one-third the only symptom may be spraying of the urinary stream. Fistulas near the bladder are difficult to repair and are discussed in Chapter 4. If a low urethrovesical fistula gives sufficient symptoms to require repair, the urethra should be dissected from the surrounding scar tissue and closed with as little tension as possible and the fascia and mucosa closed similarly beneath it. Relaxing vertical incisions placed laterally may be helpful in avoiding tension on the suture line.

Recurrence is usually due to incomplete removal of the sac. Reoperation may be extremely difficult because of scar tissue.

Stress incontinence may occur as a result of loss of support of the urethrovesical junction. Suprapubic urethrovesical suspension may be necessary.

Urethral stricture results from removal of too much of the floor of the urethra and resultant tight urethral closure. Stricture produces inability to void or slow voiding with a narrow urinary stream. Strictures can usually be dilated with Hegar or similar dilators (up to 8 or 10 mm diameter) in the office using topical anesthesia (1% lidocaine). Since there is a tendency

for strictures to re-form, dilatation will have to be repeated at least once or twice and then as the patient's symptoms indicate. .

Urinary tract infection may be persistent and difficult to treat (see Chapter 4).

Marsupialization of Diverticulum. Marsupialization involves opening the diverticulum and sewing the edges to the vaginal mucosa, creating a new external urinary meatus. Complications may arise if it is performed in the upper one half to two thirds of the urethra; they consist of stress incontinence (Coddington and Knab, 1983) and alteration in the direction and type of urinary flow. The new position of the meatus in the vagina may also predispose the urinary tract infection, especially after coitus.

Urethroplasty. Urethroplasty may be performed after conservative measures in the management of painful coitus, which is followed almost invariably by urethritis or cystitis (starting with honeymoon cystitis), have failed and when an anatomic defect is seen in which the external urinary meatus is displaced intravaginally or incorporated in the hymeneal ring. The operation consists of freeing the urethra and external urinary meatus from its vaginal attachments by dividing them transversely and suturing them vertically. Tissue is thus interposed between the urethra and the vagina (Hirschhorn, 1965; Smith et al, 1982) (Fig. 5–5). Complications consist of (1) incision of the urethra; this is closed with fine absorbable inverting sutures and (2) recurrence, which requires adequate preoperative determination that the anatomic deformity is the cause of the problem and thorough freeing and advancement of the urethra with a mucosal flap.

OPERATIONS ON THE CERVIX

Operations involving the cervix are the most common gynecologic procedures. They include:

1. Biopsies.
2. Therapeutic procedures, such as electrocauterization, cryotherapy and laser therapy.
3. Conization.
4. Dilatation and curettage and other transcervical procedures.
5. Closure of an incompetent cervix (cerclage), usually performed during pregnancy and rarely between pregnancies (see Chapter 8).

Biopsies

A biopsy may be taken from an obviously abnormal area of the cervix, such as an exophy-

Table 5–1. Complications of Urethral Diverticulectomy in 414 Reported Cases*

Complication	No.	Per Cent
Fistula	15	4
Recurrence	18	4
Stress incontinence	10	2
Stricture	5	1
Recurrent urinary tract infection	19	5

*Adapted from Ginsberg DS, Genadry R: Suburethral diverticulum in the female. *Obstet. Gynecol. Surv.* 39:1, 1984.

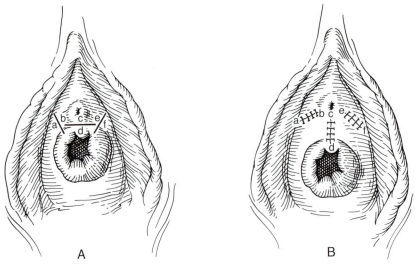

Figure 5–5. Reconstruction of anterior hymeneal ring. A, Incisions. B, Closure of incisions in opposite directions.

tic carcinoma, or may be done under colposcopic guidance. Included in the same category are excision or avulsion of cervical polyps and endocervical curettage. The latter may be an independent procedure or part of a colposcopic study of the cervix or of an evaluation of the endometrium. The only complications are discomfort to the patient and bleeding. Discomfort is almost always minor and is absent in many instances. Local anesthesia is often only partially effective and may cause as much discomfort as taking the biopsy. Bleeding is usually not severe if the biopsy is small, although it may be greater in the presence of carcinoma. It can usually be controlled by pressure with a cotton sponge, followed by insertion of a cotton or lamb's wool tampon, which is left in place for three to four hours. Application of Monsel's solution (ferric subsulfate) or use of electrocautery may be useful. However, these agents destroy the superficial layers of the cervix. This may be important if a further diagnostic procedure such as conization is needed in the near future. Often, however, a second procedure is best delayed until the biopsy site has healed, usually at least four to six weeks later. Severe continued bleeding may rarely require packing with 2-inch iodoform gauze and/or sutures, perhaps with anesthesia.

Therapeutic Procedures

Advances in screening (cytology) and diagnosis (colposcopy) over the past 50 years have greatly changed the treatment of cervical le-

sions. First, intraepithelial carcinoma, or carcinoma in situ, was recognized as a separate entity from invasive cancer. Then the progressive nature of intraepithelial disease from mild dysplasia through invasive carcinoma was appreciated. Thus, instead of treating only the end stage, invasive carcinoma, by radiation or radical excision, it became possible to manage precancerous lesions with a reasonable chance of arresting the process. Current methods of treating cervical intraepithelial neoplasia include electrocauterization, cryotherapy, laser therapy and conization. Hysterectomy is rarely indicated.

ELECTROCAUTERIZATION

Prior to the recognition of dysplasia, electrocauterization was extensively employed to treat cervical erosions. In fact, postpartum cauterization was thought to reduce the subsequent development of carcinoma. Recently it has fallen into disuse because of the development of newer techniques. Cauterization may be performed in linear radial fashion or to the flat surface of the cervix with various instruments. Complications are few. If the cervix is not carefully exposed, there is a danger of burning the vagina or even the vulva. There is some pain, but it is usually slight. The smell is unpleasant, and the smoke should be removed by suction. Chanen and Rome (1983) reported that 47 of 1864 patients (2.5%) undergoing electrocoagulation diathermy for cervical intraepithelial neoplasia had significant complications. Twenty-six (1.4%) had bleeding, which required admission to hospital and conservative treatment with bedrest and transfusions; nine (0.5%) developed cervical stenosis, which reponded to dilatation; and 12 (0.6%) developed acute pelvic infection, which was managed successfully by antibiotics.

CRYOTHERAPY

In the past 15 years cryotherapy has become the most widely used treatment for cervical intraepithelial neoplasia. Many instruments have been developed and techniques of use differ. The cryoprobe may be placed on the cervix for five to seven minutes for a single freeze or treatment may be repeated in a cycle of freeze three minutes, thaw four to five minutes and freeze three minutes. Some authors prefer to freeze once until the iceball extends 4 to 5 mm outside the probe. A double freeze extending 3 mm beyond the lesion with a four minute thaw interval appears to be more effective than a single freeze. In a randomized prospective study of 142 patients with mild or moderate dysplasia Schantz and Thormann (1984) reported a recurrence rate of 6.2% following a double freeze compared with 16.3% following a single freeze.

Intraoperative complications of cryotherapy are few and consist of mechanical problems with the equipment, pain and freezing the vaginal wall. It is well to be familiar with the instrument before using it and to know how to deal with malfunction. Pain is described by patients as similar to a menstrual cramp, usually not severe. Freezing the vagina may occur when exposure of the cervix is difficult. It can be obviated by separating the vaginal wall from the cervix by a wooden tongue blade during the freeze. No serious consequences result unless the vaginal freezing is continued and deep.

Discharge is an early postoperative complication, that occurs in all patients. It is usually thin, profuse and sometimes malodorous, and it lasts two to three weeks. No treatment is necessary unless it persists. The patient is advised to avoid douches and intercourse and to use pads rather than tampons. Bleeding occasionally accompanies the discharge, but is usually no more than spotting. It is less likely to occur if the cryotherapy is performed within a few days after the end of menstruation.

Late complications are few. Cervical stenosis was reported by Thormann and Schantz (1980) to occur in 6 of 145 patients (4%). Complications with regard to subsequent pregnancy have not usually been reported (Hemmingsson, 1982). The main concern has been recurrence of the

Table 5–2. Persistence or Recurrence of CIN after Cryosurgery

Authors	CIN 1 and 2 (%)	CIN 3 (%)
Ostergaard (1980)	6.7	19.6
Hatch et al (1981)	16.6	24
Stuart et al (1982)	6.9	17.2
Creasman et al (1984)	6.4	17.7

intraepithelial neoplasia. Data on this subject vary. Richart and co-workers (1980), in a multi-institutional study of 2839 patients treated by cryotherapy and followed for 1 to 14 years, found recurrence in 22 or 0.8%, with no difference in the rate for CIN 1, CIN 2 or CIN 3. While these figures are impressive, the report does not indicate how patients were selected for inclusion in the study, nor the quality control used in the pathologic or cytologic diagnoses. On the other hand, representative reports from single institutions are not so optimistic (Table 5–2). In particular, the recurrence rate in CIN 3 is reported to be considerable. Peckham and associates (1982) reported that when carcinoma in situ was diagnosed at their institution the recurrence rate after cryotherapy was considerably higher, i.e., 20%, as compared to 9.3% in patients with severe dysplasia. When recurrence is detected by Papanicolaou smear or other diagnostic procedure during a regular follow-up examination, it has rarely been found to be invasive, and treatment (repeated cryosurgery, conization or hysterectomy) has usually been curative. The most serious complication has been that recurrences have not been detected and have progressed to invasive cancer because of failure of the patient to return or when invasive carcinoma develops because the original cryotherapy was inadequate treatment for a more advanced and undiagnosed lesion (Sevin et al, 1979). The main points in the prevention of recurrence are (1) thorough initial diagnostic examination, (2) adequate freezing using a double freeze technique and obtaining a 3 to 4 mm iceball around the probe at each freezing and (3) inclusion of all the abnormal area in the freezing, even if it is necessary to repeat the procedure at the same sitting.

LASER THERAPY

The carbon dioxide laser was first described in 1967 and has been available for about 10 years. Its advantages are that small specific areas of abnormal tissue can be treated, the depth of tissue evaporation can be carefully controlled and thermal damage to adjacent normal tissue is small. As with cryotherapy several instruments have been developed, each with different technical attributes. The principles and possible hazards of laser therapy are described by Bellina and Bandieramonte (1984). The function of the instrument is all important to the success of the therapy.

Laser therapy appears to be well established in the treatment of vaginal and probably of vulvar intraepithelial neoplasia and of condylomata acuminata. Its place in the management of cervical intraepithelial neoplasia has yet to be determined. Vaporization of small areas, in contrast to the mass effect of electrocauterization or cryotherapy, was at first thought to be important. However, the concept of ablating the whole squamocolumnar junction to prevent recurrence has recently had increased support. Laser therapy has therefore been used to perform what is in effect a therapeutic conization. It has also been used, but with less clear rationale, for diagnostic conization.

Few intraoperative complications of laser therapy have been reported. Except in very experienced hands, the procedure is lengthy. Potentially, laser is capable of severe tissue destruction if not carefully controlled. There is also danger of reflected laser beam injury to the eyes of the patient and attendants; thus glasses, contact lenses or goggles are necessary for all involved in the therapy. Although laser therapy of the cervix is usually performed without anesthesia, pain may be considerable. Using a mail questionnaire, Lowles and co-workers (1983) found that 42% of 239 women reported pain to be moderate or severe, 44% reported it to be very slight or mild and 15% had no pain at all.

Early postoperative complications may be somewhat more common after laser therapy (7.4%) than after cryosurgery (0.6%) (Ferenczy, 1985). They include serosanguineous discharge, pain, bleeding and pelvic inflammatory disease. The discharge is less in amount and of shorter duration than that occurring after cryosurgery. Pain occurs in some women after laser therapy for vulvar disease. The reported incidence of bleeding varies from 1.2% to 10.2% (Table 5–3); it appears to vary with the depth of the laser vaporization and the power used. Bleeding can usually be managed by applying Monsel's solution, packing or the use of laser cauterization. Sutures and transfusions are very rarely needed. Following laser therapy the cervix heals in six to eight weeks, a somewhat longer period than after cryotherapy.

Table 5–3. *Bleeding* after Laser Therapy for CIN*

Authors	No. of Cases	Per Cent with Bleeding
Bellina et al (1981)	256	1.2
Baggish (1982)	364	10.2
Rylander et al (1984)	328	7.9
Reid (1984-85)	119	1.7

*Usually described as bleeding sufficient to require treatment. Minor spotting or blood-tinged discharge appears to be much more common.

Late complications such as cervical stenosis or interference with the ability to conceive have not been reported, but long-term follow-up data are not yet available. The squamocolumnar junction may be more visible after laser therapy than after cryotherapy, thus facilitating follow-up examinations of the junction and the endocervix. The rate of persistence or recurrence of cervical intraepithelial neoplasia after laser therapy appears to be similar to or somewhat better than that following cryotherapy. In a randomized series of 101 patients Kwikkel and Helmerhorst (1985) noted no significant difference in success rates between cryosurgery and laser treatment for CIN 1, CIN 2 or CIN 3. However, the size of the lesion treated was of importance, and Ferenczy (1985) noted that the CO_2 laser produced better results than cryosurgery for lesions over 3 cm in diameter or extending up to 5 mm into the endocervical canal. In a series reported by Townsend and Richart (1983) treatment in 200 patients was alternated between cryotherapy and laser therapy with 7% failure in the former and 11% in the latter.

Conization

From 1950 to 1970 conization of the cervix was frequently performed for tissue diagnosis following an abnormal Papanicolaou smear. The widespread use of colposcopy, colposcopically directed biopsy and endocervical curettage has made it possible in many instances to identify the source of the abnormal cells, to define the severity of the lesion and to treat it locally. This has sharply reduced the incidence of conization in most centers. However, it is still necessary for diagnosis when (1) the intraepithelial lesion extends into the cervical canal, (2) the endocervical curettage reveals atypical epithelium or cells, (3) there is a marked discrepancy between the cytologic, colposcopic and histologic findings and (4) the lesion is so large or irregular that office biopsy specimens may not be representative of the worst areas. It is also an important therapy for cervical intraepithelial neoplasia, because it combines treatment with diagnosis and provides information about the completeness of removal that is not available when cryotherapy or laser therapy is used.

The principle of the operation is to remove a cone-shaped portion of the cervix with the narrow end in the cervical canal. The shape of this piece of tissue, shallow and wide or deep and narrow, depends on the previous colposcopic findings, which should always be available prior to conization. Painting the cervix with Schiller's iodine solution delineates an iodine-negative area, which helps to determine the extent of excision. Hemostasis can be assisted by ligating the descending branch of the uterine artery with angle sutures placed in the lateral aspects of the cervix. The injection of dilute neosynephrine (0.005%) or adrenalin (1:200,000) into the substance of the cervix causes vasoconstriction and reduces blood loss from small vessels. However, reactive dilatation may predispose to postoperative bleeding. After excision of the cone, endocervical curettage and, if indicated, endometrial curettage, the raw cervix is closed by Sturmdorf's inverting sutures (Fig. 5–6), coagulated electrically, left open or packed with gauze. Conization can be performed safely in an ambulatory surgical center.

The chief intraoperative complication is hemorrhage. This is sometimes due to the angle sutures not being placed deeply enough. They should be replaced. Individual arterial bleeders may be ligated. Even after Sturmdorf's sutures and additional lateral sutures have been placed, bleeding may continue. Usually it can be controlled by using thrombogenic material such as Gelfoam or Avitene or by tight packing. Occasionally, all stitches must be removed and replaced. Perforation of the cul-de-sac is reported to have occurred in 5 of a series of 1833 cases but in none of the last 1500 cases (Bjerre and Eliasson, 1976). This is likely only with very extensive conization.

Early postoperative complications consist of bleeding and infection. Bleeding occurs most often in the first 24 hours or 5 to 15 days later. The incidence may be as high as 13% (Luesley et al, 1985). Claman and Lee (1974) found that bleeding occurred less often if the conization was performed in the first seven days of the menstrual cycle. When postoperative bleeding occurs, it is particularly distressing if the patient

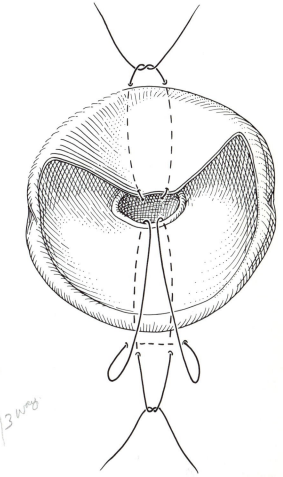

Figure 5–6. Hemostatic closure of coned cervix with Sturmdorf sutures. Anterior suture tied down; posterior suture in place.

is at home and apparently recovering well from the procedure. Bleeding is often small in amount at first and then increases rapidly. Immediate examination is essential with adequate light and equipment at hand. Bleeding points may be clamped and ligated, but this is often difficult. If it cannot be done or bleeding is in the form of a generalized ooze, the vagina should be packed firmly with 2-inch plain or iodoform gauze. An indwelling urinary catheter is usually necessary. The pack is left in place for no more than 24 hours. Intravenous fluids and blood are given as indicated. If blood soaks through the pack quickly or recurs after removal of the pack, vaginal examination should be performed under anesthesia and the cervix resutured by angle or Sturmdorf's sutures. Occasionally the bleeding may be so severe that hysterectomy or even ligation of the uterine or hypogastric arteries may be necessary. Infection in the form of fever and foul discharge occurs rarely. The discharge should be cultured and appropriate antibiotics given.

The late complications of conization consist of cervical stenosis and possible effects on sexual function, conception, pregnancy, labor and delivery. Stenosis occurs in 2.7% (Bjerre and Eliasson, 1976) to 17% (Luesley et al, 1985). The latter authors reported it to be commonest among women who had had long cones removed. The primary symptom is dysmenorrhea, and the stenosis is often obvious upon inspection. It is treated by passing a small dilator through the external os. This may have to be repeated one or more times. Because of this possibility it is advisable to check the patency of the external os at the first postoperative visit. Late stenosis in the postmenopausal woman has been described by Krieger and McCormack in patients followed for a long time (1968).

Sexual function does not appear to be affected by conization (Kilkku et al, 1982). Nor is fertility a problem (Buller and Jones, 1982). There are conflicting reports on the obstetric consequences of conization. Moinian and Andersch (1982) compared obstetric outcome in 414 patients before and after conization. They found no differences in the incidence of early spontaneous abortion but some increase in late spontaneous abortion. Cervical incompetence was present in 18% of patients conceiving after conization (19 subsequent pregnancies) and this required cerclage, with two late spontaneous abortions, two preterm deliveries and 15 term deliveries. This finding was not confirmed by Buller and Jones (1982). Moinian and Andersch (1982) also noted that in six patients (6%) labor was terminated by cesarean section because of a rigid scarred cervix. A possible explanation for the finding of cervical incompetence may relate to the size of the cone removed (Leiman et al, 1980). Thus, when tissue is removed in the region of the internal os, premature dilatation may be more likely. These authors also pointed out, however, that in their series cervical dystocia appeared to be related to the removal of a small cone.

Following conization it may be difficult to obtain adequate Papanicolaou smears and/or to perform adequate colposcopy because the squamocolumnar junction has receded up the endocervical canal. Trimbos and co-workers (1983) reported that this occurred in 30% of all patients who had had conization; a lower incidence occurred when the cervix was left open and bleeding points cauterized without sutures.

In the author's experience this figure is high. In any case, endocervical curettage may be a necessary part of thorough follow-up.

Early data comparing cold-knife conization with laser conization suggested that complications may be less with the latter technique. However, adequate prospective studies are needed.

The Vaginal Approach to Intrauterine Disease

It is often important to obtain a sample of the endometrium and to determine the size and configuration of the uterine cavity. This can be done by suction/aspiration or by dilatation and curettage (D & C).

SUCTION/ASPIRATION

Suction/aspiration has become widely used in recent years because it is relatively simple and inexpensive and has proved to be accurate. The procedure involves (1) endocervical curettage, (2) determining the depth of the uterine cavity from the external cervical os to the fundus, by using a malleable metal instrument, or the suction tube itself and (3) obtaining the endometrial sample. A variety of instruments are available. The author's preference is for a rigid tube 3 mm in diameter, which permits the contours of the cavity to be explored.

The complications of suction/aspiration are inability to insert the tube through a tight or stenosed cervix, pain, bleeding and very rarely perforation of the uterus (see later section). Koss and associates (1984) were able to obtain fragments of endometrium in 93% of 2586 first attempts at suction/aspiration. The same authors noted pain extending beyond 48 hours in 1.1% and bleeding beyound 24 hours in 2.1% of 4340 patients sampled. Intraoperative pain can be reduced by local (paracervical) anesthesia, but the slight discomfort of this and the time taken reduce its value.

DILATATION AND CURETTAGE

Dilatation and curettage enables a more complete sampling of the endometrium and a better determination of its shape and size. The procedure may be performed satisfactorily in many patients under local anesthesia to the cervix itself and with a paracervical block. General anesthesia is better for the apprehensive patient or for one in whom a thorough examination is required. Overnight hospitalization is seldom needed; patients usually can be discharged within several hours after the operation. The steps followed in a D & C include (1) endocervical curettage, (2) determining the depth of the uterine cavity (as described earlier), (3) dilating the cervical canal using, for example, Pratt dilators progressively up to size No. 8 or No. 9, (4) curetting the endometrial cavity thoroughly and (5) using polyp forceps to remove loose tissue and polypoid material.

Intraoperative complications of D & C include pain, stenosis of the cervical canal, perforation of the uterus and bleeding. Pain occurs when (1) the cervix is grasped with a tenaculum, (2) the endocervix is curetted, (3) the cervix is dilated and (4) when the top of the uterine cavity is scraped. Local anesthesia will largely eliminate pain when the endocervix is curetted and when the cervix is dilated, but some discomfort results from the grasping of the cervix and scraping of the top of the uterine cavity. This can be somewhat allayed by intravenous diazepam and/or fentanyl.

Stenosis of the cervical canal may be present when operations have been performed on the cervix or radiation has been administered previously, and the external os may be very small and hard to find. Use of a fine probe and a small hemostat may help to open the canal.

The uterus may be perforated by the sound, the dilators or the curette. Perforation is an important complication because D & C is very frequently performed. Actually, perforation was found to occur in only 0.63% of 2991 diagnostic curettages reported by McElin and co-workers (1969). Rarely, the appearance of bile-stained fluid, omentum (fat) or intestine in the material obtained by curettage or with the polyp forceps may be diagnostic of a perforation. If any of these are observed, immediate laparotomy is indicated, and a thorough search should be made for injury to intestine or mesentery. Perforation is usually recognized by the fact that the perforating instrument can suddenly be inserted far further than one anticipated. The patient's general condition (possible shock) and the amount of bleeding should be promptly assessed. If these findings are reassuring, an educated guess should be made as to the site of the perforation—through the fundus, at the cervico-uterine junction or laterally into the broad ligament. If possible, an attempt should be made to obtain sufficient tissue for diagnosis, avoiding the area of perforation. Occasionally, laparoscopy may be helpful if there is doubt about perforation and as a guide to obtaining

endometrial tissue without enlarging the perforation or involving other intraperitoneal organs. The patient should then be carefully observed for 24 to 48 hours for bleeding and signs of intraperitoneal injury or infection (peritonitis, fever). Prophylactic antibiotics such as a second generation cephalosporin should be given for 24 to 72 hours. An important step in minimizing the possibility of perforation is to examine the patient prior to any instrumentation so as to determine the size and position of the uterus.

The conservative management of uterine perforation may have to be modified if evidence of injury to intestine or bladder is definite or begins to develop, if bleeding is excessive (more likely with perforation into the broad ligament) or if cancer is present in the uterus. In the first case, abdominal rigidity, rebound tenderness and diminished peristalsis will be present. Laparotomy is indicated to inspect the intestine and perform the necessary repair (see Chapter 4); laparoscopy is of little value at this time because it is impossible to view all the intestine through the laparoscope. At laparotomy the perforation of the uterus is sutured. Hysterectomy is necessary only if bleeding is excessive and repair impossible.

If the bladder is injured, urine may be scanty and contain blood. Extravasation of urine will cause suprapubic pain and distension; the patient's pulse may be rapid and she may be in shock. Immediate exploration, closure of the perforation and suprapubic or transurethral drainage of the bladder are needed.

If a frozen section diagnosis of endometrial cancer and its histologic differentiation can be obtained at the time of perforation and the disease appears to be limited to the corpus (without spread to the cervix), hysterectomy, bilateral salpingo-oophorectomy and appropriate node biopsies may be performed to prevent continued spread of malignant cells into the peritoneal cavity. If there is doubt about the diagnosis it is best to wait.

If perforation has been managed conservatively and a prompt diagnosis is necessary, it is probably best to wait at least four weeks before repeating the dilatation and curettage and then to use great caution, avoiding, if possible, the site of the perforation. It is uncertain whether a perforation makes rupture of the uterus more likely during subsequent pregnancy, labor and delivery. However, the hole in the uterine wall is usually small and probably should not be a reason for cesarean section, unless other indications are present.

Excessive bleeding may be due to laceration

of the uterine artery or one of its branches. Laparotomy is indicated with ligation of the uterine or, if a large hematoma prevents its identification, of the internal iliac artery. Trying to control the bleeding from below by blind clamping is dangerous because of possible injury to the ureter. Intrauterine packing may only push the bleeding further laterally, creating a larger broad ligament hematoma and giving the operator a false sense of security. Occasionally bleeding from the uterus may be profuse following evacuation of a hydatidiform mole, the products of conception or a retained placenta. Intravenous oxytocics in adequate doses are essential. Rarely, coagulation defects and anomalous uterine vessels or arteriovenous communications may produce serious postoperative bleeding. Inability to control these may necessitate hysterectomy.

Early postoperative complications relate to the condition for which the D & C was performed. For example, bleeding and infection are rare following diagnostic curettage, but may be more commmon after curettage for incomplete abortion (see Chapter 8).

The most important late complication that may follow any kind of curettage is the development of intrauterine adhesions or synechiae (Asherman's syndrome). In 2981 cases collected by Schenker and Margalioth (1982) an underlying cause was identified in 1856 patients (62%). Pregnancy and puerperal factors were present in 91% of these, while trauma of various sorts without pregnancy accounted for the remaining 9% of whom almost half or 44% had genital tuberculosis. It has always been assumed that especially vigorous curettage, by removing almost all the endometrium and some of the subjacent tissue, has been a contributing cause, but this is difficult to substantiate. Recently, increasing numbers of cases with intrauterine adhesions have been discovered as women with unexplained fertility have been studied hysteroscopically. Among these patients, a history of curettage was associated with a significantly higher incidence of adhesion formation (Taylor et al, 1981).

Symptoms of intrauterine adhesions include primary sterility and menstrual disorders (often hypomenorrhea or amenorrhea). The diagnosis is made by hysteroscopy and/or hysterosalpingogram. Treatment is somewhat controversial but, in principle, consists of lysis of adhesions through the hysteroscope or by curettage, insertion of an IUD (if available) for several weeks, together with the use of conjugated estrogens for at least one month. Schenker and

Margalioth (1982) report that 90% of 49 patients so treated had normal menses; 84% became pregnant and 67% carried their pregnancies to term. However, the success rate may depend upon the underlying disease. Pregnancy loss and complications are generally reported to be higher than normal.

OTHER TRANSCERVICAL PROCEDURES

Transcervical procedures have also been used to (1) insert drains for the treatment of dysmenorrhea, (2) place radioactive substances in the uterine cavity and cervical canal and (3) drain pyometra. The first procedure is no longer used. The second is covered in Chapter 14. Pyometra is rare. It occurred in 35 cases among 16,729 patients (0.2%) treated at St Mary's Hospital, Manchester, England from 1965 to 1968 (Whiteley and Hamlett, 1971). When it is found, a tube drain is placed and sewn to the cervix or a small Foley catheter is used. Drainage is continued for three to five days. Complications include infection and recurrence of pyometra. Infection is shown by the development of persistent generalized or lower abdominal pain, tenderness and fever. It is treated by broad spectrum antibiotics (e.g. cephoxitin); prophylactic use of these is probably advisable. Recurrence occurred in 31% of Whiteley and Hamlett's patients. Drainage is again necessary. If curettage was not performed when the pyometra was found, the underlying condition, not necessarily cancer (less than 20%), is still present and diagnostic curettage needs to be performed as soon as drainage has ceased.

HYSTEROSCOPY

Hysteroscopy, and more recently, microhysteroscopy have been increasingly used in the past 10 years for direct visualization of the endometrial cavity. Local anesthesia is commonly employed. A variety of instruments have been developed (see review by Taylor and Hamou, 1983). Media used for visualization include Hyskon (32%) (Dextran with a molecular weight of about 70,000 in 10% dextrose), 5% dextrose in water and CO_2. The current uses of hysteroscopy are to examine and remove a biopsy specimen of focal intrauterine lesions that might be missed by dilatation and curettage and to treat intrauterine adhesions, excise small tumors (submucous leiomyomata) and manage congenital abnormalities such as uterine septa.

Intraoperative complications are rare (Valle, 1983; Taylor and Hamou, 1983). They include technical problems with the equipment, pain, inability to traverse the cervical canal because of stenosis, bleeding, cervical laceration and uterine perforation and, rarely, intravascular absorption of Dextran used for intrauterine instillation (Zbella et al, 1985). Bleeding is usually minor and seldom prevents completion of the examination. After hysteroscopic procedures such as myomectomy, insertion of a Foley catheter is an effective way of controlling persistent bleeding. Perforation is managed as described previously for dilatation and curettage. To help prevent perforation observation should be begin in the upper cervical canal, and the instrument should be advanced only when the field of vision is adequate. Extensive intrauterine manipulation may increase complications. Postoperative complications include shoulder pain resulting from intraperitoneal CO_2, which may be lessened by performing hysteroscopy with the patient in a slight Trendelenburg position. Infection occurs very rarely (Taylor and Hamou, 1983).

REFERENCES

Addison WA, Livengood CH III et al: Abdominal sacral colpopexy with mersilene mesh in the retroperitoneal position in the management of posthysterectomy vaginal vault prolapse and enterocele. *Am. J. Obstet. Gynecol.* 153:140, 1985.

Baggish MS: Management of cervical intraepithelial neoplasia by carbon dioxide laser. *Obstet. Gynecol.* 60:378, 1982.

Barnhill DR, Hoskins WJ, Metz P: Use of the rhomboid flap after partial vulvectomy. *Obstet. Gynecol.* 63:444, 1983.

Beecham CT, Beecham JB: Correction of prolapsed vagina or enterocele with fascia lata. *Obstet. Gynecol.* 42:542, 1973.

Bellina JH, Bandieramonte G: *Principles and Practice of Gynecologic Laser Surgery.* New York, Plenum Press, 1984.

Bellina JH, Wright VC et al: Carbon dioxide laser management of cervical intraepithelial neoplasia. *Am. J. Obstet. Gynecol.* 141:828, 1981.

Bjerre B, Eliasson G: Conization as only treatment of carcinoma in situ of the uterine cervix. *Am. J. Obstet. Gynecol.* 125:143, 1976.

Buller RE, Jones HW III: Pregnancy following cervical conization. *Am. J. Obstet. Gynecol.* 142:506, 1982.

Burgio KL, Robinson JC, Engel BT: The role of biofeedback in Kegel exercise training for stress urinary incontinence. *Am. J. Obstet. Gynecol.* 154:58, 1986.

Burgio KL, Whitehead WE, Engel BT: Urinary incontinence in the elderly: bladder-sphincter biofeedback and toileting skills training. *Ann. Int. Med.* 103:507, 1985.

Capen CV, Irwin H et al: Vaginal removal of the ovaries in association with vaginal hysterectomy. *J. Reprod. Med.* 28:589, 1983.

Carenza L, Vilani C: Schauta radical vaginal hysterectomy. *Clin. Obstet. Gynecol.* 25:913, 1982.

Chanen W, Rome RM: Electrocoagulation diathermy for cervical dysplasia and carcinoma in situ: a 15-year survey. *Obstet. Gynecol.* 61:673, 1983.

Claman AD, Lee N: Factors that relate to complications of cone biopsy. *Am. J. Obstet. Gynecol.* 120:124, 1974.

Coddington CC, Knab DR: Urethral diverticulum: a review. *Obstet. Gynecol. Surv.* 38:357, 1983.

Craig GA, Jackson P: Sexual life after vaginal hysterectomy. *Br. Med. J.* 1:97, 1975.

Creasman WT, Hinshaw WM, Clarke-Pearson DL: Cryosurgery in the management of cervical intraepithelial neoplasia. *Obstet. Gynecol.* 63:145, 1984.

Cutner LP: Female genital mutilation. *Obstet. Gynecol. Surv.* 40:437, 1985.

Dewhurst CJ: Children with ambiguous genitalia. In Huffman JW, Dewhurst CJ, Caprano VJ (Eds.): *The Gynecology of Childhood and Adolescence*, Ed. 2. Philadelphia, W. B. Saunders Company, 1981.

Ellenbogen A, Agranat A, Grunstein S: The role of vaginal hysterectomy in the aged woman. *J. Am. Geriatr. Soc.* 29:426, 1981.

England GT, Randall HW, Graves WL: Impairment of tissue defenses by vasoconstrictors in vaginal hysterectomies. *Obstet. Gynecol.* 61:271, 1983.

Evans TN, Poland ML, Boving RL: Vaginal malformations. *Am. J. Obstet. Gynecol.* 141:910, 1981.

Ferenczy A: Treating genital condyloma during pregnancy with the carbon dioxide laser. *Am. J. Obstet. Gynecol.* 148:9, 1984.

Ferenczy A: Comparison of cryo- and carbon dioxide laser therapy for cervical intraepithelial neoplasia. *Obstet. Gynecol.* 66:793, 1985.

Francis WJA, Jeffcoate TNA: Dyspareunia following vaginal operations. *J. Obstet. Gynaecol. Br. Comm.* 68:1, 1961.

Ginsburg DS, Genadry R: Suburethral diverticulum in the female. *Obstet. Gynecol. Surv.* 39:1, 1984.

Goldman J, Ovadia J, Feldberg D: The Neugebauer-LeFort operation: a review of 118 partial colpocleises. *Eur. J. Obstet. Gynecol. Reprod. Biol.* 12:31, 1981.

Hatch KD, Shingleton HM et al: Cryosurgery of cervical intraepithelial neoplasia. *Obstet. Gynecol.* 57:692, 1981.

Hemmingsson E: Outcome of third trimester pregnancies after cryotherapy of the uterine cervix. *Br. J. Obstet. Gynaecol.* 89:675, 1982.

Hirschhorn RC: Urethral-hymeneal fusion: a surgically correctable cause of recurrent cystitis. *Obstet. Gynecol.* 26:903, 1965.

Hudson CN: The use of transposition flaps in vaginal surgery. *J. Obstet. Gynaecol. Br. Comm.* 73:299, 1966.

Ingram JM: Further experience with suprapubic drainage by trocar catheter. *Am. J. Obstet. Gynecol.* 121:865, 1975.

Ingram JM: Nonsurgical technique corrects vaginal agenesis and stenosis. *Contemp. Obstet. Gynecol.* 19:46, 1982.

Kilkku P, Gronroos M, Punnonen R: Sexual function after conization of the uterine cervix. *Gynecol. Oncol.* 14:209, 1982.

Koss LG, Schreiber K et al: Detection of endometrial carcinoma and hyperplasia in asymptomatic women. *Obstet. Gynecol.* 64:1, 1984.

Krieger JS, McCormack LJ: Graded treatment for in situ carcinoma of the cervix. *Am. J. Obstet. Gynecol.* 101:171, 1968.

Kwikkel HJ, Helmerhorst ThJM et al: Laser or cryosurgery for cervical intraepithelial neoplasia: a randomized study to compare efficacy and side effects. *Gynecol. Oncol.* 22:23, 1985.

Leiman G, Harrison A, Rubin A: Pregnancy following conization of the cervix: complications related to cone size. *Am. J. Obstet. Gynecol.* 136:14, 1980.

Lowles IE, Al-Kurdi M, Hare MJ: Women's recollection of pain during and after carbon dioxide laser treatment to the uterine cervix. *Br. J. Obstet. Gynaecol.* 90:1157, 1983.

Luesley DM, McCrum A et al: Complications of cone biopsy related to the dimensions of the cone and the influence of prior colposcopic assessment. *Br. J. Obstet. Gynaecol.* 92:158, 1985.

McCall ML: Posterior culdoplasty: surgical correction of enterocele during vaginal hysterectomy; a preliminary report. *Obstet. Gynecol.* 10:595, 1957.

McElin TW, Bird CC, Reeves BD: Study of uterine perforations occurring during 2991 instances of diagnostic curettage. *Int. J. Gynecol. Obstet.* 7:243, 1969.

Moinian M, Andersch B: Does cervix conization increase the risk of complications in subsequent pregnancies? *Acta Obstet. Gynecol. Scand.* 61:101, 1982.

Montz FJ, Stanton SL: How to use the suprapubic bladder catheter. *Contemp. Obstet. Gynecol.* 25:31, 1985.

Morton KE, Dewhurst CJ: Human amnion in the treatment of vaginal malformations. *Br. J. Obstet. Gynaecol.* 93:50, 1986.

Nichols DH: Sacrospinous fixation for massive eversion of the vagina. *Am. J. Obstet. Gynecol.* 142:901, 1982.

Ostergaard DR: Cryosurgical treatment of cervical intraepithelial neoplasia. *Obstet. Gynecol.* 56:231, 1980.

Peckham BM, Sonek MG, Carr WF: Outpatient therapy: success and failure with dysplasia and carcinoma in situ. *Am. J. Obstet. Gynecol.* 142:323, 1982.

Reid R: Symposium on cervical neoplasia. V. Carbon dioxide ablation. *Colposcopy and Gynecologic Laser Surgery* 1:291, 1984–85.

Richart RM, Townsend DE et al: An analysis of "long-term" follow-up results in patients with cervical intraepithelial neoplasia treated by cryotherapy. *Am. J. Obstet. Gynecol.* 137:823, 1980.

Rivlin ME: Clinical outcome following vaginal drainage of pelvic abscess. *Obstet. Gynecol.* 61:169, 1983.

Rock JA, Reeves LA et al: Success following vaginal creation for mullerian agenesis. *Fertil. Steril.* 39:809, 1983.

Rock JA, Jones HW Jr: Vaginal forms for dilatation and/or to maintain vaginal patency. *Fertil. Steril.* 42:187, 1984.

Rock JA, Zacur HA: Pregnancy success following surgical correction of imperforate hymen and complete transverse vaginal septum. *Obstet. Gynecol.* 59:448, 1982.

Rothman D: The use of peritoneum in the construction of a vagina. *Obstet. Gynecol.* 40:835, 1972.

Rylander E, Isberg A, Joelsson I: Laser vaporization of cervical intraepithelial neoplasia. *Acta Obstet. Gynecol. Scand. Suppl.* 125:33, 1984.

Schantz A, Thormann L: Cryosurgery for dysplasia of the uterine ectocervix. A randomized study of the single- and double-freeze techniques. *Acta Obstet. Gynecol. Scand.* 63:417, 1984.

Schenker JG, Margalioth EJ: Intrauterine adhesions: an updated appraisal. *Fertil. Steril.* 37:593, 1982.

Sevin BU, Ford JH et al: Invasive cancer of the cervix after cryosurgery. Pitfalls of conservative management. *Obstet. Gynecol.* 53:465, 1979.

Smith PJB, Roberts JBM, Ball AJ: Honeymoon cystitis: a simple surgical cure. *Br. J. Urol.* 54:708, 1982.

Stanton SL: Investigation of incontinence. In Stanton SL, Tanagho E (Eds.): *Surgery of Female Incontinence.* New York, Springer-Verlag, 1980.

Stuart GCE, Anderson RJ et al: Assessment of failures of cryosurgical treatment in cervical intraepithelial neoplasia. *Am. J. Obstet. Gynecol.* 142:658, 1982.

Swartz WH, Tanaree P: T-tube suction drainage and/or prophylactic antibiotics. *Obstet. Gynecol.* 47:665, 1976.

Symmonds RE, Williams TJ et al: Posthysterectomy enterocele and vaginal vault prolapse. *Am. J. Obstet. Gynecol.* 140:852, 1981.

Taylor PJ, Cumming DC, Hill PJ: Significance of intrauterine adhesions detected hysteroscopically in eumenorrheic infertile women and role of antecedent curettage in their formation. *Am. J. Obstet. Gynecol.* 139:239, 1981.

Taylor PJ, Hamou JE: Hysteroscopy. *J. Reprod. Med.* 28:359, 1983.

Thormann L, Schantz A: A minor complication of cryosurgery—occlusion of the cervical canal. *Acta Obstet. Gynecol. Scand.* 59:377, 1980.

Townsend DE, Richart RM: Cryotherapy and carbon dioxide laser management of cervical intraepithelial neoplasia: a controlled comparison. *Obstet. Gynecol.* 61:75, 1983.

Turner UG, Edlich RF, Edgerton MT: Male transsexualism—a review of genital surgical reconstruction. *Am. J. Obstet. Gynecol.* 132:119, 1978.

Trimbos JB, Heintz APM, Van Hall EV: Reliability of cytological follow-up after conization of the cervix; a comparison of three surgical techniques. *Br. J. Obstet. Gynaecol.* 90:1141, 1983.

Valle RF: Hysteroscopy for gynecologic diagnosis. *Clin. Obstet. Gynecol.* 26:253, 1983.

Ward GD, Sutherst JR: Pruritus vulvae: treatment by multiple intradermal alcohol injections. *Br. J. Dermatol.* 93:201, 1975.

Whiteley PF, Hamlett JD: Pyometra—a reappraisal. *Am. J. Obstet. Gynecol.* 109:108, 1971.

Williams EA: Congenital absence of the vagina—a simple operation for its relief. *J. Obstet. Gynaecol. Br. Comm.* 71:511, 1964.

Wiser WL, Morrison JC et al: Management of bladder drainage following vaginal plastic repairs. *Obstet. Gynecol.* 44:65, 1974.

Woodruff JD, Genadry R, Poliakoff S: Treatment of dyspareunia and vaginal outlet distortions by perineoplasty. *Obstet. Gynecol.* 57:750, 1981.

Word B: New instrument for office treatment of cyst and abscess of Bartholin's gland. *J. Am. Med. Assoc.* 190:777, 1964.

Worth AM, Dougherty MC, McKey PL: Development and testing of the circumvaginal muscle ratings scale. *Nurs. Res.* 35:166, 1986.

Zacharin RF, Hamilton NT: Pulsion enterocele: long-term results of an abdomino-perineal technique. *Obstet. Gynecol.* 55:141, 1980.

Zbella E, Moise J, Carson SA: Noncardiogenic pulmonary edema secondary to instillation of 32% dextran 70. *Fertil Steril.* 43:479, 1985.

COMPLICATIONS OF ABDOMINAL OPERATIONS

6

MICHAEL NEWTON

LAPAROSCOPY

Introduction

Laparoscopy has become the second commonest gynecologic operation after dilatation and curettage. The idea of inspecting the intraperitoneal organs through a lighted telescope is not new. In fact, endoscopy of the abdomen, later termed peritoneoscopy, was introduced as early as 1901 and was later used sporadically in Europe and to a lesser extent in the United States (Gunning, 1974). In the last 20 years technologic advances, particularly fiberoptic illumination, have made the procedure relatively free from mechanical problems and easier to use. Although complications are uncommon, the very frequency of the procedure makes them especially important.

Laparoscopy is performed with the patient in the supine position. Her head is lowered and her legs are flat or slightly raised and abducted. The bladder should be empty. It is helpful to insert a canula into the uterine cavity to permit the position of the uterus to be varied. Pneumoperitoneum is produced by injecting gas, usually CO_2, through a small needle (Veress). This is inserted at the lower border of the umbilicus, subcostally on the left or lateral to the umbilicus. Laparoscopes with different lenses and of different sizes are available. In the more common closed procedure, a trocar is inserted blindly into the peritoneal cavity at the site of the needle puncture and the laparoscope is passed through the trocar's sleeve. In open laparoscopy it is inserted through the skin, fascia and peritoneum under direct vision, and the edges of the fascia and subcutaneous tissue are tightened around the laparoscope by sutures to prevent the escape of gas. Although a good view of the peritoneal contents may be obtained by a single puncture, and, indeed, intraperitoneal procedures may be performed through this using an operating laparoscope, a second incision is often made in the midline

143

2 to 3 cm above the symphysis pubis. Through this incision a metal rod or probe is inserted to move the intestine, omentum and pelvic organs and provide a better view. Suction tips and operating instruments can also be inserted through this puncture. After the procedure, the gas is expressed and the skin closed.

Laparoscopy may be used for diagnostic or operative purposes. The commonest operative procedures include tubal occlusion, biopsy, aspiration of fluid, recovery of eggs for in vitro fertilization, division of adhesions or cauterization of endometriotic implants. Also described are more complicated procedures such as opening and suturing the fimbriated end of the tube, using laser cauterization or removing small subserosal leiomyomata or even the appendix. Complications may be divided into those that are common to both diagnostic and operative procedures and those that relate to specific operations. Complications will be described primarily in relation to closed laparoscopy, but a section on the open technique is appended.

General Complications

The overall incidence of complications is difficult to determine because different definitions and methods of data collection are used. Mortality rates are probably less than 8 per 100,000 laparoscopies (of all types). Deaths are due to hemorrhage, gas emboli, injury to intraperitoneal organs, cardiovascular collapse, hypoventilation or sepsis; most of these are preventable (Ohlgisser et al, 1985). Complications were found to occur in 4.6% of diagnostic laparoscopies and 3.7% of laparoscopies for sterilization in the 1975 survey by the American Association of Gynecologic Laparoscopists (Phillips et al, 1977).

PREOPERATIVE COMPLICATIONS

Certain conditions may place patients at high risk for complications of laparoscopy. These relate (1) to the general condition of the patient, such as the presence of cardiac or respiratory disease or a large hiatal hernia, which may contraindicate general anesthesia, pneumoperitoneum or the use of the Trendelenburg position that is usually required or (2) to conditions that preclude adequate intraperitoneal visualization. These include obesity, which makes the insertion of the Veress needle and the trocar

more difficult, prior operations with known or strongly suspected adhesions, acute peritonitis or hemoperitoneum. None of these conditions absolutely precludes laparoscopy if the information needed is vital and cannot be obtained in any other way. Thorough evaluation of the patient's status and the risks and benefits involved is essential. For example, in a high-risk patient laparoscopy for evaluation of possible recurrent cancer might be more acceptable than laparoscopic confirmation of the diagnosis of mild or moderate endometriosis.

INTRAOPERATIVE COMPLICATIONS

Anesthesia. Both general and local anesthesia can be used. Occasional complications are encountered with each. Complications of general anesthesia are often related not only to the anesthesia itself but also to the electrical system, the associated pneumoperitoneum and the head-down position required for thorough examination of the pelvic organs. They include, in order of frequency, cardiac arrhythmias, circulatory insufficiency, hypercarbia, gas embolism, regurgitation or aspiration and pneumothorax. Local anesthesia has few of these risks, but patient discomfort may be present and the decreased pneumoperitoneum compatible with local anesthesia may lead to poor visualization. Anesthetic problems are covered in greater detail in Chapter 14.

Equipment. Complications due to inadequate function of the equipment can generally be avoided. This means that the nursing personnel should be familiar with its operation, and the equipment should be checked after and before each use. The operator should understand the principles of use, and back-up equipment should always be available.

All equipment should be adequately sterilized. Although laparoscopy is performed through a "clean" surgical field, contamination may occur from many sources. Also, it may be necessary to use the same equipment repeatedly during the same day. After detailed bacteriologic studies Corson and Block (1979) recommended soaking the equipment in fresh alkaline glutaraldehyde or 10% formaldehyde and dialdehyde (Cidex) for 15 minutes after the operations for the day have been concluded, for 15 minutes before the next day's cases and for 15 minutes between cases. These or similar precautions should be scrupulously observed.

Technique. Complications caused by technical errors appear to occur less frequently as experience with the procedure grows. They may occur, however, even among experienced operators and include:

1. Bleeding at the site of puncture of the Veress needle or trocar.

2. Failure to enter the peritoneal cavity.

3. Inability to induce pneumoperitoneum.

4. Perforation of intestine or mesentery with the Veress needle or trocar.

5. Perforation of an intraabdominal vessel with either instrument, with bleeding.

Abdominal wall bleeding on insertion of the insufflating needle or trocar seldom occurs when the puncture is made at the inferior margin of the umbilicus, since this is an avascular area. It is also infrequent with punctures in the left upper quadrant. If lateral punctures are made, as may happen when there are midline scars from previous operations, it is important to avoid the epigastric artery at the lateral margin of the rectus muscle. Incisional bleeding can usually be controlled by pressure either externally or by the trocar itself as it is inserted. Rarely, open exploration may be indicated if there is an enlarging hematoma.

Failure to enter the peritoneal cavity may be due to incorrect insertion of the Veress needle or trocar or to intraperitoneal adhesions. Necessary precautions with insertion of the Veress needle include:

1. Holding up the abdominal wall and thrusting the needle toward the hollow of the sacrum.

2. Injecting and aspirating with a syringe filled with 5 ml of saline and then observing for disappearance of a drop of saline from the hub of the needle toward the peritoneal cavity.

3. Insufflating only at a safe low pressure of less than 20 mm Hg.

4. Inserting the trocar with a twisting motion, recognizing penetration of each layer (fascia and peritoneum) separately.

If the free peritoneal cavity is not entered, insufflated gas may flow into the subcutaneous or preperitoneal space or within the abdomen into intestine or small intraperitoneal pockets sealed off by adhesions. In all instances the pressure of the entering gas will be high. Subcutaneous insufflation usually results in recognizable emphysema and crepitation. The air can usually be expressed easily. Preperitoneal air may also cause emphysema, although it may be more difficult to recognize and express. The trocar should not be inserted until pneumoperitoneum has been obtained.

Intestinal perforation with the Veress needle can be recognized by aspiration of intestinal contents and by high pressure on insufflation. A fecal odor appears only if the large intestine (not the small intestine) has been entered. Because of the small size of the Veress needle such a puncture usually does not have serious consequences, and gas insufflated into the intestine in moderate amounts will usually pass through, although perforation by excessive insufflation is possible. If perforation of the intestine with the Veress needle is strongly suspected, a different site should be used for puncture and the trocar should not be inserted until a satisfactory pneumoperitoneum has been obtained. Demonstrated or strongly suspected intestinal injury with the trocar is an indication for immediate laparotomy and closure of the perforation. The same is true if a serious trocar injury to the mesentery is suspected.

Intraabdominal bleeding may be a complication of inserting the Veress needle or the trocar, more likely the latter. Vessels in the mesentery or major arteries or veins (aorta or iliac vessels) may be injured. Blood may well up through the Veress needle, may obscure the view with the laparoscope or may be seen to collect rapidly in the pelvis. If the blood loss is considerable, the patient's blood pressure may fall and her pulse rise. Prompt laparotomy is indicated. An adequate vertical incision should be made and the bleeding point identified as soon as possible and controlled at first with pressure from finger, sponge stick or long tape sponges. Then, with adequate retraction, the exact point and extent of the laceration should be identified. If a major vessel such as the aorta is injured, pressure above and below the laceration by sponges or vascular clamps, if available, together with use of the suction tip, permits the laceration to be closed with fine arterial silk. Consultation with a vascular surgeon is advisable. Once the artery or vein is repaired the pelvis should be examined to answer the questions for which the laparoscopy was originally performed.

Insertion of the second probe may rarely injure the bladder or cause bleeding. These complications can be avoided by emptying the patient's bladder prior to the operation and by visualizing the point of insertion by transillumination with the previously inserted laparoscope.

Unsuccessful or "failed" laparoscopy performed by the closed technique is estimated to occur in 7.5 per 1000 cases, even with experienced surgeons. The usual cause is failure to enter the peritoneum with the Veress needle or trocar. Dodson (1984) suggests that in such situations the open method of laparoscopy be used and reports three successful cases.

Early Postoperative Complications

Early postoperative complications include intestinal injury, bleeding and infection. Intestinal injury may not have been appreciated at the time of laparoscopy. After a varying asymptomatic interval the patient complains of abdominal pain. Tenderness, rebound tenderness and diminished peristalsis develop and are accompanied over a 24-hour-period by fever and leukocytosis. Suspicion of injury indicates continued postoperative monitoring of vital signs, including repeated blood counts and abdominal x-rays to exclude increasing amounts of free air. Exploratory laparotomy should be performed as soon as the diagnosis is established; procedures used at that time are covered in Chapters 3 and 4.

Bleeding may occur at the site of abdominal wall puncture or intra- or retroperitoneally. If incisional bleeding can be identified, removal of sutures and resuture under local or general anesthesia is necessary. Deeper bleeding may be difficult to distinguish from bowel injury; decreasing hematocrit or paracentesis positive for blood may be present. Progressive bleeding is an indication for exploratory laparotomy and identification and control of the bleeding vessels.

Infection may occur within the peritoneal cavity either de novo or as an exacerbation of a prior peritonitis, salpingitis or other infection. It is difficult to differentiate from intestinal injury because pain and fever occur in both. With infection a broad spectrum antibiotic may improve the patient's condition within a few hours, while in intestinal perforation this may not be the case. Bladder infection may follow catheterization and is managed by urinary antibiotics after obtaining a urine culture (see Chapter 4).

Since most laparoscopies are now performed with only a brief (few hours) stay in a hospital or surgicenter, careful postoperative observation is essential. Normally the patient recovers from the anesthesia and the procedure with minimal discomfort and no change in vital signs.

Persistent pain, elevation of pulse or temperature, hypotension or hypertension indicates the need for continued monitoring and may herald one of the complications listed previously.

Intraoperative and Early Postoperative Complications of Specific Laparoscopic Procedures

It is often difficult to determine from published reports whether a given complication relates to laparoscopy itself or to the associated procedures.

Tubal Occlusion

Tubes may be occluded by electrocoagulation, silastic bands or clips. Complications arise from the manipulation involved and the type of occlusion employed. Table 6–1 shows the potential complications of the different techniques.

Electrothermal injury is most common with bipolar fulguration and rare with unipolar fulguration. It is absent with the use of bands or clips unless bleeding points have to be coagulated. The dangers of coagulation are (1) injury to neighboring structures, particularly intestine, (2) electrical injury to a large area of the tube or mesosalpinx and (3) major malfunctions such as explosions.

Electrical burns of the intestine result from the direct application of the current to the bowel wall. If such an injury is recognized at operation, it may appear as a whitened area on the serosa; this does not usually require laparotomy. If the serosa is separated and the muscularis, mucosa or even the lumen of the intestine is seen, laparotomy is indicated. The burned area should be oversewn and inverted with transversely placed interrupted silk sutures. If the injury is not recognized at the time of the laparoscopic procedure, the patient's immediate postoperative course is usually uncomplicated. However, the burned area may undergo necrosis, and two to seven days later

Table 6–1. Possible Complications of Laparoscopic Tubal Occlusion

Technique	Electrothermal Injuries	Ectopic Pregnancy	Technical Problems	Pain	Bleeding from Mesosalpinx
Unipolar fulguration	+	+	Low	Low	+
Bipolar fulguration	Rare	+	Low	Low	+
Silastic bands	0	Low	+	+	+
Hulka clips	0	Very low	+	+	Very low

perforation may occur. The patient develops abdominal pain and fever and the signs of peritonitis. Immediate laparotomy is indicated with appropriate repair of the perforation. Resection and anastomosis is often necessary because necrosis may extend beyond the area of obvious involvement. Soderstrom and Levy (1986) recommend resection of the bowel at least 4 cm beyond the site of perforation.

When silastic bands (Falope ring) or clips are used there is danger of applying them to the wrong structure, e.g., the infundibulopelvic ligament, round ligament or even intestine. The bands can usually be removed by the laparoscopic forceps. Bands may be lost from the end of the applicator, but can usually be retrieved laparoscopically. Postoperative pain may be somewhat greater after the use of bands.

Bleeding from the mesosalpinx may occur with all techniques. It is usually visible at the time and is often related to traction on the tube. When possible the bleeding points should be visualized and coagulated. If bleeding continues, laparotomy is indicated.

Late postoperative complications of laparoscopic tubal occlusion are discussed later in this chapter with those following open procedures such as abdominal, minilaparotomy and vaginal tubal ligation.

LAPAROSCOPIC BIOPSY

Laparoscopic biopsy specimens may be taken from the ovary, especially as part of an endocrine-infertility work-up, or from other peritoneal sites as part of an evaluation for primary or recurrent pelvic cancer.

Ovarian biopsy may be difficult to perform because of problems in obtaining adequate exposure. The technique described by Cibils (1975) is helpful. Bleeding sometimes complicates ovarian biopsy procedures but can usually be controlled by coagulation. There appear to be no long-term complications of one or more small ovarian biopsy procedures.

Intraperitoneal laparoscopic biopsy is often used in patients with gynecologic cancer to evaluate the effect of treatment, usually chemotherapy, prior to or sometimes instead of laparotomy. Occasionally, it is used in the initial evaluation of the patient. The special complications are failure to enter the free peritoneal cavity owing to prior adhesions or tumor, perforation of the intestine at entry and hemorrhage from bleeding biopsy sites. Also, metastases from ovarian cancer have been reported

to occur in the trocar incision later (Lacey et al, 1978). These complications (except the last) can be obviated by appropriate selection of the puncture site, proper visualization of the biopsy area and possibly by the use of small instruments such as the Needlescope (Berek et al, 1981). Since laparotomy is often part of the evaluation proposed to the patient, it is easy to proceed to this if the peritoneal cavity cannot be entered, bowel perforation is suspected or hemorrhage occurs as a result of biopsy.

OTHER LAPAROSCOPIC PROCEDURES

Laparoscopy has been used to divide adhesions or cauterize endometriotic implants. Complications are more likely to be encountered if thick adhesions are cut. Cauterizing implants increases the risk of burning the intestine. Extended procedures such as myomectomy or laparoscopic suspension of the uterus (Paterson et al, 1978) have also been described. Complications are likely to increase when intraperitoneal manipulations are performed without direct visualization of the structures involved.

Open Laparoscopy

Open laparoscopy can be performed in two ways, both of which avoid, at least in part, the difficulties caused by the blind insertion of the Veress needle and the trocar. In one technique a special blunt laparoscope (Hasson, 1971) is inserted under direct vision after all layers of the abdominal wall are incised in the region of the umbilicus; gas is then insufflated directly through the sleeve of the laparoscope and its escape is prevented by tying fascial sutures to the instrument. In another method a similar incision is made and the peritoneal cavity is entered with a finger. A conventional laparoscope is used and escape of gas can be prevented by a subcutaneous purse-string suture tied around the sleeve (Grimes, 1981). In a modification of this method, the fascia is merely scratched, and a standard laparoscope is inserted blindly in the usual manner without prior gas insufflation. In 1982 only 4% of the laparoscopies reported by the American Association of Gynecologic Laparoscopists were by the open technique (Phillips et al, 1984). A personal survey (Penfield, 1985) of 10,840 open laparoscopies showed wound infections and bowel lacerations to be the commonest complications (1.7 and 0.5/1000, respectively). In addition, the time taken to enter the peritoneal cavity, especially in an obese patient, may present a problem. Otherwise complications are similar to those with closed laparoscopy.

OPERATIONS ON THE UTERUS

Hysterectomy

INTRODUCTION

An estimated 670,000 hysterectomies were performed in United States hospitals in 1985, (National Hospital Discharge Survey, 1985). Both the number and the rate per 100,000 women rose between 1971 and 1975, but they have fallen somewhat since then (Easterday, 1983). These figures, higher than those in other countries, have given rise to considerable professional and public scrutiny. Of particular concern, therefore, are the complications that may result and the possible methods of avoiding them and ways of reducing the number of these operations.

About 75% of hysterectomies are performed by the abdominal route and 25% by the vaginal route. Although the complications differ somewhat and are indicated here and in Chapter 5, those of abdominal hysterectomy are more important simply because this approach is used more frequently.

DEFINITION OF PROCEDURE

Abdominal hysterectomy may be performed through a lower vertical or transverse incision, depending on the size of the uterus and the preference of the surgeon. After preliminary exploration of the peritoneal cavity, modified by the disease being treated, the uterus is grasped either by a tenaculum on the fundus or by clamps at the cornua and pulled upward. The round and infundibulopelvic ligaments or the utero-ovarian ligaments if the ovaries are to be conserved are divided and ligated on each side. The bladder is pushed down from the anterior surface of the cervix. The uterine artery is skeletonized, divided and ligated, and the cardinal ligaments are divided and ligated close to the cervix, pushing off the rectum posteriorly and the bladder anteriorly until the vagina is reached. The vagina is entered laterally and divided at its apex, and the uterus is removed. The vagina may be closed or left open with a circular locked hemostatic stitch around it. The

pelvic peritoneum and abdominal wall are then closed.

Many modifications of the operation have been described and may be needed as circumstances dictate. One of the chief points of difference is the use of the intrafascial (Jaszczak and Evans, 1982) or extrafascial technique. In the former the fascia overlying the cervix and rectum is divided and peeled down, enabling the lateral clamps to be placed "intrafascially" and closer to the cervix. Recently the use of automatic staples has been described for the division of the paracervical tissue and the vagina. Although operating time may possibly be saved by these devices, they are difficult to use lateral to the cervix when the normal anatomic relationships are distorted. A good length of vagina is also needed for their application. The use of metal staples in the vaginal cuff is not acceptable because of possible coital trauma to the male partner, but the newer absorbable staples do not have this disadvantage (Beresford, 1984).

INCIDENCE OF COMPLICATIONS

The exact frequency and severity of complications during and soon after abdominal hysterectomy are difficult to ascertain because of the differences in the indications for operation, in operative skills and in supportive medical and hospital facilities. Large multihospital surveys also tend to report outcome results rather than specific complications, for example, the number of patients transfused, given anticoagulants or reoperated for complications rather than the amount of blood lost, the type of thrombotic episode or the exact reason for reoperation. In spite of these biases data collected in a collaborative study and reported by Dicker and associates (1982) give an overall view of the incidence of complications (Table 6–2). No deaths were reported in this study. However, a gen-

Table 6–2. Complications of Abdominal Hysterectomy (Operative and Early Postoperative)

Complication	Incidence/ 1000 Operations
Hemorrhage requiring transfusion	323
Febrile morbidity	154
Atelectasis	59
Urinary tract injury	5
Deep venous thrombosis and embolism	4
Intestinal tract injury	3

erally accepted figure is 1 to 2 deaths per 1000 abdominal hysterectomies.

INTRAOPERATIVE COMPLICATIONS

Intestinal Tract. The prevention and management of intestinal injuries are covered in Chapter 3. In many hysterectomies the location of the colon and its relationship to the uterus must be identified early in the operation in order to avoid injury to the colon (Fig. 6–1).

Hemorrhage. Incisional bleeding is covered in Chapter 3. A special site for bleeding during the initial phases of hysterectomy is the upper attachments of the bladder and the bladder wall as it is pushed down off the front of the cervix. This bleeding can usually be controlled with pressure from a sponge as the operation proceeds.

Inside the peritoneal cavity bleeding is most likely to occur from the ovarian vessels (if the ovaries are being removed), from the uterine artery or from abnormal vessels supplying ovarian or uterine tumors or inflammatory masses. The ovarian artery is best secured by dividing the peritoneum lateral to it, skeletonizing it and placing a proximal ligature and distal suture ligature on the pedicle after division. If the vessel slips from the clamp or ligature, it may retract; it is essential to find it and ligate it, keeping the ureter under observation throughout.

The uterine artery is usually secured as it turns upward along the lateral aspect of the cervix. It is isolated as well as possible and clamped with a curved instrument such as a Heaney clamp. One well-placed suture ligature is usually sufficient. Two are inadvisable; whenever a needle is placed blindly under a clamp lateral to the uterus, there is a chance of piercing another blood vessel or including the ureter.

As the paracervical tissue is clamped and divided, severe bleeding may occur from descending branches of the uterine artery or from large veins. It is important to take small bites of tissue and use clamps that do not slip off. Heaney clamps are satisfactory but are sometimes too big. Straight Ochsner's clamps, which are often used, may slip. Boettcher's clamps are useful.

Distortion of the anatomic structures by tumors may alter the position of the uterine artery; also, new arteries and veins may supply the tumor. It is therefore essential to do all the dissection with as good exposure as possible. If a bleeding vessel cannot easily be identified and controlled, it may be necessary to pack off the bleeding area and identify and ligate the uterine artery as it leaves the internal iliac artery. When major life-threatening hemorrhage occurs, ligation of the internal iliac artery may be necessary. This should usually be done on both sides. It will not stop the bleeding immediately, but will slow it down so that pressure and use of hemostatic substances will stop it. See Chapter 3 for the management of these and related bleeding problems.

Urinary Tract. During abdominal hysterec-

Figure 6–1. Relationship of the colon to the uterus and the left ovary.

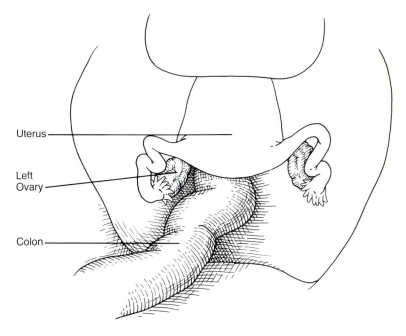

Uterus

Left Ovary

Colon

tomy injury to the bladder is most likely to occur (1) when the incision is made or when the bladder is pushed down off the front of the lower uterine segment and cervix, especially if a previous operation, particularly a cesarean section, has resulted in the bladder being fixed or adherent to the anterior peritoneum or the uterus; and (2) when the vaginal cuff is being closed or bleeding vessels close to the bladder wall are being secured. The prevention, diagnosis and management of these bladder injuries are covered in Chapter 3.

Injury to the ureter is especially likely during hysterectomy when a large uterine tumor, an inflammatory mass or endometriosis obscures the landmarks deep in the pelvis or as the paracervical tissues are being divided where the ureter lies close to the cervix. The important thing is to be aware of the possibility of injury, to recognize it when it occurs and to take every care to avoid it. When there is a large mass in the pelvis, the ureter should be identified above it and kept in sight as the dissection proceeds downward. Although adventitial tissue should be left on the ureter when possible, holding it with a Babcock clamp greatly facilitates dissection. When the cervix is being removed, it is essential to place successive clamps inside the previously sutured paracervical tissue, so as to push the ureters laterally. If injury by clamping, incision or division occurs, procedures outlined in Chapter 3 should be followed. Unless the gynecologist is familiar with these procedures, he should obtain urologic consultation.

Neurologic Complications. Neuropathy is reported by Dicker and co-workers (1982) to occur in 2 per 1000 women undergoing abdominal hysterectomy. Such injury is most likely to involve the femoral nerve, which may be compressed by continuous pressure from a self-retaining retractor on the psoas muscle. If the pulsations of the femoral artery are felt with the retractor in place, the femoral nerve is probably not being compressed. The consequences of injury to the femoral and other nerves are discussed in Chapters 3 and 4.

EARLY POSTOPERATIVE COMPLICATIONS

The early complications of abdominal hysterectomy are, in general, similar to those following any major gynecologic operation. They are covered in detail in Chapter 4. However, hemorrhagic, infectious, urinary and gastrointestinal complications are of special relevance.

Hemorrhage. Bleeding in the first 24 hours after abdominal hysterectomy may arise from (1) the uterine artery or its branches, (2) the uterine veins or their tributaries, (3) the ovarian vessels if the ovaries have been removed, (4) the vaginal cuff, (5) the bladder or (6) deep in the pelvis from the internal iliac vein or its tributaries. Hemorrhage is more likely to follow difficult procedures when intraoperative bleeding has been hard to control.

The diagnosis is relatively easy if blood appears vaginally; it is more difficult if the bleeding is intraperitoneal or retroperitoneal. The chief sign is hypotension so long as other causes of decreased blood pressure have been excluded. The steps in diagnosis are summarized in Table 6–3. Persistent hypotension despite transfusion, low venous pressure (less than 5 cm H_2O) and low urinary output point to continuing blood loss. Abdominal girth may increase. Obtaining blood from paracentesis in the right or left lower quadrant may be diagnostic.

Prompt reoperation is indicated once the diagnosis of hemorrhage has been well established. The incision is reopened and the stitches removed. Adequate exposure is essential. An attempt should be made to identify the bleeding vessel and ligate or clip it. If this cannot be done, the uterine or the internal iliac artery may be isolated and ligated. When generalized oozing is present a coagulation defect must be suspected. Hemostatic substances and even packing with a 5-yard gauze roll may be necessary (see Chapter 3).

Infection. Infection is a potential sequela of abdominal hysterectomy, since it is classified as a clean-contaminated operation because an infected organ, the vagina, is entered and transected. Also, abdominal hysterectomy may be performed soon after vaginal procedures, which may facilitate inflammation and infection in the uterine cavity and parametria. This does not appear to occur after simple biopsy of the cervix or dilatation of the cervix and curettage of the endometrial cavity. When a simple abdominal (or vaginal) hysterectomy follows conization of the cervix, morbidity is increased (DeCenzo et

Table 6–3. Diagnosis of Hemorrhage Following Abdominal Hysterectomy

1. Hypotension verified.
2. Exclude causes other than bleeding.
3. Transfuse 1 to 2 units packed red cells rapidly.
4. Measure venous pressure and urine output.
5. CBC, platelets, coagulation factors.
6. Measure abdominal girth.
7. Perform paracentesis.

al, 1971), more so if the cone-hysterectomy interval is less than 14 days. Because of these findings many authors recommend that simple hysterectomy be performed within 48 hours or deferred until four weeks or more after conization, unless there is an urgent reason for performing it sooner. The same reasoning may apply to endocervical curettage, which probably has the same potential as conization for disseminating infection into the paracervical tissue. On the other hand, radical hysterectomy following conization does not seem to be followed by increased infectious morbidity (Orr et al, 1982), possibly because of the wide excision of potentially infected parametrial tissue.

Infection is often defined in terms of febrile morbidity, i.e. a temperature of 100.4°F (38° C) or more on any two days after operation, exclusive of the first 24 hours. Using these criteria, the incidence of infection has been reported to be 32.3% after abdominal hysterectomy (Dicker et al, 1982), higher than the 15.3% rate reported by the same authors following vaginal hysterectomy. This is surprising because vaginal hysterectomy involves longer operative contact with vaginal flora. In approximately half the febrile patients no source could be identified, whereas in one quarter it was due to infection of the pelvis, vaginal cuff or abdominal incision. The remainder were primarily due to urinary tract infections. When infection was determined by documented evidence of sepsis at specific sites, it occurred after 18% of abdominal hysterectomies as compared with 8% of vaginal hysterectomies (Shapiro et al, 1982).

The appropriate studies for a patient with postoperative fever and the differential diagnosis of postoperative infection after abdominal hysterectomy, together with their management by antibiotics and other measures, are similar to those necessary for any major gynecologic procedure. They are discussed in Chapter 4.

Prophylactic antibiotics have been shown to be effective in lowering infection rates after abdominal as well as after vaginal hysterectomy. A variety of drugs and dosage systems have been suggested. First generation cephalosporins were initially used. Now second generation cephalosporins such as cefoxitin are likely to give better coverage, and metronidazole has also been recommended because of its effectiveness against *B. fragilis*. A suggested dosage schedule for cephoxitin is 1 gm (intravenously) immediately before operation, 1 gm six hours later and 1 gm 12 hours after the initial dose. Three 2-gm doses of cefoxitin over 12 hours reduced the major infection rate to 12% from the 32% observed in a control group. However, febrile morbidity was similar in both groups (Hemsell et al, 1983). One preoperative 2-gm dose of cefoxitin may be as effective as three doses (Hemsell et al, 1984). Two 2-gm doses of metronidazole, one before and one after operation, also provide effective prophylaxis against infection and were reported to be better than suction drainage through the vagina (Poulsen et al, 1984). Prophylaxis is particularly important when the chance of infection is increased by a previous operation such as conization of the cervix.

Gastrointestinal Tract. Gastrointestinal complications occurring in the first seven days after any abdominal operation include perforation, fistula formation, pneumoperitoneum, acute gastric dilatation, ileus and intestinal obstruction. None is specific for hysterectomy for benign conditions, and they are covered in Chapter 4.

Urinary Tract. During abdominal hysterectomy it is important that the bladder be empty to permit its dissection from the lower uterine segment and cervix and to enable urine output to be measured during the operation. This is best done by inserting a urethral catheter as the patient is being prepared in the operating room. Continuation of drainage and measurement of output remain important in the first 24 hours or more after operation. Since the patient is unlikely to be able to void spontaneously because of the effects of anesthesia and incisional pain, it is customary although not strictly necessary to leave the urethral catheter in place for at least 24 hours.

The monitoring of urinary output and the management of complications affecting the ureter, bladder and urethra are no different from those occurring after any major abdominal operation in gynecology and obstetrics. They are covered in detail in Chapter 4.

LATE POSTOPERATIVE COMPLICATIONS

Vaginal Vault. When the uterus has been removed, the vagina may be closed or left open. In the former situation, a continuous suture or interrupted single or figure-of-eight sutures are used. In the latter, in order to permit drainage from the pelvis, a continuous hemostatic locked suture is placed around the vaginal cuff. When a straight or T-tube drain is left in the pelvis and brought out through the vagina, either a locked stitch is placed in the cuff or only the lateral angles are closed. Healing of the vaginal vault takes four to six weeks, and there is little difference in the healing time for different methods of closure. Absorbable sutures (preferably the polyglycolic type) should generally be used. Non-absorbable sutures may cause lack of expandability of the vaginal apex. Wire sutures or staples should not be used.

Slight vaginal bleeding is common up to about 14 days after abdominal hysterectomy. It is most likely due to absorption and loosening of the cuff sutures with lysis of clots in small vessels. No immediate treatment is needed unless the bleeding becomes heavy. Later bleeding, either spontaneous or following intercourse or douching, is likely to be due to granulation tissue at the vaginal apex. This has been reported to be present in as high as 37% of cases (Howkins and Williams, 1968). It can easily be seen as a polypoid red protrusion from the cuff. If there is doubt as to its nature, it should be avulsed with an Allis forceps and submitted for pathologic examination. It can usually be successfully treated by cauterization with silver nitrate; this may have to be repeated once or twice. Fairlie and Al-Hassani (1973) noted a reduction in the incidence of vault granulation to 27% with the use of a continuous Lembert suture of Dexon to close the vagina. Occasionally the red bleeding area is more solid, cannot be avulsed or does not respond to silver nitrate. In a woman whose tubes and ovaries were conserved, this may be a prolapsed tube. The biopsy specimen will show tubal mucosa. The tube may be removed vaginally by opening the cuff and excising it. An abdominal approach may be necessary. Very rarely ectopic pregnancy, due to conception just before hysterectomy, may be found in the tube. Bleeding from the cuff may also be due to endometriosis in the scar. Again, biopsy is essential.

When the cervix has been removed, the vagina is somewhat shortened and the apex becomes less expansile. This is not so marked for the usual abdominal hysterectomy for benign disease as it is for a radical hysterectomy when the upper one third of the vagina is removed. Treatment is primarily by patient education, changing positions of intercourse so that less discomfort is experienced and insuring adequate lubrication, either by prolonging foreplay or adding lubricant such as surgical jelly. With repeated coitus some lengthening takes place. At the time of hysterectomy for a benign condition it is important to leave the vagina as long as possible.

Eversion of the vagina may follow hysterectomy. A protuberant mass that may contain intestine is seen on pelvic examination. Repair is described in Chapter 5. It is difficult because of the lack of ligamentous support in the pelvis.

Rarely the apex of the vagina may perforate suddenly with resulting protrusion of intestine. Exploratory laparotomy is urgently indicated.

Residual Ovary. When one or both ovaries are preserved at the time of abdominal hysterectomy they may cause symptoms later because of their position, hormonal changes or the development of cysts or tumors.

When the attachments of the ovaries to and their support from the uterus are removed, there is a greater tendency for them to fall into the cul-de-sac. Dyspareunia may then result, particularly with deep thrusting. This may be mitigated by changing positions for intercourse, e.g., using the side, woman-above or knee-chest position. It may be prevented by suturing the stump of the utero-ovarian ligament to the round ligament so as to suspend the ovary out of the pelvis (Fig. 6–2). This must be done without kinking the infundibulopelvic ligament.

When both ovaries have been removed at the time of hysterectomy in a woman who is experiencing menstrual cycles, the production of ovarian hormones ceases abruptly, and premature menopause occurs (see later section). Even if both ovaries are preserved there may also be hormonal effects. Stone and co-workers (1975) studied 22 women after abdominal (9 patients) or vaginal (13 patients) hysterectomy. Compared with 11 control subjects who had undergone only laparoscopy, women whose ovaries had been preserved at hysterectomy and who were in both the follicular and luteal phases of their cycles showed a significant fall in plasma estradiol levels on the second postoperative day; those who were in the luteal phase of their cycle also showed a significant fall in plasma progesterone. These changes are most likely to be caused by alteration in blood flow, either from loss of the supply from the uterine artery or from temporary compromise of the blood flow to the ovary itself (Janson and Jansson, 1977).

If both ovaries have functioned normally and appear grossly normal when preserved at hysterectomy, the subsequent hormonal pattern appears to differ little from the usual sequence of events. Thus, in seven patients Corson and associates (1981) found no difference from controls in estradiol or progesterone levels. The age of "menopause" in such patients is difficult

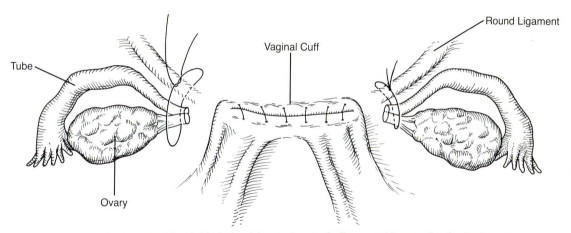

Figure 6–2. *Attachment of the right uterine tube and ovary to the round ligaments after hysterectomy.*

to determine without detailed laboratory studies (which have not been reported), but, based on clinical signs such as hot flashes, seems to be similar to that in women whose uteri remain intact. When only one ovary is preserved, hormonal production continues, although it is more likely to be abnormal with a greater number of anovulatory, marginal or inactive cycles (Beavis et al, 1969). Presumably if ovarian function has been erratic prior to hysterectomy or if the ovaries appear abnormal, if they have had procedures performed on them or if their blood supply remains compromised postoperatively, function might be altered, but information on these points is lacking.

The possible development of cysts or tumors in the preserved ovary or ovaries is a matter of concern. Since ovarian cancer is difficult to diagnose and has a low overall five year survival rate of only about 30%, it is distressing to discover it in a residual ovary. The chance of a woman with intact ovaries and uterus developing carcinoma of the ovary is about 1.1% during her lifetime and about 0.9% after the age of 40. There is no reason to suppose that hysterectomy will alter this incidence. Benign cysts and tumors may also develop in a retained ovary. Funt and co-workers (1977) noted that operation was performed for ovarian enlargements in 1.4% of 922 women who had had hysterectomies, at a mean of three years previously, with preservation of the ovaries when they were 20 to 50 years of age. The total risk, therefore, of ovarian cysts and tumors, benign and malignant, developing after hysterectomy is 2 to 3%. Whether the incidence is lessened by preserving only one ovary is not known. Studies of this subject have not shown statistically significant differences. A rough calculation indicates that if 100,000 women are subjected to hysterectomy with preservation of one or both ovaries, about 1000 will develop ovarian cancer of whom 700 will die; about 1500 will develop a benign ovarian cyst or tumor of whom perhaps one will die. Thus, ovaries will need to be removed in 143 women at the time of hysterectomy to save one woman from subsequent death by ovarian cancer. Whether this is an appropriate cost-benefit ratio has to be decided for the individual woman, in part on the basis of the consequences of castration.

If a cyst or tumor is detected on pelvic examination in one or both remaining ovaries, the same indications for operation exist as if the uterus were still present. In a premenopausal woman a small (less than 5 cm) cyst can be observed for six to eight weeks, since it may be functional in nature (follicular or corpus luteum cyst). Earlier operation is indicated if the tumor is solid. In a postmenopausal woman the discovery of a cystic or solid tumor of any size is an indication for removal, since the chance of malignancy is much greater. Ultrasonography may be helpful when the pelvic examination is difficult because the patient is obese or resistant. Occasionally laparoscopy may be needed for diagnosis.

In the absence of an enlarged ovary, pelvic pain and/or dyspareunia may be due to the abnormal position of the residual ovary (fixed in the pelvis or attached to the vaginal cuff). Removal may sometimes be indicated under these circumstances. Once a laparotomy has been performed, there is little reason for preserving any portion of a diseased ovary, even in the younger woman, because of the possibility of recurrent difficulty.

Psychological Complications. Much has been

written about the emotional sequelae of hysterectomy (Wijma, 1984). It is a difficult subject to study and it is not surprising that most investigators fail to consider many factors. The following possible sources of bias must be taken into account.

1. *The age of the woman at operation, her cultural background and socioeconomic status.* It is generally agreed that hysterectomy poses a more difficult problem for women under the age of 40. Even if the operation is urgently necessary, it means an unexpected cessation of reproductive life. Cross-cultural studies of the effect of hysterectomy are limited. In Hispanic-American families loss of the uterus and the ability to conceive may be very important to the husband and, therefore, to the wife (Williams, 1973). This is also likely to be true in other cultures. Socioeconomic status may not be very important (Roopnorinesingh and Gopeesingh, 1982).

2. *The woman's and her family's previous response to stress.* Response to one kind of major stress may foreshadow response to another. However, hysterectomy is a different stress from any other, because of the reproductive and sexual implications. Nevertheless, the patient's psychiatric background may be important in her overall reaction to hysterectomy (Ananth, 1978). Moreover, patients who have poor support from family and friends have more emotional complications (Webb and Wilson-Barrett, 1983).

3. *The disease for which hysterectomy was performed.* A hysterectomy performed for cancer may have very different implications for the patient than one performed primarily for sterilization. In the former, concern about recurrence and possible death is paramount; in the latter there may be second thoughts about the necessity of the operation. Asymptomatic patients for whom the operation was unexpected present more problems postoperatively (Tang, 1985).

4. *Removal of one or both ovaries.* The effect of removing both ovaries at the time of hysterectomy obviously affects the hormonal milieu and might, therefore, be expected to have emotional as well as physical effects. Even if both ovaries are preserved, there is often evidence of temporary ovarian dysfunction as indicated by the previously described hormonal studies and the occurrence of hot flashes in one third of such patients (Roopnorinesingh and Gopeesingh, 1982). When only one ovary remained, the same authors found the postoperative incidence of hot flashes to be 50%.

5. *The physical complications of the operation.* If a woman has a major complication of hysterectomy, such as hemorrhage requiring reoperation, severe infection or pulmonary embolism, her emotional response to the procedure may be altered. Even a minor complication such as wound separation, vaginal bleeding or a lower urinary tract infection may have emotional consequences, at least in the first few weeks after the operation.

6. *Use of matched controls.* A major operation of any sort may have emotional sequelae. Therefore, women undergoing hysterectomy should be compared with control women having a procedure of similar severity; cholecystectomy has often been used. Moreover, the comparison should be prospective rather than retrospective.

7. *Time after the operation.* The psychologic effects of hysterectomy may not be manifested immediately after the operation. Studies that do not continue for two and preferably more years may miss important sequelae.

Symptoms that may have a predominantly psychologic background (although somatic components must be recognized) include hot flashes, weight changes, psychourinary symptoms, loss of energy, depression and loss of libido. Physician visits for these symptoms were found to be more common in 2,332 women who had had hysterectomies in the province of Manitoba during 1974 than in 2,533 age-matched women who had had cholecystectomies. This difference was found to be highly significant for psychologic, urinary and menopausal problems (Roos, 1984).

Hot flashes may be defined as a sudden sensation of warmth, especially over the upper chest, neck and face, followed by perspiration in the same area. Since they are primarily the result of oophorectomy, they are considered later.

Weight gain is popularly supposed to accompany menopause and, by inference, hysterectomy. If oophorectomy has been performed, it is possible but unlikely that the hormonal changes may be causative. However, it seems more probable that the enforced or self-directed inactivity that often follows hysterectomy, together with a normal intake of calories, is responsible. Appropriate explanation and dietary control are indicated.

Long-term urinary complications of hysterectomy have received little attention. Although mostly physical in nature, they may have emotional components. They may consist of repeated bladder infections often initiated by catheterization at the time of the operation, stress incontinence related to the loss of support of the urethrovesical angle (Richards, 1974) or urethritis due to lack of estrogen. Detailed urinary tract investigation is indicated, as outlined in Chapter 4. Treatment is given for specific problems. Reassurance and further counseling may be important if no specific disorders are found.

Loss of energy and decreased ability to work are reported by some authors to follow hysterectomy (see review by Newton and Baron, 1976). Again, loss of ovarian function might contribute to this, but clearly many other factors may be involved.

The occurrence of depression following hysterectomy has been widely described and its frequency debated. Possible reasons for it have been adduced from ancient writings on the centering of emotions on the womb, psychoanalytic theories on the loss of femininity and environmental factors such as lack of estrogen or lowered plasma tryptophane levels (Ananth et al, 1982). Previous psychiatric problems appear to predispose to depression or similar postoperative sequelae. Thirty to more than 50% of patients with preoperative depression or other psychiatric difficulties are reported to have depression or similar problems postoperatively (Ananth, 1978). Apart from this, depression followed hysterectomy in as many as 33% of patients when compared with a rate of 7% in age- and operation-matched controls (Richards, 1973). These observations have been confirmed by others who have followed patients for two or more years after operation. However, the problems of defining depression, both subjectively and objectively, and determining its extent and the possible importance of cultural differences are emphasized by the finding of Kav-Venaki and Zakham (1983) that there was no difference in depression between post-hysterectomy and post-cholecystectomy patients in Israel when a Depression Adjective Check List was used. This is clearly a subject that needs further investigation, taking into account all the possible sources of bias.

Sexual Complications. Changes in sexual response, most commonly loss of libido, are consistently reported in 30 to 40% of women who have had hysterectomies (Zussman and Zussman, 1981), with somewhat greater frequency after removal of both ovaries. In a study of 171 patients who had undergone hysterectomy without removal of the ovaries Sakai and coworkers (1983) found that vaginal lubrication decreased in 46% and remained unchanged or increased in 42%. Loss of feelings of femininity,

which occurred in 52% of patients, was commonly associated with lack of lubrication. Interestingly 27% noted loss of uterine sensation, and the majority of these women complained of a decrease in the ability to climax. Those who felt no loss of uterine sensation reported no difficulty in achieving orgasm. Many of the biases mentioned previously affect any study in this field. Factors responsible for decreased libido may be primarily psychosexual or in part pathophysiological. Examples of the former might be long standing aversion to intercourse with lack of orgasm, a change in the partner's attitude or a feeling of lessened femininity. The latter might include decrease in comfort due to the smaller capacity of the vagina, dyspareunia from prolapse of an ovary or hormonal changes resulting from oophorectomy.

Many women are reluctant to mention sexual complications, at least in the early weeks after hysterectomy, often attributing them to the physical stress of the operation. Therefore, in order to make a diagnosis and manage the problem appropriately, the gynecologist should:

1. Include a sexual history in his preoperative evaluation of the patient. This means using non-directive questions and listening with sensitivity.

2. Involve the patient's partner in the preoperative discussion, when possible.

3. Inquire about sexual problems postoperatively, attaching equal importance to them and to primarily physical symptoms such as incisional pain, urinary frequency or constipation.

4. Continue follow-up for a sufficient period of time to detect any long-term sexual dysfunction.

5. Be aware of and use consultants or agencies to whom the patient and her partner can be referred if preliminary discussions indicate the need for extensive counseling.

Other. Pregnancy has been reported to occur following hysterectomy. Among the 28 cases collected by Winslow and associates (1969), 15 had apparently had total hysterectomies. In seven of these fertilization had occurred prior to hysterectomy (avoidable by operating in the proliferative phase of the cycle). Eight had occurred later. Among these, seven followed vaginal and one abdominal hysterectomy. No viable infants were delivered. These extraordinary circumstances occur when the ovaries are preserved and when a communication remains or develops between a tube and the vagina. The diagnosis requires great perspicacity. Treatment is by operative removal of the pregnancy.

Late gastrointestinal (intestinal obstruction, fistula), urinary (ureteral obstruction, fistula, recurrent infection) and other complications are not specific for hysterectomy and are covered in Chapter 4.

Overview. Abdominal hysterectomy remains a major operation that has a very low but fairly constant mortality and significant morbidity, the exact incidence of which is not clearly known and may be underestimated. National differences in the performance of the operation have repeatedly been noted, with more occurring in North America than in Europe (Easterday et al, 1983; van Keep et al, 1983). Many hysterectomies performed in the United States appear to be elective or semi-elective, that is to say they are done at an elective time for the convenience of the patient or her physician. Richards, (1978) for example, indicated that 76.5% of 340 hysterectomies performed by four gynecologists in a suburb of Denver were elective. An underlying reason for many elective hysterectomies is still likely to be sterilization.

Because of the overall number of hysterectomies and the morbidity (and mortality) involved, careful evaluation of the indications for the procedure as well as attention to the management of complications is important. This problem was epitomized 40 years ago by Miller (1946) in his address at the the 50th Anniversary of the Chicago Lying-in Hospital, entitled "Hysterectomy—Therapeutic Necessity or Surgical Racket?" In the province of Saskatchewan, surveillance of the indications for hysterectomy resulted in a fall of 32.8% in the number of hysterectomies performed in that province between 1970 and 1974. Similar concerns have resulted in the development of programs (primarily by insurance companies) that require the patient to seek a second opinion prior to having a major procedure such as a hysterectomy performed. On the local hospital level audit of hysterectomies and anonymous discussion of the results of these studies is an important measure for control of unjustified operations. The effect of these measures on the appropriateness, cost and number of hysterectomies remains to be determined.

Subtotal (Supracervical) Hysterectomy

In 1946 Miller reported on a survey of 246 hysterectomies performed in 1944 at 10 different hospitals in three midwestern states. Of the 234 abdominal operations 72 or 31% were sub-

total hysterectomies. Nowadays subtotal hysterectomy is seldom performed in the United States unless removal of the cervix would endanger the patient's life.

In subtotal hysterectomy the uterus is transsected at or below the junction between the corpus and the cervix uteri after the uterine arteries on each side are ligated. The top of the cervix is then covered with pelvic peritoneum.

The operative and early postoperative complications of subtotal hysterectomy do not differ from those occurring after total hysterectomy. Indeed, they may be less severe, because there is less dissection near the bladder, ureters or rectum. Later the cervix is subject to the same disorders as if the whole uterus were present. These include chronic cervicitis, cervical intraepithelial neoplasia, polyps or prolapse. Management of these disorders is similar to that when the body of the uterus is present, i.e., annual cytologic studies, diagnostic colposcopy, biopsy and, if necessary, conization. Persistence or increase in these problems, e.g., marked prolapse, is an indication for cervicectomy. This can usually be performed vaginally, often without entering the peritoneal cavity. If invasive carcinoma develops in the cervical stump (0.1 to 1.9%), it is more difficult to handle surgically in Stage I because of the absence of the uterus to provide traction or radiotherapeutically in any stage because of the difficulty of inserting radioactive sources into the short cervix, thereby compromising radiation dosage.

Subtotal hysterectomy does not seem to add long-term urinary or sexual complications; in fact, it may be followed by less difficulty. Kilkku and associates (1981) noted that urinary symptoms (pollakiuria, nocturia, dysuria or pressure sensation) were less frequent in a series of 105 patients who had had subtotal hysterectomy compared with 107 who had total hysterectomy, one year after operation. The same authors found no significant difference in libido or coital frequency after the two operations. There was, however, a greater reduction in frequency of orgasm after total as compared with subtotal hysterectomy (Kilkku, 1983; Kilkku et al, 1983).

Other Operations

MYOMECTOMY

Myomectomy means removal of one or more myomata (leiomyomata) from the uterus. It is usually performed abdominally, although a prolapsed or cervical myoma may be removed vaginally. Removal through the hysteroscope or the laparoscope has also been described. Abdominal myomectomy is indicated when large and symptomatic myomata are present in a young woman who is anxious to retain her reproductive capacity or when the myomata may be contributing to infertility (inability to conceive or repeated abortions) and there is no other apparent cause for this.

Preoperative complications consist primarily of irregular bleeding and anemia. The former should be studied by obtaining an endometrial sample for pathologic examination. The latter is managed by dietary measures or, in severe cases (hemoglobin less than 8 gm/dl), by preoperative transfusions.

Intraoperative complications during myomectomy include (1) hemorrhage, (2) injury to the uterotubal junction and (3) incision of the endometrial cavity. Many techniques of minimizing blood loss have been described. The uterine artery may be compressed by a clamp (Bonney's clamp) or by a rubber tourniquet placed around the upper end of the cervix by perforating the broad ligament lateral to the uterine artery. Some authors recommend releasing this constriction every 10 minutes. Compression of the uterine artery may not be easy because of the distortion of the uterus by the myomata, and bleeding may also be encountered as the broad ligament is pierced. Vasoconstrictors such as pitressin (20 units in 20 ml of saline or neosynephrine 0.005%) may be injected into the uterine wall. The possible circulatory effects of these drugs must be taken into account. When the vasoconstrictors wear off, renewed bleeding may occur. Using the CO_2 laser for myomectomy may reduce blood loss (McLaughlin, 1985), but the expense of the equipment and the training required may be disadvantageous. A good approach is to make a vertical incision on the anterior surface of the uterus at the top of the fundus, proceed rapidly with the procedure and secure adequate hemostasis with sutures, avoiding uterine artery compression and vasoconstrictors (except) in rare instances (Buttram and Reiter, 1981). Injury to the uterotubal junction may occur if the uterus is greatly distorted by myomata. It can be minimized by making the uterine incision(s) in an anteroposterior direction and by resuturing them carefully. Entering the endometrial cavity is often not necessary and should be avoided if possible. If it occurs, it is best not to put sutures through the endometrium.

The immediate postoperative complications

of myomectomy consist primarily of hemorrhage. If this occurs within the uterus, vaginal bleeding may be seen and an enlarging, painful, tender lower abdominal (uterine) mass noted. If the bleeding is intra- or extraperitoneal, similar symptoms and signs may be present as after a total hysterectomy. A D & C may be a useful preliminary diagnostic procedure, but in either case reexploration may be needed with control of the arterial blood supply to the uterus and/or hysterectomy.

Late postoperative complications include (1) menstrual changes, (2) regrowth of myomata, (3) infertility and abnormalities of pregnancy and (4) intraperitoneal adhesions.

When myomata have been removed without entering the endometrial cavity being entered and normal ovarian function remains, menstrual abnormalities related to the operation are rare. They may be more common if the cavity has been entered, but firm data on this are lacking.

Myomata recur in about 15% of patients (range 4 to 30%) after myomectomy, according to data from 18 series totaling 3,206 patients reported from 1926 to 1980 and collected by Buttram and Reiter (1981). Sixty-nine per cent of patients in whom myomata recurred (338 out of 493), 10% of all patients reported, received major treatment subsequently by hysterectomy, second myomectomy or radiation therapy.

Difficulty in conceiving, abortion, premature labor and fetal wastage all occur following myomectomy, although most reports indicate considerable improvement after the operation. A special concern has been the possibility of rupture of the pregnant uterus prior to or during labor. Using as an analogy rupture of a classical cesarean section scar, post-myomectomy rupture has been thought more likely to occur when the endometrial cavity has been entered and to occur unexpectedly in the latter half of pregnancy as frequently or more frequently than during labor. This has encouraged many authors to recommend cesarean section if the endometrial cavity has been entered at the time of myomectomy. However, abdominal delivery may not be necessary unless there are other indications, provided that the pregnancy and labor progress normally and that there is no premonitory uterine pain.

Good data on the incidence of adhesions and intestinal obstruction following myomectomy are not available. It seems logical to suppose that omentum and intestine might adhere to the uterine scar and that posteriorly the tubes and ovaries might become attached. Therefore, attempts to prevent such adhesions are appropriate. They include:

1. Closing the uterine serosa with fine synthetic absorbable sutures or using subserosal sutures.

2. Suspension of the uterus, if retroflexed, by bringing the round ligaments through the rectus muscles and attaching them to the anterior rectus sheath (modified Gilliam suspension).

3. Pulling the bladder up and attaching it over the lower part of the uterine incision. The only problem about this is the danger of entering the bladder should a subsequent cesarean section or hysterectomy be necessary.

4. Covering the uterine incision with omental or peritoneal grafts or the round ligament. These procedures may add more sutures and other possible sites for adhesions.

5. Insertion of 32% Dextran 70 (Hyskon) into the peritoneal cavity at the time of closure. The advantages and disadvantages of this are discussed elsewhere. Present data show that it may be helpful, provided there are no contraindications such as a coagulation defect (see Chapter 3).

Uterine Suspension

Uterine suspension is performed infrequently nowadays. It used to be recommended for prolapse or for women whose uteri were retroflexed and who were felt to have dysmenorrhea and pelvic pain as a result of this. It is now only occasionally indicated to prevent the uterus from becoming adherent to the tubes and ovaries after operations for endometriosis or after myomectomy. The principal operative techniques include attachment of the round ligaments to the anterior rectus sheath (modified Gilliam procedure), fixation of the round ligaments to the back of the uterus (Baldy-Webster procedure) or plication of the uterosacral ligaments. Complications are primarily those of any transperitoneal procedure. In addition, injury to the ureter may occur when the uterosacral ligaments are plicated. Retroflexion may recur when the round ligaments are used, since they may stretch again.

Metroplasty

Repair of the uterus is occasionally performed if a major congenital anomaly that affects menstruation or reproductive capacity is present.

Such operations include unification of a bicornuate uterus (Strassmann), incision of a uterine septum and closure of the uterus (Tompkins) or wedge resection of a septum (Jones). Other procedures include excision of a rudimentary uterine horn that is obstructed and dilated. The chief intraoperative complication is bleeding, which may be controlled in the same way as for a myomectomy. The early and late postoperative complications are similar to those that follow myomectomy. In a series of 18 patients who were randomly assigned to undergo either the Jones' or Tompkins' metroplasty, the pregnancy outcome was similar in both, but the Tompkins' procedure was easier and resulted in decreased blood loss and shorter operative time (DeCherney and Tarlatzis, 1984). Cesarean section is usually advised for delivery and is probably necessary because of the extent of the uterine incisions and the possibility of uterine rupture. One additional complication may be cervical incompetence. This is especially likely to occur if the cervix (or one of two cervices if two are present) has been incised or weakened by removal of a low septum that leads to a double cervix or by wide excision of a rudimentary horn at its junction with the cervix.

OPERATIONS ON THE TUBES

Unilateral Salpingectomy

Ectopic pregnancy is the primary reason for surgical removal of one tube. Complications of this procedure are covered in Chapter 8.

Bilateral Salpingectomy

There is no indication nowadays for complete removal of both tubes as a separate procedure. However, partial salpingectomy is a very common method of sterilization. It may be performed after delivery or abortion or as an interval procedure. For the former, either a curved incision at the lower border of the umbilicus or a vertical midline incision between the symphysis pubis and the umbilicus is made. For the latter, a lower midline vertical incision or a transverse incision at the pubic hairline (minilaparotomy) is made, in addition to the laparoscopic techniques described previously. The operation may also be performed vaginally through the cul-de-sac (posterior colpotomy).

Several different techniques of tubal ligation (non-laparoscopic) have been described. The commonest is the Pomeroy technique in which a loop of tube is elevated with a Babcock clamp at about its midpoint. The medial and lateral sections of the tube are then ligated by tying them together under the clamp with a single catgut ligature. The central portion is then excised. In Uchida's operation the medial and lateral portions of the tube are ligated separately. The medial end is buried between the leaves of the mesosalpinx and the lateral end is exteriorized outside the mesosalpinx. In the similar Irving procedure the medial end of the tube is buried in the posterior aspect of the uterus beneath the peritoneum. Excision and ligation of the fimbriated ends of the tubes (fimbriectomy) has also been used, especially in vaginal tubal ligations. The Pomeroy technique requires the least manipulation and is therefore less likely to lead to intraoperative bleeding.

INTRAOPERATIVE COMPLICATIONS

Vertical Midline Incision. Intraoperative complications are similar to those of any laparotomy (see Chapter 3). Identification and exposure of the tube, the most important problem, is usually not difficult and can be facilitated by extending the incision, if necessary.

Transverse Lower Incision (Minilaparotomy). Minilaparotomy has been widely used in recent years as a quick and convenient method of sterilization, especially in parts of the world where laparoscopic equipment is not available. Although general anesthesia is commonly given in the US, local anesthesia with or without intravenous analgesics may be used. Since the objectives are speed, a small incision and convenience for the patient, several preoperative and intraoperative precautions are necessary.

1. Obesity, pelvic masses, prior bladder operations or known adhesions, especially with a fixed retroflexed uterus, due to pelvic inflammatory disease or endometriosis are relative contraindications to the procedure.

2. The bladder should be empty, since the peritoneal cavity is entered close to it.

3. An instrument such as a Rubin's cannula or other uterine elevator should be inserted into the uterus prior to the laparotomy so that the uterus can be mobilized to expose the tubes.

4. Appropriate retractors should be available so that the tubes can be more easily identified.

5. The Trendelenberg position is very helpful.

Many of these precautions were described in detail by Brenner and Dingfelder (1976) and more recently by Lee and Boyd (1980).

Failure to identify the tubes and accomplish the ligation occurred in 3.8% of Lee and Boyd's (1980) patients managed with local anesthesia. In one, general anesthesia was used subsequently with success and in the other seven local adhesions and enlargement or retroversion of the uterus were present. Extension of the incision, by converting it into a normal Pfannenstiel's incision, usually permits completion of the operation.

Bleeding may occur if the mesosalpinx is torn as the tube is pulled up. If the bleeding cannot easily be controlled by clamp and ligature, the incision should be extended to permit better exposure.

Vaginal Approach. In the vaginal approach the posterior cul-de-sac is opened, the uterus is displaced to the right or left with a long narrow retractor and the tubes are brought into view and pulled down with a Babcock clamp. The same problems of exposure, identification of the tube and bleeding occur as with the abdominal approach. If exposure is difficult, it is best to resort promptly to an abdominal (vertical midline) incision to complete the operation; all patients undergoing vaginal tubal ligation should be informed in advance of the (remote) necessity of such an abdominal incision.

EARLY POSTOPERATIVE COMPLICATIONS

Minilaparotomy, according to a World Health Organization Task Force Report (Wilson, 1982) on 791 women from eight different cities around the world, was accompanied by major complications in 1.5%. These included pelvic inflammatory disease requiring hospitalization, incisional problems requiring reoperation, injury to other organs or excessive bleeding. Minor complications (no further operation needed) occurred in 12.3%. These included immediate bleeding, injury to the uterus, injury to other organs, pelvic inflammatory disease, incision-related problems and urinary tract infection. Reports of pain were difficult to evaluate because of the varying cultural background of the patients, but 120 (15.2%) patients complained of pain immediately after the operation. Lower figures (2.5%) for overall complication rates were reported by Lee and Boyd (1980). In another series of 800 patients, 32% of whom were considered to be at high risk, 7.1% had incisional complications and 2.1% had postoperative fever (Domenzain et al, 1982). In six patients the fever was found to be due to salpingitis and in six to cystitis. Incisional problems such as hematoma or seroma may give rise to pain but can usually be managed expectantly. Postoperative fever should be investigated to determine its cause (see Chapter 4).

Vaginal tubal ligation avoids the complications of bleeding in the abdominal incision and, to some extent, of pain. However, pelvic infections are more common (4.5% of 799 patients reported by Brenner, 1981). Management is by appropriate antibiotics. Data are not available on the long-term sequelae of such infections.

Long-term Effects of Tubal Occlusion (Sterilization)

PREGNANCY

All methods of tubal occlusion (by laparoscopy or laparotomy) have failures (subsequent pregnancies). It is often difficult to determine the exact pregnancy rate from published reports, because the series are small or the follow-ups short. Bhiwandiwala and associates (1982), using life-table pregnancy rates in a study of 12,218 women from various countries, found the cumulative failure rate at 12 months following interval tubal occlusion to be 0.23/100 women for electrocoagulation and 0.44/100 for tubal rings placed laparoscopically. The same authors make a distinction between technical failure and method failure. In the former the planned technique could not be carried out, and the surgeon had to adopt another. This happened in 69% of the failures, whereas in 31% sterilization was incomplete, leading to the possibility of future pregnancy. Technical failures were significantly lower in the electrocoagulation group than in the laparoscopy/tubal ring group. Method failure rate was 0.26/100 women sterilized by laparoscopy/electrocoagulation techniques, compared with 0.47/100 women sterilized by tubal rings. Mumford and co-workers (1980) compared the cumulative failure rate at 12 months after interval tubal occlusion and found it to be 0.52/100 women after the laparoscopy/tubal ring method, 0.43 after the minilaparotomy/tubal ring method and 0.36

after minilaparotomy/Pomeroy ligation in a total of 5,414 women. Vessey and co-workers (1983) used the Pearl formula (pregnancies per 100 woman-years of exposure) and found that laparoscopy/electrocauterization had a Pearl index of 0.26, laparoscopy/tubal rings and clips 0.21 and laparotomy (all procedures) 0.11 with an overall rate of 0.16. Using a titanium silicone rubber clip applied by laparoscopy or minilaparotomy, Filshie and co-workers (1981) reported a total (technical and methodologic) failure rate of 0.55/100 women.

In summary, worldwide experience suggests that a certain number of technical failures will occur with all methods because of spontaneous reanastomosis (Soderstrom, 1985), whereas some may depend upon operator experience and choice of method. Two thirds of these technical failures can be corrected at the time of operation by using another method. Overall failure rates can be expected to average 0.2 to 0.5/1000 women over a 12-month period. Some increase in the number of pregnancies is likely to occur later. For example, Vessey and co-workers (1983) noted a Pearl index of 0.10 more than 12 months following sterilization and 0.37 prior to 12 months after operation.

Some failures are due to "luteal phase pregnancies." These can be avoided by performing the operation only in the early postmenstrual (proliferative) phase of the menstrual cycle and by careful preoperative examination, including a pregnancy test.

Some authors have reported a high incidence of ectopic pregnancy among tubal occlusion failures. For example, Vessey and co-workers (1983) reported that 7 out of 16 post-sterilization pregnancies were ectopic, the majority occurring more than 12 months after the procedure. McCausland (1982), from a pathologic review of 42 tubes removed after previous laparoscopic coagulation, suggests that thermal injury to the endosalpinx of the proximal part of the tube may be more likely to lead to fistula formation and the possibility of ectopic pregnancy than the fibrosis that occurs when the distal part of the tube is electrocoagulated.

REPRODUCTIVE FUNCTION

Earlier studies indicated the likelihood of adverse menstrual changes after tubal occlusion. With improved methodology, such as that described by Fortney and co-workers (1983), the long-term effects of sterilization on reproductive function have been found to be few. The majority of women report no changes in menstrual pattern. When changes occur they are in equal proportion in opposite directions, and many can be attributed to discontinuation of oral contraceptives or intrauterine devices used prior to sterilization (DeStefano et al, 1983; Bhiwandiwala et al, 1984). Moreover, Bhiwandiwala and co-workers (1984) found no increase in abnormal menstrual function whether tubal sterilization was performed by unipolar coagulation, bipolar coagulation, silastic bands or other methods, although DeStefano and co-workers (1983) noted that significantly more women had an increase in menstrual pain after unipolar coagulation than after the other procedures. Nevertheless, some doubts still remain about the circulatory and possible hormonal effects of tubal occlusion, as shown by the work of El-Minawi and associates (1983), which demonstrated postoperative uterovaginal and ovarian varicosities and pelvic venous spaces. Studies by Manzanilla-Sevilla and co-workers (1978), however, indicated no changes in pelvic arterial perfusion. The risk of hysterectomy within 15 months of tubal sterilization is low, 1.6%, but long-term follow-up is necessary (Kendrick et al, 1985).

PSYCHOLOGICAL SEQUELAE

Much was written 10 to 30 years ago about the possible emotional complications of sterilization. In a typical study Khorana and Vyas (1975) noted that the vast majority of patients, 92%, expressed satisfaction with the operation. Women who were persuaded to accept sterilization for medical reasons were more likely to regret the procedure, but those who underwent it voluntarily were usually satisfied. This would appear to be still true. However, with increasing divorce and remarriage, women may desire to become pregnant by their new partners and regret the previous operation. Thus, there has been considerable concern about the possibility of reversing tubal ligation. This question is further discussed later.

MORTALITY AND OTHER IMPLICATIONS

Peterson and co-workers (1982), extrapolating from 29 deaths reported after sterilization from 1977 to 1981, estimated that the case fatality rate was 3.6/100,000 procedures, giving a possible 108 deaths in the US during the period of surveillance. Twenty-one of these 29 deaths occurred after interval sterilization; of these six were due to the complications of anesthesia, six to sepsis, three to hemorrhage and six to myo-

cardial infarction or other circulatory complications.

These mortality figures indicate that the chance of dying from tubal occlusion is slight but present, although it is likely that improvements in anesthetic and other techniques will reduce mortality further. However, they are also relevant to a debate of importance, but currently decreasing interest—is hysterectomy preferable to tubal ligation for sterilization? The present answer appears to be no. Mortality from hysterectomy is estimated to be 100 to 200/100,000 operations (extrapolated from Easterday et al, 1983), 30 to 60 times higher than that for tubal ligation. Moreover, on an economic basis, the initial cost of tubal sterilization is less, although long-term costs following the two procedures are extremely difficult to determine. By comparison, the mortality, major complications, failures and cost of vasectomy for the male partner are far less (Smith et al, 1985).

Tuboplasty

Operations to restore tubal patency have become much more common in the past 15 years partly because of the development of microsurgical techniques and partly because of the desire for renewed fertility by women who have had their tubes occluded and have been divorced but now want to conceive by their new partners.

Several types of tubal reconstruction are possible: (1) simple lysis of adhesions (salpingo-ovariolysis), (2) salpingostomy (opening the occluded lateral end of the tube), (3) anastomosis of the lateral and medial parts of the tube, (4) implantation of the tube into the cornu of the uterus, (5) fimbrioplasty (reconstruction of the fimbriated end of the tube when it has been excised), and (6) combinations of these procedures.

Since the sole objective of tuboplasty is to restore fertility, the avoidance of preoperative complicating factors and precise intraoperative techniques are of the greatest importance. Early and late postoperative complications may occur as with any laparotomy.

PREOPERATIVE COMPLICATIONS

Contraindications to tuboplasty that make the operation impractical or dangerous to the patient's health include:

1. Age (over 40).
2. Major illnesses such as severe heart disease, hypertension or diabetes.

3. Uterine or ovarian tumors.

4. Dense sclerotic adhesions in the pelvis from pelvic inflammatory disease, endometriosis or previous operations.

5. Genital tuberculosis.

6. Acute pelvic inflammatory disease.

Relative contraindications may arise from the infertility studies, which are an essential preliminary to operation. Data from the history are helpful. If the patient has previously had a tubal ligation, it is important to identify the procedure used. For example, removal of the fimbria by fimbriectomy, unipolar electrocauterization, or loss of a large part of the tube with less than 4 cm remaining (Rock et al, 1982) makes success less likely.

Tubal reconstruction will fail if other than tubal factors are responsible for the woman's infertility, i.e., anovulation. The fertility of her husband also needs assessment, because if he is producing no living spermatozoa, the couple should consider in advance the possibility of artificial insemination, in vitro fertilization (IVF) or adoption.

Preoperative evaluation of the tubes themselves by hysterosalpingogram and diagnostic laparoscopy is essential, since these studies may reveal unsuspected adhesions or insuperable kinking of the tubes.

INTRAOPERATIVE COMPLICATIONS

Infection is a major cause of tuboplasty failure. Therefore, aseptic precautions must be scrupulously observed and prophylactic antibiotics given (see Chapter 2). During operation, hemorrhage and trauma to the tubes and surrounding tissues must be avoided by (1) careful dissection, (2) continuous irrigation with lactated Ringer's solution or a balanced salt solution containing 5000 units of heparin per liter, (3) fine electrocoagulation of bleeding points, and (4) use of magnification, fine sutures and small instruments. During the operation, attention must also be paid to trying to prevent postoperative adhesions (1) by the use of cortisone either systemically or by injection into the uterus and tubes during and after operation; the effectiveness of this is in question, and (2) by injecting a Dextran solution such as Hyskon into the peritoneal cavity at the end of the procedure (see Chapter 3). Early postoperative laparoscopy may be one way of decreasing the number of adhesions. Trimbos-Kemper and co-workers (1985) performed laparoscopy during the second year after tubal reconstructive procedures and found significantly fewer adhesions

in those who had laparoscopy on the eighth day after operation as compared with those who had not had an early postoperative laparoscopy.

POSTOPERATIVE COMPLICATIONS

Since the anticipated end result of tuboplasty is pregnancy, failure to conceive or pregnancy wastage are important late complications. Prior to the use of microsurgical techniques, pregnancy rates were low (10 to 30%). More optimistic results have recently been reported. Siegler and associates (1985), in a collective review of seven series of cases, totalling 767 patients, noted an overall success rate of 67.7%. Success varies according to the procedure performed. Thus, Gomel (1983) reports pregnancy rates of 83% for tubo-tubal anastomosis, 62% for tubo-cornual reimplantation, 56% for salpingo-ovariolysis and 42% for salpingostomy. Hulka's (1982) successes are lower, being 44%, 20%, 32% and 40% respectively. It is expected that more data will soon become available as increasing numbers of reproductive endocrinology centers are now performing microsurgical tuboplasties.

Since some scarring and alteration in function of the tubes must inevitably follow tuboplastic procedures, the incidence of ectopic pregnancy is high. For example, Gomel (1983) reports an incidence of 9% after salpingostomy, 6.2% after tubocornual implantation and 1.7% after tubo-tubal anastomosis. Because of the frequency of this complication, the patient should be made aware of it before operation.

Once tuboplasty has failed, a second procedure is not likely to be successful. Lauritsen and associates (1982) reported that 16% of patients having a second tuboplasty conceived as compared with 59% of those having the operation for the first time.

OPERATIONS ON THE OVARIES

Oophorectomy

The complications of operations in which one or both ovaries are removed at the time of hysterectomy have been partly reviewed previously (see page 152). In the young woman part or all of one ovary may be removed for a benign or borderline cyst or tumor.

PARTIAL OOPHORECTOMY

The decision to remove part of an ovary is made at the operating table after consideration of the intraabdominal findings, the patient's age and preferences for preservation of ovarian function and gross examination of the ovary itself. Thus, in the presence of polycystic ovarian disease, apparently thin-walled cysts with no surface projections, benign cystic teratomas and perhaps with some solid tumors that clearly appear benign, the lesion is carefully dissected off the remaining normal ovarian tissue and then sent for pathologic examination by frozen section if necessary. If it is benign, the remaining ovarian tissue is reconstructed.

The chief intraoperative problems are bleeding from the ovary and the difficulty of restoring the ovary to near normal shape and appearance. Individual bleeding vessels can be ligated with 30 or 40 vicryl sutures, and venous oozing usually ceases as the ovary is closed. When considerable ovarian tissue remains, closure can be done with two layers of continuous 30 or 40 polyglycolic sutures. When there is only a thin shell of ovarian tissue, a plicating stitch can be used, according to the method described by Schreier and Alexander (1959) after Bonney's original description (Fig. 6–3). It is important not to constrict or kink the infundibulopelvic ligament.

The postoperative complications of ovarian cystectomy are similar to those that follow any laparotomy. The frequency of recurrence of cysts is difficult to determine because of their great variety.

UNILATERAL OOPHORECTOMY

Intraoperatively no special complications occur during unilateral oophorectomy. Postoperatively, with one ovary remaining, menstrual function and ability to conceive remain normal in most instances. When premenopausal patients with one ovary or parts of one or both ovaries were followed, Ranney and Chastain (1978) found that 52 of 243 (21%) patients required reoperation for gynecologic causes. Twenty patients in this series (at the time of reporting) had gone through menopause at an average age of 49.4 years, indicating continuing normal hormonal function.

BILATERAL OOPHORECTOMY

Removal of both ovaries, for various reasons and usually accompanied by hysterectomy, may occur prior to the perimenopausal years (before age 45), during that era (age 45 to 55) or postmenopausally (over age 55).

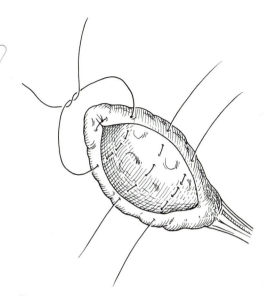

Figure 6–3. Closure of the right ovary by using a plicating stitch.

In the premenopausal period, loss of ovarian function has specific short-term and long-term complications in most, although, surprisingly, not all women. The short-term effects consist primarily of hot flashes, insomnia and irritability. These may be compounded by a variety of symptoms such as depression or tiredness, which may be related to environmental, nutritional or other changes occurring at the same time. Long-term effects include loss of secondary sexual characteristics and cardiovascular or bone changes. Breasts and labia may atrophy, skin dryness is noted and the vaginal mucosa becomes reddened, thinner and drier with delayed lubrication on sexual arrousal in some women. Urinary symptoms such as urethritis and even incontinence may occur. The risk of non-fatal myocardial infarction in women undergoing bilateral oophorectomy before the age of 35 was found to be 7.2 times that of premenopausal women as a whole (Rosenberg et al, 1981), whereas Johansson and co-workers (1975) noted an increase in coronary vascular occlusion up to age 70 and increases in serum cholestrol and triglyceride levels in women castrated between 15 and 30 years of age. Bone changes consist of osteoporosis and an increased tendency for fractures. Aitken and co-workers (1973a), assessed bone density in the third metacarpal bone and found that oophorectomy before the age of 45 was associated with a significantly increased incidence of osteoporosis within three to six years of operation. As a corollary, estrogens (mestranol) given within two months of operation prevented subsequent bone mineral loss (Aitken et al, 1973b). Estrogens started even three to six years after the operation caused a highly significant increase in bone mineral content.

In perimenopausal women, short-term complications are similar to those in younger women, but the long-term complications are not so apparent. The incidence of vascular and bone disease does not seem to differ from that seen in women who have gone through natural menopause.

Postmenopausal women will sometimes have similar early complications, indicating cessation of continuing production of estrogens at the time of operation. Long-term effects are similar to those following natural menopause.

MANAGEMENT AFTER OOPHORECTOMY

No replacement therapy is required after unilateral oophorectomy. The management of short-term and the prevention of long-term symptoms after bilateral oophorectomy depend on the reason for the oophorectomy and the age of the patient.

When bilateral oophorectomy has been performed for benign disease in the premenopausal woman and the uterus is no longer present, hormones should be given and continued at least until the expected age of natural menopause (50 years) both to ameliorate symptoms and to prevent the later development of osteoporosis. Long-term therapy with estrogens after the expected age of natural menopause may continue to protect against osteoporosis, but this is not yet proved. A good general diet, exercise, sunshine and adequate intake of calcium are important. The postmenopausal woman should obtain 1500 mg of calcium daily. Table 6–4 shows the amounts of calcium in commonly consumed foods. It is not easy to obtain the required calcium, especially if the woman does not eat dairy products. Lactose intolerance may further reduce calcium intake. Therefore, supplementary calcium intake of 500 to 1000 mg daily should be recommended (Keyler and Peterson, 1985).

The need for prophylaxis of osteoporosis is equally important in women whose ovaries have been removed premenopausally and who have received no replacement estrogen therapy. This is true especially if they have other risk factors (Table 6–5). Such patients may have no symptoms, but should be screened by single-beam absorbtiometry, which measures density in the radius, or by the more sensitive dual-beam

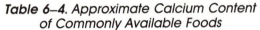

Table 6–4. Approximate Calcium Content of Commonly Available Foods

Foods	Mg Calcium (approximate)
Milk (8 oz)	290
Yogurt (plain, low fat, 8 oz)	415
Cheese (average, 3 oz)	200
Salmon (canned with bones, 3 oz)	167
Sardines (canned with bones, 3 oz)	372
Almonds (2 oz)	132
Leafy green vegetables (various, ½ cup)	150–200
Orange (1 medium)	50
Beans (various, 3 oz)	50–100

absorbtiometry, which measures density in the lumbar spine. These measurements have been used in various ways to indicate the risk of fracture (Wahner, 1985). If this is appreciable, hormone replacement, as described later, is advisable. Repeated absorbtiometry, preferably both single- and dual-beam studies, should be obtained at one or possibly more six-month intervals to help determine the rate of bone loss, if any. Currently, the expense, complexity and unavailability of these valuable studies limit their application.

In women without uteri, hormonal replacement by estrogens alone is appropriate. Conjugated estrogen, 0.625 mg daily, is sufficient. It is best taken at night and can be given for the first 25 days of the month, for three weeks out of four or for five days out of seven. Continuous estrogen intake may result in soreness of

Table 6–5. Risk Factors for Developing Osteoporosis*

Primary or Idiopathic	Secondary
Unavoidable	Medical conditions
Family history	Chronic renal failure
Menopause	Gastrectomy and
Phenotype: short,	intestinal bypass
slender	Malabsorption
Race: white and Oriental	syndromes
Avoidable	Endocrinopathies
Nutritional factors	Adrenocortical excess
Calcium	Diabetes
Vitamin D	Hyperparathyroidism
Bone robbers	Hyperthyroidism
Acidifying foodstuffs	Medications
Alcohol	Antacids (with
Caffeine	aluminum)
Fiber	Anticonvulsants
Protein	Steroids
Salt	Thyroid extracts > 3
Physical inactivity	gr/day
Smoking	

*From Notelovitz M: Using devices that measure bone mass. *Contemp. Obstet. Gynecol.* (Technology 1985) 25:61, 1985. Reprinted with permission.

the breasts in some women; there appears at present to be no definite danger of neoplasia in the breasts or other organs from this regimen. A similar effect can be obtained by other routes of administration—vaginally (conjugated estrogens), percutaneously (estradiol) (Holst et al, 1983) or subdermally (estradiol) (Lobo et al, 1980); these methods may be more troublesome for the patient in the long run. There would appear to be no need to add a progestin to the estrogen unless the uterus is present, when it is needed to avoid overstimulation of the endometrium. Then a progestin, e.g., medroxyprogesterone acetate (10 mg daily) should be added from the 15th through the 25th day of each month.

The use of replacement hormones after oophorectomy or abdominal radiation therapy for malignant disease is less clearly defined. The growth or regrowth of cancer of the cervix, vagina or vulva does not appear to be related to estrogens. These hormones can, therefore, be given safely, for example, to young women treated for carcinoma of the cervix by radiation therapy. Cancer of the endometrium is often estrogen-dependent, but a retrospective study by Creasman and co-workers (1986) suggests that estrogen replacement therapy after definite treatment does not increase the rate of recurrence. It is uncertain if the regrowth of cancer of the ovary or fallopian tube is stimulated by estrogen, but widespread opinion is against the use of estrogens in these circumstances, at least soon after operation. In patients with these cancers progestins have been shown to be an acceptable substitute, at least in preventing hot flashes, although their long-term effect on bone is uncertain (Lobo et al, 1984). Progestins can be given by mouth as medroxyprogesterone acetate (20 mg daily) or megestrol (20 to 40 mg daily) or by injections of depomedroxyprogesterone acetate (50 to 150 mg) once every two to four months.

It should be noted that a variety of non-hormonal medications can be used with varying effectiveness when treatment of symptoms is important and hormone therapy is felt to be contraindicated. These include diet, exercise, additional vitamin B or E, a variety of mood-affecting drugs and continued emotional support; in fact, these may often be considered as the first steps in therapy.

Transposition of Ovaries

Young women who are about to receive pelvic radiation for Hodgkin's disease, carcinoma of the cervix or other pelvic disorders are often anxious to retain ovarian function and/or reproductive capacity. In such cases one or both ovaries may be transposed (1) to the midline (back of the uterus) or (2) upward and laterally just beneath the inferior pole of the kidney and lateral to the psoas muscle. Alternatively the ovary may be exteriorized under the skin.

The technique of midline transposition is described by Donaldson (1981). This operation is most appropriate when no midline pelvic radiation is to be used. It can be performed in the course of a staging procedure or as a separate operation. The patency of the tubes is preserved, and the sites of the ovaries are identified by using wire sutures to attach them to the back of the uterus. In eight patients, Donaldson (1982) reported that the dose to ovaries that were transposed to the midline averaged 460 rads (slightly more than 10% of the total dose) when lateral pelvic radiation was given with central shielding. This dose is considerable, but less than the 500 to 800 rads thought to be necessary to abolish ovarian function. Pregnancy occurred in 21 patients in Donaldson's series who underwent pelvic radiation (some having received chemotherapy in addition). Fifteen of the 21 patients delivered one or more healthy infants at term.

Lateral transposition is described by Nahhas (1981). It is most appropriate when midline as well as lateral pelvic radiation is to be given. If pregnancy is desired, the difficulty of transposing the fallopian tubes and ensuring their patency somewhat limits the procedure's usefulness. Lateral transposition is estimated to reduce the dose of radiation received to 1 to 3% of that given to the pelvis (Nahhas, 1981). Other possible complications include torsion of the ovarian pedicle or the development of a cyst or tumor in the transposed ovary.

Exteriorization of the ovary under the skin laterally, with preservation of blood supply, was described by Kovacev (1968) in 38 women. Twenty-eight of 30 patients followed periodically retained ovarian function, but cysts developed in five, and these required repeated aspiration.

INFERTILITY

In the past, ovaries were transplanted into the cornu of the uterus in women whose tubes had been removed or irremediably blocked, in the hope that ovulation would occur directly into the uterus and be followed by fertilization (Estes' procedure). Twenty-seven cases were reported by Beyth and Polishuk (1979); none resulted in pregnancy, although collected series from the older literature showed a 10.4% pregnancy rate (28 out of 269 operations). The Estes operation is outdated by in vitro fertilization procedures.

OTHER PELVIC OPERATIONS

Presacral Neurectomy

Division of the presacral nerve(s) used to be a common operation for dysmenorrhea. Now it is seldom performed and usually only as an adjunct to conservative operations for endometriosis if the patient has had significant dysmenorrhea unrelieved by antiprostaglandins. Presacral neurectomy consists of excising a 2-cm band of tissue in front of the sacral promontory and between the ureters. Intraoperative complications include damage to the ureters and the inferior mesenteric vessels and hemorrhage from the middle sacral vein(s), which lies close to the front of the sacrum. Immediate postoperative complications are similar to those for other laparotomies. Late complications consist primarily of failure to alleviate menstrual pain. This occurs in 25% of patients, according to Black (1964), and is related to the thoroughness with which the nerve fibers are resected. The onset of labor may not be recognized and its duration may be shortened because of reduced pain. Coitus and orgasm do not appear to be affected.

Division of Uterosacral Ligaments

Occasionally relief of dysmenorrhea may be achieved by division of the uterosacral ligaments, usually performed during other conservative procedures for endometriosis. Approximately 1 cm of the ligament is excised between ligatures. The major complication is injury to a ureter. The ureter should be identified on each side before the ligament is cut. No data are available on the failure rate of this procedure. A satisfactory response to blocking the uterosacral ligaments with local anesthesia may be a good omen for a successful operation.

OPERATIONS ON THE URINARY TRACT

Urethrovesical Suspension

Many operations have been devised for the treatment of stress incontinence. When symptoms are associated with pelvic relaxation the vaginal approach is preferred by many at first; this consists of an anterior colphorrhaphy (with or without a vaginal hysterectomy) and suspension of the urethrovesical junction from below (Beck and McCormick, 1982). If the patient's main symptom is stress incontinence with only a moderate cystocele or if stress incontinence occurs after vaginal repair, urethrovesical suspension is usually indicated either from above or by a combined approach. At the same time vaginal repair may be performed. The operations in common use and their characteristics are as follows (S = suprapubic approach; C = combined approach):

MARSHALL-MARCHETTI-KRANTZ PROCEDURE (S)

The paraurethral tissue is sewn to the back of the symphysis pubis with two or three sutures on each side. Formerly, the bladder was sewn to the posterior rectus sheath, but this is now not generally done.

BURCH PROCEDURE (S)

The tissue lateral to the urethra is sewn to Cooper's ligament (reflected part of the inguinal ligament) with two sutures on each side.

SLING PROCEDURES

Goebell-Frangenheim-Stoeckel Operation (C). A strip of fascia lata from the thigh appears to provide the most satisfactory sling. Synthetic materials, since they are not incorporated into the host tissue, do not contribute to the fibrosis, which appears to be necessary for adequate repair. The fascial strip is passed from above through the rectus muscle, around the upper part of the urethra, using a small vaginal incision, and carried back up through the opposite rectus muscle. It is secured snugly with sutures. The contraction of the recti supplies an additional tightening of the sling. In a modification of this procedure the sling may be transected below the urethra and fixed to the paraurethral tissue. Alternatively, it may exteriorized; in this case it becomes covered by mucosa within a few months.

Aldridge Procedure (C). This procedure is similar to the Goebell-Frangenheim-Stoeckel operation, but strips of anterior abdominal wall (external oblique) fascia are used, one on each side with the base near the midline. In a modification of this procedure, Zacharin (1983) passes the sling through the posterior pubourethral ligament by means of an incision between the symphysis pubis and the urethra and then fixes it to the paraurethral tissue and the vagina.

Others. In the Peyrera procedure (C) and its modifications a suture is passed blindly from a superficial suprapubic incision by means of a long needle around the urethra and back up to the abdomen. In the Stamey procedure (C) endoscopy is used to assist in suspending the paraurethral tissue to the anterior rectus sheath with No. 2 nylon sutures passed through a Dacron tube (Stamey, 1980).

Many modifications of each of the above techniques are described (Riggs, 1986). The complications of urethrovesical suspension are common to all types of procedures, but certain complications are specific to particular procedures.

INTRAOPERATIVE COMPLICATIONS

Dissection in the space of Retzius may be accompanied by venous bleeding, usually controllable by pressure. There is risk of penetrating the urethra when sutures are placed in the paraurethral tissue. It is important that a catheter be placed in the bladder and that a finger be inserted into the vagina to avoid this; if penetration of the urethra occurs, the suture should be removed and reinserted. Sutures may occasionally pull out of the symphysis pubis or Cooper's ligament. A round-bodied needle of appropriate size should be used, since a taper-point needle is likely to cause tearing. Any excess bleeding is an indication for drainage of the space of Retzius, usually with a Penrose drain placed centrally or one placed at each side through stab incisions below the transverse abdominal incision. Some authors routinely use a drain. There is some advantage to this, since bleeding may occur postoperatively even when the operative field has been dry.

Obtaining a fascia lata strip from the thigh usually presents no complications, except unfamiliarity with the use of the fascial stripper. When a strip is obtained from the abdominal fascia, careful repair is important to prevent the development of a hernia. A blind procedure such as the Peyrera operation increases the chance of accidental injury to the bladder or urethra.

EARLY POSTOPERATIVE COMPLICATIONS

Early postoperative complications are similar to those for any major abdominal or vaginal procedure (see Chapters 4 and 5). The specific problems are related to the urinary tract. Ex-

travasation of urine into the space of Retzius (or peritoneal cavity) is shown by absence of output from the suprapubic or urethral catheter. If the former is in place, it should be removed and an indwelling urethral catheter inserted. Reexploration of the space of Retzius, identification of the site of leakage, closure and drainage of the space is usually indicated, especially if a suprapubic catheter has been used.

Inability of the patient to void occurs in 10 to 15% of patients. In these cases bladder drainage must be continued. Eventually, at least six weeks later, in cases in which a sling has been used, the sling may be transected vaginally with good results, indicating that fibrosis at the urethrovesical junction is important. If a Marshall-Marchetti-Krantz or similar procedure has been used, it may be necessary to reexplore the space of Retzius and cut the sutures.

Urinary tract infection is a common sequel of continued urethral catheter drainage; it is less so with a suprapubic catheter. Oral urinary antibiotics such as trimethoprim/sulfamethoxazole should be continued. The emotional aspects of the ability to void are important, but management may not be easy.

LATE POSTOPERATIVE COMPLICATIONS

Recurrent stress incontinence is reported to occur in 10 to 20% of women after all types of operations; no one procedure is 100% successful. Many authors point out the importance of careful selection of patients in the first instance to exclude those with urgency incontinence or neurologic problems. Zacharin (1983) emphasizes the importance of clinical history, physical findings and cystoscopic studies in making the diagnosis.

Osteitis pubis occurs rarely after urethrovesical suspension. It is characterized by a dull pubic pain spreading to neighboring structures, often associated with fever and a urinary tract infection. Radiologic changes appear late and show erosion of the bone, followed by irregular superficial bone destruction. The course of osteitis pubis is prolonged—somtimes two to three years. Various treatments have been reported to be successful, including corticosteroids, anti-inflammatory agents, analgesics, local heat, bed rest and possibly antibiotics (Pent, 1972).

Abdominal Repair of Cystocele

Abdominal repair of a cystocele consists of excising a wedge-shaped piece of anterior vaginal wall at the time of abdominal hysterectomy. Intraoperative complications include bleeding when the bladder is dissected off the vagina, adequacy of exposure and danger of injury to the ureter and bladder. Macer (1978) reports a bladder flap hematoma in three of 76 patients (4%). The same author's recurrence rate, five or more years after operation, was 7.9% as compared with 21.8% when the cystocele repair was performed vaginally.

OPERATIONS ON THE INTESTINAL TRACT

Unanticipated injury to the intestinal tract (damage to the serosa or muscularis, entry into the lumen or compromise of blood supply) may occur during any gynecologic procedure. Management of these complications is covered in Chapter 3 and under the specific operations in which they occur. Operations on the intestinal tract per se do not occur often in the course of gynecologic operations except as incidental or emergency procedures and during exenteration or operations for ovarian cancer. They include incidental appendectomy, excision of Meckel's diverticulum, intestinal resection and colostomy.

Appendectomy

Elective appendectomy is often performed at the time of hysterectomy or other gynecologic procedure. Since acute inflammation is seldom present in such cases, the infectious complications that follow appendectomy for acute appendicitis do not usually occur (Cooperman, 1983). In fact, reports of complications related to incidental appendectomy per se are rare. Bleeding from the mesoappendix may occur and require reexploration. Perforation of the appendiceal stump is also a possibility. Finally, adhesions to the stump or mesoappendix may cause later intestinal obstruction.

Repeated recommendations that appendectomy should be performed at the time of hysterectomy and other obstetric-gynecologic procedures, including cesarean section, have been made in the past 75 years. When directors of residency programs in obstetrics and gynecology were polled in 1975–76, 66% favored appendectomy at the time of uncomplicated hysterectomy (Hays, 1977). A commonly advanced

reason is the possibility of acute appendicitis developing later. This is not very likely. It is estimated that 6% of the population will develop appendicitis during a lifetime, but since its highest incidence is in males between the ages of 20 and 30 the chance of the disease developing in women after the age of 40 to 50 (when most hysterectomies are performed) must be considerably less, perhaps 1 to 2%. Another and better reason is the possible discovery of abnormalities in the removed appendix. Waters (1977) reported that 22% of removed appendices that were closely studied showed sufficient pathologic changes to justify excision. About a quarter of these or 6% of the total specimens had significant disease such as endometriosis, carcinoid tumor, metastatic carcinoma or tuberculosis.

There is good reason to perform incidental appendectomy if the organ appears abnormal or is likely to be involved in the disease process being treated, e.g., inflammatory disease, endometriosis or ovarian cancer. If the appendix is grossly normal, appendectomy is appropriate if (1) preoperative consent has been obtained; (2) the gynecologic operation has not been unduly prolonged or complicated; and (3) the appendix is easily accessible, i.e., not fixed behind the cecum or ileum. Appendectomy should be performed at the end of the procedure. It is important to ligate the vessels in the mesoappendix carefully and to check for bleeding before closing the abdomen. The base of the appendix should be ligated. There is no advantage to invaginating the stump (Engstrom and Fenyo, 1985).

Meckel's Diverticulectomy

Meckel's diverticulum is found in about 2% of the population at about two feet from the ileocecal junction. It is appropriate to look for it in the course of gynecologic surgery. However, removal is generally not indicated unless the diverticulum has a narrow base or appears to contain ectopic tissue (gastric mucosa, tumor). When it is to be removed an elliptical incision is made around its base with rubber-shod clamps placed across the intestine above and below to prevent spillage of intestinal contents. The diverticulum is excised and the defect is closed transversely in two layers. Complications are similar to those of any other intestinal closure (see Chapter 4).

Intestinal Resection

Intestinal resection, apart from that performed in the course of operations for malignant disease, may be necessary in rare cases of pelvic inflammatory disease or endometriosis. The same complications occur after such procedures as after intestinal anastomoses for obstruction. These are covered in Chapter 4. When resection has to be performed unexpectedly a complicating problem is that the bowel has not usually been cleansed mechanically nor have antibiotics been given preoperatively. Therefore, the use of antibiotics (intravenously) during and after operation is important.

Colostomy

Colostomy may occasionally be planned as part of an exenteration or to divert the fecal stream in the management of rectovaginal fistula. It may also be indicated when colonic obstruction occurs in ovarian cancer and rarely in pelvic inflammatory disease or endometriosis. It may be unexpectedly necessary when the bowel has not been prepared and diverticular disease is found in the descending or sigmoid colon or injury occurs as the colon is being dissected off a pelvic mass.

Colostomies may be of two types, loop or end. The loop colostomy is made in the transverse colon and is brought out through the skin in the left (preferably) or right upper quadrant of the abdomen. It is indicated in emergencies, in poor risk patients or when subsequent closure is likely. An end colostomy is constructed at the lower end of the descending colon or in the sigmoid colon and is brought out in the left lower quadrant. It is used when the stoma is expected to be permanent. When possible, the end of the colon should be opened and everted ("matured") by sewing the mucosa to the intestinal wall below it and then to the skin (Fig. 6–4). The distal end may be brought out as a mucous fistula well away from the stoma, e.g., at the lower end of the vertical incision, or it may be closed and dropped back into the pelvis.

INTRAOPERATIVE COMPLICATIONS

The transverse colostomy is prepared by pulling a loop of transverse colon through the rectus muscle and the other layers of the abdominal wall and securing it externally by inserting a rod or suitable device placed through the mesentery beneath the colon. The intestine may be opened immediately or after a delay of 24 hours if it is feared that heavy fecal contamination of the peritoneal cavity may occur. Finding the colon may present some difficulty through a small (transverse) incision; the taeniae are the important signs for identification. The hole in the peritoneum, rectus muscle and fascia must be large enough so that a small finger can be inserted beside the loop after it has been brought out.

In forming an end colostomy a problem is

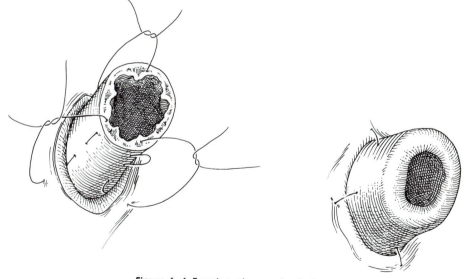

Figure 6–4. Eversion of an end colostomy.

sometimes encountered in freeing enough length of colon so that at least one inch projects outside the skin. This may necessitate mobilizing the entire descending colon by dividing the lateral peritoneal attachment up to the splenic flexure. However, freeing the splenic flexure, if it is necessary, must be done carefully because its attachments to the spleen may be torn, leading to intractable bleeding from the spleen. As the colon is brought out, a space will be left lateral to the mesentery through which small intestine could potentially herniate. When possible the mesentery should be sutured to the lateral peritoneum so as to close the hole completely. If it cannot be closed, no sutures should be used, since a large hole is less dangerous than a small one. Finally, difficulty in closing a midline incision is sometimes encountered after a colostomy unless the peritoneum of the incision is pulled sharply medially as the transperitoneal hole for the colostomy is being made.

EARLY POSTOPERATIVE COMPLICATIONS

Complications of colostomies and other intestinal stomas, especially those occurring soon after operation are relatively frequent (Table 6–6). According to Pearl and associates (1985), they occur somewhat more frequently after gynecology-oncology procedures than after general surgical procedures (37% compared to 30%).

Necrosis. This is usually due to interference with the blood supply of the colon either because the intestine is stretched through and constricted by the abdominal wall or because its blood supply has been ligated during the preparation of the stoma. When inspected on the first postoperative day the stoma appears

Table 6–6. Local Complications of Intestinal Stomas*

Type	No. (% of Total)
Skin irritation	83 (42.1)
Necrosis	27 (13.7)
Retraction	26 (13.2)
Parastomal infection	25 (12.7)
Stenosis	13 (6.6)
Prolapse	10 (5.1)
Bleeding	6 (3.1)
Hernia	5 (2.5)
Evisceration	2 (1.0)
Total	197 (100)

*From Pearl RK, Prasad L et al: Early local complications from intestinal stomas. *Arch. Surg.* 120:1145, 1985. Reprinted with permission.

black. The extent of the necrosis is not usually clear. Sometimes the original discoloration improves. No treatment is effective. Necrosis may presage later retraction of the stoma.

Retraction of the Stoma. A transverse loop colostomy may retract beneath the abdominal wall soon after the operation if the rod comes out inadvertently or is removed too soon (before the seventh day). The loop can occasionally be grasped with a Kelly hemostat and pulled out and the rod reinserted. If that is not possible, the patient must be placed under anesthesia and the loop must be found and pulled out as soon as possible. Attempts to minimize retraction have included using a tongue of skin or a biodegradable (Biethium) bridge sewn to the fascia (Jenkinson et al, 1984). Similarly, an end colostomy may retract because of necrosis. It must be pulled out quickly in a similar manner.

Bleeding. Bleeding from vessels beneath the skin or in the muscle may appear externally or spread under the skin, giving rise to a hematoma. No treatment is indicated unless the bleeding is severe and continuous. Then, with the patient under anesthesia, a search must be made to find and ligate the bleeding vessel.

Infection. The subcutaneous tissue around the stoma is a common potential site for infection. When this is suspected, the patient should receive broad spectrum antibiotics unless she is already receiving them. Warm compresses may be helpful.

Appliance Malfunction. The most difficult complication of a colostomy is the patient's adjustment to it. It represents a major change in her physiology, one that she did not want, hoped would not occur and is reluctant to accept. The situation is worse if the colostomy was entirely unexpected. This means that the procedure should be mentioned in advance even if it is a very remote possibility. If it is likely, an experienced enterostomal therapist should see the patient before the operation, mark the best site for the stoma and explain in encouraging terms how the patient will be able to cope with the colostomy. After the operation early participation in colostomy care by the patient herself and a concerned family member with the aid of the enterostomal therapist is important. Stomas and individuals vary, and the patient has to recognize that her early concern about the apparatus and its adjustment to her needs will eventually make her more comfortable. Also to be considered in this context are the important questions of irrigation, diet, odor and gas. These problems are dis-

Table 6–7. Complications of Colostomy*

Complication	Sigmoid (end) 104 cases		Transverse (loop) 80 cases	
	No.	*Per Cent*	*No.*	*Per Cent*
Stricture	19	18	0	0
Hernia	18	17	12	15
Bleeding	15	14	8	10
Diarrhea	14	13	4	5
Obstruction	6	6	2	2
Prolapse	4	4	7	9
Retraction	4	4	1	1
Perforation	3	3	0	0
Abscess	2	2	12	15
Constipation	2	2	1	1
Evisceration	1	1	1	1
Gangrene	1	1	1	1
Fistula	0	0	1	1
Miscellaneous	4	4	3	4

*Adapted from Hedberg SE, Welch CE: Complications in surgery of the colon and rectum. In Hardy JD (Ed.): *Complications in Surgery and their Management*, Ed. 4. Philadelphia, W. B. Saunders, 1981.

cussed in detail by Rowbotham (1981). Discussion with others who already have stomas can be extremely helpful.

LATE COMPLICATIONS

Later complications occurring after loop and end colostomy are shown in Table 6–7. It should be noted that hernias, strictures, retraction, obstruction and diarrhea are more common with end colostomy, whereas prolapse and abscess formation are more common with loop colostomy. Minor hernia beside the colostomy requires no treatment; major protrusion may require operation with, in the case of transverse colostomy, separation of the proximal and distal loops. Similarly, prolapse of significant proportions may need excision of redundant bowel. Stricture can be ameliorated by daily dilatation by the patient using a finger cot. Eventually, if the stricture becomes severe, causing obstruction, and cannot be dilated, surgical revision is necessary. The end stoma is pulled out and resutured, the fascial opening being enlarged. Stricture is unlikely with a loop colostomy. An important complication is the position of the stoma. If it is close to the rib cage, at the waist or too low, it will be difficult to manage. This is why preoperative determination of the site is important. Surgical revision may be necessary, if an appliance cannot be worn satisfactorily.

Temporary (usually transverse loop) colostomies can be closed 6 to 12 weeks later if the primary reason for them has disappeared. At operation, after bowel preparation the colon is completely freed from its fascial and peritoneal attachments, closed in two layers (see Chapter 3) and dropped back into the peritoneal cavity. Following closure wound infection is relatively common, averaging 13% but varying by type of wound closure, according to a review by Berne and co-workers (1985).

REFERENCES

Aitken JM, Hart DM et al: Osteoporosis after oophorectomy for non-malignant disease in premenopausal women. *Br. Med. J.* 2:325, 1973a.

Aitken JM, Hart DM, Lindsay R: Estrogen replacement therapy for prevention of osteoporosis after oophorectomy. *Br. Med. J.* 3:515, 1973b.

Ananth J: Hysterectomy and depression. *Obstet. Gynecol.* 52:724, 1978.

Beavis ELG, Brown JB, Smith MA: Ovarian function after hysterectomy with conservation of the ovaries in premenopausal women. *J. Obstet. Gynecol. Br. Comm.* 76:969, 1969.

Beck RP, McCormick S: Treatment of urinary stress incontinence with anterior colporrhaphy. *Obstet. Gynecol.* 59:270, 1982.

Berek JS, Griffiths CT, Leventhal JM: Laparoscopy for second-look evaluation in ovarian cancer. *Obstet. Gynecol.* 58:192, 1981.

Beresford JM: Automatic stapling techniques in abdominal hysterectomy. *Surg. Clin. North Am.* 64:609, 1984.

Berne TV, Griffith CN et al: Colostomy wound closure. *Arch. Surg.* 120:957, 1985.

Beyth Y, Polishuk WZ: Ovarian implantation into the uterus (Estes operation): clinical and experimental evaluations. *Fertil. Steril.* 32:657, 1979.

Bhiwandiwala PP, Mumford SD, Feldblum PJ: A comparison of different laparoscopic sterilization occlusion techniques in 24,439 procedures. *Am. J. Obstet. Gynecol.* 144:319, 1982.

Bhiwandiwala PP, Mumford SD, Feldblum PJ: Menstrual pattern changes following minilap/Pomeroy, minilap/ring and laparoscopy/ring sterilization: a review of 5982 cases. *Int. J. Gynecol. Obstet.* 22:251, 1984.

Black WT Jr: Sympathectomy in the treatment of dysmenorrhea: a second look after 25 years. *Am. J. Obstet. Gynecol.* 89:16, 1964.

Brenner WE: Evaluation of contemporary female sterilization methods. *J. Reprod. Med.* 26:439, 1981.

Brenner WE, Dingfelder JR: Sterilization by minilaparotomy in not recently pregnant patients. *Int. J. Gynecol. Obstet.* 14:35, 1976.

Buttram VC, Reiter RC: Uterine leiomyomata: etiology, symptomatology, and management. *Fertil. Steril.* 36:433, 1981.

Cibils L: *Gynecologic Laparoscopy.* Philadelphia, Lea & Febiger, 1975.

Cooperman M: Complications of appendectomy. *Surg. Clin. North Am.* 63:1233, 1983.

Corson SL, Block S: Sterilization of laparoscopes. Is soaking sufficient? *J. Reprod. Med.* 23:49, 1979.

Corson SL, Levinson CJ et al: Hormonal levels following sterilization and hysterectomy. *J. Reprod. Med.* 26:363, 1981.

Creasman WT, Henderson D et al: Estrogen replacement therapy in the patient treated for endometrial cancer. *Obstet. Gynecol.* 67:326, 1986.

DeCenzo JA, Malo T, Cavanagh D: Factors affecting cone-hysterectomy morbidity. *Am. J. Obstet. Gynecol.* 110:380, 1971.

DeCherney AH, Tarlatzis B: Equal success following the Tompkins procedure or Jones procedure for habitual abortion due to an intrauterine mullerian anomaly. *Fertil. Steril. (Abstracts)* 41:71S, 1984.

DeStefano F, Huezo CM et al: Menstrual changes after tubal sterilization. *Obstet. Gynecol.* 62:673, 1983.

Dicker RC, Scally J et al: Hysterectomy among women of reproductive age—Trends in the United States, 1970–1978. *J. Am. Med. Assoc.* 248:323, 1982.

Dodson MG: The treatment of failed laparoscopy using open laparoscopy. *Int. J. Gynecol Obstet.* 22:331, 1984.

Domenzain ME, Gonzalez MA, Teran J: Minilaparotomy tubal sterilization: a comparison between normal and high-risk patients. *Obstet. Gynecol.* 55:199, 1982.

Donaldson SS: The preservation of ovarian function in patients undergoing pelvic irradiation: indications and technique. In Ballon SC (Ed.): *Gynecologic Oncology: Controversies in Cancer Treatment.* Boston, GK Hall & Co., 1981.

Dyck FJ, Murphy FA et al: Effect of surveillance on the number of hysterectomies in the province of Saskatchewan. *N. Engl. J. Med.* 296:1326, 1977.

Easterday CL, Grimes DA et al: Hysterectomy in the United States. *Obstet. Gynecol.* 62:203, 1983.

El-Minawi MF, Mashhor N, Reda MS: Pelvic venous changes after tubal sterilization. *J. Reprod. Med.* 28:641, 1983.

Engstrom L, Fenyo G: Appendicectomy: assessment of stump invagination versus simple ligation: a prospective randomized trial. *Br. J. Surg.* 72:971, 1985.

Fairlie EJ, Al-Hassani SSM: The Lembert suture in the prevention of vaginal vault granulation after total abdominal hysterectomy. *J. Obstet. Gynaecol. Br. Comm.* 80:839, 1973.

Filshie GM, Casey DM et al: The titanium/silicone rubber clip for female sterilization. *Br. J. Obstet. Gynecol.* 88:655, 1981.

Fortney JA, Cole LP, Kennedy KI: A new approach to measuring menstrual pattern change after sterilization. *Am. J. Obstet. Gynecol.* 147:830, 1983.

Funt MI, Benigno BB, Thompson JD: The residual adnexa—asset or liability? *Am. J. Obstet. Gynecol.* 129:251, 1977.

Gomel V: An odyssey through the oviduct. *Fertil. Steril.* 39:144, 1983.

Grimes EM: Open laparoscopy with conventional instrumentation. *Obstet. Gynecol.* 57:375, 1981.

Gunning JE: The history of laparoscopy. *J. Reprod. Med.* 12:222, 1974.

Hasson HM: A modified instrument and method for laparoscopy. *Am. J. Obstet. Gynecol.* 110:886, 1971.

Hays RJ: Incidental appendectomies; current teaching. *J. Am. Med. Assoc.* 238:31, 1977.

Hedberg SE, Welch CE: Complications in surgery of the colon and rectum. In Hardy JD (Ed.): *Complications in Surgery and their Management,* Ed. 4. Philadelphia, W. B. Saunders, 1981.

Hemsell DL, Heard ML et al: Single-dose cefoxitin prophylaxis for premenopausal women undergoing vaginal hysterectomy. *Obstet. Gynecol.* 63:285, 1984.

Hemsell DL, Reisch J et al: Prevention of major infection after elective abdominal hysterectomy: individual determination required. *Am. J. Obstet. Gynecol.* 147:520, 1983.

Holst J, Cajander S et al: Percutaneous estrogen replacement therapy. Effects on circulating estrogens, gonadotropins and prolactin. *Acta Obstet. Gynecol. Scand.* 62:49, 1983.

Howkins J, Williams DK: Vault granulations after total abdominal hysterectomy. *J. Obstet. Gynaecol. Br. Comm.* 75:84, 1968.

Hulka JF: Adnexal adhesions: a prognostic staging and classification system based on a five-year survey of fertility surgery results at Chapel Hill, North Carolina. *Am. J. Obstet. Gynecol.* 144:141, 1982.

Janson PO, Jansson I: The acute effect of hysterectomy on ovarian blood flow. *Am. J. Obstet. Gynecol.* 127:349, 1977.

Jaszczak SE, Evans TN: Intrafascial abdominal and vaginal hysterectomy: a reappraisal. *Obstet. Gynecol.* 59:435, 1982.

Jenkinson LR, Houghton PWJ et al: The Biethium bridge—an advance in stoma care, *Ann. R. Coll. Surg. Engl.* 66:420, 1984.

Johansson BW, Kaij L et al: On some late effects of bilateral oophorectomy in the age range 15–30 years. *Acta Obstet. Gynecol. Scand.* 54:449, 1975.

Kav-Venaki S, Zakham L: Psychological effects of hysterectomy in premenopausal women. *J. Psychosom. Obstet. Gynecol.* 2:76, 1983.

Kendrick JS, Rubin GL et al: Hysterectomy performed within 1 year after tubal sterilization. *Fertil. Steril.* 44:606, 1985.

Keyler D, Peterson CD: Oral calcium supplements. *Postgrad. Med.* 78:123, 1985.

Khorana AB, Vyas AA: Psychological complications in women undergoing voluntary sterilization by salpingectomy. *Br. J. Psychiatry* 127:67, 1975.

Kilkku P: Supravaginal uterine amputation vs. hysterectomy: effects on coital frequency and dyspareunia. *Acta Obstet. Gynecol. Scand.* 62:141, 1983.

Kilkku P, Gronroos M et al: Supravaginal uterine amputation vs. hysterectomy. *Acta Obstet. Gynecol. Scand.* 62:147, 1983.

Kilkku P, Hirvonen T, Gronroos M: Supravaginal uterine amputation vs. abdominal hysterectomy: the effects on urinary symptoms with special reference to pollakisuria, nocturia and dysuria. *Maturitas* 3:197, 1981.

Kovacev M: Exteriorization of ovaries under the skin of young women operated upon for cancer of the cervix. *Am. J. Obstet. Gynecol.* 101:756, 1968.

Lacey CG, Morrow CP et al: Laparoscopy in the evaluation of gynecologic cancer. *Obstet. Gynecol.* 52:708, 1978.

Lauritsen JG, Pagel JD et al: Results of repeated tuboplasties. *Fertil. Steril.* 37:68, 1982.

Lee RM, Boyd JAK: Minilaparotomy under local anesthesia for outpatient sterilization; a preliminary report. *Fertil. Steril.* 33:129, 1980.

Lobo RA, March CM et al: Subdermal estradiol pellets following hysterectomy and oophorectomy. *Am. J. Obstet. Gynecol.* 138:714, 1980.

Lobo RA, McCormick W et al: Depo-medroxyprogesterone acetate compared with conjugated estrogens for the treatment of postmenopausal women. *Obstet. Gynecol.* 63:1, 1984.

Macer GA: Transabdominal repair of cystocele; a 20 year experience, compared with the traditional vaginal approach. *Am. J. Obstet. Gynecol.* 131:203, 1978.

Manzanilla-Sevilla R, Gonzalez-Iniguez R et al: Tubal sterilization and ovarian perfusion; selective arteriography in vivo and in vitro. *Int. J. Gynecol. Obstet.* 16:137, 1978.

McCausland A: Endosalpingosis ("endosalpingoblastosis") following laparoscopic tubal coagulation as a etiologic factor of ectopic pregnancy. *Am. J. Obstet. Gynecol.* 143:12, 1982.

McLaughlin DS: Metroplasty and myomectomy with the CO_2 laser for maximizing the preservation of normal tissue and minimizing blood loss. *J. Reprod. Med.* 30:1, 1985.

Miller NF: Hysterectomy: therapeutic necessity or surgical racket? *Am. J. Obstet. Gynecol.* 51:804, 1946.

Mumford SD, Bhiwandiwala PP, Chi I-Cheng: Laparoscopic and minilaparotomy female sterilisation compared with 15,167 cases. *Lancet* 2:1066, 1980.

Nahhas WH: The preservation of ovarian function in patients undergoing pelvic irradiation: indications and technique. In Ballon SC (Ed.): *Gynecologic Oncology: Controversies in Cancer Treatment.* Boston, GK Hall & Co., 1981.

National Center for Health Statistics. National Hospital Discharge Survey, 1985.

Newton N, Baron E: Reactions to hysterectomy: fact or fiction? *Primary Care* 3:781, 1976.

Notelovitz M: Using devices that measure bone mass. *Contemp. Obstet. Gynecol.* (Technology 1985) 25:61, 1985.

Ohlgisser M, Sorokin Y, Heifetz M: Gynecologic laparoscopy: a review article. *Obstet. Gynecol. Surv.* 40:385, 1985.

Orr JW Jr, Shingleton HM et al: Correlation of perioperative morbidity and conization to radical hysterectomy interval. *Obstet. Gynecol.* 59:726, 1982.

Paterson MEL, Jordan JA, Logan-Edwards R: A survey of 100 patients who had laparoscopic ventrosuspensions. *Br. J. Obstet. Gynaecol.* 85:468, 1978.

Pearl RK, Prasad L et al: Early local complications from intestinal stomas. *Arch. Surg.* 120:1145, 1985.

Penfield AJ: How to prevent complications of open laparoscopy. *J. Reprod. Med.* 30:660, 1985.

Pent D: Osteitis pubis: a review. *Obstet. Gynecol. Surv.* 27:645, 1972.

Peterson HB, DeStefano F et al: Mortality risk associated with tubal sterilization in U. S. hospitals. *Am. J. Obstet. Gynecol.* 145:125, 1982.

Phillips J, Hulka B et al: Laparoscopic procedures: the American Association of Gynecologic Laparoscopists' membership survey for 1975. *J. Reprod. Med.* 18:227, 1977.

Phillips JM, Hulka JF, Peterson HB: American Association

of Gynecologic Laparoscopists' 1982 membership survey. *J. Reprod. Med.* 29:592, 1984.

Poulsen HK, Borel J, Olsen H: Prophylactic metronidazole or suction drainage in abdominal hysterectomy. *Obstet. Gynecol.* 63:291, 1984.

Prasad ML, Orsay CP et al: A survey of technical considerations in the construction of intestinal stomas. *Am. Surg.* 51:462, 1985.

Ranney B, Chastain D: Ovarian function, reproduction and later operations following adnexal surgery. *Obstet. Gynecol.* 51:521, 1978.

Richards BC: Hysterectomy: from women to women. *Am. J. Obstet. Gynecol.* 131:446, 1978.

Richards DH: Depression after hysterectomy. *Lancet* 2:430, 1973.

Richards DH: A post-hysterectomy syndrome. *Lancet* 2:983, 1974.

Riggs JA: Retropubic cystourethropexy: a review of two operative procedures with long-term follow-up. *Obstet. Gynecol.* 68:98, 1986.

Rock JA, Bergquist C et al: Tubal anastomosis following unipolar cautery. *Fertil. Steril.* 37:613, 1982.

Roopnarinesingh S, Gopeesingh T: Hysterectomy and its psychological aftermath. *West. Indian Med. J.* 31:131, 1982.

Roos NP: Hysterectomies in one Canadian province: a new look at risks and benefits. *Am. J. Public. Health* 74:39, 1984.

Rosenberg L, Hennekens CH et al: Early menopause and the risk of myocardial infarction. *Am. J. Obstet. Gynecol.* 139:47, 1981.

Rowbotham JW: Managing colostomies. *CA* 31:336, 1981.

Sakai K, Yamamoto T, Kamiya H: Female sexual response after hysterectomy. *Nippon Sanka Fujinka Gakkai Zasshi* 35:757, 1983.

Schreier PC, Alexander A: Ovarian cystectomy for benign dermoid cysts. *Miss. Doctor* 37:83, 1959.

Shapiro M, Munoz A et al: Risk factors for infection at the operative site after abdominal or vaginal hysterectomy. *N. Engl. J. Med.* 307:1661, 1982.

Siegler AM, Hulka J, Pereta A: Reversibility of female sterilization. *Fertil. Steril.* 43:499, 1985.

Smith GL, Taylor GP, Smith KF: Comparative risks and costs of male and female sterilizations. *Am. J. Public Health* 75:370, 1985.

Soderstrom RM: Sterilization failures and their causes. *Am. J. Obstet. Gynecol.* 152:395, 1985.

Soderstrom RM, Levy BS: Bowel injuries during laparoscopy; causes and medicolegal questions. *Contemp. Obstet. Gynecol.* 27:41, 1986.

Stamey TA: Endoscopic suspension of the vesical neck for urinary incontinence in females. *Ann. Surg.* 192:465, 1980.

Stone SC, Dickey RP, Mickal A: The acute effect of hysterectomy on ovarian function. *Am. J. Obstet. Gynecol.* 121:193, 1975.

Tang GW: Reactions to emergency hysterectomy. *Obstet. Gynecol.* 65:206, 1985.

Trimbos-Kemper TCM, Trimbos JB, van Hall EV: Adhesion formation after tubal surgery: results of the eighth-day laparoscopy in 188 patients. *Fertil. Steril.* 43:395, 1985.

van Keep PA, Wildemeersch D, Lehert P: Hysterectomy in six European countries. *Maturitas* 5:69, 1983.

Vessey M, Huggins G et al. Tubal sterilization: findings in a large prospective study. *Br. J. Obstet. Gynaecol.* 90:203, 1983.

Wahner HW: Assessment of metabolic bone disease: review of new nuclear medicine procedures. *Mayo Clin. Proc.* 60:827, 1985.

Waters EG: Elective appendectomy with abdominal and pelvic surgery. *Obstet. Gynecol.* 50:511, 1977.

Webb C, Wilson-Barrett J: Self-concept, social support and hysterectomy. *Int. J. Nurs. Stud.* 20:97, 1983.

Wijma K: Psychological functioning after non-cancer hysterectomy: a review of methods and results. *J. Psychosom. Obstet. Gynaecol.* 3:133, 1984.

Williams MA: Cultural patterning of the feminine role: a factor in the response to hysterectomy. *Nurs. Forum* 12:378, 1973.

Wilson E: Minilaparotomy or laparoscopy for sterilization: a multicenter, multinational randomized study (WHO Task Force on Female Sterilization). *Am. J. Obstet. Gynecol.* 143:645, 1982.

Winslow HC, Strasbaugh N, Mervine ND: Pregnancies following hysterectomy. *Penn. Med.* 72:45, 1969.

Zacharin RF: Abdominoperineal urethral suspension in the management of recurrent stress incontinence of urine—a 15-year experience. *Obstet. Gynecol.* 62:644, 1983.

Zussman L, Zussman S: Sexual response after hysterectomy-oophorectomy: recent studies and reconsideration of psychogenesis. *Am. J. Obstet. Gynecol.* 140:725, 1981.

COMPLICATIONS OF RADICAL ONCOLOGIC OPERATIONS

7

JOHN R. LURAIN
MICHAEL NEWTON

Complications occur more commonly in operations done for the treatment of gynecologic malignancies than for benign diseases. This is due to the more radical nature of the procedures needed to encompass the disease and the disease processes per se. With extension of the limits of dissection closer to intestinal, urinary and vascular structures, injury or damage to these organ systems is more likely to occur. The malignant lesions may also be adherent to tissues beyond the reproductive tract or distort the anatomy so as to make their removal more difficult and dangerous. In this chapter complications of some radical operations will be delineated, as well as ways to minimize and deal with these complications. Specifically, complications involving radical hysterectomy, radical vulvectomy, pelvic exenteration, operations for removal of advanced ovarian cancer and para-aortic lymph node dissection will be examined. Since many of the complications of radical procedures are similar to those of less serious operations, the reader is referred to Chapter 4 for a general account of postoperative complications.

RADICAL HYSTERECTOMY

See P 148 Hysterec

Radical hysterectomy (Type III hysterectomy) involves removal of the uterus and upper one third of the vagina along with the parametrial and paravaginal tissues out to the pelvic sidewalls. It is usually combined with removal of the pelvic lymph nodes from the common iliac artery down to the femoral canal and the obturator nerve. This operation is performed mainly for cure of early cancer of the cervix, Stage IB. Occasionally the operation is appropriate treatment for a small central recurrence or for persistent disease following radiation therapy for cervical cancer.

Although Wertheim (1912) described the procedure and presented a series of 500 operative cases in the early 20th century, the high

175

operative mortality rate (18.6%) and the 31.5% major surgical complication rate precluded its ready application to the treatment of cervical cancer. Radiation therapy remained the primary treatment modality until Bonney (1935) in England and Meigs (1944) in the U.S. showed that radical pelvic surgery could be as safe and effective a form of treatment as radiation for early cervical cancer.

Operative mortality from radical hysterectomy has declined sharply from almost 20% in Wertheim's report to less than 1% in most recent series. This decline has largely been the result of improvements related to anesthesia, blood banking and transfusion therapy and antibiotic therapy to prevent and treat infection. Since 1944, operative mortality rates have been reported between 0 and 2.7% (Table 7–1). Most mortalities are presently related to postoperative thromboembolism. Other less frequently reported causes are complications secondary to intraoperative and postoperative hemorrhage and infection. Prophylactic mini-dose heparin or intraoperative and postoperative pneumatic calf compression may decrease the reported 2 to 5% incidence of thrombophlebitis and associated embolization. Use of prophylactic antibiotics and proper drainage of the pelvis appear to decrease the incidence of serious infections.

Complications occur in approximately 30% of patients undergoing radical hysterectomy. However, only about 5 to 12% are major complications that can be specifically attributable to the procedure itself. Most complications peculiar to radical hysterectomy involve the ureter, bladder and lymphatic system.

Ureteral Injury and Ureterovaginal Fistula

The ureter is especially liable to injury during radical hysterectomy because it runs directly through the parametrial and paracervical tissue on its way to the bladder. The surgeon must completely dissect the ureter out of its bed in Wertheim's tunnel, being careful not to injure it or strip its blood supply, which runs up and down the ureter in its adventitia. Care must be taken not to clamp or hold the ureter with any rigid object that would compromise its blood supply, leading to later necrosis and fistula formation. The risk of ureteral injury or complication is increased by the presence of pelvic endometriosis, pelvic inflammatory disease and co-existing pregnancy, all of which distort the anatomy, and by prior irradiation, which compromises the blood supply and makes the dissection more difficult (Green et al, 1962).

Intraoperative injury to the ureter occurs in up to 2% of procedures and requires immediate correction. When the ureter is inadvertently crushed or ligated, prompt removal of the clamps or ligature usually is sufficient treatment. The extent of ureteral damage is dependent upon the size of the damaged area and the elapsed time before recognition of the injury. Revascularization with return of normal color and propagation of peristalsis through the traumatized segment after release of the clamp or ligation signifies minimal damage, and no further treatment is necessary. If the injury is felt to be more extensive, a silastic catheter should be used to stent the ureter for about 10 days. If the viability of the ureter is seriously ques-

Table 7–1. Complications of Radical Hysterectomy and Pelvic Lymphadenectomy Performed for Treatment of Early Stage Carcinoma of the Cervix

Author(s)	Year	No. of Patients	Operative Mortality (%)	Urinary Fistulas (%)*		Bladder Atony (%)	Lympho-cyst (%)
				U/V fistula	V/V fistula		
Liu and Meigs	1955	473	1.7	– (9.5)	–	–	–
Christensen et al	1964	394	0.5	8.8	–	21.0	–
Brunschwig and Barber	1966	438	1.1	11.1	11.4	–	–
Blaikley et al	1969	257	1.95	3.89	–	–	–
Ketcham et al	1971	84	2.7	3.6	4.8	8.3	–
Park et al	1973	150	0.6	0	0	0.6	2.6
Hoskins et al	1976	224	0.89	2.2	0.45	–	0.4
Morley and Seski	1976	208	1.4	4.8	0.5	3.8	–
Webb and Symmonds	1979b	610	0.3	2.5	2.3	11.0	2.9
Sall et al	1979	349	0	2.0	0.9	0.9	1.7
Benedet et al	1980	241	0.4	7.5	1.7	–	1.2
Langley et al	1980	284	0	5.6	11.4	4.9	–
Lerner et al	1980	108	0	0.9	–	5.6	0.9

*U/V = ureterovaginal; V/V = vesicovaginal.

tioned, complete excision of the damaged area with either direct ureteral anastomosis or vesical reimplantation should be performed. Ureteral transection requires repair by either end-to-end reanastomosis or reimplantation into the bladder, depending on the site of injury. Generally, transections above the midplane of the pelvis are handled by end-to-end ureteroureterostomy. The ends should be fish-mouthed and repair performed with one layer of interrupted through-and-through 3-0 absorbable sutures over a silastic stent. If the ureter has been divided within 5 cm of the bladder, reimplantation into the bladder is preferable. Mobilization of the bladder by a vesicopsoas hitch procedure may facilitate approximation. In a ureteroneocystostomy, the ureter is brought through the bladder wall just above the trigone. A mucosa-to-mucosa anastomosis is performed, and the periureteral tissue is attached to the outside of the bladder using interrupted 3-0 absorbable sutures. All ureteral anastomoses should be drained retroperitoneally.

Ureteral complications, mainly ureterovaginal fistulas, used to be the most frequent and serious problems following radical hysterectomy. In the last decade or more, the incidence of ureteral fistulas and strictures has been reduced from 5 to 15% to less than 1% by the application of several techniques: (1) closure of the vaginal cuff and drainage of the retroperitoneal spaces by means of suction catheters to reduce infection, (2) suspension of the ureter to the superior vesical artery and (3) catheter drainage of the bladder postoperatively until adequate bladder function returns.

Avoidance of postoperative collections of blood, serum and lymph and subsequent infection beneath the pelvic peritoneal closure is important in preventing postoperative ureteral fistulas and strictures. These accumulations, with or without infection, tend to compromise the blood supply, distort the anatomy and interfere with ureteral function. Optimal hemostasis and lymph stasis, which have been improved with the use of clips in pelvic node dissection, as well as suction catheter drainage of the retroperitoneal spaces for five to seven days, together with prophylactic antibiotic therapy are all indicated in an effort to avoid or minimize these complications.

Green (1966) has suggested suspending the ureters to the anterior division of the hypogastric arteries at the conclusion of the operative procedure. This technique, theoretically, may improve ureteral peristalsis, decrease vulnera-

bility of the ureter to damage from pelvic infection, and prevent ureteral kinking or stricture. The ureter is gently elevated in comfortable approximation to the superior vesical and internal iliac arteries and its adventitia is sutured to the adventitia of the vessels along several centimeters of their course using fine 5-0 absorbable sutures. Using this technique in 284 consecutive radical hysterectomies, Green reported only three ureterovaginal fistulas, no postoperative ureteral strictures and a marked reduction in the incidence of transient, asymptomatic hydroureter and hydronephrosis as documented by postoperative intravenous pyelogram.

Adequate bladder drainage postoperatively until the return of significant bladder function seems to be important in reducing the incidence of ureteral complications. Following radical hysterectomy, the bladder becomes hypotonic because of the disruption of its autonomic nerve supply. Keeping the bladder adequately drained postoperatively, usually for two to six weeks, until bladder function returns, takes pressure off the lower, most vulnerable portions of the dissected ureters, thereby allowing local healing and revascularization to proceed undisturbed. Green and co-workers (1962) demonstrated a two-fold decrease in ureteral complications with prolonged postoperative bladder drainage. A logical approach to this problem is to place a suprapubic bladder catheter at the time of surgery and to remove it when the patient is able to void spontaneously with repeatedly low residual urine volumes.

Ureterovaginal fistula often presents 7 to 14 days postoperatively as a sudden, profuse watery vaginal discharge with a characteristic uriniferous odor. Premonitory signs and symptoms such as unexplained fever, vague pelvic discomfort and the development of a mass or induration above or lateral to the vaginal apex usually precede the development of the fistula. The presence of a ureteral rather than a vesical fistula can be easily established by first instilling methylene blue into the bladder and making certain that dye does not appear in the vagina, and then ascertaining that an intravenous injection of indigo carmine does produce dyed urine in the vagina. Intravenous pyelography may be helpful in establishing the presence and location of the ureteral fistula and in determining whether obstruction exists. Cystoscopy with attempted retrograde catheterization of the ureters is the most important procedure and should be done promptly. The site of the fistula can be determined more precisely, and, hopefully, a silastic catheter can be passed through the fistulous ureter into the renal pelvis to splint the ureter. This technique is successful in about 30% of patients. The splinting ureteral catheter is left in place for 14 to 21 days, resulting in healing of the fistula in most cases.

If a ureteral catheter cannot be passed and the ureterovaginal fistula remains open, surgical repair is necessary. Renal function and drainage usually remain excellent in the presence of a ureterovaginal fistula, allowing two to three months to elapse before surgical correction is undertaken. Stricture and subsequent infection can occur, however, resulting in kidney damage or loss, which has been reported to occur in as many as 18 to 33% of cases. The surgical management of a postoperative ureteral fistula or stricture involving the lower ureter is best handled by ligation of the ureter below the fistula and implantation of the ureter proximal to the fistula into the bladder (ureteroneocystostomy). No splinting of the ureter is necessary. If the ureter is damaged above the mid-pelvis, the damaged segment should be excised and an end-to-end ureteral reanastomosis (ureteroureterostomy) performed over a silastic stent. The operative site should be drained using a soft retroperitoneal suction drain, and the bladder should be drained, preferably through a suprapubic catheter, for 10 to 14 days.

Bladder Injury and Vesicovaginal Fistula

Despite the extensive dissection and mobilization of the bladder that is required during radical hysterectomy, bladder injury and vesicovaginal fistulas are uncommon. Intraoperative bladder injury ranges in incidence from 0.4 to 3.7%. Bladder lacerations or injuries that are recognized and repaired primarily rarely result in any sequelae. Vesicovaginal fistulas have been reported to occur in 0 to 7% of patients undergoing radical hysterectomy. These fistulas are most often seen in patients who have had prior uterine surgery or radiation therapy. The diagnosis can be established by instilling methylene blue dye solution into the bladder and observing its immediate appearance in the vagina. Cystoscopy confirms the diagnosis, size and location of the fistula. Once the diagnosis is made, bladder catheter drainage is continued in an attempt to get a small fistula to heal spontaneously. In general, a waiting period of

two to four months is allowed before surgical correction is attempted in order to optimize local tissue conditions for healing and successful repair. Except in cases in which radiation therapy complicates the development of the vesicovaginal fistula, a standard vaginal repair is possible and usually successful. In patients who have received radiotherapy, a transvesical or possibly a transvaginal approach with interposition of a pedical graft from the omentum, another part of the bladder or the bulbocavernosus fat pad is usually desirable. Postoperative bladder catheter drainage should continue for two weeks.

Bladder Dysfunction

Postoperative bladder dysfunction has become the most important complication of radical hysterectomy now that the incidence of fistulas and serious infections has been greatly reduced (Forney, 1980; Kadar et al, 1983). Injury to the nerve supply of the bladder is inevitable if a radical hysterectomy is performed properly. This results in all patients being unable to void properly for a variable period the after operation. Up to 50% experience permanent loss of bladder sensation and need to strain or use suprapubic pressure to empty their bladders. This represents only a minor inconvenience to most of these patients. However, at least 5% of patients develop severe disability, including incontinence, enuresis and complete inability to void. The severity of the disability seems to be directly related to the extent of the inferolateral dissection of the cardinal and uterosacral ligaments. Severe bladder dysfunction can largely be prevented by conserving the more lateral and inferior portions of the pelvic ligaments. The obvious implication is that cases selected for radical hysterectomy should be chosen so that the operation is performed on small lesions (< 3 cm) that are confined to the cervix, where adequate surgical margins can be obtained without resecting the entire cardinal ligaments at the pelvic sidewalls down to the pelvic floor, thereby not compromising the cure rate or bladder function. Postoperative bladder drainage with a suprapubic catheter allows for evaluation of the return of bladder function and measurement of residual urine volumes in order to determine when urinary bladder drainage is no longer required. This evaluation is accomplished without prolonged unnecessary bladder drainage, repeated catheterizations or increased risk of infection.

Lymphatic Complications

Postoperative lower extremity edema and pelvic lymphocysts have been reported after radical hysterectomy and pelvic lymphadenectomy. The incidence of postoperative lymphedema is much higher in those patients who have the procedure combined with external pelvic irradiation. There is also a positive correlation between the extent of the pelvic lymph node dissection and the development of lymphedema. Undoubtedly, postoperative pelvic infection is also a significant variable. Lymphocysts have been noted in up to 3% of patients. With the use of retroperitoneal suction drains and clips to aid in decreasing lymphatic drainage after pelvic lymphadenectomy, the incidence of retroperitoneal accumulation of lymphatic fluid in the area of dissection has decreased markedly. If a lymphocyst develops despite these precautions, it may produce no symptoms and present only as a mass situated laterally in the pelvis, or it may be associated with infection or ureteral obstruction. The lymphocyst may be drained by placement of a retroperitoneal suction catheter directly or under computerized tomographic or ultrasonographic guidance. The catheter should be left in place on suction until drainage virtually ceases; this may take up to four to six weeks for large cysts.

Infection

Infection following radical hysterectomy can be a major complication. Sites of infection include the wound, the pelvis and vaginal cuff, the peritoneal cavity and the urinary tract. Serious infections and overall morbidity have been remarkably decreased by the use of perioperative prophylactic antibiotics, closure of the vagina and retroperitoneal suction drainage (Sevin et al, 1984). There appears to be no increase in infection or morbidity when radical hysterectomy is performed between three days and four to six weeks after cone biopsy of the cervix, as has been documented when a simple hysterectomy follows a cone biopsy during this time period (Webb and Symmonds, 1979a; Orr et al, 1982). This is probably due to the wider extent of the dissection away from the cervix in a radical hysterectomy.

RADICAL VULVECTOMY

Radical vulvectomy with excision of the inguinal and femoral lymph nodes has been the primary operative treatment for carcinoma of the vulva. This is a major procedure often performed in older women who are relatively poor operative risks. Complications are likely to occur and include: (1) breakdown and necrosis of the skin incisions with or without infection; (2) hemorrhage; (3) lymphangitis; (4) thrombophlebitis; (5) leg edema; (6) vaginal relaxation and urinary incontinence and (7) dyspareunia (Table 7–2).

Incisional Complications

Skin necrosis and separation, especially in groin incisions, is by far the most common complication. Although in the majority of cases skin loss is minimal, large areas of skin flap may become necrotic. This problem is aggravated by collections of blood, lymph or serum developing below the flaps, excessive undermining of the skin edges and closure of the wound under tension. The most likely place for breakdown to occur is at the center of the lower abdominal incision over the symphysis pubis, extending outward and downward from this

Table 7–2. Complications of Radical Vulvectomy and Bilateral Groin Dissection

Author(s)	Year	No. of Patients	Complications (%)				
			Wound Breakdown	Lymphedema/ Lymphangitis	Thrombo- phlebitis	Pelvic Relaxation	Sexual Dysfunction
Green et al	1958	100	45	26	7	12	–
Rutledge et al	1970	151	53	32	–	3	–
Boutselis	1972	60	48	47	1.7	15	8
Figge and Gaudenz	1974	50	20	28	5	24	–
Benedet et al	1979	154	19	5	–	<1	<1
Iversen et al	1980	262	5.7*	1.5	–	0.8	–
Calame	1980	58	70	65/10	–	17	–
Podratz et al	1983	175	85	69/13	9	11	13

*Severe only.

point. The extent of this problem usually cannot be determined until at least seven days after the operation, usually after the skin sutures or staples have been removed, although a preliminary idea of the likelihood of breakdown can be obtained from the color of the skin edges shortly after the operation. If they are dusky, at least superficial slough of the skin is likely to occur; however, if the color is normal, primary wound healing cannot necessarily be predicted. This complication can be minimized in a number of ways. The underminded skin flaps should be a full thickness of skin and fat to prevent interference with the vascular supply. Undermining of the skin flaps should be performed only to the extent necessary to dissect the lymph nodes adequately and approximate the wound edges without tension. Use of a "butterfly" or "trapezoid" incision that removes a strip of groin skin together with the underlying nodes (Green et al, 1958), a vertical midline inverted tennis racket incision (Goldberg et al, 1979), separate groin incisions (Hacker et al, 1981) or myocutaneous flaps (Chafe et al, 1983) have all been advocated to diminish the frequency of this problem. Particular care should be taken after completion of the groin dissection to trim off any devascularized skin before the incision is closed. Fluorescence with fluorescein and ultraviolet light may be of help in outlining devascularized areas. Tension when suturing the skin edges should be avoided. Pressure dressings applied over the skin flaps also aggravate the problem. Suction wound drainage is essential; it will help in preventing both pressure and infection resulting from hematomas and seromas developing beneath the skin flaps. Suction drains should be placed under the skin in both groins, brought out through separate stab incisions and maintained for a minimum of four to five days. The wound edges should be kept clean and dry. If necrosis occurs and the skin edges separate, the incision should be cleansed with hydrogen peroxide and packed with fine mesh gauze three times daily. Debridement should be carried out once the lines of demarcation between viable and dead tissue become obvious. Some purulent discharge and localized inflammation often accompany this complication. Antibiotics appropriate to the organisms cultured from the wound should be given. More severe cellulitis or, rarely, necrotizing fasciitis may occur. Inflammation and infection tend to compromise skin flap viability further so prophylactic antibiotics are commonly used in addition to the usual surgical principles of good skin preparation, hemostasis,

aseptic technique and wound drainage in an attempt to reduce this problem. Healing of open groin or vulvar wounds usually takes several weeks. Honey has been suggested to aid wound healing (Cavanagh et al, 1970), but is not recommended. Secondary closure or skin grafting is rarely necessary or desirable. While healing is taking place, the patient should be encouraged to eat properly, remain reasonably active, and care should be continued at home when the wound is clean and granulating.

Postoperative Hemorrhage

Hemorrhage from the groin incisions is rare but usually arises from rupture of the femoral artery or vein. This life threatening complication is usually associated with wound breakdown and infection and occurs two to three weeks postoperatively. Emergency compression of the bleeding point, transfusion and, if the femoral artery is involved, replacement by a graft are necessary. Transplanting the sartorius muscle over the exposed vessels at the time of surgery guards against this problem.

Lymphangitis

Lymphangitis involving the lymph vessels that previously drained into the inguinal nodes from the leg, buttock and lower part of the abdomen is a rare complication. It may occur many months after operation and is apt to be recurrent. It is characterized by high fever, malaise and pain, swelling and erythema in the affected area. Bed rest and antibiotics are usually successful treatment. Administration of long-acting penicillin monthly for six months after operation may be effective prophylaxis against lymphangitis.

Thrombophlebitis

Thrombophlebitis is probably the most serious of the common complications that accompany radical vulvectomy and groin dissection. It is clinically recognized in up to 9% of patients postoperatively and accounts for the majority of immediate postoperative deaths. Considering the overall impact on morbidity and mortality of thrombophlebitis, all known effective measures should be employed to decrease this risk. These include the use of prophylactic preoperative mini-dose subcutaneous heparin, intermittent calf compression and early ambulation.

The use of prophylactic anticoagulation has been reported to increase the incidence of hematoma or seroma formation and subsequent wound breakdown, but this complication should be weighed against the potential mortality from pulmonary embolism.

Seroma

Seroma formation below the groin flaps has been reported to occur in about 10% of patients. Clipping or ligating the lymphatic vessels at the base of the femoral triangle and in the femoral canal may reduce the risk. Suction drainage beneath the groin incisions has reduced the incidence of this complication. If a seroma or lymphocele develops after the drains have been removed, repeated aspirations with a needle or reinsertion of a suction drain for several weeks will usually result in the resolution of the problem.

Edema of the Leg

Edema of the leg is a very common late complication of groin dissection, occurring in the majority of patients to some degree. This most commonly takes the form of minimal edema of the thighs. Severe lymphedema of the lower extremities occurs in less than 5% of patients. The incidence of this complication is increased by severe breakdown of the groin incisions and the use of pre- or postoperative pelvic irradiation. Frequent elevation of the legs, the use of elastic stockings and occasional diuretics will help reduce the degree of swelling. The edema usually subsides after 9 to 12 months as the lymph finds other channels for its return.

Pelvic Relaxation and Incontinence

Pelvic relaxation and urinary incontinence may follow radical vulvectomy. This is due largely to excision of the supporting perineum as well as interference with the nerve and vascular supply of the perineal musculature. Plication of the levator muscles to build up the perineum is an important prophylactic measure that should be taken at the time of operation. Usually up to half the urethra can be removed and continence maintained. If partial urethral resection is necessary to remove the cancer or if a cystourethrocele exists, it is advisable to perform an anterior colporrhaphy with placement of plicating sutures at the urethrovesical junction to help ensure continence and maintain anterior vaginal wall support. Surgical correction of vaginal and uterine prolapse with or without associated urinary incontinence is difficult, and the prolapse has a high recurrence rate.

Sexual Dysfunction

Sexual dysfunction (see later section) following radical vulvectomy may be due to removal of the clitoris and labia, which normally supply sexual stimulation, to actual constriction of the introitus by scar tissue or to the emotional response of the patient or her partner to the operation. Clitoral excision often results in the loss of the ability to achieve orgasm, but this is not universal. Less radical procedures that preserve the clitoris may now be appropriate treatment for early cancers. Introital stenosis can usually be prevented during radical vulvectomy by extending the dissection high up the rectovaginal septum, which allows good mobility of the vagina when it is being sutured to the perineal incision. Once constriction of the introitus due to contracture of scar tissue is present, a surgical procedure using a vertical incision at the fourchette closed transversely or a Z-plasty will usually enlarge the vaginal opening sufficiently to allow nonpainful coitus. When emotional factors predominate as the cause of postoperative dyspareunia the problem is more complex.

PELVIC EXENTERATION

Exenterative procedures in gynecology are usually performed for locally recurrent or persistent cervical or vaginal cancer after adequate radiation therapy. These procedures are generally done with curative intent; if metastatic disease is found outside the pelvis, if malignancy is fixed to bone or the muscles of the lateral pelvic sidewall or if the pelvic nodes contain cancer, the disease is judged unresectable and the operation is abandoned. Anterior exenteration includes radical hysterectomy, vaginectomy and total cystectomy with the formation of a urinary conduit. Posterior exenteration includes radical hysterectomy, vaginectomy and resection of the rectosigmoid with a sigmoid colostomy. Total pelvic exenteration involves radical hysterectomy, vaginectomy, total cystectomy, resection of the rectosigmoid and formation of a urinary conduit and colostomy. Total exenteration remains the most commonly performed procedure; posterior exenteration is almost never indicated. With the application of modern radiotherapeutic techniques, there are fewer indications for these procedures. In selected patients, however, pelvic exenteration may provide the patient her only chance for survival. Cure rates of approximately 30 to 40% are reported.

The operative mortality rate for pelvic exenteration varies in recent reports from 1.4 to 24%, but is usually now about 5 to 10% (Table 7–3). This relatively high mortality is related directly to the severity and number of complications occurring during and after the procedure. The overall complication rate usually exceeds 50%, and patients who do have complications most often have multiple problems. Complications encountered in such radical surgery relate to fluid and electrolyte alterations, blood loss, protracted anesthesia, sepsis, urinary diversion, intestinal anastomosis, complications resulting from the denuded evacuated pelvis and loss of sexual function. Most of these problems have been solved, or improvements have been made in the past decade that have contributed to decreased mortality and morbidity.

Fluid and electrolyte problems are well managed by newer concepts and improved monitoring techniques, e.g., Swan-Ganz catheters. Operative mortality and morbidity (especially cardiopulmonary complications) are inversely related to operating time and blood loss during surgery. The use of gastrointestinal staplers has shortened the operative time significantly. Hypogastric artery ligation, performed in an attempt to reduce operative blood loss, does not significantly alter blood loss but does increase pelvic complications, probably as a result of pelvic devascularization. Sepsis can now usually be controlled by appropriate antibiotics. Preoperative mechanical and antibiotic bowel preparation as well as prophylactic perioperative systemic antibiotics help to prevent postoperative infections.

Urinary Complications

Urinary diversion is usually accomplished by implanting the ureters into an isolated segment of ileum (anterior exenteration) or transverse or sigmoid colon (total exenteration). Pyelonephritis and hyperchloremic acidosis are two potential problems with urinary conduits. Using an isolated segment of ileum or colon and keeping the segment of bowel relatively short (12 to 15 cm) prevents urine from being stored and thereby reduces chloride absorption and ureteral reflux. Strictures at the site of the ureterointestinal anastomosis may occur, leading to obstruction, pyelonephritis and uremia. The most serious complication of urinary diversion with exenteration is the development of a urinary leak or fistula (Orr et al, 1982b). This occurs in 4 to 16% of cases, depending on the type of intestinal segment, the presence of prior pelvic irradiation and the use of ureteral stents. Most fistulas and strictures occur when an irradiated ileal segment is used for the urinary conduit, rather than a portion of the transverse colon or suprapelvic sigmoid colon. The use of silastic ureteral stents, over which the ureteral-intestinal anastomosis is more easily performed, protects the anastomotic site from leakage and stricture and decreases the fistula rate. The ureteral stents are transfixed loosely to the conduit wall by fine chromic catgut sutures that give way, allowing the stents to be extruded by ureteral peristalsis in 14 to 21 days. Strictures and fistulas can be detected by intravenous pyelogram or loopogram. Revision of the anas-

Table 7–3. Complications of Pelvic Exenteration

Author(s)	Year	No. of Patients	Complications (%)				
			Surgical Mortality	Urinary Fistula	Bowel Fistula	Bowel Obstruction	Pelvic Abscess
Brunschwig	1967	318	17	–	–	–	–
Symmonds et al	1975	198	8.1	4	13	12	4
Karlen and Piver	1975	87	14	9	26	14	9
Morley and Lindenauer	1976	70	1.4	5.7	7	17	–
Rutledge et al	1977	296	13.5	–	–	–	–
Curry et al	1981	37	5.4	16	19	19	3
Averette et al	1984	92	24	12	16	5.4	3.3

tomosis is often necessary, but because of the high mortality from reoperation and the possibility of spontaneous closure of some fistulas, observation with maximal medical support is usually indicated initially. Urinary leaks may also occur from the proximal end of the conduit. The use of the gastrointestinal stapler probably decreases this likelihood, although urinary conduit calculi have been reported in association with stapled conduit closures.

Gastrointestinal Complications

Gastrointestinal complications remain a significant cause of perioperative morbidity and mortality (Orr et al, 1982a). They account for up to 60% of all nonmalignant indications for reoperation after exenteration. These complications are increased by performing an intestinal anastomosis in previously irradiated small bowel and failure to enclose the denuded pelvic cavity. Orr and co-workers (1983) demonstrated that avoidance of a small bowel anastomosis by means of a colon conduit, use of an omental pedicle to bring new blood supply into the pelvis and keep small bowel from becoming adherent to the pelvic floor and hyperalimentation reduced the risk of small bowel obstruction and fistula. The usual site of bowel obstruction and fistula is the terminal ileum. These complications are more common in patients who have sutured compared with stapled anastomoses. The most common procedure for treatment of these distal small bowel obstructions and fistulas is bypass, usually an ileotransverse enterocolostomy, and isolation of the involved bowel segment, which has a lower overall morbidity than resection. Rectovaginal fistulas are a significant risk (20 to 30%) when extensive dissection of the rectovaginal septum is undertaken during anterior exenteration. Because of this recognized problem, anterior exenteration should probably only be performed if adequate margins of resection can be obtained without extensive dissection of the rectovaginal septum, allowing preservation of the blood supply to the irradiated rectum. The development of a small bowel or rectal fistula in the immediate postoperative period is associated with a high mortality (approximately 50%), usually relating to the need for reoperation. Management of a fistula should include localization of the fistulous site (radiographically if necessary), institution or continuation of hyperalimentation, attempts to control pelvic sepsis if present and early surgical intervention.

Closure of the Pelvic Cavity

Closure of the pelvic cavity continues to be a problem, although recent improvements have been made. The use of some form of pelvic reconstruction, usually an omental lid or alternately an isolated colonic segment, peritoneal graft, myocutaneous flap or synthetic mesh, has signficantly reduced the complication rate by preventing the small bowel from falling down on the new pelvic floor, resulting in obstruction, fistula formation or herniation. Jakowatz and co-workers (1985) reported a reduction in complications, especially small bowel obstruction and fistula and infection, from 82 to 48% with the use of pelvic reconstruction in patients undergoing exenteration who had received prior pelvic irradiation.

Perineal Incision Complications

Complications related to the perineal wound are of concern because of the size of the cavity, the malodorous discharge and chronic infection that result, the time it takes the wound to heal and the loss of vaginal function. In the woman who was sexually active, creation of a neovagina is an important part of the rehabilitation process. Three satisfactory techniques are the use of gracilis myocutaneous flaps at the time of exenteration, application of a split-thickness skin graft into the perineal defect three to six weeks postoperatively, and vulvovaginoplasty (Williams' procedure) (see page 189).

OVARIAN CANCER SURGERY

Surgery is the most important aspect of the management of ovarian cancer. Surgical exploration confirms the diagnosis of ovarian cancer, defines the stage of the disease and provides the initial treatment. It may also be used to determine the response to adjuvant therapy and can sometimes be valuable for resection of recurrent or residual tumor or relief of bowel obstruction. In approximately 60 to 70% of cases of epithelial ovarian cancer, the tumor has spread beyond the ovary at diagnosis, and widespread intraabdominal carcinomatosis is present. The most important prognostic factor for these advanced ovarian cancers is the amount of residual disease remaining after the initial operation. The surgeon must be prepared to resect the primary cancer and as much of the metastatic disease as possible with acceptable morbidity. This usually involves total omentectomy, bilateral salpingo-oophorectomy, hysterectomy and resection of as many of the peritoneal implants as possible, including at times segmental resection of small or large bowel. A maximal effort should be made if it is determined that it would be possible to resect all tumors with a diameter greater than 2 cm. The presence of large para-aortic lymph nodes, masses involving the lesser omentum, splenic pedicle and porta hepatis, and parenchymal liver metastases contraindicate radical cytoreductive surgery. Using these criteria, optimal cytoreduction can usually be achieved in 65 to 75% of patients, leading to an improved quality of life, a better response to chemotherapy and prolonged survival (Griffiths et al, 1979; Wharton and Herson, 1981).

Preoperative and Postoperative Care

When performing such extensive operations on patients with advanced intraabdominal cancer, one can expect intraoperative and postoperative complications. These complications can be minimized, however, by proper preoperative and postoperative care. Bowel surgery may be required in up to 10% of primary operations for ovarian cancer in order to optimize surgical clearance of metastatic disease. Bowel preparation, both mechanical and antibiotic, will reduce the morbidity associated with these procedures. Patients with advanced ovarian cancer often have an associated weight loss and are nutritionally depleted, which is caused in part by extrinsic compression of the bowel and impaired small bowel function secondary to mesenteric plexus involvement. Pre- or postoperative intravenous or jejunal hyperalimentation is indicated in malnourished patients. The risks of infection and pulmonary embolization can be reduced by the use of prophylactic systemic antibiotics and subcutaneous, low-dose heparin plus intermittent pneumatic calf compression, respectively. The patient's electrolytes and hematologic values should be in a range to allow her to tolerate major surgery. Typing and cross matching of adequate amounts of blood are important. Postoperatively, intensive cardiopulmonary monitoring may be necessary, especially in those patients from whom massive ascites were removed at surgery. The potential for rapid intraoperative fluid shifts and the third spacing of fluid during the first 48 hours after the operation are indications for central cardiovascular monitoring using a Swan-Ganz catheter. Careful attention to fluid and electrolyte status and serum protein and hemoglobin levels is imperative.

Mortality and Morbidity

Although it has been clearly demonstrated that maximal cytoreductive surgery is the most important contributor to increased survival in advanced ovarian cancer, there is limited information regarding the morbidity and mortality associated with cytoreductive procedures. Hacker and co-workers (1983) noted major complications in 8 of 31 patients (26%) who had optimal cytoreduction for Stage III ovarian cancer. There were no deaths related to the operative procedure. Complications included wound dehiscence (2), prolonged ileus for more than seven days (2), congestive heart failure (1), pneumonia (1), fever of unknown etiology (1) and hemorrhage (1). The incidence and type of complications did not differ between patients undergoing optimal versus suboptimal resection in this series. The authors did not provide information on febrile morbidity or minor complications. Chen and Bochner (1985) reported postoperative morbidity in two thirds of 60 patients undergoing maximal cytoreductive surgery. Of these 40 patients, 53% (32) had febrile morbidity, including urinary tract infection (14), wound infection (9), atelectasis or pneumonia (7), hematoma (1) and phlebitis (1). Two patients were brought back to the operating room because of inadequate hemostasis. One patient developed a sigmoidcutaneous fistula, which was later successfully corrected. One death occurred in a patient with chronic hypertension who succumbed to renal failure three weeks postoperatively. Four other patients had prolonged oliguria (less than 300 ml of urine/24 hours) for varying periods of time. Most of these complications were of a transient or minor nature, such as wound or urinary tract infections and atelectasis, while serious morbidity was encountered in only 6.7% of patients.

From these reports, it is apparent that the morbidity and mortality of primary cytoreductive surgery for advanced ovarian cancer are acceptable. Most morbidity is associated with pulmonary, cardiovascular, bowel and wound problems. Attention to pre- and postoperative care will minimize most of these potential problems, enhancing the desirability and safety of aggressive primary tumor reductive surgery.

Complications of Operations For Recurrent Disease

Operations performed for relief of intestinal obstruction due to recurrent or progressive ovarian cancer, on the other hand, are associated with high morbidity and mortality. In a series of 23 patients reported by Castaldo and co-workers (1981), there were 22 complications in 10 patients, including 3 postoperative deaths, 4 wound infections, 4 recurrent small bowel obstructions, 3 episodes of sepsis, 3 enterocutaneous fistulas, 2 wound dehiscences, 2 pulmonary emboli and 1 patient with gastrointestinal bleeding. Piver and co-workers (1982) reported major complications occurring in 19 (31%) of 60 patients undergoing surgery for ovarian cancer–induced intestinal obstruction. Nine patients (15%) died of postoperative complications. Most major complications were related to the intestinal tract including fistulas, anastomotic leaks and short bowel syndrome with severe diarrhea. Krebs and Goplerud (1983) had an operative mortality rate of 12% in a series of 104 operations performed for surgical correction of bowel obstruction due to ovarian carcinoma. Fatal complications included intestinal anastomosis disruptions (4), gastrointestinal hemorrhage (2), sepsis (1), pulmonary embolism (1), myocardial infarction (1) and persistent bowel obstruction (2). In all of these reports, morbidity and mortality were highest in those patients who had received prior radiotherapy, patients with multiple sites of obstruction that required more than one intestinal anastomosis, patients over 65 years of age, patients with severe nutritional deprivation and patients with advanced recurrent cancer whose life expectancy was less than two months. Proper selection of patients, use of gastrointestinal stapling devices and hyperalimentation as an adjunct to surgery will help to decrease the morbidity and mortality in this high risk group of patients.

PARA-AORTIC LYMPHADENECTOMY

Para-aortic lymphadenectomy has become a more common surgical procedure in gynecologic oncology with the recognition of spread of gynecologic malignancies out of the pelvis to this area in the absence of apparent disease spread elsewhere. Approximately 30% of women with locally advanced cervical carcinoma (Stages IIB to IVA) have aortic lymph node metastases. Women with Stage I endometrial cancer with large or poorly differentiated tumors, deep myometrial invasion or occult cervical involvement have a significantly increased risk of para-aortic nodal metastases. When ovarian adenocarcinoma is clinically limited to the ovary (Stage I), approximately 10% of women have subclinical aortic node metastases; this incidence increases to over 30% when intraperitoneal disease spread is present. Para-aortic lymphadenectomy is, therefore, a valuable adjunct to staging in women with cancers of the cervix, endometrium and ovary in order to determine proper subsequent management.

Complications Related to Associated Radiation Therapy

Many of the complications resulting from para-aortic lymphadenectomy are related to the subsequent use of external extended-field radiation therapy (Piver et al, 1981). A transperitoneal para-aortic lymph node dissection frequently results in segments of ileum or jejunum becoming adherent to the posterior parietal peritoneum overlying the aorta and vena cava where the peritoneum was opened or to the undersurface of the incision. This restricts the normal intestinal mobility and, therefore, leads to higher radiation dosage to the adherent segment of small intestine, and may result in obstruction or fistula formation. Use of a paramedian J-shaped abdominal incision with a retroperitoneal approach to the para-aortic nodes for cervical cancer before the use of external radiation therapy has significantly reduced these complications (Berman et al, 1977). Unfortunately, para-aortic lymphadenectomy performed at the time of primary surgery for endometrial and ovarian carcinoma requires a transperitoneal approach.

Venous Complications

The vena cava may be easily injured during a para-aortic lymphadenectomy because of its thin wall and the presence of small vessels coming out of its anterior surface. Small lacerations can usually be controlled by using one hand to apply pressure over the defect with a sponge stick and repairing the rent with fine cardiovascular sutures of 3-0 or 4-0 silk as the defect is slowly uncovered. Small injuries may actually resolve with only pressure applied to the area for a couple of minutes. Larger injuries to the vena cava should be initially controlled with laparotomy packs; adequate blood replacement should be assured and help obtained before proceeding further. Occlusion of the vena cava above and below the defect and the use of suction to keep the field dry, will usually allow for repair of the defect as noted earlier. Vascular clamps applied to the vena cava should be avoided, if possible, since they may worsen the injury. Extensive injury to the vena cava below the level of the renal veins may require ligation of the vena cava above and below the damaged area, using heavy nonabsorbable sutures without repair. This may be the only method of preventing excessive blood loss and reducing the risk of subsequent pulmonary embolism from clot formation at the site of the vena caval damage. Ligation of the infrarenal portion of the vena cava produces minimal morbidity, but this procedure should not be performed above the level of the renal veins. Injury to the vena cava above the renal vessels must always be repaired.

Arterial Complications

The aorta is infrequently injured during para-aortic lymphadenectomy because of its thick wall. If injury does occur, aortic vascular clamps are placed above and below the injured area, and the defect is repaired with interrupted cardiovascular sutures in order to achieve close intimal approximation. Large defects that cannot be repaired by simple everting sutures require saphenous vein or synthetic graft patching (Bergan et al, 1976).

Injury or inadvertent ligation of the inferior mesenteric artery may occur at the time of para-aortic node dissection. If this happens, it is important to ascertain whether there is arterial backflow between the middle and left colic arteries. Ligation of the inferior mesenteric artery can usually be performed with minimal morbidity, but reimplantation into the aorta should be considered if adequate backflow is not demonstrated in order to prevent ischemia to the descending colon and rectosigmoid. The addition of postoperative radiotherapy to the pelvis may also add to the morbidity of inferior mesenteric artery ligation.

Miscellaneous Complications

Postoperative complications of para-aortic lymphadenectomy are most commonly related

to the lungs, wound and intestine (Piver and Barlow, 1974; Lagasse et al, 1980). Prolonged ileus, probably as a result of the extensive packing of the intestine that is required to expose the retroperitoneal area, is a frequent complication.

PSYCHOSOCIAL AND SEXUAL COMPLICATIONS

The psychosocial and sexual complications of operations and treatments for genital cancer in women differ from those resulting from the therapy of benign diseases in four aspects. First, the disease itself has major psychosocial and sexual effects which complicate management at all stages from diagnosis to terminal care. Second, therapy is often more radical, more urgent and more threatening to the identity and function of the woman herself. Third, pain and death are important complications of the disease itself and of its therapy. Fourth, several different types of treatment may be used, i.e., various combinations of surgery, radiation therapy and chemotherapy. Their effects may be cumulative and often difficult to identify separately. In this section the management of the whole patient and of the complications of operations will be emphasized. The specific complications of chemotherapy and radiation therapy are covered elsewhere (Chapters 13 and 14).

The Impact of Gynecologic Cancer

PSYCHOSOCIAL

The Patient. During the course of gynecologic cancer several events cause significant stress to the patient. These include diagnosis, treatment, follow-up, recurrence and, in some cases, terminal course and death. The reaction of the patient and her family to the disease as a whole and to these specific events depends on her personality, prior response to stress and the family constellation.

Studies of the behavioral responses to cancer include the evaluation of such characteristics as mood and affect (Gottschalk, 1984) or depression (Endicott, 1984). The subject is reviewed in detail by Friedenbergs and co-workers (1982). These investigations often relate to cancer in general and are not specific to gynecologic cancer. They usually involve the use of more or less sophisticated psychometric tests that are not easily available to the physician who has primary responsibility for the management of the patient. However, perceptive observation of the patient with gynecologic cancer will indicate that she frequently reacts to the disease and the various events connected with it by denial, anger, bargaining, depression or acceptance (Newton, 1972). These responses are similar to those described by Kubler-Ross (1969). They do not necessarily occur over a specific period of time or in that order, as Kubler-Ross implied, but may be detected in rapid succession or in varying order during a single or several interviews.

The Patient's Family and Friends. Patients with cancer have difficulty communicating with others about their problems. One of the many fears of patients with early disease is that they will be rejected or abandoned by their loved ones (Wortman, 1984). This need for support becomes greater if the treatment is difficult or prolonged or if the disease recurs.

Family and friends are usually concerned when a patient whom they love or know has cancer. The fact that the cancer involves the reproductive tract adds another dimension, because a woman's reproductive and sexual functions are fundamental to family life. Family concern is expressed in many ways—anxiety, desire to protect or wish to support. Often the family's reaction mirrors the patient's and may go through the same processes of denial, anger, bargaining, depression and acceptance. Inevitably there are both positive and negative feelings. The latter may take the form of lack of concern, over-concern, reluctance to inconvenience themselves in a crisis and hostility to the patient and her problems.

Quality of Life. "Satisfaction with living" and "quality of life" are terms widely used in respect to patients with cancer. Unfortunately, they are terms that everybody understands but nobody can define well. Nevertheless, it is important to measure the components of quality of life so as to form an estimate of the cancer patient's status as a whole. This is especially true since many of the powerful current operative, radiotherapeutic and chemotherapeutic treatments prolong life but are associated with significant side effects. Performance scales of physical activity have classically been considered as representative of the quality of life. However, these do not measure body functions (symptoms), ability to do productive work or family (social) relationships. In developing a functional living index for cancer (FLIC) Schipper and co-workers (1984) point out that a

measure of the quality of life of patients with cancer should be (1) cancer-specific; (2) oriented to everyday living; (3) self-administered; (4) of general applicability and easy interpretability; (5) repeatable; (6) sensitive to various levels of illness from the clinically well to the terminally ill patient and (7) valid and reliable. The disadvantages of even a relatively simple evaluation tool such as the FLIC are the time and expertise required to apply it repeatedly over the course of a patient's disease. Moreover, it and similar studies may not be entirely applicable to women with gynecologic cancer; in fact, medical data on patients so studied are frequently fragmentary. However, the questions contained in the FLIC (Table 7–4) provide a continuing basis for patient evaluation by the physician or oncology nurse.

Table 7–4. Functional Living Index: Cancer*†

1. Most people experience some feelings of depression at times. Rate how often you feel these feelings.
2. How well are you coping with your everyday stress?
3. How much time do you spend thinking about your illness?
4. Rate your ability to maintain your usual recreation or leisure activities.
5. Has nausea affected your daily functioning?
6. How well do you feel today?
7. Do you feel well enough to make a meal or do minor household repairs today?
8. Rate the degree to which your cancer has imposed a hardship on those closest to you in the past two weeks?
9. Rate how often you feel discouraged about your life.
10. Rate your satisfaction with your work and your jobs around the house in the past month.
11. How uncomfortable do you feel today?
12. Rate in your opinion, how disruptive your cancer has been to those closest to you in the past two weeks.
13. How much is pain or discomfort interfering with your daily activities?
14. Rate the degree to which your cancer has imposed a hardship on you (personally) in the past two weeks.
15. How much of your usual household tasks are you able to complete?
16. Rate how willing you were to see and spend time with those closest to you in the past two weeks.
17. How much nausea have you had in the past two weeks?
18. Rate the degree to which you are frightened of the future.
19. Rate how willing you were to see and spend time with friends in the past two weeks.
20. How much of your pain or discomfort over the past two weeks was related to your cancer?
21. Rate your confidence in your prescribed course of treatment.
22. How well do you appear today?

*Items are scored from 1 to 7 by the patient.
†From Schipper H, Clinch J et al: Measuring the quality of life of cancer patients: functional living. *J. Clin. Oncol.* 2:472, 1984. Reprinted with permission.

PSYCHOSEXUAL

The usual initial symptoms of gynecologic cancer (except for ovarian cancer) directly involve sexual and reproductive function. They include vaginal bleeding, discharge and, in the case of vulvar cancer, a lump on the external genitalia. For the young woman anxious to have children they pose an immediate threat to her ability to reproduce; this threat is not present for the woman who has completed her family or is postmenopausal. If the woman is sexually active, her desire for coitus sharply decreases in most instances, although her sexual needs may persist. Her response to the situation will vary according to her age, sexual history and relationship with her partner if she has one. The immediate response of the partner will also vary. Apart from concern at the illness of a loved one, he may feel guilty, particularly if bleeding has followed intercourse; also, he may feel that continuing vaginal intercourse may worsen his partner's condition, and occasionally he may fear that he will develop cancer.

Any type of major therapy, irrespective of the specific organ involved, discourages and even interdicts coitus for a varying time, depending upon the specific treatment. If treatment is prolonged, or recurrence occurs, initial fears are compounded. Moreover, both members of the couple may find it difficult to admit or discuss the problem. These difficulties may vary with different cultures (O'Hoy and Tang, 1985).

The Effects of Specific Therapy

HYSTERECTOMY AND BILATERAL SALPINGO-OOPHORECTOMY

Removal of the uterus, tubes and ovaries is part of the primary treatment of cancer of the corpus uteri, tube or ovary. The psychosexual consequences are similar to those following the same operation performed for benign disease. The only difference may be in the use of replacement therapy after bilateral oophorectomy. Since some endometrial and ovarian cancers are positive for estrogen receptors, there is a possible theoretical objection to the use of estrogens as replacement therapy. This seems logical if some tumor has been left behind at operation. However, if the tumor has been completely removed, there would seem to be little or no risk. If estrogen therapy is of concern, medroxyprogesterone acetate suspension (Depo-Provera) 150 to 200 mg intramuscularly

every two to four months is effective in reducing hot flashes (see Chapter 6).

RADICAL HYSTERECTOMY

Most reports of large series of patients treated by radical hysterectomy for carcinoma of the cervix have been concerned with major physical complications. Sexual sequelae are seldom mentioned. Nevertheless, these are of obvious importance since up to 90% of patients adequately treated for early (Stage I) carcinoma of the cervix now survive for more than five years without evidence of disease. Further, patients evaluated for sexual complications have sometimes received radiation therapy in addition to radical hysterectomy, so it is difficult to separate the effects of each treatment (see Chapter 14). Among 15 patients in the lower socioeconomic classes, Vincent and co-workers (1975) found that 27% reported a decrease in desire for intercourse and 47% a decrease in the frequency of coitus.

These changes may have physical and psychologic causes. Two major physical factors are delay in the return of bladder function and shortening of the vagina. The former frequently requires that the patient wear an indwelling catheter for four to six weeks. During this time, however, the vaginal apex is healing and vaginal coitus is contraindicated. Sometimes prolonged catheterization is needed and this may continue to inhibit vaginal intercourse although the apex of the vagina is healed, and it may necessitate other methods of sexual expression. An occasional late problem is stress incontinence during coitus. Improvement in perineal muscle tone and emptying the bladder immediately prior to intercourse can improve this symptom.

If a radical hysterectomy is properly performed, the vagina is usually shortened. This presents difficulty in coitus at first. Bleeding may occur, and this causes concern because the male partner feels that he has injured the woman and she fears a recurrence of her disease because she has same symptom that originally led to the diagnosis. Eventually the vagina will stretch, although often not to its original depth. Methods of reducing the chance of bleeding and discomfort include adequate lubrication, rear entry, adduction of the female partner's thighs and use of other erotic zones.

Psychologic factors may affect both partners. An extreme reaction by the male partner is desertion or divorce. Data are lacking on how often this occurs, either early or later after operation. A lesser reaction is continued absence of vaginal intercourse, which may result from the fears of both partners. The patient may be afraid of undoing the effects of treatment or causing recurrence. The partner may be afraid of hurting or causing symptoms similar to those that occurred prior to diagnosis and possibly acquiring cancer himself or being affected by radiation if the patient has had that kind of treatment. The therapy of these problems is discussed below.

EXENTERATION

Pelvic exenteration is most commonly performed for cancer of the cervix, occasionally for cancer of the vagina or advanced cancer of the vulva and rarely for recurrent cancer of the corpus uteri. Outside the gynecologic field it is also performed for cancer of the rectum or bladder. The operation, whether anterior (removal of bladder in addition to uterus, cervix and vagina), posterior (removal of rectum with uterus, cervix and vagina) or total (removal of all the pelvic organs) often has major complications and severe physical, psychological and sexual results.

When exenterations were first reported by Brunschwig (1948), emphasis was placed on the fact that this operation was the patient's only chance for survival. Anatomic changes were, and indeed still are, regarded as secondary. However, in the past 15 years, the postoperative death rate has fallen to less than 10% and the number and type of complications, although high, are usually manageable. Thus, more attention has been paid to the long-term effects of the procedures and on the woman's quality of life and her sexuality.

The psychologic and sexual complications are magnified because (1) the disease is known by the patient to have recurred; (2) a major alteration has occurred in the patient's body appearance and image; (3) one or two abdominal stomas result (more often two since total exenteration is more commonly performed than anterior or posterior exenteration) and (4) the operation involves partial or complete loss of the vagina and the surrounding muscles.

Most reports on the effect of stomas cover few patients because of the infrequency of the procedure even on large gynecologic services. Vera (1981) describes in detail the impact of stomas. Initial reactions, present in 50% or more of the patients, include uncertainty about care, shock, disgust or puzzlement. Stomas decrease physical, social and sexual activities in one third to one half of the patients for a variety

of reasons. Stomas prove to be inconvenient because of leakage or skin problems in over half the patients. Hurney and Holland (1985) divide the psychosocial problems of ostomy patients into (1) physical—practical problems of handling stoma function and appliances; (2) emotional—impaired self-esteem, depression, anxiety and fear of sexual undesirability and (3) interpersonal—impaired sexual function or fears about it, strain on family and work relationships and social isolation.

Removal of the vagina makes normal coitus impossible. With an exenteration procedure the importance of this is overshadowed at first by the severity of the operation. However, when the vagina is removed without the formation of stomas, as occurs in young women with DES-related clear cell adenocarcinoma of the vagina, the problem is more acute. Unless the procedure has been performed for cancer of the vulva, the clitoris and labia are usually retained. Moreover, in anterior or posterior exenteration part or all of the posterior or anterior vaginal wall respectively may be left in place. In any case, the construction of a neovagina is an important part of the operative procedure or the early postoperative care. The various techniques have been reviewed by Magrina and Masterson (1981). The chief methods are as follows:

1. Insertion of a vaginal obturator at or shortly after operation and use of this until the vagina has epithelialized. Estrogen cream may facilitate healing.

2. Use of a split-thickness skin graft at various times after operation, with the operative cavity being preserved at the end of the operation or soon afterwards by a soft mold or created later by upward dissection from the perineum.

3. Use of a segment of intestine.

4. Vulvovaginoplasty, creating a pouch from the labia (see Chapter 5).

The sexual complications of exenteration are a product of the whole operation, the stoma and the absent or reconstructed vagina. Clearly, sexual activity is reduced. Andersen and Hacker (1983), in one of the few studies on this subject, found that postexenteration patients reported a reduction in sexual activity below that of anatomically normal women with sexual dysfunction. Four of 15 patients continued to be sexually active, four were not active and did not wish to be while seven were dissatisfied with their inactivity. These proportions may vary in different circumstances, e.g., age, educational level or socioeconomic status, but information on these differences is scanty.

VULVECTOMY

Loss of even a small portion of the vulvar tissue can be extremely distressing, especially to younger women, in whom intraepithelial carcinoma is now being found more frequently. Apart from possible pain on intercourse, the disfiguration, readily visible with a mirror, is embarrassing and detracts from the patient's self-image as a woman. The use of laser therapy has improved this situation, since there is less residual scarring.

In radical vulvectomy, with or without inguinal and/or pelvic lymphadenectomy, the labia, mons and clitoris are removed, and the introitus may be narrowed. Healing may be prolonged. In women whose coital function has ceased, the changes may have no sexual effects, although the anatomic changes themselves may be of equal concern. For younger women removal of the area of sexual stimulation as well as constriction of the introitus is a major sexual complication.

A small study of the sexual effects of vulvectomy in 15 relatively young Danish women (average age 48.9 years, range 32 to 60 years) showed a sharp decrease in coital activity and in acceptance of such activity. Reduced libido and sexual arousal and increased orgiastic dysfunction and dyspareunia were also reported by the majority of women. Both patients and their partners noted depression and reduced acceptance of the woman's body (Moth et al, 1983).

Management

The management of the psychosocial and sexual complications of gynecologic cancer therapy involves recognition, prevention and treatment. Because of the complexity of the diseases and their treatments, management includes a wide range of interactions between the patient and her family and the individual physician and other members of the therapeutic team.

THE PHYSICIAN AND THE PATIENT

The physician who tells the patient about the diagnosis should recognize that this may be the most important interview during the patient's illness. The following guidelines are worth considering:

1. Knowledge of the patient's previous response to stress may be helpful.
2. Information on her social and family history may give some clues as to her likely reactions.

3. The diagnosis should be presented clearly, in language the patient can understand, not in medical jargon, with emphasis on the hopeful aspects.
4. The patient's response may be any one or a mixture of the five reaction patterns mentioned previously.
5. Opportunity for the patient to express her feelings or ask questions is essential.

Just as with physical or pharmacologic procedures, complications of the patient's response to the knowledge that she has cancer must be recognized and managed. For example, if one of the responses predominates, it may presage further emotional problems. Immediate and continued denial may mean that the information given should be repeated and that further time is needed for her to understand what has happened. An opportunity for that discussion must be provided. Anger and bargaining often prolong the initial discussion, and patience is needed to encourage the patient to see some positive aspects of the situation.

THE PHYSICIAN AND THE PATIENT'S FAMILY

The patient's family and social environment must be included in the initial work-up and planning for the patient. To deal with the disease alone, without including the people and circumstances with which the patient interacts, makes management much more difficult.

It is important to appreciate the part played by the woman in the family. For example, an elderly man who married a younger woman and expected that she would "take care of him" in his old age may be greatly disturbed to learn that she has cancer, since it may mean that his support is deserting him. Looking after her may not have been his underlying reason for marriage. Children who have been raised protectively and managed by their mother throughout their childhood and adult lives may find it difficult to conceive of looking after her.

Discussion should be held with the family to assess the degree of their concern and include them in the plans for treatment and follow-up. When there are many family members, they may have different expectations. The person(s) who will have the most to do with the patient, i.e., bringing her for treatment or looking after her postoperatively, is the most important.

For the patient with a close supportive family, friends, acquaintances and co-workers may be less significant because of the tendency of the cancer patient to withdraw into a close family circle. Such friends may be important in the management of complicated responses because of their well-meant attempts to advise the patient and particular members of the family on the basis of their own experiences or information they may have received from the media or other sources.

A complicating factor to be considered in the woman's response to cancer is the absence of close family members. Then attempts must be made to recruit the help of neighbors, friends, co-workers or church members. It is here that the team approach to management is particularly helpful.

Reactions of family and friends to continuing problems of treatment and recurrence follow similar patterns. The persistent demands of the patient's illness sap the initial kindly support, particularly when the helping family members have problems within their own group such as small children, other sickness or work demands. Then wider support needs to be found.

SEXUAL COUNSELING

Sexual problems require specific attention. They are best managed by a combination of preoperative and postoperative counseling. It is not usually possible for a woman to fully appreciate the effect of the operation in advance. However, it is important to provide special interview time prior to the operation at which the patient's sexual attitudes, behavior and expectations can be discussed. The patient's partner should be included, when possible. Postoperatively, emphasis should be placed on the anticipation of complete recovery (if this is realistic) but with the recognition that sexual function may be different and need adjustment. Since resumption of vaginal coitus must often be delayed for physical reasons, it is important to give or imply permission for other kinds of sexual behavior during this interval, i.e., caressing or mutual oral-genital or other stimulation. If the couple are close, signs of affection are particularly meaningful to the woman at this time.

Follow-up is especially necessary if preoperative information has not been given or has not been understood. Before discharge and at follow-up visits the patient should be given an opportunity to voice her concerns about coitus. Questions can be asked and replies given more freely if the surgeon who performed the operation or a team member whom she knows is able to see her. It is best if the husband or partner can participate in this discussion. At this time, also, it is advisable to determine if

more intensive counseling is likely to be needed. It is important that such counseling be given by someone who appreciates the character and significance of the operation.

SEXUAL COUNSELING FOR SPECIFIC OPERATIONS

Sexual problems following radical hysterectomy are chiefly related to the disease itself and to the shortness of the vagina. Sexual counseling primarily involves encouraging the patient to accept herself as a whole woman and discussing practical methods of dealing with the vaginal length (see earlier discussion).

Management of sexual disability following exenteration requires initially that the counselor:

1. Begin discussion before operation.
2. Recognize that the patient's sexual confidence and body image have been disrupted and that she may be worried and frustrated and feel inadequate.
3. Understand that incomplete information may have been given to the patient and her partner about the sexual consequences of the operation, and that, even if information has been given, its significance may not have been understood or appreciated.
4. Permit the patient to discuss her sexual activity, asking directive questions if necessary. For example, sexual dreams and even feelings of a phantom vagina may be significant.
5. Evaluate the importance of sexual behavior to the patient before and after the operation. Obviously, if a sexual relationship was not previously part of her life, whether she is single or married, elaborate discussion of the subject may not be necessary.

After clarification of the above issues the following points should be considered in advising her.

1. Support if she wishes to achieve normal coitus i.e., reconstruction of the vagina.
2. Encouragement of self-confidence and acceptance of normal sexual feelings.
3. Explanation of the pleasure and acceptability of sexual stimulation of other parts of the body, such as breasts or other areas.
4. Information about methods of dealing with or hiding the stomas during intercourse. Attempts at intercourse in the stoma are not advisable, although manual stimulation of the stoma may be erotic for some women.
5. Participation of the partner in combined and/or separate counseling sessions.

After radical vulvectomy it often takes a long time for the introitus to heal, thus adding to the disfiguration caused by the operation. Stenosis is another serious consequence. It is important for the surgeon to be alert to this during operation by freeing the vagina from the rectum as high as possible and everting the vaginal mucosa. Postoperatively dilatation and the use of a Z-plasty at the introitus may be helpful. Practical suggestions for women who wish to maintain sexual activity include an adequate explanation of what was done, emphasis on other zones of sexual stimulation, provision of artificial external lubrication with water-soluble jelly and possible changes in coital position.

Multidisciplinary Approach to Management

The Need for a Multidisciplinary Approach

Current patterns of medical care may of themselves be responsible for psychosocial complications. The classic concept of one physician managing a patient with cancer from diagnosis through treatment to cure or death is now seldom possible. The disease and its treatment have become too complex. The sequel, however, is all too frequently encountered in the United States. In one variation of this theme, a patient with lower abdominal discomfort is found by her family physician to have a pelvic tumor. She is referred to a gynecologist who recognizes that the tumor has to be removed. At operation he finds an ovarian cancer that has spread outside the pelvis to the omentum and peritoneal surfaces. He removes the pelvic organs, obtains a diagnosis and then refers the patient to a radiation therapist. The radiation therapist treats the patient's whole abdomen with external radiation. The patient does well for a time but the disease then recurs. The radiation therapist refers the patient to a medical oncologist for further management. When the disease appears to be persistent after a course of chemotherapy or complications occur, the patient has nowhere to go. Which of her various specialists should she consult?

The concentration of patients with gynecologic cancer in tertiary centers has not necessarily improved coordination of care. Although close in location, the various specialists may be just as far apart as their colleagues outside such centers. The size of the institution, the changing housestaff and often the distance of the patient from her home exaggerate fragmentation of care and cause the patient additional stress.

Medical personnel other than physicians are now having increasing contact with patients and responsibility for significant portions of their cancer care. Examples are nurses on the inpatient hospital floors and in physicians' offices, social workers, dietitians, home care support specialists and chaplains, to name a few. This multitude further confuses patients and detracts from continuity of care.

The need for many experts in managing gynecologic cancer will not disappear. The problem then is how to coordinate that care to the benefit of the patient and her family.

Functions of Caregivers

Analysis of the roles of those who participate in the care of the gynecologic cancer patient is essential if all are to make the best use of their special skills.

The physician who coordinates the patient's care plays an important role in preventing and managing complications. It is ideal if that physician has special knowledge and experience in the complete care of the patient with gynecologic cancer, but it is essential that he or she is accustomed to managing such patients on a regular and not an occasional basis. Such a physician is usually a gynecologist or, preferably, a gynecologic oncologist. His expertise lies in what he has been trained to do—make diagnoses, plan medications and treatment, perform operations or prescribe chemotherapy (or radiation therapy) and conduct follow-up examinations. He has neither the time nor, frequently, the skill to deal with the varied medical problems and with all the questions that an informed patient may ask, or to arrange help at home for her and her family. But if he is to be an effective leader of the interdisciplinary team, he must recognize the contribution of the other physicians and professionals involved and coordinate their efforts. He must serve as the "continuing physician" for the consultants such as the radiotherapist, medical oncologist, urologist and others, as well as making sure that other members of the team are familiar with the progress of the patient's disease and her treatment.

Several types of specialization have taken place in nursing with regard to cancer and gynecologic cancer in particular. Examples are the gynecologic oncology nurse, nurse clinician or clinical nurse specialist. Such a nurse serves many functions—continuity of care, explanation and education and administration of chemotherapy and other treatment (Chamorro, 1981). Other nurses are specialists in certain aspects of gynecologic cancer, especially in tertiary centers, such as operating room, postoperative care, home care or enterostomal therapy.

A social worker is an integral part of any gynecologic oncology caregiving group. There are some patients whose families, by their closeness, can give all the help that is needed. Young women with children or older women with others depending on them or who have no family support need social work help early in the course of their disease to assist them in coping with domestic, environmental and financial stresses.

Examples of other professionals who function effectively in specific segments of patient care include chaplains, dietitians, pharmacists and others. Their contact with patients may be brief but is none the less important, if only because any of them may be the single person with whom the patient communicates well and from whom she seeks information and support.

DECISION POINTS IN THERAPY

An interdisciplinary approach is not needed for all patients throughout the course of their disease. For example, a patient with Stage IA, G1 adenocarcinoma of the corpus uteri who has a supportive family may be almost completely managed by her gynecologic surgeon or gynecologic oncologist and his oncology nurse. When she is in the hospital having definitive surgical treatment, operating room, recovery and gynecologic floor nurses play an important role but it is temporary. In a patient with more complicated disease, even with a supportive family, there are several points of decision at which she needs specific help, apart from that given by the responsible gynecologic oncologist. These are:

1. Diagnosis. The oncology nurse may be most useful in repeating or interpreting what the physician has said and in providing additional information about the planned management.

2. Initial Treatment. The personnel involved depend on the type of treatment. For example, if radiation therapy is used, the radiation oncologist and his technicians are the primary figures. If an operation is performed, surgical, recovery room and gynecologic floor nurses (especially with a primary nursing care plan) are closely involved with the gynecologic oncology patient. But if the treatment is compli-

cated, as with radical hysterectomy or radical vulvectomy, the social worker and the home care specialist may be needed. The role of others will depend on each patient's needs.

3. Follow-up. In the uncomplicated case, the primary persons involved (in addition to the physician) will be the gynecologic oncology nurse or office assistant.

4. Complications and Recurrence. It is at these points in the disease that more caregivers become involved and continuity of care is likely to suffer. Physician consultants from various specialties such as urology or medical oncology may make important contributions. Social workers, dietitians, enterostomal therapists and home care specialists are often needed, while support from chaplains or volunteer groups may be essential. Exenteration epitomizes the need for help from many members of the caregiving group.

5. Terminal Care. Emphasis is on physicians experienced in pain relief, home and hospice caregivers and supportive team members who can help the patient and her family adjust to approaching death and help the family adjust to bereavement.

COORDINATION OF MULTIDISCIPLINARY CARE

Care is given and coordinated by meetings and documented by records. Meetings mean contact between people in which both parties or groups participate; one does not simply tell or instruct the other. Of necessity meetings often occur by telephone, but those that mean the most take place face to face. Meetings may take place in the traditional way between professionals and patients, between professionals or between patients themselves.

Meetings Between Professionals and Patients. These are most relevant at the points of decision mentioned before, but they may also be important at times that seem less critical or stressful. A meeting is different from taking a history or trying to ascertain in depth a patient's feelings. It is a separate event at which a mutual decision has to be reached regarding the next steps in the course or management of the patient's disease. Both professionals (whether physician, nurse or other) and patients have objectives to be realized. The physician wishes to clarify the diagnosis without making the situation appear hopeless, to lay out the alternatives in treatment and give his opinion as to what should be done. The patient has to assimilate the shock of the diagnosis, to consider the implications of the possible treatments and, eventually, to plan for the future. The same kind of transaction occurs when the oncology nurse or social worker meets with the patient. The difficulties that professionals have with such meetings are the time that they take and the desire to reach a firm conclusion as soon as possible. However, the patient often needs time to get used to what she has been told and to participate actively in planning. Sometimes, therefore, an inconclusive end is inevitable and, indeed, beneficial; arrangements must be made to continue the dialogue.

An important aspect of the professional-patient interaction is the provision of appropriate instructional literature and information on sources of help available to patients and their families.

A variant of the one-on-one meeting between professional and patient is a family conference. This may be useful when the patient has many relatives who are anxious to know what is happening or who hold differing ideas on how to help the patient. The objectives are similar to those of one-on-one meetings, except that the professional point of view may be expressed by more than one person and from a different angle, e.g., by the physician and the social worker. Family conferences are difficult to arrange because relatives may have to come from different places; leaving out one or two may cause later difficulties.

Meetings Between Professionals. The simplest meeting of professionals is between physician and nurse. In this each communicates with the other what they have learned about the patient or have told her. For example, the physician may say that he has talked to a patient about radical hysterectomy for carcinoma of the cervix, but that she does not seem to have a clear idea of what this involves and repetition by the nurse would be helpful. Or the nurse may indicate that the patient seems not to understand the implications of a radical vulvectomy in regard to recovery time and that further information should be given by the physician on that point.

When more professionals are involved, multiple one-on-one meetings are inappropriate. In such situations a patient care conference can be very effective. The essentials of this meeting as we have conducted it are:

1. It is held regularly, once a week at a set time. More frequent conferences may be suitable in some circumstances.

2. All the relevant caregivers are invited to attend. This includes physicians, the oncology nurse, gynecology floor nurses, the social worker, representatives of home and supportive care groups, a member of the psychiatric liaison service, dietitians, the chaplain, the pharmacist, the enterostomal therapist and somtimes others.

3. The primary discussion centers on inpatients, but follow-ups on outpatients are given by various members.

4. Each inpatient's medical history is presented by a physician (staff or resident), nursing data are given by the nurse primarily involved and input is provided by other members of the group who have seen the patient.

5. There is free discussion—the most important feature.

6. A decision is reached as to how to proceed with further care, who is to do what and how to follow up the management plans.

7. General topics relevant to patient care are discussed as they arise during the meeting. These have included such subjects as dealing with stomas, hyperalimentation or sexuality problems, handling families with differing ideas on the patient's care, dealing with personal feelings about resuscitation and dying patients or settling jurisdictional conflicts between different caregivers.

8. A note is entered in the patient's chart, when appropriate or feasible, indicating that discussion took place at the conference and outlining the agreed plans for future management.

Similar meetings between smaller groups of professionals can be held at other times and in different circumstances, as for example with outpatient office caregivers. However, such conferences should always be focused on sharing information and making plans for further management.

Meetings Between Patients. These include therapeutic group discussions, facilitated group discussions and self-help groups. The first two are primarily planned by professionals, although the professional input is more directive in therapeutic group discussions. Self-help groups are organized by patients usually without professional contributions.

Therapeutic counseling groups, such as that reported by Ferlic and co-workers (1979), have usually included patients with a variety of cancers. For patients with gynecologic cancer, Cain and co-workers (1986) found that thematic counseling, whether on an individual or group basis (led by a social worker), resulted in greater psychosocial and sexual benefits than standard interactive counseling between caregivers and patients. The themes covered in each counseling session included (1) the nature of cancer, (2) the causes of cancer, (3) the impact of treatment on body image and sexuality, (4) relaxation, (5) diet and exercise, (6) relating to caregivers, (7) talking with family and friends and (8) goal setting. Limitations of organized counseling sessions of this kind are that, for the group sessions at least, an extra, often difficult, visit to a medical center may be needed, and that patients with different gynecologic cancers may have very different psychosocial and sexual problems. Moreover, it is difficult to include in these groups patients with advanced or recurrent disease, who may actually need the most help, because of the discouraging effect their conditions may have on the others attending.

Our own limited experience has been with facilitated groups. At the Chicago Lying-In Hospital a convenient conference room was available adjacent to the outpatient clinic. Patients gathered prior to being seen by the physicians. Coffee was provided and one of the chaplains and/or the oncology social worker was present to facilitate discussion and answer questions. Talk flowed easily even among patients with different diseases and backgrounds. A second venture was the development of a patient support group at Prentice Women's Hospital of Northwestern Memorial Hospital during 1982–83. This was held once a week in a conference off the gynecology floor. All inpatients were invited to attend. An experienced nurse and a woman chaplain facilitated the initial meetings. Attendance varied according to the number of patients on the inpatient unit at the time. Fruitful discussion was held on such subjects as how to tell one's family about the cancer.

Several questions remain in regard to the development and function of therapeutic and facilitated groups. Where and how often should they be held? Who serves as the best director or facilitator? Should family members be invited? Much further study is required on these matters.

Self-help groups in special areas may be very supportive, for example, for women who have stomas. By their very nature self-help groups do not advertise themselves. They are often pioneered by one or more individuals who have or have had a specific disease (Brown and Griffiths, 1986). Information on such groups and their development is hard to obtain; in Chicago useful data have been collected by the Self Help Center (1986).

Records. The importance of records in coordinating care cannot be overestimated. A unit record system is essential for a tertiary care institution as are the means to make the individual record promptly available. When outpatient care is given outside the center, there must be a reliable method of transmitting data and summaries of records in both directions. It is important that nurses and other professionals include in the patient's record data on their observations, discussions with patients and treatments given. Comments on the treatment plan should involve only the expertise of the individual concerned or be the result of an agreed plan of therapy developed at a meeting. Agreement should be reached on a given gynecologic oncology service as to how notes should be written, on the importance of brevity and on the necessity of avoiding comments critical of any aspects of care.

Pain

Pain in gynecologic cancer may be due to physical causes inherent in these tumors and their growth (Table 7–5) It may also depend upon the site or origin of the disease. The subject is reviewed in general by Foley (1985).

PAIN FROM SPECIFIC CANCERS

Vulvar cancer causes no or minimal pain in the early stages. Treatment by surgery (radical vulvectomy and inguinal lymphadenectomy) may result in persistent postoperative pain in the incision and pain in the legs due to edema. If external radiation therapy is used, local skin reaction over the vulva and perineum can cause continued discomfort. Advanced vulvar cancer can cause pain in the groin, due to enlarged lymph nodes. Progressive local disease and ulceration can cause severe (and terminal) pain.

Vaginal cancer, in the early stages, usually causes no pain except for possible dyspareunia. Treatment by radiation with resulting fibrosis may cause persistent pelvic pressure and rectal pain.

Cervical cancer is painless in the early stages. As spread into the parametrium and uterosacral ligaments occurs pain may be noted in the back

Table 7–5. Physical Causes of Pain in Patients with Gynecologic Cancer

Initial extent of lesion
Effects of treatment
Local progression
Distant spread

or, depending on the nerves involved, extending into the back or front of the legs. Surgical treatment (radical hysterectomy) results in postoperative pain that is usually self-limited. Following radical hysterectomy, the discomfort of a full bladder is often felt as pain in the back, because of bladder denervation. Radiation therapy per se does not usually result in pain, although pelvic fibrosis, ureteral obstruction or radiation enteritis may cause specific pain related to these organs. If pain in the back or legs develops during treatment it is very likely to be caused by recurrent disease.

Cancer of the corpus uteri also causes no pain in the early stages. Surgical treatment and radiation therapy cause no more than the usual acute postoperative pain. Local recurrence in the vagina does not usually cause pain, and distant metastases or recurrence are also unlikely to cause pain unless, for example, extensive spread has occurred to the lungs or to the bone.

Cancer of the ovary (and the tube) may cause some pain initially, especially if the tumor is very large or has undergone an accident such as torsion or hemorrhage. Postoperative pain is self-limited. However, recurrence usually involves the peritoneal cavity and intestines, and the pain of intestinal obstruction or distension due to recurrence may be difficult to distinguish from that due to postoperative adhesions. Distant metastases or recurrence, for example, to the lung or pleura, may occasionally cause pain in the organ involved.

Psychologic causes may be an important component of gynecologic cancer pain. They can be related to background and environmental events and must be taken into account in every patient (see later section).

EVALUATION

Nature of Pain. Acute pain is typical of the postoperative state, occurring in patients with and without cancer. Chronic pain is more characteristic of cancer and its sequelae. Table 7–6 shows the difference between the types of pain and indicates that chronic pain, by virtue of its several symptoms and signs, calls attention to the needs of the whole patient. The occurrence of one or more episodes of acute pain in a woman known to have chronic pain should raise the suspicion either that there has been a sudden change in the cancer itself or that some unrelated event has occurred.

Site of Pain. The exact site of the pain and its referral should be determined as well as

Table 7–6. Comparison of Acute and Chronic Pain*

Acute Pain	Chronic Pain
Increased cardiac rate	Sleep disturbance
Increased stroke volume	Irritability
Increased blood pressure	Appetite disturbance
Papillary dilatation	Constipation
Palmar sweating	Psychomotor retardation
Hyperventilation	Lowered pain tolerance
Escape behavior	Social withdrawal
Anxiety state	Abnormal illness behavior
	(Masked) depression

*From Steinbach DA: Chronic pain as a disease entity. *Triangle, Sandoz Journal of Medical Science* Vol. 20, No. 1/2:27, 1981, Copyright Sandoz Ltd. Reprinted with permission.

possible, since these will give a clue to the underlying structures involved.

Intensity of Pain. It is difficult to determine the degree of pain except by the patient's own estimate of its severity and type. Assessment of the number of analgesic pills taken at home or in the hospital may be helpful. Detailed psychologic tests are not usually available to the average gynecologist or gynecologic oncologist and indeed their use is not very practical for the distressed patient in pain. However, the use of a visual analogue is simple and may be helpful. In one type, the patient is asked to indicate the amount of pain on a 100-mm line that extends from "least possible" to "worst possible" pain. Additional information to be obtained about pain relates to its variation during the 24 hours, its interference with activities and changes in mood related to it (Cleeland, 1984).

MANAGEMENT

Initial management of chronic pain is by the intermittent oral use of mild analgesics such as aspirin, acetaminophen, nonsteroidal anti-inflammatory agents or small amounts of codeine or oxycodone (see Chapter 13 for drugs available, their effects, complications and equivalency). However, when the patient is regularly taking 30 mg or more of codeine or its equivalent every three to four hours, then the pain itself becomes a complication that requires investigation and treatment. The search for possible causes of the pain must be thorough. Factors to be considered include (1) dependency of pain on movement, (2) presence of inflammation, ischemia or muscle spasm or (3) evidence of spinal cord or specific nerve involvement. If no obvious cause is found, the patient may either be dependent on the analgesic drug(s) or undiagnosed persistent disease may be present. In the former case, weaning may be difficult (see Chapter 13). In the latter, a program of management should be started on the following lines (Twycross, 1978):

1. When possible, oral medication should be used.

2. The dose of medication must be adjusted promptly during the first 24 to 72 hours of therapy. This usually necessitates hospital admission and careful observation.

3. Medication should be given regularly around the clock as frequently as is necessary. The interval depends upon the drug used. Missing a 2:00 AM dose may result in pain getting out of control. Many patients can receive a higher dose at bedtime so that the one in the middle of the night can be omitted.

4. The comfort of the patient with advanced disease is paramount; addiction may occur but should be regarded as much less important. Patients usually reach a dose that is acceptable to them and, indeed, this dose may wax and wane during the course of the illness.

5. The patient and her relatives must be taught in the hospital to take responsibility for managing pain. At home strict around-the-clock administration of pain medication may need to be modified, because of individual variations in pain occurrence and tolerance.

6. Morphine is a good drug for the initial management of pain. The oral dose is about three times the parenteral dose. Most patients stabilize at a dose of 10 to 30 mg every two to four hours, but doses as high as 100 mg may be needed. The initial dose depends on the amount of medication already being taken by the patient. Changing to another drug, particularly a longer-acting one such as methadone, may be helpful.

7. Other medications may be necessary to control other symptoms or the side effects of the analgesics. Common results of the regular use of morphine are initial drowsiness and confusion, especially in older women, which lasts from three to five days. Usually it does not need specific treatment. Nausea and vomiting (which may also be related to the disease itself) may require an antiemetic. Other drugs such as cortisone, anti-inflammatory drugs and muscle relaxants may be needed to control specific symptoms.

Two major symptoms accompanying pain and its treatment are constipation and depression. Constipation must be handled as soon as any appreciable amount of narcotic analgesics is given. Management is not easy. A diet containing roughage, adequate fluid, a stool softener and occasional laxatives or suppositories are necessary. Depression requires judicious use of antidepressant drugs (Gorgynski and Massie, 1981).

Various procedures on the nervous system have been suggested to handle pain in specific areas and reduce the complications of heavy doses of narcotics. These include single nerve blocks or a sympathetic (celiac axis) block. If a trial block with local anesthesia is successful, injection with alcohol or phenol may provide several months of relief. Wider pain relief may be achieved by the use of the same substances in the subarachnoid space. In special circumstances unilateral pain can be controlled by percutaneous radiofrequency cordotomy in the cervical region. Finally, there has been recent interest in the use of continuous epidural narcotics which may be administered by the patient herself at home (Malone et al, 1985). The participation of an anesthesiologist experienced in pain management is essential to the successful use of any of these techniques.

Physical therapy is an important part of pain management. Passive and active exercises can ameliorate stiffness and arthritis, which may themselves be responsible for pain. Transcutaneous nerve stimulation (TNS) consists of bursts of electrical stimulation to designated body areas applied through electrodes attached to a battery-operated unit. This can be controlled by the patient herself, thus permitting her participation in pain management. Unfortunately, the effects of this may be transient, and the patient may develop tolerance (Wall, 1985).

Mental techniques such as guided imagery, self-relaxation (biofeedback) and hypnosis may all be used to help relieve pain. Hypnosis is applicable to about two thirds of patients with cancer. Whether the trance state is induced by a hypnotist or is self-produced, the hypnotized individual, by focusing on one concept involving a change in perception, may relegate to the periphery of consciousness unwanted perceptions such as excessive pain (Spiegel, 1985).

Death

Death is the ultimate complication of operations and procedures performed for cancer. It may occur rarely during or immediately after an operation and occasionally in the postoperative phase, arbitrarily defined by many as within 30 days after the operation. Most frequently death is the end stage of the disease, often caused by a combination of the complications of treatment and the disease itself.

The unexpectedness of death at or soon after operation presents the greatest problem. Even if the risk of death has been explained to the patient and her family before the operation, little can soften the immediate shock. Recapitulation of the severity of the disease, the necessity of operation and a factual statement of what happened are the best approaches. Although the gynecologist naturally feels badly at what he may regard as his "failure," he should not let this feeling cause him to imply error when none occurred. Repetition of the facts and time are required for family members to assimilate the event. If the oncology nurse or another member of the interdisciplinary group has been close to the patient, he or she may contribute by being present and re-enforcing what the gynecologist has said.

Terminal Care

Death that occurs as a late complication after operations or treatment for cancer is usually preceded by a phase of increasing disease and declining vital powers, often called the terminal phase. This may be as short as a few days or as long as a year or more. Because it presents many medical, psychosocial and environmental problems, it deserves consideration as a specific complication of the treatment of cancer. Terminal care involves diagnosis, management, the use of measures to prolong life and the care of the patient's family during this period and after the death. The attitude of caregivers toward death and dying is an important aspect of the subject.

DIAGNOSIS

Before deciding that a patient with cancer is in a terminal state, it must be established that all possible treatment has been given for primary, persistent or recurrent disease, that the cancer is progressive and that no further curative therapy is possible. It is relatively easy to determine that cancer is still present from biopsy or other diagnostic studies and to decide that all known effective treatment has been given. However, the terminal patient and her family are exposed to many new drugs or procedures that are hailed as cures by the media. The physician who has a close relationship with his patient is often queried about such "cures."

Sometimes he may know that a particular method is in the very early stages of investigation and/or is not applicable to the type of cancer that the patient has. Sometimes he may have no knowledge of the treatment described. In any case, frank and open discussion of the situation is essential. First he should repeat the evidence for the patient's disease, treatment and prognosis. Second, he should attempt to evaluate fairly the "new" treatment on the basis of his own knowledge. Third, he should not deny the patient and her family an opportunity to seek other advice or treatment. Last, he should repeatedly show them his continuing concern and desire to provide help, even if cure does not seem possible.

MANAGEMENT

Home, Hospital, Hospice. Until 100 years ago death occurred at home. Once a diagnosis of terminal cancer had been made or more likely assumed by the patient and her family, little medical help was available except sympathetic understanding and drugs to relieve pain. The patient often but by no means always had the help and support of her family. Children and adults became aware of death as being a normal though difficult human experience. With the development of new methods of supporting life by nutrition, pain relief and other techniques, it became apparent that more could often be done to relieve suffering and improve physical comfort in hospitals devoted to the care of the sick. But in recent years a change has occurred in the United States. It is clear that acute care hospitals, try as they may, often cannot provide continuous sympathetic care because of the changing personnel, the presence of other patients with acute problems and the inability of modern medical skills to overcome the inevitable progress of the disease.

The modern hospice concept was pioneered at St. Christopher's Hospital, London by Dr. Cicely Saunders. A hospice is a community hospital that cares for patients with terminal cancer and their families as in- and outpatients. Support from the hospice is provided for home care by the family but admission is available as necessary and free access is provided for the patients' families. In the United States hospices have taken two forms, one based on the St. Christopher's model and one in which the home care support is provided but hospitalization takes place when necessary at a cooperating local acute care hospital in which special beds and nursing personnel may be devoted to such terminal patients (Davidson, 1978). Currently available data indicate that full hospice care results in less anxiety and more satisfaction among patients and families than conventional home/acute hospital care. Questions of expense and efficiency of pain relief have not yet been settled (Parkes, 1985). Ideally, patients with terminal cancer should have a choice of services. At the present time hospice facilities are insufficient to fill the needs, but if the kind of home support that they provide is available, it should be utilized.

Diet, Medication and Physical Care. The day to day care of the terminal patient consists primarily of providing relief of symptoms and avoiding treatments of any sort that cause discomfort without adding significant benefit. Diet should consist of what the patient wants and can eat. Medication should relieve pain and improve symptoms such as nausea, depression or constipation. Physical care should be concentrated on position and support in bed or a chair and easy availability of necessities. But most important are the concern of caregivers, a matter of fact approach to the problem and the willingness to listen and answer questions simply and honestly. The unkindest thing to do is to ignore the patient and to regard her as a non-person. Since the question of diagnosis and curative treatment is irrelevant, discussion with her must concentrate on immediate needs, on family and on events outside herself. How far medical therapy should go in prolonging life, i.e., ordinary versus extraordinary measures, is discussed in Chapter 16.

BEREAVEMENT

Recognition of the impending death of a family member puts a great strain on the survivors. Support of them becomes an increasingly important part of terminal care. Principles of management include:

1. Providing continuity of care by one or two members of the interdisciplinary team. In the hospital this may be a physician or a specially concerned nurse. At home it may be a visiting nurse or volunteer hospice worker.
2. Appreciating family members' varying reactions. Particularly difficult to handle are denial and anger; the latter spreads in many directions. When the death is expected and understood, grieving by family members prior to it is common, even to the extent of their shunning the patient as if she were already dead; prolonged dying

makes this behavior more likely. Dealing with these feelings requires time, explanation and empathetic understanding.
3. Evaluating families or family members who are particularly vulnerable and need special support. Parkes (1978) found that the following were at high risk:
   a. Persons of low socioeconomic status.
   b. Housewives without employment outside the home.
   c. Those with young children at home (and the children themselves).
   d. Those without a supportive family or with a family that actively discourages the expression of grief.
   e. Those who show a strong tendency to cling to a patient before death and/or pine for her afterwards.
   f. Those who express strong feelings of anger or bitterness before or after the patient's death.
   g. Those who express strong feelings of self-reproach.
   This evaluation may also help to determine which members of the medical team are most likely to be able to give support.
4. Handling the immediate event of death. In the hospital it is best if information is given by someone who is very familiar with the situation, usually the physician. This person should be well acquainted with the medical and legal formalities that are required. This is particularly important if permission for autopsy is to be sought.
5. Early counseling of the bereaved. The close family are usually in a state of shock for several days. A visit after this time by a member of the interdisciplinary team may provide the bereaved with an opportunity to express grief. The family's needs for medical or other aid may also be ascertained.
6. Later counseling of the bereaved. This may be a follow-up of the first visit at a preagreed time. It may again consist of allowing the expression of grief and the counselor may be able to encourage the family to step forward in their new lives.

CARE OF THE CAREGIVERS

It is difficult for any physician or other caregiver to face the critical illness and death of a patient with whom he or she has been closely involved. His or her feelings are well described by Astrachan (1973). He is reminded of his own mortality, he is concerned about the ordeal of handling the death with the family, he feels a sense of failure in his own medical management of the case and he may personally mourn the loss of someone who has become a friend. The gynecologist may have a more difficult situation. Gallup and co-workers (1982) surveyed 3229 practicing obstetrician-gynecologists in the southeastern United States and found that only 11% of those who responded indicated that any emphasis had been placed on the care of dying patients during their residencies. However, the majority did, in fact, care for some dying patients in their practice. Additional problems that complicate the feelings of those who practice both obstetrics and gynecology and see dying patients is that much of their work is with happy events such as birth and relatively simple and successful office treatments and operative procedures. Thus a death is indeed difficult and depressing. On the other hand, gynecologic oncologists do not necessarily have this dilemma, but face the disappointment of having struggled unsuccessfully against the cancer.

The feelings of other members of the interdisciplinary team are similar. Personal involvement with the care of terminal patients on the part of the nurse, social worker or volunteer makes their grief at the patient's death more poignant, while the personal sense of failure may not be so great.

Discussions on death and dying during residencies may help to prepare obstetrician-gynecologists for these events. In the actual treatment of patients an interdisciplinary conference is the best forum to discuss the general problem as well as the individual concerns of members of the team. It is in this area that a closely knit group, in which the members are not afraid to air their feelings, can generate a great deal of mutual support. Often a liaison psychiatrist or a chaplain can serve as a catalyst to bring these feelings into open discussion.

REFERENCES

Andersen BL, Hacker NF: Psychosexual adjustment following pelvic exenteration. *Obstet. Gynecol.* 61:331, 1983.

Astrachan JM: The critically ill patient and the gynecologist. *Am. J. Obstet. Gynecol.* 116:119, 1973.

Averette HE, Lichtinger M et al: Pelvic exenteration: a 15-year experience in a general metropolitan hospital. *Am. J. Obstet. Gynecol.* 150:179, 1984.

Benedet JL, Turko M et al: Radical hysterectomy in the treatment of cervical cancer. *Am. J. Obstet. Gynecol.* 137:254, 1980.

Benedet JL, Turko M et al: Squamous cell carcinoma of the vulva: results of treatment, 1938–1976. *Am. J. Obstet. Gynecol.* 134:201, 1979.

Bergan JJ, Dean RH, Yao JST: Vascular injuries in pelvic cancer surgery. *Am. J. Obstet. Gynecol.* 124:562, 1976.

Berman ML, Lagasse LD et al: The operative evaluation of patients with cervical carcinoma by an extraperitoneal approach. *Obstet. Gynecol.* 50:658, 1977.

Blaikley JB, Ledarman M, Pollard W: Carcinoma of the cervix at Chelsea Hospital for Women, 1935–1965. Five year and ten year results of treatment. *J. Obstet. Gynaecol. Br. Comm.* 76:729, 1969.

Bonney V: The treatment of carcinoma of the cervix by Wertheim's operation. *Am. J. Obstet. Gynecol.* 30:815, 1935.

Boutselis JG: Radical vulvectomy for invasive squamous cell carcinoma of the vulva. *Obstet. Gynecol.* 39:827, 1972.

Brown T, Griffiths P: Cancer self help groups: an inside view. *Br. Med. J.* 292:1503, 1986.

Brunschwig A: Surgical treatment of carcinoma of the cervix, recurrent after irradiation or combination of irradiation and surgery. *Am. J. Roentgenol. Rad. Ther. Nucl. Med.* 99:365, 1967.

Brunschwig A: Complete excision of pelvic viscera for advanced carcinoma; a one-stage abdominoperineal operation with end colostomy and bilateral ureteral implantation into the colon above the colostomy. *Cancer* 1:177, 1948.

Brunschwig A, Barber HRK: Surgical treatment of carcinoma of the cervix. *Obstet. Gynecol.* 27:21, 1966.

Cain EN, Kohorn EL et al: Psychosocial benefits of a cancer support group. *Cancer* 57:183, 1986.

Calame RJ: Pelvic relaxation as a complication of the radical vulvectomy. *Obstet. Gynecol.* 55:716, 1980.

Castaldo TW, Petrilli ES et al: Intestinal operations in patients with ovarian carcinoma. *Am. J. Obstet. Gynecol.* 139:80, 1981.

Cavanagh D, Beazley J, Ostapowicz F: Radical operation for carcinoma of the vulva. A new approach to wound healing. *J. Obstet. Gynaecol. Br. Comm.* 77:1037, 1970.

Chafe W, Fowler WC Jr et al: Radical vulvectomy with use of tensor fascia lata myocutaneous flap. *Am. J. Obstet. Gynecol.* 145:207, 1983.

Chamorro T: The role of a nurse-clinician in joint practice with gynecologic oncologists. *Cancer* 48:622, 1981.

Chen SS, Bochner R: Assessment of morbidity and mortality in primary cytoreductive surgery for advanced ovarian carcinoma. *Gynecol. Oncol.* 20:190, 1985.

Christensen A, Lange P, Neilsen E: Surgery and radiotherapy for invasive cancer of the cervix: surgical treatment. *Acta Obstet. Gynecol.* 43:59, 1964.

Cleeland CS: The impact of pain on the patient with cancer. *Cancer* 54:2635, 1984.

Curry SL, Nahhas WA et al: Pelvic exenteration: a 7-year experience. *Gynecol. Oncol.* 11:119, 1981.

Daly JW, Pomerance AJ: Groin dissection with prevention of tissue loss and postoperative infection. *Obstet. Gynecol.* 53:395, 1979.

Davidson GW: *The Hospice: Development and Administration.* Washington, Hemisphere Publishing Corp., 1978.

Endicott J: Measurement of depression in patients with cancer. *Cancer* 53:2273, 1984.

Ferlic M, Goldman A, Kennedy BJ: Group counselling in adult patients with advanced cancer. *Cancer* 43:760, 1979.

Figge DC, Gaudenz R: Invasive carcinoma of the vulva. *Am. J. Obstet. Gynecol.* 119:382, 1974.

Foley KM: The treatment of cancer pain. *N. Engl. J. Med.* 313:84, 1985.

Forney JP: The effect of radical hysterectomy on bladder physiology. *Am. J. Obstet. Gynecol.* 138:374, 1980.

Freidenbergs I, Gordon W et al: Psychosocial aspects of living with cancer: a review of the literature. *Int. J. Psychiatry Med.* 11:303, 1982.

Gallup DG, Labudovich M, Zambito PR: The gynecologist and the dying cancer patient. *Am. J. Obstet. Gynecol.* 144:154, 1982.

Goldberg MI, Belinson JL et al: Surgical management of invasive carcinoma of the vulva utilizing a lower abdominal midline incision. *Gynecol. Oncol.* 7:296, 1979.

Gorzynski JG, Massie MJ: How to manage the depression of cancer. *Your Patient and Cancer* August:25, 1981.

Gottschalk LA: Measurement of mood and affect in cancer patients. *Cancer* 53:2236, 1984.

Green TH Jr: Ureteral suspension for prevention of ureteral complications following radical Wertheim hysterectomy. *Obstet. Gynecol.* 28:1, 1966.

Green TH Jr, Meigs JV et al: Urologic complications of radical Wertheim hysterectomy: incidence, etiology, management, and prevention. *Obstet. Gynecol.* 20:293, 1962.

Green TH Jr, Ulfelder H, Meigs JV: Epidermoid carcinoma of the vulva: an analysis of 238 cases. Part II. Therapy and end results. *Am. J. Obstet. Gynecol.* 75:848, 1958.

Griffiths CT, Parker LM, Fuller AF Jr: Role of cytoreductive surgical treatment in the management of advanced ovarian cancer. *Cancer Treat. Rep.* 63:235, 1979.

Hacker NF, Berek JS et al: Primary cytoreductive surgery for epithelial ovarian cancer. *Obstet. Gynecol.* 61:413, 1983.

Hacker NF, Leuchter RS et al: Radical vulvectomy and bilateral inguinal lymphadenectomy through separate groin incisions. *Obstet. Gynecol.* 58:574, 1981.

Hoskins WJ, Ford JH Jr et al: Radical hysterectomy and pelvic lymphadenectomy for the management of early invasive cancer of the cervix. *Gynecol. Oncol.* 4:278, 1976.

Hoskins WJ, Ford JH Jr et al: Gastrointestinal complications associated with pelvic exenteration. *Am. J. Obstet. Gynecol.* 145:325, 1983.

Hurney C, Holland J: Psychosocial sequelae of ostomies in cancer patients. *CA* 35:170, 1985.

Iversen T, Aalders JG et al: Squamous cell carcinoma of the vulva: a review of 424 patients, 1956–1974. *Gynecol. Oncol.* 9:271, 1980.

Jakowatz JG, Porudominsky D et al: Complications of pelvic exenteration. *Arch. Surg.* 120:1261, 1985.

Kadar N, Saliba N, Nelson JH: The frequency, causes and prevention of severe urinary dysfunction after radical hysterectomy. *Br. J. Obstet. Gynaecol.* 90:858, 1983.

Karlen JR, Piver MS: Reduction of mortality and morbidity associated with pelvic exenteration. *Gynecol. Oncol.* 3:154, 1975.

Ketcham AS, Hoye RC et al: Radical hysterectomy and lymphadenectomy for carcinoma of the uterine cervix. *Cancer* 28:1272, 1971.

Krebs HB, Goplerud DR: Surgical management of bowel obstruction in advanced ovarian carcinoma. *Obstet. Gynecol.* 61:327, 1983.

Kubler-Ross E: *On Death and Dying.* Toronto, McMillan, 1969.

Lagasse LD, Creasman WT et al: Results and complications of operative staging in cervical cancer: Experience of the Gynecologic Oncology Group. *Gynecol. Oncol.* 9:90, 1980.

Langley II, Moore DW et al: Radical hysterectomy and pelvic lymph node dissection. *Gynecol. Oncol.* 9:37, 1980.

Lerner HM, Jones HW III, Hill EC: Radical surgery for the treatment of early invasive cervical carcinoma (Stage IB): review of 15 years' experience. *Obstet. Gynecol.* 56:413, 1980.

Liu W, Meigs JV: Radical hysterectomy and pelvic lymphadenectomy: a review of 473 cases including 244 for primary invasive carcinoma of the cervix. *Am. J. Obstet. Gynecol.* 69:1, 1955.

Magrina JF, Masterson BJ: Vaginal reconstruction in gynecologic oncology: review of techniques. *Obstet. Gynecol. Surv.* 36:1, 1981.

Malone BT, Beye R, Walker J: Management of pain in the terminally ill by administration of epidural narcotics. *Cancer* 55:438, 1985.

Meigs JV: Carcinoma of the cervix—the Wertheim operation. *Surg. Gynecol. Obstet.* 78:195, 1944.

Morley GW: Infiltrative carcinoma of the vulva: results of surgical management. *Am. J. Obstet. Gynecol.* 124:874, 1976.

Morley GW, Lindenauer SM: Pelvic exenteration therapy for gynecologic malignancy. *Cancer* 38:581, 1976.

Morley GW, Seski JC: Radical pelvic surgery versus radiation therapy for Stage I carcinoma of the cervix (exclusive of microinvasion). *Am. J. Obstet. Gynecol.* 126:785, 1976.

Moth I, Andreasson B et al: Sexual function and somatopsychic reactions after vulvectomy. A preliminary report. *Danish Med. Bul.* 30 (Suppl. 2):27, 1983.

Newton M: Psychosomatic crises in gynecologic cancer. In Morris N (Ed.); *Psychosomatic Medicine in Obstetrics and Gynecology: Proceedings.* Karger, Basel, 1972.

O'Hoy KM, Tang GWK: Sexual function following treatment for carcinoma of the cervix. *J. Psychosom. Obstet. Gynaecol.* 4:41, 1985.

Orr JW Jr, Shingleton HM et al: Correlation of perioperative mobidity and conization to radical hysterectomy interval. *Obstet. Gynecol.* 59:726, 1982a.

Orr JW Jr, Shingleton HM et al: Urinary diversion in patients undergoing pelvic exenteration. *Am. J. Obstet. Gynecol.* 142:883, 1982b.

Park RC, Patow WE et al: Treatment of Stage I carcinoma of the cervix. *Obstet. Gynecol.* 41:117, 1973.

Parkes CM: Psychological aspects. In Saunders CM (Ed.): *The Management of Terminal Disease.* London, Arnold, 1978.

Parkes CM: Terminal care: home, hospital or hospice? *Lancet* 1:155, 1985.

Piver MS, Barlow JJ: Para-aortic lymphadenectomy in staging patients with advanced local cervical cancer. *Obstet. Gynecol.* 43:544, 1974.

Piver MS, Barlow JJ, Krishnamshetty R: Five-year survival (with no evidence of disease) in patients with biopsy-confirmed aortic node metastasis from cervical carcinoma. *Am. J. Obstet. Gynecol.* 139:575, 1981.

Piver MS, Barlow JJ et al: Survival after ovarian cancer induced intestinal obstruction. *Gynecol. Oncol.* 13:44, 1982.

Podratz KC, Symmonds RE et al: Carcinoma of the vulva: analysis of treatment and survival. *Obstet. Gynecol.* 61:63, 1983.

Rutledge FN, Smith JP, Franklin EW: Carcinoma of the vulva. *Am. J. Obstet. Gynecol.* 106:1117, 1970.

Rutledge FN, Smith JP et al: Pelvic exenteration: analysis of 296 patients. *Am. J. Obstet. Gynecol.* 129:881, 1977.

Sall S, Pineda AA et al: Surgical treatment of Stages IB and IIA invasive carcinoma of the cervix by radical abdominal hysterectomy. *Am. J. Obstet. Gynecol.* 135:442, 1979.

Schipper H, Clinch J et al: Measuring the quality of life of cancer patients: functional living. *J. Clin. Oncol.* 2:472, 1984.

Self Help Mutual Aids Groups—Chicago Metropolitan Area. Evanston, IL, The Self Help Center, 1986.

Sevin BU, Ramos R et al: Antibiotic prevention of infections complicating radical abdominal hysterectomy. *Obstet. Gynecol.* 64:539, 1984.

Spiegel D: The use of hypnosis in controlling cancer pain. *Cancer* 35:221, 1985.

Sternbach DA: Chronic pain as a disease entity. *Triangle* 20:27, 1981.

Symmonds RE, Pratt JH, Webb MJ: Exenterative operations: experience with 198 patients. *Am. J. Obstet. Gynecol.* 121:907, 1975.

Twycross RG: Relief of pain. In Saunders CM (Ed.) *The Management of Terminal Disease.* London, Arnold, 1978.

Vera MI: Quality of life following pelvic exenteration. *Gynecol. Oncol.* 12:355, 1981.

Vincent CE, Vincent B et al: Some marital-sexual concomitants of carcinoma of the cervix. *South. Med. J.* 68:552, 1975.

Wall R: Cancer pain management. *Infect. Surg.* 4:194, 1985.

Webb MJ, Symmonds RE: Radical hysterectomy: influence of recent conization on morbidity and complications. *Obstet. Gynecol.* 53:290, 1979a.

Webb MJ, Symmonds RE: Wertheim hysterectomy: a reappraisal. *Obstet. Gynecol.* 54:140, 1979b.

Wertheim E: The extended abdominal operation for carcinoma uteri: based on 500 operative cases. *Am. J. Obstet. Dis. Women Child.* 66:169, 1912.

Wharton JT, Herson J: Surgery for common epithelial tumors of the ovary. *Cancer* 48:582, 1981.

Wortman CB: Social support and the cancer patient. *Cancer* 53:2339, 1984.

COMPLICATIONS OF OBSTETRIC OPERATIONS

8

EDWARD R. NEWTON

The obstetrician plays a unique and difficult role in the care of the pregnant woman. Of all the branches of medicine, only obstetrics must consider two patients in one treatment plan. The specter of diethylstilbestrol continues to remind us of the magnitude of tragedy caused by disregard for the fetus. The formulation of a treatment plan is hampered by the incomplete knowledge of normal physiologic differences between pregnant and non-pregnant women. Unfortunately, even less is known about fetal physiology and the consequences of maternal disease in pregnancy. Despite the tremendous advances in perinatal medicine, we are still limited to indirect assessment of fetal status, using ultrasound, electronic fetal monitoring, hormonal tests, amniocentesis or fetoscopy. Arguments rage as to which is the best method of indirect measurement. The safest observation is that all have significant error and many have both defined and unrecognized risks of intervention that must be considered in any management plan.

In this "scientific" age of obstetrics, often forgotten but tremendously important aspects of obstetrics are the emotional or psychosocial implications. Pregnancy, labor, delivery and the early neonatal experience play integral roles in the establishment of the mother-infant bond. Irreparable disruption of this bonding has frightening social implications. Highly social primates such as humans depend on early training by interested parents for smooth integration into society. It is, therefore, important for the obstetrician to examine the emotional and psychosocial complications as well as the physical complications in his treatment plan.

If the obstetrician is to play this unique and difficult role successfully, he must be knowledgeable of the risks as well as benefits of the proposed treatment or test. This knowledge of the risks will allow the obstetrician to educate patients better who, in turn, can provide better informed consent, thus reducing the accelerating medicolegal risk of obstetrics. Should a complication occur, he must also institute the appropriate management in order to prevent further damage to the mother or infant.

The purpose of these chapters is to provide a reference for the clinician. The general format will be to start with a general introduction and to discuss the problems of diagnosis. A brief description of the procedure aimed at reducing specific complications will be given. The intraoperative and postoperative complications will be described with suggestions about prevention and treatment.

GENERAL STATISTICS

Mortality statistics are the crude rulers by which governments, lawyers and epidemiologists measure the quality of obstetric care in different populations.

Standard definitions are as follows:

1. Stillbirth rate: number of intrauterine fetal deaths per 1000 infants born. These infants must weigh at least 500 grams and/or measure 25 cm crown to heel in length.

2. Neonatal death rate: number of neonatal deaths per 1000 live births. A neonatal death is a death occurring within the first 28 days of life. An early neonatal death is a death occuring within seven days of birth.

3. Maternal death rate: number of maternal deaths (defined as death of a woman during or within 42 days of cessation of pregnancy) per 100,000 live births. A direct maternal death is a death arising from an obstetric complication of pregnancy, e.g., postpartum hemorrhage. An indirect death is one occurring as a result of a preexisting disease aggravated by pregnancy, e.g., mitral stenosis.

4. Perinatal mortality rate: the total number of stillbirths plus neonatal deaths per 1000 births.

By any criterion and regardless of cause, there has been a dramatic fall in maternal mortality in the United States in the last 30 years. Table 8–1 depicts the fall in maternal death rate over time. Although many factors are related to the decline, the five major ones are antibiotics, improved antepartal surveillance, safer cesarean section, improved and judicious use of anesthesia, and improved blood banking facilities. Current causes of maternal mortality are listed in Table 8–2. Sepsis, hemorrhage and toxemia contributed the largest proportion of maternal deaths prior to 1970. As

Table 8–1. Maternal Death Rate*

Year	Maternal Death Rate
1935	582.1
1945	207.2
1955	47.0
1965	31.6
1975	12.8
1978	9.9
1982	7.9
1983	8.3
1984	5.7

*From Facts of Life and Death. No. (PHS) 79-1222, 1979. *National Center for Health Statistics*, Monthly Vital Statistics Report, Vol 33(12) March 26, 1985.

there has been improvement in the prevention and treatment of these problems, the role of iatrogenic causes of maternal death has become larger. Even now a recent review of maternal deaths associated with abortion revealed that only 14% of deaths were totally unavoidable or non-preventable (Selik et al, 1981). Embolism is now the leading cause of maternal death. This is strongly related to surgical intervention.

With a backdrop of undeniable improvement in maternal mortality, recent articles have sharpened the focus on two issues: the accurate reporting of maternal deaths and the emerging concept of reproductive mortality.

The national maternal death rate is compiled by the United States government by using primarily maternal death certificates. The use of maternal death certificates alone is inadequate in the study of maternal death. This type of surveillance fails to identify 18 to 73% of maternal deaths (Cates et al, 1984), and some causes are underrepresented. When Rubin and co-workers (1981) in Georgia linked maternal death certificates with live birth certificates, maternal mortality for the years 1975 to 1976 was increased by 27%. A majority of the unreported deaths were related to complications of

Table 8–2. Causes of U.S. Maternal Mortality*

	Per Cent
Embolism	19.8
Hypertensive disease	17.0
Hemorrhage	13.4
Infection	8.0
Cerebrovascular accident	4.3
Anesthesia/analgesia complication	4.0
Abortion	16.5
Other	17.0

*Data from Kaunitz AM, Hughes JM et al: Causes of maternal mortality in the United States. *Obstet. Gynecol.* 65:605, 1985.

operative delivery, i.e., anesthetic death and pulmonary embolism. Data from state maternal death committees confirm the margin of error in reporting maternal deaths. Furthermore, a National Center for Disease Control (CDC) review of local hospital and state records was able to double the number of maternal deaths secondary to abortion (Cates et al, 1978; Cates and Grimes, 1981). These specific epidemiologic studies and techniques have increased the maternal death rate associated with live births and abortions. Future reviews of maternal deaths associated with stillbirth, spontaneous abortion and ectopic pregnancy will further increase the maternal mortality rate. Specific review of causes of death may also change the traditional order of importance.

Accurate measures of maternal mortality are vitally important to the risk versus benefit assessment of various methods of fertility control. A growing concept in epidemiology is reproductive mortality. This statistic is a composite of deaths from contraceptive methods, abortion, ectopic pregnancy and other complications of pregnancy. The importance of this figure is highlighted by data showing that in England since 1975 more women have died from complications of pregnancy prevention than from late ($\geq$20 weeks) maternal mortality (Beral, 1979). Sachs and co-workers (1982) reported similar data for the United States in 1975. Table 8–3 depicts the distribution of reproductive mortality. In 1975, total deaths from abortion and contraception exceeded other maternal deaths. This trend will continue, with an increasing proportion of deaths related to fertility control.

The perinatal mortality rate has also shown a significant decline in recent years. Table 8–4 depicts the trend in the United States since 1955. Williams and Chen (1982) closely examined the sources of the decline in perinatal mortality rate in California in the 1970s. They concluded that 81% of the fall was secondary to

Table 8–3. Reproductive Mortality— U.S.A. 1975*

Pregnancy related	Number
Ectopic	50
Abortion	49
Other maternal deaths	428
Contraception related	
Oral contraception	452
Intrauterine device	6
Sterilization	14
Total	999

*From Sachs BP, Lande PM et al: Reproductive mortality in the United States. *J. Am. Med. Assoc.* 247:2789, 1982. Copyright 1982, American Medical Association. Reprinted with permission.

improved birth weight specific mortality rates and 19% was secondary to improvement in birth weight distribution. Birth weight specific changes reflect improvement of neonatal and obstetric practice. Neonatal intensive care, increased use of cesarean delivery and fetal monitoring (Williams and Hawes, 1979; Williams and Chen, 1982, Lee et al, 1980) have been cited as sources of this improvement. Changes in birth weight distribution are a reflection of changes in socioeconomic status and distribution of preventive care, especially in the prevention of premature birth. Differences in birth weight distribution are a major reason for the lower rank that the United States has in world statistics on perinatal mortality. Erikson and Bjerkedal (1982) compared the perinatal statistics in Norway (rank 5th) to those in the United States (rank 16th). They concluded that the United States' statistics are better in birth weight specific rates than those of Norway. However, in the United States more infants are delivered under 2,500 grams (6.55% vs. 5.08%) and this adversely affects the rank order of the United States. Immaturity, respiratory distress, asphyxia, infection and congenital abnormalities account for 90% of perinatal mortality. Table 8–

Table 8–4. Perinatal Mortality in U.S.*

Year	Perinatal Mortality	Neonatal Death Rate	Stillbirth Rate
1955	36.2	19.1	17.1
1965	33.9	16.2	17.7
1975	22.3	10.7	11.6
1977	19.6	9.8	9.8
1982	18.6	7.7	8.9
1983	–	7.3	–
1984	–	6.9	–

*From Facts of Life and Death. No. (PHS) 79-1222. *National Center for Health Statistics*, Monthly Vital Statistics Report, 33(12) March 26, 1985.

Table 8–5. *Causes of Perinatal/Neonatal Death*

	Iowa* 1978–1979 (%)	St. Margaret's Hospital† Boston, Mass. 1978–1982 (%)
Immaturity‡	23.8	24.7
Asphyxia	14.8	25.6
Infection	12.4	7.3
Respiratory distress	17.9	12.6
Congenital abnormality	21.1	17.7
Other	10.0	12.1
Number	459	453

*Data from Hein HA, Brown CJ: Neonatal mortality review; a basis for improving care. *Pediatrics* 68:504, 1981.
†Data from Newton ER et al: Obstetric diagnosis and perinatal mortality. *Am. J. Perinatol.* In Press.
‡Iowa less than 750 grams. St. Margaret's Hospital 24 weeks or less or clinically defined between 24 and 26 weeks.

5 depicts causes of perinatal/neonatal mortality in two populations. In addition to defining the causes of neonatal death in a large population (Iowa), Hein and Brown (1981) reviewed the level of neonatal care in relationship to the cause of death. They concluded that an unwarranted number of potentially salvageable infants died at Level I and II hospitals. For example 70% of infants who died of respiratory distress died in Level I and II hospitals. Hein and Brown (1981) make a strong argument for the transfer of high risk mothers to Level III care. The widespread practice of maternal transport will improve the birth weight specific death rate. The birth weight distribution will be improved to a lesser extent. Again, a word of caution is warranted with perinatal statistics. There is good evidence that perinatal death is underreported. McCarthy and co-workers (1980) reported a comparison of state vital statistics to hospital records in Georgia from 1974 to 1977. They concluded that 21% of neonatal deaths are not reported and suggested that this is a conservative estimate. Forty percent of these unreported cases were fetuses that weighed more than 1500 grams. Similar estimates of underregistration are affected by geographic area, marriage status, race and failure of hospitals and morticians to file death certificates.

In conclusion, several general observations can be made. One, maternal mortality has fallen dramatically, but the reproductive mortality statistics will better assess the risk of reproduction in a risk versus benefit analysis. Two, perinatal mortality has also shown a dramatic fall. In the United States most of the decline has been secondary to improved obstetric and neonatal care within birth weight specific categories. Until there is improvement of preventive care, the United States will continue to rank below many other countries because of its higher incidence of low birth weight infants.

THERAPEUTIC ABORTION

In the last 30 years the obstetrician-gynecologist has been assigned another responsibility, reproduction control. More specifically, the specialist is responsible for the complications of contraception and pregnancy termination. The specialist's role in contraception is discussed in Chapter 13. The role in pregnancy termination is a major change in the philosophy of medical care. Historically, technical skill has been used to relieve the suffering of disease. Pregnancy, wanted or unwanted, is not a disease and in the case of elective termination, the technical skill is used for social purposes. The impact of this role is amplified by the fact that late second trimester abortion has a higher death-to-case ratio than continuing the pregnancy.

Procedures

An excellent description of the techniques and intraoperative concerns is provided by Hern (1983).

First Trimester Abortion

Suction Curettage. Suction curettage is the method of choice, and, as with any surgical procedure, however minor, careful and knowlegeable performance is the key to safety. Ideally, the patient should have had a recent cervical culture for *N. gonorrhoeae*, and the cervix should have had gentle, prolonged dilatation with either preoperative laminaria or 1 to 3 mg intravaginal prostaglandin E_2. The complications of laminaria are relatively minor but may include bleeding, pelvic infection and cervical trauma. Prostaglandins generally produce less morbidity but can result in severe cramping, nausea and fever.

Under sterile conditions with paracervical block anesthesia the following technique is used:

1. Careful sizing of the uterus. If there is any concern as to the actual size, ultrasound may be used as an adjunct.

2. Adequate visualization of the cervix and stabilization with a wide-mouthed Jacob's tenaculum. Single tooth tenacula should be avoided as they lacerate the pregnant cervix. Adequate cervical priming will also reduce cervical laceration.

3. The cervical canal is then dilated gently with tapered Pratt dilators. The maximum size dilator should be roughly equal to the size of cannula to be used.

4. After adequate dilatation, a cannula is introduced without suction to the top of the fundus. The size of cannula should be roughly equal to the length of gestation. One should avoid using a cannula greater than 10 to 12 mm if possible for fear of damaging the internal cervical os. The cannula may be straight or angulated. However, an angulated cannula describes a much wider arc in the 360 degree rotation during the procedure. In early gestation (i.e., smaller cavities), this is a disadvantage.

5. Suction is applied to the curette. The pump must generate pressure of at least 60 to 70 mm Hg and have an airflow greater than 90 ml per minute. With suction the curette is rotated 360 degrees and slowly withdrawn in increments of 1 to 2 cm. The curette is reintroduced in this fashion two or three times.

6. The uterine cavity is lightly curetted with a Sims curette (No. 2 to No. 6).

7. The products are then examined for fetal tissue. Repeat suction curettage is then performed.

8. Oxytocin (30 units in 1000 ml D5/1/2 NS at 0.3 units/minute intravenously) is now given to cause the uterus to contract. Methergine, 0.2 mg every six hours, may be given orally for 24 to 48 hours after the procedure for reduction of blood loss.

9. Prior to ending the procedure, ovum or sponge forceps are introduced closed into the endometrial cavity, opened and, with a twisting motion, removed. This is repeated several times

to ensure that loose products of conception (POC) are removed.

10. The patient is observed postoperatively for two to four hours for complications.

11. The products of conception must be first examined by the surgeon and then sent to the pathologist for histologic studies.

Sharp Curettage. With the ready availability of adequate suction equipment, sharp curettage should rarely be performed. The preparation of the patient is similar, and again slow careful dilatation with tapered dilators is indicated. Often sharp curettage involves greater dilatation than suction curettage. At this point, closed ovum forceps are gently introduced, opened and then withdrawn with a twisting motion. This removes the bulk of the POC. This procedure may be repeated two or three times. Using a dull curette the placental site is located and the remaining tissue is gently removed. After the curettage, the ovum forceps are again introduced to remove any loose POC.

The technical disadvantages of sharp versus suction curettage are:

1. Increased length of the procedure with subsequently more blood loss.

2. Increased risk of retained products.

3. Possible wider cervical dilatation.

4. Increased risk of uterine perforation.

5. Possible damage to the basal layer of of the endometrium with possible future placental abnormalities.

SECOND TRIMESTER ABORTION

Dilatation and Evacuation. The factors enabling safe dilatation and evacuation (D & E) are:

1. Accurate sizing of the uterus with adjunctive use of ultrasound.

2. Adequate preparation including a cervical culture for *N. gonorrhoeae* and a test for *Chlamydia*, Papanicolaou's smears and cervical priming with laminaria or prostaglandin.

3. Adequate instruments.
   a. Adequate suction (over 70 mm Hg and over 100 cc/min airflow).
   b. Specialized instruments.
   c. Atraumatic Bierer forceps for grasping the anterior cervical lip.
   d. Adequately sized tapered dilators (Pratt).
   e. A 16-mm suction cannula.
   f. Ovum forceps with broad, serrated jaws for traction (Sopher or Bierer vulsellum forceps).

g. A 14-mm (Evans') or a 16-mm (Sims') curette to remove large tissue fragments with low risk of trauma to the endometrium.

4. Gradual acquisition of operative skill starting with early second trimester (13-14 weeks) abortions.

5. Recognition of coexistent medical or surgical problems.

6. Local anesthesia with a paracervical block augmented with analgesics and sedatives is the safest choice for pain control. Local anesthesia allows the patient to report unusual symptoms and reduces serious complications.

After removing the laminaria, the cervix must be examined for adequate dilatation. The cervix should be dilated to a diameter in millimeters equal to the number of menstrual weeks plus two. If preoperative dilatation is not sufficient, tapered dilators should be used to dilate the cervix adequately. The membranes are ruptured with serrated forceps. Starting with amniotomy is thought to reduce the risk of amniotic fluid embolism. Rupture of membranes and uterine contractions will bring the fetal parts to the lower uterine segment. If the gestation is 15 menstrual weeks or less, a suction curette (No. 12 or greater) may be used. Longer gestations (equal to or more than 16 weeks) require that fetal and placental tissue be removed first. Intravenous oxytocin (20 to 30 units) is started at the introduction of the cannula to maintain a contracted uterus and reduce blood loss. Occasionally the fetal head is difficult to extract. The clinician can place his hand on the patient's abdomen to guide the tissue into the lower uterine segment (Hanson's maneuver). If this technique fails, more aggressive attempts should not be used for fear of perforation. A prostaglandin suppository (20 mg of prostaglandin E_2) may be a valuable adjunct, to complete the abortion after failed dilatation and evacuation. After the removal of the products of conception the cavity lining should be curetted using a large curette to identify and remove retained placental tissue. The patient must be observed for two to four hours postoperatively for hemorrhage.

Instillation Procedures. Intrauterine instillation of saline, urea, or prostaglandin F_2 alpha or a combination of these agents is used for abortion if gestation is greater than 18 weeks. All these agents induce labor. The expulsion time varies between 6 and 36 hours; prostaglandins work the fastest. Preoperative cervical priming with laminaria or a vaginal prostaglandin will reduce induction time. The key points are maintaining sterility and avoiding intravascular injection of agents.

After cervical priming and a preoperative ultrasound, the amniotic cavity is entered with a large gauge spinal or Touhy needle (18 gauge or larger; see Chapter 9). Free flow of clear amniotic fluid is essential prior to instillation of agents. Removal of amniotic fluid before instillation is important only in late second trimester abortion. This can be accomplished using a sterile three-way stopcock. After the instillation the patient is observed closely in the recovery room for one to two hours. Once contractions are of good quality or membranes are ruptured, the patient is returned to the labor room.

Frequently (20 to 50%) retained tissue is a problem with amnio-infusion. After passage of the fetus the oxytocin rate may be increased. There is little chance of lower uterine segment rupture because of the dilated cervix. If the placenta has not passed within two hours, manual removal is necessary. Under sterile conditions with adequate pain relief, the patient is placed in the dorsal lithotomy position, prepared and draped. A closed sponge forceps is gently introduced into the uterus, and the placenta is removed in pieces. A dull curette may be used for more adherent pieces. After manual removal, the patient must be observed for six hours in the recovery room. Prophylactic broad spectrum antibiotics are indicated because of the surgical intervention.

Complications

GENERAL MORTALITY AND MORBIDITY

Maternal death is the worst complication of abortion. The primary causes of death are listed in Table 8–6. In 55 deaths due to legal abortion in the United States between 1975 and 1977, Selik and co-workers (1981) identified five major contributors to death: delay in seeking abortion until after the 12th week of gestation (47%), incomplete emptying of the uterus by the physician (16%), perforation of the uterus (16%), failure to refer to another physician when appropriate (11%), and the use of an instillation procedure instead of dilatation and evacuation for abortions performed at less than 17 weeks (11%). Most deaths involved more than one factor.

The role of delay in seeking abortions is illustrated in Figure 8–1. The figure depicts the

Table 8-6. Deaths Associated with Legal Abortions by Primary Cause in the United States, 1972-1975*

Primary Cause	Percent
Infection	26.9
Embolism	26.0
Anesthesia	15.4
Hemorrhage	9.6
Coagulopathy	6.7
Pre-existing heart disease	3.9
Cerebrovascular accident	1.9
Electrolyte imbalance	1.9
Other	7.7

*From Grimes DA, Cates W: Complications of legally induced abortion: a review. *Obstet. Gynecol. Surv.* 34:177–191, © by Williams & Wilkins, 1979. Reprinted with permission.

death-to-case ratio per week of gestation. The graphs highlight two salient management goals. First, once the decision has been made, there should be no delay in the performance of abortion. Second, a dilatation and evacuation procedure should be the treatment of choice for early second trimester abortions of gestations at or before 18 weeks. Late second trimester abortions should still involve intraamniotic instilla-

tion of abortifacients such as saline, prostaglandins or urea.

Sepsis is the leading cause of death in legal abortion. Incomplete abortion and perforation are the chief initiating events in fatal septic outcome. Epidemiologic evidence also supports a strong component of patient responsibility. The single woman under 25 years of age is the most likely patient to succumb from infection following abortion. Delay in seeking abortion, fear involving parents and delay in seeking medical attention when postoperative infection occurs are listed as behavioral aspects associated with septic death from legal abortions (Selik et al, 1981).

To the average patient a 1:50,000 risk of death is extremely remote. However, what concerns her is the short and long-term morbidity. Two predominant factors increase the morbid risk of abortion; advanced gestational age and abortion technique. The risk of a major medical complication increases sevenfold (0.3% to 2.26%) with advancing gestational age (Grimes and Cates, 1979). The risk of unintended surgery (laparoscopy ± laparotomy) after first trimester suction curettage is 0.39%, after dil-

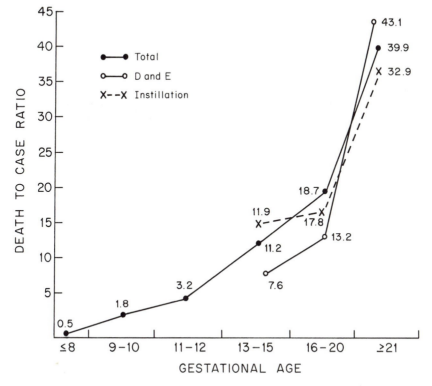

1. Deaths per 100,000 abortions

Figure 8-1. Delay in seeking abortions. Death to case ratio for legal abortion by gestational age (1972-1976).

atation and evacuation 0.21% and after instillation procedures 0.4% (King et al, 1980; Peterson et al, 1983; Karfrissen et al, 1984). The risk of hysterectomy occurring as a complication of curettage and instillation is 0.14% and 0.43%, respectively (Grimes, Flock et al, 1984).

Table 8–7 reveals a point of acceleration after 12 weeks' gestation in terms of major morbidity. Accurate estimation of gestational age is especially important after 11 weeks. One study revealed that 5% of pregnancies thought to be less than 12 weeks are actually at 13 or more weeks of gestation (Burnhill, 1979). Accurate dating by documentation of the date of a pregnancy test, careful pelvic examination by an experienced clinician, and an ultrasound screening for amenorrhea longer than 11 weeks should reduce the frequency of underestimation. Abortion technique, often related to gestational age, again, influences major complication rates (Table 8–8). Suction curettage has one fifth the morbidity risk of instillation procedures. Abdominal procedures have a relative risk ratio to other abortion methods of about 40.

PERIOPERATIVE COMPLICATIONS

Uterine Perforation. Uterine perforation is a much feared complication of therapeutic abortion (Grimes, 1984). The incidence of perforation is presented in Table 8–9. Those patients who have a therapeutic abortion complicated by perforation have a risk of death at least 150 times greater than the risk of death in patients without a perforation (Grimes et al, 1981; Grimes et al, 1983). The signs of uterine perforation are sudden loss of resistance to the uterine instrument, presence of any type of

Table 8–7. Major Complication Rates of Abortions by Gestational Age*

Gestational Age	Major Complication Rate/100 Abortions
6	.36
7–8	.27
9–10	.45
11–12	.77
13–14	1.37
15–16	1.91
17–20	2.16
21–24	2.26

*From Grimes DA, Cates W: Complications of legally induced abortion: a review. *Obstet. Gynecol. Surv.* 34:177–191, © Williams & Wilkins, 1979. Reprinted with permission.

Table 8–8. Major Complication Rate of Abortions by Procedure*

Type of Procedure	Major Complication Rate/100 Abortions
Suction curettage	0.4
Sharp curettage	0.9
Instillation of abortifacient	1.9
Hysterotomy	14.9
Hysterectomy	16.1

*From Grimes DA, Cates W: Complications of legally induced abortion: a review. *Obstet. Gynecol. Surv.* 34:177–191, © Williams & Wilkins, 1979. Reprinted with permission.

extrauterine tissue, intraoperative or postoperative hemorrhage, postoperative sepsis and persistent postoperative pelvic pain.

Berek and Stubblefield (1979) described the anatomic location of 20 perforations occurring during abortion. Eighty percent occurred in the cervix or lower uterine segment. These resulted in lacerations of the uterine artery in 40% of cases. Critical in their description was the fact that cervical or lower uterine perforations may present up to several days postoperatively and may not be easily diagnosed by laparoscopy. If perforation is suspected during the procedure, the procedure should cease and a laparoscopy should be performed. Adjacent pelvic organs should be systematically examined for trauma. Small non-bleeding perforations should merely be observed. Then the abortion may be completed with laparoscopic visualization. Laparoscopy should be considered in the postoperative patient presenting with signs of sepsis, persistent hemorrhage and persistent pelvic pain.

Major diagnostic or therapeutic surgery is a serious concern in uterine perforation. The incidence of major operative intervention (laparotomy) is presented in Table 8–10, which combines data from Nathanson (1972b), Lauersen and Birnbaum (1973), Freiman and Wulff (1977), and Ben-Baruch and co-workers (1982). Forty-four percent of perforations diagnosed by laparoscopy resulted in laparotomies (Figure 8–2).

Hemorrhage. The frequency of significant hemorrhage varies according to gestational age, technique and definition. Abortion at 12 weeks or less is accompanied by an 0.6 to 3.9% risk of hemorrhage (see Table 8–9). Prostaglandin and saline abortion techniques have a higher incidence of hemorrhage than dilatation and evacuation. The difference in frequency of hem-

Table 8–9. Method of Abortion and Risks of Morbidity

| Method | No. of Patients | Complications* | | | | |
		Hemorrhage	Infection	Cervical Laceration	Perforation	Transfusion
Menstrual† Extraction	2,101	3.9	1.3	0	0	0.09
Suction‡	148,021	0.6	0.8	0.2	0.2	0.05
Dilatation and Evacuation§	27,532	0.8	1.0	0.9	0.30	0.2
Saline Instillation‖	18,675	1.8	2.4	0.5	0.05	0.9
Prostaglandin Plus Urea Instillation¶	2,802	6.2	5.3	1.3	0	0.3

*Rate/100 abortions.
†Data from Atienza MF, Berkman RJ et al: *Am. J. Obstet. Gynecol.* 121:490, 1975; Irani KR, Henriques ES et al: *Obstet. Gynecol.* 46:596, 1975; Hale RW, Kobana TY et al: *Am. J. Obstet. Gynecol.* 134:213, 1979; Munsick RA: *Obstet. Gynecol.* 60:738, 1982.
‡Data from Nathanson BN: *N. Engl. J. Med.* 286:403, 1972a; Tietze C, Lewit S: *Stud. Fam. Plann.* 3:97, 1972; Hodgson JB: *Adv. Plan. Parenthood* 9:52, 1975; Cates W et al: *Am. J. Epidemiol.* 106:200, 1978.
§Data from Grimes DA, Schulz KF et al: *N. Engl. J. Med* 298:1141, 1977a; Peterson WF, Berry FN et al: *Obstet. Gynecol.* 62:185, 1983; Kafrissen ME, Schulz KF et al: *J. Am. Med. Assoc.* 251:916, 1984.
‖Data from Grimes DA, Schulz KF et al: *Obstet. Gynecol.* 49:612, 1977b.
¶Data from Kafrissen ME, Schulz KF et al: *J. Am. Med. Assoc.* 251:916, 1984.

orrhage with technique is closely related to advanced gestational age and termination by instillation techniques. Instillation techniques also have a 7 to 30% chance of incomplete abortion (Grimes et al, 1977b; Kafrissen et al, 1984). Retained products of conception and poor post-evacuation uterine tone are major causes of hemorrhage with abortion. Local anesthesia, post-suction curetting and the use of perioperative oxytocic agents are specific ways to reduce these complications.

The evaluation of uterine hemorrhage is confused by inconsistent definitions and poor methods of estimating the amounts of blood lost. The definitions of uterine hemorrhage in the references used for Table 8–9 vary from 100 to 500 ml. Physicians' estimates of blood loss are notoriously poor. They are made more inaccurate by differing proportions of the products of conception to blood. The frequency of transfusion would be expected to reflect the degree of hemorrhage. In general, the rate of transfusion is one-fifth to one-tenth the incidence of re-

ported hemorrhage. However, the rate of transfusion may not accurately estimate the incidence of significant hemorrhage. The younger patient can tolerate a much lower postoperative hemoglobin level than an older, sicker patient. The surgeon is also less likely to transfuse an outpatient. Post-abortion anemia has not been studied and may represent a significant long-term morbid complication for women of childbearing age. Woodward (1984) has described a method of estimating second trimester blood

Table 8–10. Major Surgical Intervention After Uterine Perforation*

Intervention	No.	Percent
Laparoscopy/laparotomy	51	44
Laparotomy with repair of defect	27	23
Hysterectomy	10	12
Repair of omental or bowel damage	9	11

*116 patients.

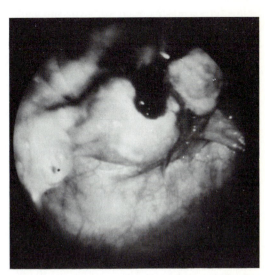

Figure 8–2. Uterine perforation. Laparoscopic demonstration of fundal perforation by a uterine dilator.

loss by using total volume of tissue and fluid weight (gm) and fetal foot length (mm).

Cervical Injury. The risk of cervical injury is proportional to the gestational age; the greater the dilatation needed, the greater the risk of injury. Trauma may result from the tenaculum tearing through the cervical lip. As bleeding may be quite profuse, a figure of 8 absorbable suture may be used. Deep laceration approaching one third of the length of the cervix must be repaired in layers with fine synthetic absorbable suture. Persistence of a cervicovaginal fistula will result in mucorrhea, metrorrhagia, dyspareunia and a risk of premature delivery with subsequent pregnancy.

The mechanics of cervical dilatation are described by Hulka and co-workers (1974). The internal os provides a majority of the resistance and the resistance is greater at 0.9 cm. The greater the force needed to dilate the cervix, the more likely is a cervical laceration or uterine perforation (Johnstone et al, 1976; Schulz et al, 1982). A variety of techniques are used to reduce these risks. Slow, steady gradual dilatation with tapered Pratt dilators is the most widely used technique. Blunt-ended Hagar dilators require greater force and have been implicated in later cervical incompetence. Another technique is to soften and dilate the cervix with laminaria or by administration of a prostaglandin preoperatively. Laminaria slowly dilate the internal os by swelling as water is absorbed. The major disadvantages of natural laminaria is the length of time needed for complete swelling (6 to 9 hours). New synthetic laminaria may reduce the maximum swelling time to three to four hours and maintain uniform mechanical properties under stress (Wheeler and Schneider, 1983). An additional risk of hydrophilic dilators is that of infection. They should be used with caution in patients at high risk for pelvic inflammatory disease. A documented recent negative gonorrhea culture and chlamydia test would be helpful in this high risk group. On the other hand, the use of small amounts of vaginal prostaglandins preoperatively would reduce the infection risk and has been shown to be effective in the reduction of cervical resistance (Lauersen et al, 1982).

Anesthetic Complications. Complications of anesthesia account for 15.4% of maternal deaths related to abortion (see Table 8–6). The leading causes of anesthetic related abortion deaths from 1972 to 1977 were drug overdose and hypoxia secondary to hypoventilation (Peterson et al, 1981). In this study, local anesthesia seemed to have a lower death-to-case ratio than general anesthesia even when gestational age factors and concomitant operative procedures (tubal ligation) were controlled. However, a prospective randomized clinical trial (Andolsek et al, 1977) suggests similar major complication rates between paracervical and general anesthesia. The character of the major complications was different. General anesthesia was associated with higher rates of cervical injury, bleeding and perforation. Paracervical anesthesia had higher rates of retained products of conception.

The prevention of iatrogenic mortality and morbidity secondary to anesthesia rests with proper selection of patients, use of correct drug dosage, and meticulous administration of the smallest effective doses of anesthesia. A complete array of resuscitative equipment and drugs is essential in abortion. Training of medical and paramedical personnel in cardiopulmonary resuscitation is essential in facilities performing abortion. The specific management of local anesthestic overdose is discussed in Chapter 15.

Liveborn Infant. A complication of late second trimester abortion is the delivery of a liveborn infant with the possibility of survival. Perinatal centers are recording 30 to 50% survival at 26 weeks and occasional survival at 24 weeks. As many as 50% of gravidas have unreliable dates, and second trimester ultrasound has an error of one to two weeks. Thus, a fetus thought to be 23 weeks may turn out to be at 25 weeks and viable. The incidence of liveborn infants is related to technique. Saline instillation is more fetocidal. However, live births occur with saline instillation at a rate of 0.17 per 100 abortions, with an occasional long-term survival. Hysterotomy has an incidence of 0.85 per 100 abortions (Stroh and Hinman, 1976). The Hastings Institute estimated that in 1974 there were six to seven infants born after second trimester abortions who grew to maturity (Grimes and Cates, 1979).

If the clinician is surprised with a liveborn infant of possible viability, many difficult medical, legal and ethical problems arise. The fetus should be treated supportively until a neonatologist can determine viability. The obstetrician will expose himself to legal liability if he should interfere with supportive care.

Hypernatremia. The infusion of hyperosmolar saline solution has been associated with hypernatremia as a complication. The incidence is about 0.01 per 100 abortions (Grimes and Cates, 1979). The symptoms are sharp abdominal pain, hyperesthesia, backache, headache, irritability and agitation. These symptoms should alert the clinician to the possibility of intravascular injection of saline. At this point the infusion should be immediately terminated and the patient observed. Transient cases of hypernatremia of greater than 160 mEq/L may cause no discernible adverse effects. The possibility of amniotic fluid embolism should be entertained if symptoms progress. The rapid infusion of 1000 ml of 5% dextrose in water should rapidly improve hypernatremia. The use of hypertonic saline in midtrimester abortion in patients with cardiac disease, hypertension, hemoglobinopathy, congenital coagulopathy and neurologic or renal diseases is contraindicated.

Water Intoxication (Hyponatremia). Water intoxication during abortion is an entirely preventable iatrogenic complication. Most women with water intoxication have been given a high dose oxytocin infusion in an electrolyte-free solution over a long period of time. The antidiuretic properties of oxytocin are shown with a reduction of urine output after 15 units and reach a maximum at 45 units. The clinical manifestations of water intoxication (hyponatremia) include oliguria, weakness, muscular irritability, headache, depressed sensorium, coma, convulsion and death. Central nervous system symptoms occur with a serum sodium level below 120 mEq/L. Preventive techniques such as recording intake and output, intermittent cessation of oxytocin infusion, the use of an electrolyte solution instead of a salt-free solution and intermittent evaluation of the serum sodium level are the first concerns in management. Usually mild hyponatremia can be treated with cessation of oxytocin, because oxytocin has a short half-life. Within an hour the urine output should increase. The presence of convulsions or coma with a serum sodium of less than 120 mEq/L demands more aggressive management. This requires the use of a potent intravenous diuretic (furosemide) to induce diuresis, followed by hourly replacements of sodium and potassium lost in the urine. Replacement of sodium and potassium is accomplished by using 3% saline with added potassium. Hyponatremia should be corrected within six to eight hours.

SHORT-TERM POSTOPERATIVE COMPLICATIONS

Febrile Morbidity. Approximately 0.75 per 1000 patients undergoing first trimester suction curettage will have an elevation of temperature greater than 38 degrees Celsius for over 24 hours. Corresponding figures for second trimester terminations are 1.0% for dilatation and evacuation, 2.4% for saline instillation and 5.3% for prostaglandin induction plus urea instillation (see Table 8–9). Factors known to increase infectious morbidity are low socioeconomic class, length of induction, abortion method and the presence of virulent organisms such as gonococcus, chlamydia or beta hemolytic streptococcus. Retained placenta, uterine hematomas and uterine perforation increase the risk dramatically.

Adequate evacuation under sterile conditions is a cornerstone of reducing infectious morbidity. The technique of a thorough vacuum aspiration followed by curettage check and reaspiration reduces retained tissue or blood. A culture for *N. gonorrhoeae* and a chlamydia test prior to abortion are warranted; 1 to 4% of the population seeking abortions will have positive cervical cultures. These organisms will increase postabortal infection rates two to four times (Osser and Persson, 1984; Burkman et al, 1976). Grimes, Schultz and Cates (1984) reviewed the literature on the efficacy of prophylactic antibiotics on postabortal infection. If the cervical cultures are negative, a 24 hour course of tetracycline perioperatively seems to be effective. If cultures have not been performed a full course of tetracyclines is recommended. The choice of tetracycline covers both gonococcus and chlamydia. The recommended dosage is 1.5 gm oral tetracycline two to three hours prior to the procedure and 500 mg every six hours afterward for four days. If the cultures are positive the patient should be treated prior to abortion.

Retained Products of Conception. The frequency of retained tissue varies with techniques of abortion. Suction curettage has a 0.4 to 0.6% risk of retained products of conception (Grimes and Cates, 1979). Instillation procedures have a 7 to 30% risk of retained placenta for more than two hours after expulsion of the fetus. Dilatation and evacuation has a 0.51 to 0.90% risk of retained placenta (Grimes et al, 1977; Kafrissen et al, 1984). Retained products have a tremendous impact on the development of postoperative complications. Of 18 women who died from dilatation and evacuation procedures in the United States between 1972 and 1978, seven died from complications of sepsis and hemorrhage from incomplete abortion (Cates and Grimes, 1981). Incomplete abortion increases the risk of death from sepsis 50 times

(Grimes et al, 1981). Apart from the increasing death-to-case ratio secondary to sepsis and hemorrhage, a large part of the more common morbidity is a result of retained tissue. Retained tissue provides a nidus for local infection, which then leads to pelvic sepsis. Retained tissue prevents the normal hemostatic role of the contracted uterus and thus leads to prolonged postoperative bleeding.

The intraoperative diagnosis of incomplete evacuation has usually relied upon an estimation of the volume of tissue obtained. The following procedures are critical for the proper evaluation of the completeness of a first trimester suction curettage. Successive washes of the gauze bag containing tissue should remove most of the blood. The water is then squeezed out and the tissue is separated into decidual, fetal and placental tissue. The surgeon must identify all fetal parts in more advanced gestations. Any question of completeness of a first trimester suction curettage should indicate a repeat curettage. After the procedure the gestational tissue should be weighed; any amount less than 15 gm indicates that the patient should be followed more closely.

Another technique especially helpful in gestations less than eight weeks is to float the tissue in 200 ml of tap water. Placental tissue will appear as soft, fluffy, feathery, villous tissue adherent to obvious membranes (Fig. 8–3). When gross inspection fails to identify distinct placenta, particulate matter is prepared as a wet mount and examined under the microscope using low power with high contrast. Placental villi are characteristic. The villi are shaped like clubs and do not have visible capillaries. Decidua will have prominent capillaries and may show endometrial glands (Fig. 8–4) (Lindahl and Ahlgren, 1986; Munsick, 1982).

When the latter technique fails to identify trophoblastic tissue or the tissue weighs less than 15 gm, there are four possible explanations: ectopic pregnancy, false positive pregnancy tests, failed abortion and very early gestation. The immediate management should include a quantitative serum beta human chorionic gonadotropin (hCG) determination, frozen section pathologic examination of the tissue, culdocentesis and education of the patient. The patient should be informed of the serious implications of a possible ectopic pregnancy, and she should be instructed to return in three to four days for follow-up on the serum hCG and the final histology. She should have access to immediate medical care and must provide information as to where she may be reached.

As many as 2 to 4% of first trimester suction curettages are performed on non-pregnant patients. This may represent the false positive rate of pregnancy tests (Hale et al, 1979; Munsick, 1982). Clearly the method of testing is important; a slide test may be inaccurate secondary to proteinuria, blood or medication. However, the serum beta hCG level is rarely inaccurate.

Ectopic Pregnancy. Ectopic pregnancy is a feared complication of abortion. Between the years 1972 and 1978 the CDC identified 10 maternal deaths from ectopic pregnancy after

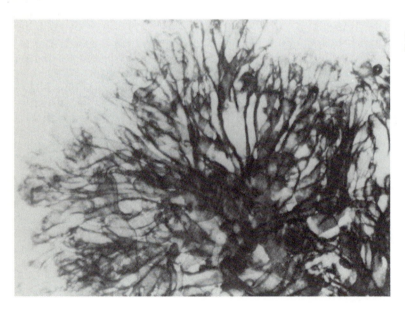

Figure 8–3. *Wetmount microscopic appearance of placental villi.*

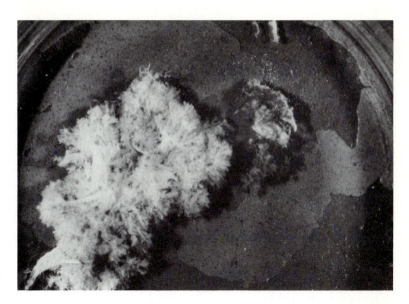

Figure 8–4. Products of conception in water. Fluffy villi (left) *and shaggy decidua* (right).

legally induced abortion (Rubin et al, 1980). During this time there were 122 maternal deaths associated with abortion; 8% of these deaths were secondary to ectopic pregnancy. The incidence of ectopic pregnancy after abortion is 3.3 to 3.7 per 10,000 procedures. In 1979 there were about 500 ectopic pregnancies associated with legally induced abortions. Ectopic pregnancy must be ruled out in the patient with a positive pregnancy test when no products of conception are identified pathologically. Clinical identification of villi at the time of abortion needs to be reemphasized. Reliance on a delayed pathologic examination may fail to prevent death from ectopic pregnancy (Rubin et al, 1980). Seven of ten patients died after the tissue was sent for permanent section. Three died within three days of the procedure, before the final report returned to the clinic. Four patients died because an attempt to contact the patient about the histologic findings failed.

Failed Abortion. Failed abortion is a risk of suction curettage procedures at less than 12 weeks' gestation and composes approximately 70% of cases where minimal tissue or no villi are found, excluding false positive pregnancy tests. Failed abortion occurred 46 times in 65,045 first trimester abortions (0.071%) (Fielding et al, 1978; Kaunitz et al, 1985). The risk is related to gestational age; the relative risk of failed abortion at less than eight weeks is 4.8 to 6 times that of an abortion at eight weeks or more gestation.

The management of failed abortion should include a quantitative beta hCG test and, if positive, a good quality ultrasonographic examination. An intrauterine pregnancy should be first treated with repeat suction curettage. If this fails or if the ultrasound shows no intrauterine pregnancy, the patient needs a laparoscopy. If the fallopian tubes are normal, the primary diagnosis is a pregnancy in an anomalous uterus. Valle and Sabbagha (1980) reported that 7 of 25 patients with failed abortion had uterine anomalies. They recommended hysteroscopy as the next step in the patient with a failed abortion and normal fallopian tubes as demonstrated by laparoscopy. After localization of the pregnancy the termination can be completed. Occasionally the pregnancy will be in a blind uterine horn and will require laparotomy.

Occasionally early termination (gestation less than 7 weeks) will produce minimal tissue with occasional villi. In a reliable asymptomatic patient an alternative to laparoscopy may be serial quantitative beta hCG determinations and close observation. The fall in human chorionic gonadotropin (hCG) after first trimester therapeutic abortion was determined by Lähteenmäkz (1978). He noted that the mean serum concentration of hCG-LH (luteinizing hormone) fell to 10% of the initial value by 1.8 days, to 1% by 6.1 days and to 0.1% by 14 days. Data from Marrs and co-workers (1979) suggest that an hCG greater than 750 mIU/ml on the eighth postoperative day may indicate a significant amount of retained tissue. The rate of fall seems to be related to technique as well as to the initial hCG level (Steier et al, 1984); hysterotomy, hysterectomy and instillation procedures cause a more rapid decline. Failure of the beta hCG level to fall should initiate an endeavor to rule out ectopic pregnancy or retained placenta.

Hormonal studies after abortion have highlighted another short-term problem with abortion, the risk of pregnancy. Ovulation as measured by LH peak, progesterone level, temperature charts or endometrial biopsy occurs as early as the 14th day (usually, 20 to 22 days) after first trimester abortion (Boyd and Holmstrom, 1972; Obel and Madsen, 1980). An LH peak can occur even though the hCG level is elevated as high as 35 mIU/ml. The first menses will occur between 2 and 10 weeks post-abortion (usually, 4.3 to 5.2 weeks). These data suggest that the patient be cautioned about pregnancy, and contraception should be initiated prior to the two week postoperative checkup.

Embolism. Embolism accounted for 27% of abortion deaths between 1972 and 1975 in the United States (see Table 8–6). Embolism includes the traditional thrombotic type (37%), amniotic fluid embolism (52%) and air embolism (11%). Thromboembolism seems to be related to preexisting risk factors, history of thrombophlebitis, obesity, use of oral contraceptives, type A blood, use of general anesthesia and concurrent sterilization (Kimball et al, 1978). Death from thromboembolism is a late complication, averaging 15.6 days after the procedure. Thus, the incidence of thromboembolism as a complication is probably underestimated. Specific preventive objectives are identification of the high risk patient, use of local anesthetics, use of prophylactic heparin in high risk patients and avoidance of oral contraceptive pills prior to two to four weeks postoperatively.

Amniotic fluid embolism is a significant risk of abortion performed at greater than 12 weeks' gestation (Guidotti et al, 1981). Although originally described with saline abortion, it can be associated with all methods. Concurrent use of oxytocin seems to increase this risk. The exact incidence is hard to determine because the diagnosis is difficult to make unless the patient dies. The cardinal symptoms are hypoxia, cyanosis, disseminated intravascular coagulation (DIC) and cardiovascular collapse. At least some of the coagulopathy reported with second trimester abortions is caused by small non-fatal emboli. The reported incidence of coagulopathy with saline and/or urea instillation is 0.12 to 0.3 per 100 abortions (Grimes and Cates, 1979). Serial measurements of the coagulation system indicate an increase in coagulopathy with periods of increased uterine activity.

Air embolism has resulted from reversal of suction with the vacuum extractor. This is a totally preventable complication and underlines the responsibility of the surgeon to check his equipment. Air embolism may also occur spontaneously.

LONG-TERM COMPLICATIONS

Perinatal Loss. The relationship of abortion to subsequent pregnancy outcome is a very real and common issue to both the obstetrician and the patient. Induced abortion is a highly emotional and guilt-ridden time for the patient, and it is only natural for her to question its importance in any future obstetric or gynecologic complications. One of the more common questions a perinatologist answers is whether previous abortion caused current perinatal problems. The literature is replete with studies showing adverse effects. Table 8–11 lists the reported adverse effects of induced abortion.

The reader is directed to two recent reviews for details of the literature and explanations for divergent conclusions (Br. Med. J., 1981; Bracken, 1978). In summary, there are major weaknesses in all current studies. They are:

1. Failure to control for confounding maternal factors such as smoking, socioeconomic class, previous and concurrent medical problems, previous pregnancy history, previous gynecologic history.

2. Failure to control for abortion technique.

3. Reliability of reporting previous abortion.

4. Failure to control for complications of previous abortion.

5. Failure to control for repeat aborters.

6. Lack of follow-up on subsequent pregnancies after index pregnancy.

Recent studies have shown improvement in terms of these weaknesses, especially confounding maternal variables. They have demonstrated within the limits of their own respective methodologic weakness that a single vacuum aspiration abortion, at less than 10 weeks' gestation

Table 8–11. Long-term Complications of Induced Abortion

Menstrual irregularities
Infertility
Spontaneous abortion
Ectopic pregnancies
Prematurity
Low birth weight
Rh sensitization
Placenta previa
Antepartum bleeding

and with no postoperative complications, has no significant lasting adverse effect. Otherwise the following adverse effects are probably valid:

1. Dilatation and curettage, an older technique, has an increased likelihood in subsequent pregnancies of prematurity, low birth weight, second trimester abortion and defective placentation (placenta previa and retained placenta).

2. Forced cervical dilatation of the cervix to greater than 10 to 12 mm will increase the risk of premature delivery. The efficacy of the slow dilatation by laminaria or vaginal prostaglandins has not been established, but theoretically these techniques will help.

3. Induced abortion complicated by retained products of conception, infection and repeat curettage probably increases the risk of infertility, ectopic pregnancy and defective placentation.

4. Repeated abortions may have more than additive risk of long-term complications.

5. The adverse effects of abortion may be additive to other risk factors; e.g., previous exposure to diethylstilbesterol or previous abortion.

In counseling the patient as to the long-term risk of abortion, it is important to discriminate between a statistical risk versus a real risk for that patient. For example, if a technique or complication was unequivocally shown to increase by a factor of three the risk of premature delivery, her subsequent pregnancy still has an 80 to 85% chance of term delivery. By the same token, an obstetric patient who relates her previous therapeutic abortions to a current obstetrical crisis must be counseled that abortion is by no means the only factor.

Rhesus Sensitization. Freda and co-workers (1970) have shown the risk of sensitization is less than 1% at gestations less than six weeks, 2% at eight weeks and greater than 9% for abortions at 12 weeks or beyond. All Rhesus antigen negative, unsensitized women having abortions should be given RhoGAM. For abortions at gestations less than 12 weeks a 50 microgram dose is adequate. The use of RhoGAM after abortion in the United States was reported to be as low as 42% (Grimes et al, 1977). A utilization rate of 50%, assuming a 5% risk of sensitization of at risk patients, will result in about 5,000 new cases of Rhesus sensitization at current rates of therapeutic abortion. This is a highly significant medical, economic and social long term risk of abortion.

Psychosomatic Aspects of Induced Abortion. In the last 25 years there has been a dramatic change in opinion as to the psychologic effects of abortion. Prior to 1960, the general feeling was that therapeutic abortion either magnified the "normal" depression associated with termination of pregnancy or led to neurosis or psychosis. Unfortunately, this opinion was based on a few often-quoted articles that suffered from faulty research design, non-specific results and biased conclusions.

Hubbard, (1977) in a review of the literature, proposed four criteria for acceptable research on the psychologic impact of abortion:

1. Use of control versus test groups.

2. Pre- and post-abortion psychologic evaluation.

3. Standardized data gathering procedures.

4. Predetermined criteria for evaluation.

Recent studies with improved research design have shown that most patients (92 to 96%) adjust well to abortion. Even patients with psychiatric histories cope with the crisis without long-term sequelae. However, abortion is still approached by most women with considerable emotional stress and anguish. Approximately one quarter of women find the decision to abort very difficult (Bracken, 1977). Their anxiety relates to the following factors: lack of support for the abortion from significant others, inadequate coping mechanism to deal with the stress of decision making, being married, strong moral beliefs against abortion and a fear of the surgical procedure.

The need for adequate counseling would seem to be justified by the conflicts and difficulties in decision making. In addition, counseling makes sense from a medical point of view. Counseling has been implicated in reducing anxiety associated with the pain of the procedure, especially when the operator has less experience. The counselor can warn the physician about a patient who is highly anxious at the start of the procedure and is more likely to experience pain. Counseling has been associated with an increased acceptance of contraception and post-abortion follow-up. Finally, adequate counseling is necessary in special situations such as repeat abortion.

The goal of pre-abortion counseling should be to ensure that the client has made a rational and informed decision. Janis and Mann (1977) have devised decision counseling to help counselors improve the quality of their client's decision making. The following are the criteria that a counselor may use to judge the overall quality of the client's decision process.

1. Has the client examined a wide range of options or courses of actions, including carrying

the pregnancy to term with subsequent adoption?

2. Has the client examined the motivation behind her decision?

3. Has the client carefully weighed the risks as well as the benefits that could follow from each alternative?

4. Has the client searched out new information relevant to weak areas of knowledge?

5. Has the client assimilated the new knowledge in respect to all the choices?

6. Has the client made detailed provisions for implementing the chosen course of action with special attention to contingency plans that might be required if various complications were to materialize?

SPONTANEOUS ABORTION

Spontaneous abortion is defined as the unintentional loss of a pregnancy of less than 20 weeks' gestation with a fetal weight less than 500 gm. At least 10 to 25% of documented pregnancies will end with a spontaneous abortion. The frequency varies with the scrutiny of the population observed and the sensitivity of the pregnancy test, i.e., serum β hCG determination versus slide test. This incidence represents an estimated 800,000 spontaneous abortions yearly. Most major textbooks in obstetrics and gynecology recommend that most if not all spontaneous abortions be followed by a dilatation and curettage. Despite the tremendous medical, social and economic impact, complications of therapy have not been adequately studied.

The major cause of spontaneous abortion in the first trimester (less than 12 weeks) is chromosomal or structural abnormalities incompatible with life. Boue and co-workers (1975) found that 61% of spontaneous abortions at less than 12 weeks were fetuses that were chromosomally abnormal. Mikano (1970) suggested that an additional 20% of aborti will have severe structural defects unexplained by chromosomal abnormalities. Thus, structural malformation and chromosomal abnormality account for about 80% of abortions at less than 12 weeks. The rest may be explained by a variety of factors such as point mutuation, infection or hormonal inadequacies. Genetic abnormality may not be manifested by structural or chromosomal abnormalities but by metabolic or functional abnormalities from the point mutations of genes. Infections such as mycoplasma, chlamydia, viral infection (herpes) and gonorrhea, play a role in the loss of a chromosomally and structurally normal abortus at less than 12 weeks' gestation. Insufficient corpus luteum function is also implicated in recurrent first trimester abortions.

Most discussions of spontaneous abortion combine abortions at 12 weeks or less with those of the second trimester (13 to 20 weeks). However, second trimester spontaneous abortions have a different incidence, etiology, management and prognosis. Between 15 to 30% of spontaneous abortions occur between 12 and 20 weeks. In contrast to first trimester abortion, chromosomal or structural abnormality plays a much smaller role. After a developmental age of nine weeks (LMP 11 weeks previously) less than 10% show structural or chromosomal abnormality (Mikano, 1970). Mullerian duct abnormalities (incompetent cervix), infection (myocoplasma) and placental abnormalities (previa, abruptio) play a much larger role.

The management of early abortion (less than 12 weeks) depends, by definition, on its clinical presentation. These definitions are as follows:

1. Threatened abortion: uterine bleeding with or without cramping and *not* associated with cervical dilatation, rupture of membranes, or a falling serum hCG level.

2. Inevitable abortion: intrauterine bleeding with cervical changes, rupture of the membranes or negative pregnancy test after a previously positive test.

3. Incomplete abortion: partial passage of products of conception.

4. Complete abortion: complete passage of products of conception.

5. Missed abortion: products of conception are retained for prolonged periods (4 to 6 weeks).

6. Habitual abortion: three or more consecutive abortions.

Problems and Complications of Diagnosis

About 20 to 30% of pregnancies will have first trimester bleeding and one half to two thirds of those will go on to an abortion. The prediction of eventual abortion is difficult. Clinically, those patients with strong midline cramping, heavier bleeding and the loss of pregnancy symptoms have a worse prognosis. Two relatively inexpensive tests have been used as predictors of abortion. These are ferning of the cervical mucous and the finding of over 10% of karopyknotic cells on a Papanicolaou's smear from the lateral vaginal wall. Both tests indirectly measure the biologic effects of insufficient progesterone. The predictive value of these tests has not been clearly established and may not improve on the clinical history.

Hertz (1984) has examined the wide variety of expensive assays and ultrasound that have been used to try to predict abortion when first trimester bleeding is present. They include serial assay of human chorionic gonadotropin, progesterone, estrogen, human placental lactogen and concentration of pregnancy zone protein (PZP). For each of these a statistically significant association between low or falling values and poor prognosis has been shown. Although these may be helpful in the individual patient, their sensitivity is not high enough to warrant a change in management if they are abnormal. In addition, the lack of reliability and expense probably add an unjustified economic burden.

Ultrasound may provide reliable information that can be used in the management of threatened abortion. This includes the presence or absence of:

1. An intrauterine sac at more than seven weeks' gestation.

2. A fetal pole at greater than eight weeks' gestation.

3. Fetal movement or heart movement at greater than nine weeks' gestation.

4. Co-existing pelvic abnormality, e.g., adnexal masses.

5. Gestational trophoblastic disease.

Some authors relate poor prognosis to other morphologic parameters such as low gestational sac volume, low implantation of the gestational sac and double or multiple gestational sacs. The reliability of these morphologic changes are much more operator-dependent than the previously listed criteria. In centers with experienced operators and high resolution equipment, the reliability can be good, but with office ultrasonography the reliability may not be good enough to warrant a change in management, i.e., suction curettage.

Another major problem is in the sensitivity of ultrasonic criteria indicating poor prognosis. The predictive value of a positive test is a measurement of the frequency with which normal pregnancies would be terminated if all pregnancies with abnormal tests had suction curettage. In patients with threatened abortion and abnormal ultrasound criteria about 10 to 25% will continue their pregnancies (Hertz, 1984; Mantoni, 1985). On the other hand, the finding of a normal sac with fetal heart movement allows considerable optimism. The ability of the examination to predict a continued pregnancy (specificity) is greater than 90% (Duff, 1975; Hertz, 1984; Mantoni, 1985). This compares favorably with the specificity of admitting symptoms. Duff (1975) compared ultrasonographic predictions with clinical judgement. Of patients presenting with light bleeding and no contractions, 60% eventually aborted. Likewise only 60% of patients with heavy bleeding and contractions aborted.

The time-honored management of threatened abortion has been bedrest. This management will certainly not change the outcome in 60 to 80% of first trimester abortions, those with major anatomic or chromosomal abnormality. The value of bedrest in the remaining 20 to 40% is undefined. Loss from infection such as herpes, gonorrhea, mycoplasma and so forth, will not be altered by bedrest. However, focus on the reduction of activity has a decided benefit on improving patient awareness. She will pay more attention to symptoms and will be encouraged to communicate with her physician at any sign of infection, loss of tissue or excessive blood loss.

The generalized use of steroids (estrogen or progesterone) in threatened abortion is mentioned only to be condemned. The tragedy of the diethylstilbestrol (DES) story underlines this proscription. Dieckmann and co-workers (1953) clearly showed diethylstilbestrol not to be effective, and multiple authors since 1971 have shown increased incidences of vaginal cancer and pregnancy wastage in DES exposed offspring. The use of progesterone has likewise been shown not to be of value in threatened abortion by at least two double-blind trials (Goldzieher, 1964; Shearman and Garrett, 1963). These trials involved only patients with documented low progesterone levels. Despite the negative results of these and other studies using progesterone, its use has been recommended in highly selected patients such as habitual aborters with documented luteal deficiency and no other structural abnormalities (Tho et al, 1979).

First Trimester Spontaneous Abortion

PROCEDURES

The management of first trimester pregnancy wastage (missed abortion, inevitable abortion, incomplete abortion and complete abortion) must be approached with three basic principles. First, surgical intervention has risks similar to those of therapeutic abortion. Longer gestations have higher risks of cervical laceration, hemorrhage and perforation. Second, incomplete abortion with its devitalized retained tissue is an excellent nidus of infection. Third, spontaneous abortion is a crisis and a loss for the woman. She deserves emotional respect and factual knowledge as to the cause and risk of recurrence.

Suction curettage is the method of choice. Prior dilatation of the cervix by the products of conception greatly reduces the risk of cervical injury and perforation. These risks may also be reduced by using a sponge forceps or an Allis clamp to stabilize the cervix. The need for anesthesia is reduced, and consequently most procedures may be performed under analgesics or paracervical block. The suction technique and precautions are the same as described for therapeutic abortion. Key points of emphasis are adequate suction strength, adequate removal of loose products of conception, and early recognition of perforation and its complications.

Postoperatively the key to management is observation for signs of infection, excessive bleeding and extrauterine pregnancy. The patient should avoid vigorous activity (including sexual activity) until bleeding has stopped. She must be reminded that ovulation can occur as early as two weeks post-abortion and contraception counseling should be given. Unless the presence of trophoblastic tissue has been confirmed by a pathologist, the patient should be cautioned about the signs and symptoms of ectopic pregnancy. At the time of the procedure the possibility of ectopic pregnancy may be suggested by the evacuation of less than 15 gm of tissue, lateralizing pelvic pain or the presence of an adnexal mass. In these patients histologic demonstration of the products of conception is essential prior to discharge. In addition, the risk of Rh sensitization in an Rh negative woman necessitates giving RhoGAM after spontaneous abortion (see later section in this Chapter).

The anesthetic risk, surgical risk and risk of post-traumatic intrauterine synechiae mandate close scrutiny of the need for evacuation. Not all abortions need to be followed by evacuation procedures. In a reliable asymptomatic patient who demonstrates a complete abortion on gross and histologic examination, close observation may be indicated. The pelvic examination should reveal a contracted uterus without adnexal tenderness or masses. An ultrasound examination may be useful in defining a complete abortion; a linear central cavity echo in either or both the longitudinal or transverse scans of

the uterus indicates an empty uterus (Jeong et al, 1981). Cervical cultures for *N. gonorrhoeae*, group B streptococcus and chlamydia will identify those patients at risk for infection.

POSTOPERATIVE COMPLICATIONS

Sepsis. Once the cervical barrier has been broken by spontaneous dilatation or the passage of tissue, the risks of infection and hemorrhage increase greatly. Like therapeutic abortion, sepsis plays a major role in death from spontaneous abortion. In the United States between 1972 and 1980, 122 women died as a result of spontaneous abortion. Infection (56%), hemorrhage (17%), embolism (9%), anesthesia (5%) and other causes (13%) accounted for these deaths (Berman et al, 1985). In a review of behavioral aspects contributing to abortion deaths, Selik and co-workers (1981) identified five consistent factors. First, the patient delayed in consulting a physician for obvious complications or illness (22%). Second, the physician ordered inappropriate antibiotics (20%). Third, the physician delayed in diagnosing possible septic abortion (15%). Fourth, the physician delayed in emptying the uterus after incomplete abortion (10%). Fifth, perforation and patient obesity were each associated with 10% of deaths.

Death from sepsis is especially important in the group who have an intrauterine device (IUD) in place in early pregnancy. Cates and co-workers (1976) showed a risk of death 50 times greater in women with an IUD in place compared with women without an IUD. Seventeen women of 50 who died in association with spontaneous abortion were wearing IUD's. Though it appeared that the multifilament Dalkon Shield was a significant risk factor, other types of IUD were reported in these deaths. The risk of sepsis is not just a maternal risk. Foreman and co-workers (1981) noted that the presence of an IUD at the beginning of the second trimester increased pregnancy wastage ten fold. The relative risk of a septic second trimester loss was 26 to 1. The removal of the IUD in the first trimester did not increase the risk of a second trimester loss.

Asherman's Syndrome. An additional risk of a post-abortion dilatation and curettage is that of post-traumatic uterine synechiae, Asherman's syndrome. The clinical presentation is that of post-traumatic infertility, amenorrhea or hypomenorrhea and increased dysmenorrhea. Asherman's syndrome occurs primarily after postpartum or post-abortion curettage. Diagnostic dilatation and curettage has been associated with a minority of cases. The intrauterine adhesions result from a denudation of the basalis of the endometrium in combination with hypoestrogenism (postpartum) or infection. The exact frequency of this complication is not clear. Bergman (1961) noted prospectively in 91 patients with postpartum curettage that at least four had Asherman's syndrome. Klein and Garcia (1973) have reported a relationship between intrauterine adhesions of some degree and curettage within two months following pregnancy (see Chapter 5).

Late Pregnancy Risks. What are the long-term effects of first trimester bleeding? First trimester bleeding is felt to occur at the implantation or placental site. Blood clots in this location will decrease the absorptive area of the placenta much in the same way abruptio placentae does in the second and third trimesters. The expected complications are placental infarcts, intrauterine growth retardation, premature delivery, increased fetal death rate, asphyxia and increased perinatal mortality rate. Hypoxia is a known teratogen, and an increase in congenital abnormalities might be expected. Two large surveys have confirmed an increase in perinatal complications secondary to placental insufficiency in pregnancies associated with first trimester bleeding (Funderburk et al, 1980; Niswander et al, 1972). The increase in poor outcome is two to three times (15 to 30%). In women with no prior term births, a history of two prior pregnancies with adverse outcomes (abortion, premature delivery or prenatal death) and first trimester bleeding the risk of subsequent poor outcome was 61% (Funderburk et al, 1980). The role of first trimester bleeding in teratogenesis is not clear. Retrospective studies have associated first trimester bleeding with an increase in central nervous system abnormalities (Ornoy et al, 1976). However, these can be the result of prolonged hypoxic insult as well as from an acute episode occurring with first trimester bleeding. Another problem is that the defective placentation may just be an addition to a co-existing congenital malformation. Pregnancies associated with chromosomal abnormalities, (e.g., trisomy 21) are more often associated with perinatal problems, including first trimester bleeding.

Risk to Future Pregnancies. Another logical question is What is the chance of recurrence? Jansen (1982) has given an eloquent critique of the literature on recurrent spontaneous abortion. Many biases compromise reports. Most studies have not controlled variables known to increase the recurrence risk: maternal age, gravidity, history of no previous term birth, history of a previous child with birth defects, previous spontaneous abortion and infertility. The identification of the actual pregnancy is a problem. The effects of subclinical abortion, delayed menses, and therapeutic abortion will change the incidence. Most studies rely on patient recall; thus artifacts or biases can adversely affect the results. Memory artifact refers to the fact that the greater the interval between spontaneous abortion and the inquiry the less likely the patient is to remember the event. For example, questioning a 60-year-old woman will reveal a lower incidence of abortion than questioning a 30-year-old woman. Compensation artifact represents a conscious desire to modify motivation for further pregnancies according to the outcome of the previous pregnancy. For example, a woman with one spontaneous abortion may be so affected by the experience that she will not conceive again. The recurrence artifact is a statistical artifact related to the incidence of spontaneous abortion; increasing gravidity will expose a legacy of spontaneous abortion. Selection artifact refers to the bias introduced by case selection. For example, obtaining a pregnancy history from mothers admitted for delivery will eliminate the women who have never experienced a term pregnancy. Another major weakness of studies on abortion is that most include both first and second trimester abortions. As mentioned earlier, there are widely different causes of first and second trimester abortion. Second trimester abortions probably have a higher risk of recurrence than first trimester abortions. For example, the probability of recurrent pregnancy wastage in untreated incompetent cervix is approximately 80%.

Despite these weaknesses in the study of recurrence, the most widely accepted figures for recurrent abortion are 23% for a history of one previous abortion, 26% for a history of two consecutive abortions and 32% for a history of three consecutive abortions (Warburton and Fraser, 1964). From a counseling point of view, workup for a recurrent abortion should be initiated after two consecutive abortions. The workup should include a history of environmental agents, a timed endometrial sampling, a hysterosalpingogram and cervical cultures for *Mycoplasma* or *Chlamydia*. Parental karotyping is very expensive and should only be done if there is history of two abortions plus birth defects. After three consecutive abortions ka- rotyping may then be indicated. Approximately 5 to 10% of patients with three or more consec- utive spontaneous abortions will have chromo- somal defects. Fifty to one hundred individual cell chromosomes must be examined, since mosiacism is a common finding; only 5 to 10% of the cells may be abnormal.

Second Trimester Spontaneous Abortion

Second trimester pregnancy wastage is a dif- ferent entity from first trimester loss; genetic abnormality is a cause in only a minority of cases. Structural defects of the uterus, placental abnormalities and infection play a much larger role. Consequently, second trimester patients often present with histories similar to the prob- lems of the third trimester. Some of these may be self-limited and require only hospitalization and close observation (placenta previa). In oth- ers, conservative management is not going to change the outcome, and early aggressive treat- ment may be indicated (ruptured membranes).

PROCEDURE

The choices of surgical management are dil- atation and evacuation or vaginal prostaglandin induction of labor. Dilatation and evacuation has the advantage of speed and reduction of blood loss. Its disadvantages are risk of anes- thesia, risk of perforation and the need for an experienced physician and specialized equip- ment. Prostaglandins can be very effective but have the disadvantage of significant side effects and the possibility of retained placenta.

Dilatation and Evacuation. This technique is as described under therapeutic abortion. Points for special consideration are:

1. Accurate sizing of the uterus. Often it is not consistent with the date of the last men- strual period.

2. Fetal tissues may be necrotic and more friable. More care must be used with extraction. The subsequent pathologic examination is very important in terms of counseling for future pregnancies.

3. Necrotic tissue is an excellent nidus of infection. Prophylactic antibiotics are indicated.

Intravaginal Prostaglandins. The following is an appropriate protocol. The patient is typed and cross-matched for blood and transfused if the hematocrit is less than 30%. A large bore (16 gauge) IV catheter is placed with normal saline running. The patient has individualized

nursing care, and vital signs are taken every 15 to 30 minutes. One half hour prior to the insertion of prostaglandins the patient is treated with analgesics (meperidine), antiemetics (Com- pazine) and antidiarrheal (Lomotil) and antipy- retic (Tylenol) agents. A 5-mg prostaglandin E_2 is inserted vaginally as a test dose. The patient is observed for one half hour for excessive uterine activity. Then a full dose of 20 mg prostaglandin E_2 suppository is inserted every three to five hours until delivery. The most common side effects of prostaglandins are pyr- exia, nausea, vomiting, diarrhea, headache and moderate labor pain. Ninety percent of patients will be successfully delivered, with a mean interval of 8 to 10 hours. The success of induc- tion is proportional to the duration of fetal death and inversely proportional to the gestational age until 32 weeks gestation. About one half of the patients have spontaneous expulsion of the complete placenta, thus avoiding the risk of curettage. Prostaglandins should be used with extreme caution in patients with a uterine scar because of the risk of a ruptured uterus. Active intervention to remove the placenta should start two hours after the delivery of the fetus. Prior to the manual removal of the placenta, the patient should have blood readily available and a large bore intravenous catheter in place. Un- der adequate anesthesia and sterile conditions, most of the placenta should be removed with large, blunt curettes. Sharp curettes should be avoided because of risk of postoperative intra- uterine synechiae. The uterine cavity should be carefully examined for abnormalities of shape and retained tissue. Postoperative oxytocin or ergotrate should be given to control bleeding. Prophylactic broad spectrum antibiotics, e.g., cefoxitin, should be used in any type of second trimester spontaneous abortion.

COMPLICATIONS

The intraoperative and short-term complica- tions of second trimester abortion are similar to those described in the section on second trimes- ter therapeutic abortion. Infection and sepsis are somewhat greater risks in late fetal death. Of special importance are coagulopathy, Rh sensitization and maternal emotional problems that require counseling.

Fetal Death and Coagulopathy. The pro- longed retention of products of conception may be complicated by maternal coagulopathy re- gardless of gestational age. As the placenta and fetus degenerate, thromboplastic material en- ters the maternal circulation and reduces the concentrations of fibrinogen, platelets, thrombin and factors V, VIII and XIII. Normally the process is asymptomatic and slow; a significant coagulopathy rarely occurs prior to four weeks after fetal death and approximately 25% of patients will develop it then. The development of a coagulopathy may be diagnosed by weekly determinations of fibrinogen, platelet count, prothrombin time and partial thromboplastin time. A fibrinogen level less than 150 mg/dl or a platelet count less than 100,000 is an indication for evacuation of the uterus.

The decision to intervene in fetal death is not easy. Spontaneous labor usually ensues quickly after fetal death, in 75% of patients after two weeks and in 90% after three weeks. Conservative management has the disadvantages of pschologic turmoil and maternal coagulopathy. Intervention runs the risk of surgical trauma, cervical injury or uterine perforation. The advent of intravaginal prostaglandins and increased surgical experience with dilatation and evacuation have decreased the risks of intervention. A reasonable approach to fetal death is to manage the patient conservatively for three weeks with serial clotting studies. Intervention prior to three weeks is indicated for developing coagulopathy, poor patient compliance and significant psychologic abnormalities. After three weeks intervention and dilatation and evacuation (gestation less than 18 weeks), intravaginal prostaglandins (gestation of 18 to 28 weeks) or oxytocin (gestation greater than 28 weeks) is indicated.

The primary treatment of significant coagulopathy is to empty the uterus. Medical correction of clotting abnormalities is rarely necessary and is controversial. Heparin can be effective therapy in the coagulopathy associated with fetal death. Heparin is given in its usual anticoagulant doses by continuous intravenous infusion. However, in the face of active bleeding or surgical intervention (hysterotomy), heparin is probably contraindicated. In these cases the clotting abnormalities should be corrected by fresh frozen plasma and/or platelet transfusion. Pooled blood components, cyoprecipitate or fibrinogen should be avoided because of the risk of hepatitis and/or autoimmune deficiency disease.

Rhesus Sensitization. Any type of spontaneous abortion either in the first or second trimester is associated with varying degrees of fetal to maternal transfusion. The factors associated with greater risk are increasing gestational age, presence of antepartum bleeding and surgical manipulation. These facts are especially important to the Rhesus (Rh) negative unsensitized mother. The risk of sensitization with spontaneous abortion varies between 2 and 9%. All women who are Rh negative and unsensitized should receive RhoGAM prophylactically. For spontaneous abortion at less than 12 weeks, a 50 microgram dose is probably effective. After 12 weeks a 300 microgram dose is recommended. A Kleihauer-Betke test may predict more precisely the volume of fetal-maternal transfusion. The lack of utilization of RhoGAM in spontaneous abortion is a major source of Rhesus sensitization. Grimes and co-workers (1977) noted that about 20% of eligible women do not receive RhoGAM after spontaneous abortion. On a nationwide scale this translates to between 500 and 1000 new Rh sensitizations per year in the United States.

Counseling. Counseling in late second trimester abortion and fetal death is extremely important (Lewis, 1976; Kowalski, 1980; Lake et al, 1983). By the 18th to 20th week of pregnancy the fetus has become an entity; the mother has observable changes in body image and the fetus has identified itself by movement. All too often a fetal death is treated as a nonevent. The sight and touch of the baby is avoided by the parents, the body is removed quickly and quietly, the mother is isolated from "normal" mothers and medical personnel avoid discussing the issue. Such behavior may reinforce conscious and unconscious feelings of guilt and anger on the part of the parents. The parents should be encouraged to accept this fetus as an entity by seeing and touching the body. The causes and non-causes as well as the risk of recurrence should be openly discussed. Bringing the tragedy to the status of a reality will allow a more normal grief response. This therapy will reduce the risk of depression, frigidity, impotence, marital difficulties and damaging attitudes toward future children or pregnancies.

The risk of recurrence needs to be adequately examined and discussed with the parents. As much information as possible should be obtained at the time of evacuation. A minimum workup should include cervical cultures (gonorrhea, *Mycoplasma*, *Chlamydia*), manual examination of uterine contour at delivery, a pathologic examination of placenta and fetus and chromosomal studies of the fetus. Many cases will have no clear cause for fetal death. Problems such as incompetent cervix will benefit greatly from intervention.

Septic Abortion

CLINICAL PICTURE

Septic abortion conjures up images of desperate women being victimized in dark, unsterile backrooms. Fortunately this image is fading with legalized abortion. However, infection remains a common and potentially lethal complication in both spontaneous and therapeutic abortion (Grimes et al, 1981). Postoperative infection has been discussed earlier in this chapter under both spontaneous and therapeutic abortion. These sections were directed at the primary surgeon. However, all too often the obstetrician-gynecologist sees the patient late in the course of a septic complication and in a setting where he or she was not the primary surgeon. This section is designed to help the clinician manage these situations.

In most cases the history of a recent pregnancy, a recent outpatient therapeutic abortion or positive pregnancy test is clear, but should be confirmed. A negative home pregnancy test in the face of amenorrhea may suggest a false negative test, an event which occurs in 20% of tests. Without a confirmed history, any woman with pelvic infection and a menstrual history other than regular periods with moliminal changes needs a pregnancy test. A serum beta human chorionic gonadotropin (hCG) determination is recommended. In cases of instrumental trauma or abnormal pregnancy, the hCG level may be sufficiently low to be undetectable by conventional urine pregnancy tests.

Except for vaginal bleeding the presenting symptoms of septic abortion are not unlike those of pelvic inflammatory disease or septic complications of therapeutic abortion. A temperature greater than 38° C (100.4 F), lower abdominal and back pain, peritoneal pain, and heavy vaginal bleeding are the most common symptoms. When there has been a delay in seeking therapy, high fever, rigors and a foul smelling cervical discharge may be manifest. Risk factors for septic abortion are a history of recurrent pelvic inflammatory disease, current intrauterine device use and any concomitant immune system compromise, e.g., diabetes or recent cancer chemotherapy. In therapeutic abortion a history of passage of tissue after the abortion, complications of abortion or use of prophylactic antibiotics is important. Prophylactic antibiotics may significantly confuse the clinical presentation.

On physical examination the extent and complications of infection should be evaluated. Generalized peritonitis, the presence of adnexal masses and unstable cardiovascular state are important indicators of severe disease. Cardiac instability includes tachycardia (120 beats or more per minute), wide pulse pressure and orthostatic changes in both blood pressure and heart rate. Cold, sweaty, clammy skin should alert the clinician to life-threatening disease.

The microbiology of septic abortion is that of a multiorganism infection. Gram negative aerobes produce endotoxins that may cause many of the signs of shock. Anaerobes seem to be active in persistent infection. *Chlamydia*, *Mycoplasma*, and gonorrhea can also be present. Despite the multiplicity of organisms in septic abortion, there are three classes of infection that can be particularly virulent. *Staphylococcus aureus* can produce a toxic shock syndrome. Clostridial infection and beta hemolytic streptococcus can produce rapidly advancing fasciitis. The presence of these organisms should be identified early in therapy. In addition to aerobic and anaerobic cultures, a gram stain of the cervical discharge is performed. A gram stain of cervical discharge showing sheets of gram positive diplococci or club-shaped gram positive organisms with myometrial fragments should alert the clinician to streptococcal or clostridial infection.

Perforation must be suspected in all septic abortions when instrumentation has taken place. Clues to perforation include sudden severe abdominal pain during the procedure, history of difficult dilatation, fixed severely anteflexed or retroflexed uterus, inexperienced surgeons and history of second trimester therapeutic abortion. The physical signs of hemorrhage, rapidly developing generalized peritonitis and broad ligament masses should increase the suspicion of perforation. In these patients early laparoscopy may be indicated. In all patients with septic abortion, an abdominal flat plate and upright chest x-ray should be performed. These films will provide critical data concerning perforation of a viscus, intramyometrial or intrafascial gas (clostridial infection) and the presence of foreign objects.

The natural course of septic abortion follows a sequence of localized infection of the uterus that spreads to the tubes and peritoneum. Many of the systemic symptoms and eventual causes of death are only indirectly related to the bacteria. Thrombosis in the pelvic vessels from nearby infection poses a risk of pulmonary embolism. Massive activation of the complement system from bacterial endotoxins will cause uncontrolled release of cellular components such as histamines, kinins and other activators of the coagulation system. These participate in the clinically recognizable stages of septic shock. Hemorrhage is usually a common feature in death from septic abortion. The blood loss results from retained products of conception, perforation and coagulopathy from infection. Intravascular hemolysis from disseminated intravascular coagulation or *Clostridia* endotoxin contributes to the inability of the patient to relieve tissue hypoxia.

Advanced septic abortion leads to septic shock. The classification of septic shock is as follows:

1. Primary (reversible) septic shock
   a. warm hypotensive shock (early)
   b. cold hypotensive shock (late)
2. Secondary (irreversible) shock

A patient with warm hypotensive shock is characterized by skin that is flushed and warm. Usually she is alert and responsive. Her temperature is 38 to 40.5° C. She has a moderate tachycardia with a slightly widened pulse pressure (over 60 mm Hg). She shows orthostatic blood pressure and heart rate changes (greater than 15 mm Hg and 15 beats per minute). She will occasionally have rigors. Urinary output is good. Although the patient may remain in this phase for a considerable length of time, she may also rapidly pass into the more serious shock phases. Clinically, the transition often appears during a spike in the temperature. This observation tends to support the theory of endotoxic activation of the complement system.

The cold hypotensive phase of reversible shock is dramatic in its presentation. The patient appears moribund with obtunded mentation. Her skin is pale, cold and clammy. Subnormal temperature can be noted. Her blood pressure can no longer maintain adequate renal blood flow, and urinary output falls. She usually has a tachycardia of 120 to 140 beats per minute. The triad of hypotension, tachycardia and oliguria is characteristic of this phase.

In secondary irreversible shock, prolonged local tissue hypoxia results in metabolic acidosis and high blood lactate levels. Hypoperfusion and acidosis affect all organ systems including the cardiovascular system, which was previously compensating for infection. A rapid downward deterioration ensues with progressive cerebral, cardiac and respiratory dysfunction. Cardiac arrest, acute renal failure and adult respiratory distress syndrome are terminal events in these cases.

MANAGEMENT

The clinician may first see a patient in any phase of septic abortion. The first principle of management is a determination of the source and the extent of infection. Of clinical importance are signs of systemic disease: cardiovascular instability, disseminated intravascular coagulation, hemolysis or respiratory distress. The second principle, if septic shock is present, is to establish adequate surveillance systems: intravenous catheter (18 gauge or larger), Foley catheter and continuous human monitoring. Vital signs should be taken every 15 to 30 minutes. Strong consideration should be given to central venous or, preferably, pulmonary wedge pressures in patients with any cardiovascular instability. The third principle is early and adequate medical management, including broad spectrum antibiotics, fluid expansion and cardiac drugs (dopamine), to support the cardiovascular system, and the possibilities of steroid therapy in the most severe cases. The choice of antibiotic and the medical management of septic shock are discussed in Chapter 4. The fourth and most important principle is early surgical management. Antibiotic therapy without surgical management is a major mistake. The septic products of conception are relatively isolated from the antibiotics and will be a continuous source for endotoxin and blood loss. The sooner this risk is removed the more effective the management. Rapid attempts at stabilization of cardiovascular function should be initiated if necessary while the initial laboratory work is being completed. Antibiotics should be started immediately.

In a patient without previous instrumentation a suction curettage under local anesthesia is all that is needed. With prior instrumentation and possible uterine perforation laparoscopy may be indicated. Sepsis in a patient with an empty uterine cavity is highly suggestive of a perforation. These patients benefit from a repeat curettage and laparoscopy. The presence of hemolysis plus evidence of clostridial infection is a very grave sign. These patients need immediate laparotomy and hysterectomy with possible extensive debridement. The life expectancy in patients with clostridial infection with hemolysis is a matter of hours if debridement is not undertaken. Although usually less severe, extensive streptococcal infection may require aggressive surgical management with hysterectomy. The presence of a pelvic mass in septic abortion is an indication for laparotomy. The extent of surgery at this point is a very difficult question if the mass is an abscess. In terms of immediate postoperative risk a total abdominal hysterectomy and bilateral salpingo-oophorectomy has less chance of recurrent infection, pain and repeat surgery. However, it is not easy to decide to perform oophorectomy or hysterectomy in a young woman. Conservative surgery may be indicated in these cases. This entails removal of just the abscess, i.e., a unilateral or bilateral salpingectomy and conservation of the ovaries. It must be remembered that conservation of the uterus also requires evacuation of its contents with suction curettage.

A surgical principle of laparotomy, important and unique to septic cases, is the prevention of spread of infection by either the hematogenous or the intraperitoneal route. The blood supply should be isolated and clamped first, much as in a hysterectomy for cancer. This will reduce the operative blood loss and lessen dissemination of endotoxins or bacteria from manipulation of the infected tissue. Avoidance of upper abdominal exploration and effective isolation of the operative field with laparotomy sponges will reduce upper abdominal contamination. Blood and devitalized tissue can be excellent sources for continued infection. Hemostasis must be excellent, and bites of tissue should be small. If a hysterectomy has been performed, the vaginal cuff is best left open. Abscess cavities should be drained with closed suction drains.

Irrigation of the operative site should be performed in Fowler's position to avoid further peritoneal spread. Irrigation with antibiotic solution has been shown to reduce infection. Prior to closure, irrigation with a solution of 2 gm cefoxitin in 1000 ml normal saline will give surface tissue levels three to four times higher than if the antibiotic is given by the intravenous route. Infection will delay healing and will reduce the lasting strength of sutures, especially catgut. The use of polyglycolic suture for pedicles has the advantage of lasting strength. Use of the Smead-Jones technique with permanent suture is indicated in closure of the abdominal wall (see Chapter 3).

Wound infection will occur in 10 to 20% of cases. This increased risk is secondary to innoculation by septic peritoneal contents and loculated tissue fluids after closure. Delayed skin closure has been advocated by some to reduce the risk of wound infection. One method of doing this is as follows. The skin is left open with moistened sponges as packing. After one to three days the wound is inspected and if the infection is minimal or absent, the wound is closed under local anesthesia. Delayed skin closure may reduce the incidence of wound infection by 75%. Another alternative is to use subcutaneous drains for up to 24 hours postoperatively. It must be remembered that drains can act as wicks for surface bacteria. Also these drains should not come out of the center of the incision but inferior or lateral to it.

Infections of the pelvis and wound are the major concerns in the postoperative period in patients having a laparotomy for septic complications of pregnancy. Continued pelvic cellulitis requires intravenous antibiotics for at least five days and until the patient has been afebrile for 48 hours. Wound infection will depend on the skin closure. Primary skin closure in a contaminated wound will be complicated by wound infections in about 20% of cases. Briefly, wound infection is best managed by close observation for spread (fasciitis), application of local moist heat and early drainage of collections of pus (see Chapter 4). Unless there is significant cellulitis, antibiotics may not add to the efficacy of drainage.

Pelvic thrombophlebitis is a constant risk of any surgery in the pelvis. Infection increases local coagulability and causes vascular endothelial damage by direct extension and/or toxins. The hypercoagulability of normal pregnancy enhances the risk of pelvic thrombophlebitis in septic abortion. The prevention of this complication is difficult, although the use of antibiotics that cover anaerobes seems to reduce the incidence of both thrombophlebitis and abscess. Intravenous heparin is given for 10 to 14 days. Anticoagulation is documented by a partial thromboplastin time one and a half to two times the control time. The use of heparin, theoretically, will prevent the further growth and embolization of existing clots. Pulmonary embolism in the face of adequate coagulation is the major indication for surgical ligation of the vena cava and ovarian veins. In the non-pregnant patient the transcutaneous placement of an umbrella in the vena cava is both less morbid and more efficacious. However, during pregnancy, the ovarian veins dilate and can be a major source of emboli. Thus surgical ligation may be necessary (see Chapter 4).

INCOMPETENT CERVIX

Cervical incompetence (CI) is the apparent failure of the cervical sphincter (internal os) to maintain closure until term. Classically the clinical history is one or more midterm losses after painless dilatation of the cervix. Rather than contractions the patient feels pelvic pressure, vaginal discharge and urinary urgency and frequency. Delivery is rapid and relatively asymptomatic. There may be confusing findings such as spotting, contractions or rupture of membranes. Cervical incompetence must be differentiated from premature labor, abruption or amnionitis as a source of mid-trimester fetal loss. Cervical incompetence accounts for 15 to 25% of mid-trimester losses. About 0.5 to 1% of all pregnancies are complicated by incompetent cervix (Cousins, 1980).

The chief causes of cervical incompetence are trauma (30 to 50%) and congenital abnormalities of the cervix (20 to 40%). In the remaining 20% no cause can be found. Trauma includes the disruption of the internal integrity of the cervix by cone biopsy, forced cervical dilatation, forceps, precipitous delivery or vaginal breech delivery. Cervical laceration can also be a result of low vertical cesarean section or an inferior extension of a transverse uterine incision.

Stillman (1982) reports a 25 to 55% chance of an adverse pregnancy outcome and only 40 to 70% chance of a viable pregnancy in DES-exposed female offspring because of congenital abnormalities. The presence of cervico-vaginal or upper tract changes seems to increase the risk but adverse outcomes can occur with normal appearance of the cervix and vagina (15 versus 4% in controls). This could imply a role for cervical incompetence.

Complications of Diagnosis

The consequences or complications of a mistaken diagnosis of cervical incompetence is that unnecessary treatment may be given. On the other hand, if the diagnosis is made too late, treatment may be ineffective in preventing premature delivery. The crux of pre-conceptional diagnosis of cervical incompetence rests on an adequate history of previous labor experiences, abortion history, and in utero exposure to DES. Outpatient procedures that have been advocated to confirm the diagnosis of cervical incompetence include direct measurement of the cervical canal diameter (hysterosalpingogram), intracervical balloon traction tests or the free passage of a number 8 Hagar dilator through the cervical canal. Any one of these tests may raise or lower the level of suspicion but none are confirmatory for cervical incompetence.

Harger (1983) has critically reviewed diagnostic tests for cervical incompetence and has concluded that no test successfully withstands scientific scrutiny.

During pregnancy it is important to make the diagnosis prior to excessive dilatation of the cervix (greater than 3 cm) or prior to 22 weeks, and this is not easy. Since many patients are relatively asymptomatic, the obstetrician must rely on good patient follow-up and frequent cervical examinations in high risk pregnancies. High resolution ultrasonography may provide further clues in the asymptomatic patient at 18 weeks or more gestation. Brook and co-workers (1981) described a consistent finding of increased anterio-posterior diameter (over 2.57 cm) of the cervix at the level of the internal os in women with incompetent cervices when compared with controls (1.67 cm).

Complications of Management

The treatment of cervical incompetence includes medical and surgical management. The effectiveness and complications of these methods are difficult to assess because not all causes of CI are recognized nor can it always be differentiated from other causes of premature labor, and because most studies rely on retrospective data and have major biases. These weaknesses are:

1. Diagnostic criteria are frequently omitted.
2. Definitions of successful outcome vary.
3. Treatment approaches are not detailed.
4. Fetal salvage is not stated nor is it adequate, i.e., the inclusion of first trimester spontaneous abortions with prior losses. This worsens the cerclage salvage index.
5. Cases are not categorized by etiology.
6. Results include combined therapies i.e. cerclage plus bedrest plus progesterone.
7. Complication rates are not adequately presented i.e. loss secondary to the procedure or the frequency of preterm birth.
8. Statistically, the chance of subsequent preterm loss after one such loss is only 15%; after two subsequent losses the risk is 30% (Bakketeig et al, 1979). In most studies cases are not categorized by previous abortion history.
9. A common method of evaluating successful cerclage is to divide the number of surviving infants after the procedure by the number of surviving infants prior to the procedure, the infant salvage ratio. This technique does not take into account improvement of prenatal and

neonatal care in the high risk mother receiving a cerclage.

Selection bias can have a major impact even in prospective randomized studies. For example, Lazar and co-workers (1984) and Rush and co-workers (1984) showed that cerclage did not seem to affect outcome in both moderate and high risk patients in two prospective randomized trials. These two studies underline the need for scientific study of the efficacy and cost effectiveness of cerclage. The infant salvage ratio of various management schemes is shown in Table 8–12. The following sections describe the complications and weaknesses of the various managements in addition to the overall statistical weaknesses concerning management of CI.

MEDICAL THERAPY

The medical treatment of cervical incompetence has included bedrest, progesterone and the use of a pessary. The reduction of activity including bedrest is a standard part of therapy in all intervention for cervical incompetence. There has been no scientific evaluation of its efficacy but conventional wisdom suggests some good results. The risks of prolonged bedrest include failure of compliance (voluntary or involuntary), disruption of home or economic support and, probably, an increase in the incidence of pulmonary embolism. These have not been studied.

The basis for the use of progesterone is that elevated progesterone concentrations are associated with decreased isthmic and cervical diameters. Progesterone may also make the myometrium refractory to oxytocin and change the

biochemical characteristics of the cervical stroma. These theories are the basis of studies using 17α-hydroxyprogesterone caproate (Delalutin) in the prevention of midtrimester loss (Johnson et al, 1979). Although very high success rates (80 to 90%) are reported, these studies suffer from many of the methodologic weaknesses described earlier. The complications of this therapy are the theoretical inability to affect the outcome of pregnancies complicated by cervical incompetence from extensive external trauma and the risk of teratogenesis from progesterone. The teratogenic risk is largely overestimated, as outlined by Wilson and Brent (1981) in their excellent review. Furthermore, the drug is given at a stage of gestation when non-genital organ systems are already developed and have a low vulnerability to teratogens. The development of the reproductive tract is an exception. Diethylstilbestrol (DES)-induced genital tract lesions have been shown to result from exposure at 14 to 20 weeks gestation, albeit at a lower rate than at 8 to 14 weeks (Kaufman et al, 1980). It is incumbent on the advocates of progesterone to prove that natural progesterones do not cause the same reproductive tract abnormalities that DES has caused.

The use of a pessary has been advocated by some earlier authors such as Vitsky (1968). The efficacy reported is comparable to other methods (infant salvage ratio of 4.16). However, many methodologic omissions weaken the conclusions. In theory the pessary displaces the cervix posteriorly, relieves direct pressure on the cervix by elevation of the fetal head and provides vaginal reinforcement of the cervix. The major risk of a pessary is infection. A

*Table 8–12. Infant Salvage Ratios in Cervical Incompetence**

| Treatment | Before Treatment | | | After Treatment | | | Infant Salvage Ratio |
	Pregnancies (No.)	Survivors (No.)	Mean (%)	Pregnancies (No.)	Survivors (No.)	Mean (%)	
Pessary	193	42	21.8	64	58	90.6	4.16
Progesterone	414	104	25.1	74	68	91.9	3.66
Surgery							
1. Lash Procedure	355	41	11.5	77	61	99.2	6.89
2. Shirodkar Cerclage	1957	427	21.8	898	739	82.3	3.78
3. MacDonald Cerclage	751	204	27.2	292	215	73.6	2.71
4. Transabdominal Late Cerclage	185	34	18.4	107	91	85.0	4.62

*From Cousins SL: Cervical incompetence 1980: a time for reappraisal. *Clin. Obstet. Gynecol.* 23:467, 1980. Reprinted with permission.

foreign body in the vagina will certainly change the flora, perhaps to more virulent varieties. Cervical infection plays a significant role in the pathology of cervical incompetence. Once cervical incompetence progresses to a point at which the membranes are exposed to the vaginal flora, a subclinical infection of the membranes can occur. The activation of phospholipase A by bacteria or the maternal leukocytes initiates the production of prostaglandins. The local effect of prostaglandins on the cervix has been well demonstrated, i.e., softening and dilatation. This may progress with painless dilatation and exposure of a larger area of membranes, leading to subclinical chorioamnionitis. Host response with leukocyte infiltration causes an increased production of prostaglandins. The ensuing contractions and the production of cytolytic enzymes cause rupture of the membranes. Neither bedrest, progesterone nor a pessary reduces the exposure of the amnion to the vagina.

SURGICAL PROCEDURES

Most obstetricians rely on surgery in the treatment of cervical incompetence. The objective is to repair the primary anatomic defect or to reinforce cervical resistance by a circumferential suture or band. In the non-pregnant patient with anatomic defects, the procedure most often chosen is the "Lash" procedure. During pregnancy, Shirodkar's and McDonald's cerclages are often used. Occasionally patients will present in pregnancy with a congenitally short or amputated cervix, marked scarring or deep external lacerations. In these patients a transabdominal approach with cerclage at the level of the uterosacral and cardinal ligaments is the only choice.

Repair of a Uterocervical Defect or Fistula. In the non-pregnant patient, the anatomic defect most commonly identified is a deep cervical laceration. The surgical procedure is initiated with gentle reflection of the mucosa surrounding the defect. The bladder base is likely to be densely adherent to the defect. Any fistulous tract is then removed. A small endometrial biopsy at the apex of the defect will confirm the extent of the cervical lesion. The raw edges of the cervix are closed in layers of 00 polyglycolic sutures. The mucosa is then closed with interrupted simple sutures of 00 polyglycolic acid. Injury to the bladder anteriorly and to the uterine artery and ureters laterally are the most important surgical complications. A preopera-

tive intravenous pyelogram is helpful in identifying ureteral abnormalities. The bladder mucosa may be stained with methylene blue preoperatively for quick identification of a laceration. Another helpful technique is to identify the inferior reflection of the bladder on the cervix by a probe introduced through the urethra. The infant salvage ratio for reconstructive repair of the cervix is 6.9 as shown in Table 8–12.

Midtrimester Cerclage. Two operations are commonly used for the incompetent cervix during pregnancy, the McDonald and the Shirodkar procedures. McDonald's procedure is technically the easier, consisting of a simple purse string suture of a 5-mm Mersaline strip anchored with two silk sutures to the mucosa. The suture must be placed as high on the cervix as possible to be effective. This endangers the bladder anteriorly; injury can be avoided by identifying the bladder reflection with a probe. The author's practice is to place the knot posteriorly, feeling that an anterior knot irritates the bladder and increases the risk of urinary infection. However, a posterior knot makes removal somewhat more difficult. Finally, as little as possible of the Mersaline should be exposed. The suture can be a nidus of vaginal infection.

The Shirodkar procedure involves placing an encircling Dacron or Mersaline band beneath the mucosa at the level of the internal cervical os and suturing it in place. More dissection is required than with the McDonald operation. The choice between the two procedures depends largely upon the surgeon's training and experience. The McDonald suture can be placed under paracervical block, but the Shirodkar requires general or conduction anesthesia. The risks of Shirodkar's procedure are very similar to removal of a cervical fistula, with possible urinary tract and vascular injury. Increased blood loss occurs at the reflection of the mucosa. An additional problem is the increased difficulty in removal secondary to cervical scarring. This has resulted in a significantly increased cesarean section rate in the Shirodkar procedure versus the McDonald procedure (15% vs. 6%) (Harger, 1980).

Any patient who is a candidate for a cerclage procedure must be assessed for the surgical risk. Table 8–13 depicts the frequency of complications of combined cerclage procedures. About 2 to 4% of pregnancies will be lost as a result of the procedure. Chorioamnionitis, with or without ruptured membranes, causes 60% of

Table 8–13. Complications of Cerclage*

Complication	Percent	Range (%)
Postoperative rupture of membranes (PROM)	2.3	1.1–9.0
Postoperative chorioamnionitis (No PROM)	1.7	0.8–7.7
Suture displacement	4.3	3.0–13.0
Parturitional cervical laceration	3.4	0.7–13.2
Premature delivery	26.0	25.0–33.0
Cesarean section for cervical dystocia	3.5	1.4–4.3

*From Harger JH: Cervical cerclage: patient selection, morbidity and success rate. *Clin. Perinatol.* 10:321, 1983. Reprinted with permission.

the losses. About 26% of patients will deliver pre-term (28 to 37 weeks) fetuses or those small for gestational age. Displacment of the suture, requiring a decision whether or not to replace it, occurs in 5% of the cases. Premature contractions requiring tocolysis occur in 6 to 24%. Cervical dystocia from scar tissue formed by the procedure occurs in 1 to 5%.

Harger (1980) carefully reviewed the factors associated with success of the procedure and the incidence of complications. Operations performed for the classic indication, two or more painless second trimester losses, were associated with the best success. When current cervical dilatation was used as an indication it was not associated with an improvement following cerclage. Emergency cerclage, cervical dilatation greater than 3 cm and suture after 20 weeks were associated with a reduced fetal salvage rate to 50 to 60% and an increase in postoperative rupture of the membranes and chorioanmionitis.

Both cerclage procedures complicate the method of delivery. Either the suture must be cut or a cesarean section performed. It may not be easy to decide when to cut the suture, nor is cutting it simple if the suture is buried. Cesarean section adds to the morbidity of delivery, but a successful suture may help carry another pregnancy without complications.

Complications of cerclage procedures can be prevented or reduced by recognizing uterine bleeding, active labor, ruptured membranes, a widely dilated cervix, fetal anomalies and polyhydramnios as contraindications to operation. Cerclage should be performed after 12 weeks' gestation to avoid first trimester pregnancy complications. The prophylactic use of antibiotics has not been adequately studied. However, preoperative cervical cultures for *N. gonorrhoeae*, mycoplasmas, *Chlamydia* and group B streptococcus should be performed. The prophylactic use of tocolysis has not been properly studied. It would seem prudent to treat only those patients with postoperative contractions.

Late Cerclage. Occasionally the diagnosis of cervical incompetence is made late. The woman presents in late second trimester with (1) cervical effacement greater than 50%; (2) cervical dilatation greater than 4 cm; (3) herniation of intact membranes through an open cervix; (4) a live intrauterine fetus; (5) absence of established labor; (6) absence of established vaginal bleeding and (7) no clinical evidence of infection. The prognosis without treatment is hopeless. Olatunbosun and Dyck (1981) and Goodlin (1979) have argued for cerclage. The preparation for cerclage involves a reduction of the herniated forewaters by amniocentesis, Trendelenburg position and general anesthesia (uterine relaxation). Filling the bladder with 400 to 500 ml of saline may reduce the membranes without the risks of amniocentesis. The cervix is then pulled forward by four stay sutures at 3, 6, 9, and 12 o'clock. The membranes are gently pushed back by a sponge forceps and cotton balls. The cervix is then closed with large mattress sutures of single stranded nylon. Both the mentioned papers recommend prophylactic antibiotic therapy for the prevention of post-cerclage chrioamnionitis. Cultures of the cervix should be taken prior to the procedure. The combined success rate of the two studies was 14 out of 21 living children. Bedrest and hospitalization are recommended for four to five days postoperatively. Any sign of infection would be an indication for prompt pregnancy termination.

Transabdominal Cerclage. Another uncommon occurrence is the patient whose cervix is either congenitally foreshortened or so traumatized that transvaginal cerclage is not possible in pregnancy. These patients may be candidates for permanent cerclage at the level of the uterosacral and cardinal ligaments. The procedure involved is a laparotomy through either a transverse or a vertical incision. The vesico-uterine peritoneal reflection is divided transversely, and the bladder is reflected off the lower uterine segment. The increased vascularity laterally is quite apparent. A space medial to and between the ascending and descending branches of the uterine arteries is developed, using blunt dissection. A right-angled clamp with tapered jaws is ideal for this part of the procedure. Once the cardinal ligaments have been perforated bilaterally, an encircling 5-mm Mersaline band is placed around the cervix at the level of the internal os. The band is tightened snugly and tied in a square knot. The free ends are secured with 00 silk sutures. The bladder flap is then closed with a running suture of 000 chromic catgut.

This approach to the management of cervical incompetence must be reserved for a highly selected group of patients. The risks include hemorrhage from the uterine vessels or injury to the distal ureter and the need for two major procedures—permanent placement of the suture and cesarean section.

ECTOPIC PREGNANCY

The incidence of ectopic pregnancy has doubled from 1970 to 1980 in the United States (Rubin et al, 1983). A similar rise has taken place in Sweden (Westrom et al, 1981) and in the British Isles (Beral, 1975). In 1978 the incidence was 9.4 per 1000 conceptions in the United States. Thus, approximately 42,400 patients underwent surgical procedures to correct this problem and in the process were exposed to a wide variety of complications. However, this may not represent the true incidence of surgical risk. Data on the number of women with a preoperative diagnosis of ectopic pregnancy and a different postoperative diagnosis are not readily available. It is reasonable to assume that two to three surgical procedures (laparoscopy, dilatation and curettage and laparotomy) are often performed for one postoperative diagnosis of ectopic pregnancy. The postoperative diagnosis in the other cases would be one of the following: pelvic inflammatory disease, ovarian cyst, appendicitis, "normal pregnancy," or a variety of less frequent conditions. Thus, at least 100,000 women per year may be at risk for surgical complications of the diagnosis and treatment of ectopic pregnancies.

Complications of Diagnosis

Early diagnosis has the greatest influence on the surgical management and prognosis and is the key to reducing the complications of ectopic pregnancy. Thus, delays and errors in diagnosis contribute significantly to the complications.

The availability of very sensitive pregnancy tests (quantitative hCG) has been a major breakthrough in the diagnosis of early pregnancy complications. A positive pregnancy test eliminates alternative diagnoses such as pelvic inflammatory disease. Prior to the development of radioimmunoassay techniques as many as 50% of women with ectopic pregnancies had a negative slide test for pregnancy. This lack of sensitivity probably results in many "negative" laparotomies or laparoscopies. In the stable patient, diagnostic and therapeutic operations should await radioimmunoassay for hCG if the results of less expensive tests are negative.

Despite the availability of good pregnancy testing there is a dangerous disinterest in pregnancy testing for women of childbearing age. Laubach and Wilchins (1977) initiated urine pregnancy testing on all women between the ages of 12 and 50 admitted to a 300 bed acute care community hospital. In the first two years 2077 patients were screened. Forty-five percent of women with positive tests did not know that they were pregnant. Many were having extensive diagnostic x-ray workups for pelvic masses or nausea and vomiting. Brenner and co-workers (1980) found in 300 consecutive ectopic pregnancies that 50% of patients had medical consultation more than 24 hours prior to the diagnosis of ectopic pregnancy. Of these 150 patients, 38% had two or more consultations. Clearly, these statistics indicate that patients and health care providers both need education as to the signs of pregnancy and ectopic pregnancy.

Although the pregnancy test significantly simplifies the differential diagnosis, there are many other first trimester complications that mimic ectopic pregnancy and constitute diagnostic complications. Halpin (1970) found that of patients admitted for suspected ectopic pregnancy with positive pregnancy tests, 37% had a diagnosis other than ectopic pregnancy. In order to exclude other diagnoses clinical history, levels of hCG, ultrasonographic examination, uterine curettage, and culdocentesis are important.

Clinical history and physical examination are only moderately sensitive and specific. Halpin (1970) compared ectopic cases to non-ectopic cases in relation to the classic signs and symptoms of irregular bleeding, abdominal pain, abdominal tenderness and adnexal masses. These "classic" signs were about 50% sensitive and about 60% specific for actual ectopic pregnancy.

Ultrasonographic examinations are used extensively in suspected cases of ectopic pregnancy. Four prospective ultrasonographic evaluations for ectopic pregnancy (Gleicher et al, 1983; Levi and Leblicq, 1980; Kelly et al, 1979; Lawson 1978) revealed that about 75% of 792 patients had a clear ultrasonic diagnosis of ectopic pregnancy. Subsequent comparison with the final diagnosis showed a sensitivity of 74% and a specificity of 96%. The two most important findings are an intrauterine gestational sac, especially with a double sac sign, and a gestational sac outside the uterus. A diagnosis of intrauterine pregnancy virtually excludes the diagnosis of ectopic pregnancy. The risk of a combined intrauterine and extrauterine gestation is 1:10,000 to 20,000. The demonstration of a gestational sac with a fetal pole outside the uterus is a finding highly sensitive for ectopic pregnancy.

Apart from the diagnosis of pregnancy, serial measurements of hCG have been used to predict abnormal pregnancy. Kadar (1981) found that normal pregnancy beta hCG levels rose by at least 66% within a 48 hour sampling interval. No normal pregnancy was associated with a falling hCG. The rate of rise of hCG in ectopic pregnancy was less than one half of that in intrauterine pregnancies. When the lower limit of a normal rise in hCG was set at 29% for a one day sampling interval, 66% for 2 days, 114% for 3 days, 175% for 4 days, and 255% for 5 days, he found a sensitivity of 86% and specificity of 86%.

Diagnostic curettage is most helpful in ruling in spontaneous abortion or other first trimester intrauterine pregnancy complications. The key histologic finding is trophoblastic or other fetal tissue. This finding has a very high sensitivity for intrauterine pregnancy (99%). On the other hand, the classic hypersecretory endometrium (Arias-Stella reaction) is found in only 50 to 70% of ectopic pregnancies. Apart from terminating an unsuspected intrauterine pregnancy, complications of diagnostic curettage are primarily related to surgical trauma, such as cervical injury and perforation. The management of these complications is discussed earlier in this chapter.

The presence of intraabdominal blood is an important indicator used in the diagnosis of ruptured ectopic pregnancy. A transabdominal or transvaginal (culdocentesis) sampling can be used. A culdocentesis can be performed on an outpatient basis with minimal discomfort to the patient. With traction on the posterior lip of the cervix, an 18-gauge spinal needle attached to a 10-ml syringe is inserted into the cul-de-sac under local anesthesia and the contents of the cul-de-sac aspirated (see Chapter 12). Nonclotting blood is suggestive of intraperitoneal bleeding. Determination of the fluid's hematocrit is also helpful.

Culdocentesis is the most sensitive test for (ruptured) ectopic pregnancy except for laparoscopy. Collected data (Alsuleiman and Grimes, 1982; Brenner et al, 1980; Helvacioglu et al, 1979; Halpin, 1970; Webster et al, 1965; Chez and Moore, 1963) show that 1,364 of 1,451 (94%) had nonclotting blood (positive test) on culdocentesis performed with ectopic pregnancy. Among all patients seen with possible ectopic pregnancy, about 26% of those without ectopic pregnancy will have bloody fluid on culdocentesis (Halpin, 1970). Most often ruptured corpus luteum cysts are present in these cases. Hibbard (1979) noted that when the hematocrit of the fluid was less than 12%, a stable patient could be managed conservatively, until the results of a pregnancy test were obtained.

Apart from the complications of an error in diagnosis, the other side effects of culdocentesis are relatively minor. They include injury to neighboring structures, i.e., colon or pelvic vessels. A retroverted uterus may be penetrated and oftentimes gives a bloody tap. One known death has been reported from culdocentesis; in this patient a pelvic kidney was injured. These risks are best avoided by a careful pre-procedure pelvic examination. Culdocentesis should not be attempted in cases in which the uterus is fixed in the cul-de-sac.

Laparoscopy is the standard of diagnosis for unruptured ectopic pregnancy. Samuelson and Sjovall (1972) examined the sensitivity and specifity of laparoscopy in 489 cases of suspected ectopic pregnancy. They found that in 2.2% of cases the pelvic organs could not be visualized well enough for diagnosis. In technically successful and interpretable laparoscopies one ectopic pregnancy was overlooked in 166 cases (0.6%). A false diagnosis of ectopic pregnancy was made in 1.9% of cases. The total diagnostic error when laparoscopy failed as a diagnostic tool was 4.7%. The complications of laparoscopy are discussed in Chapter 6.

Procedures

SALPINGECTOMY

Salpingectomy is the most common surgical procedure for the treatment of ectopic pregnancy. Even in centers in which conservative surgery is advocated (DeCherney and Minken, et al, 1981) the incidence is 60 to 80%. A vertical rather than a transverse (Pfannenstiel) incision is preferable unless the diagnosis of ectopic pregnancy is clear, for example, after laparoscopic visualization. Many investigators, including the author, recommend cornual resection to reduce the risks of future cornual ectopic pregnancy. Support for this is largely theoretical. The special surgical complications of cornual resection are blood loss and excessive myometrial removal. Blood loss may be reduced by placing a purse string suture prior to wedging out the interstitial portion of the tube. Excessive myometrial removal may compromise intrauterine integrity in future pregnancy. Hallatt (1975) described four interstitial pregnancies among 123 repeat ectopic pregnancies, all occurring after cornual resection. Prior to closure, in all procedures for ectopic pregnancy, many authors advocate the use of adhesion reducing agents, e.g., dextran 70. The efficacy of this approach is uncertain and is discussed in Chapter 4. The use of prophylactic antibiotics is prudent because of the association of ectopic pregnancy with histologic evidence of salpingitis. Agents effective against *N. gonorrhoeae*, *Chlamydia* and *Mycoplasma* should be used in combination or alone.

In the past, ipsilateral oophorectomy has been advocated out of fear that subsequent ovulation from that ovary will increase the chances of repeat ectopic pregnancy. Regardless of the management of the ovary, the risk of repeat ectopic pregnancy is 10 to 15%. There are no controlled data to support a reduction of this risk by oophorectomy. On the other hand, there is morbidity from the additional procedure. Increased surgical adhesions and alteration in the volume of estrogen-producing tissue may add to the already dismal fertility rate in patients with a history of ectopic pregnancy.

Occasionally the surgeon entertains the possibility of hysterectomy as management. An example would be the patient with an ectopic pregnancy after tubal ligation. The actual incidence of concurrent hysterectomy varies from close to zero in more recent series to 42% at Charity Hospital in New Orleans from 1959 to 1963 (Webster et al, 1965). There is considerable morbidity associated with hysterectomy (see Chapter 6) and in the vast majority of cases the procedure is not justified. The advent of in vitro fertilization provides hope for the infertile patient who has had both tubes removed but retains her uterus.

LINEAR SALPINGOSTOMY

Linear salpingostomy is the most important procedure in conservative management of ectopic pregnancy and preservation of tubal patency in patients who desire further pregnancy, who have an unruptured tubal gestation and who are surgically stable. An incision is made on the antimesenteric border of the tube and the conceptus is shelled out using suction, scoop or a knife handle. The tubal wall is then closed in one or two layers using 5-0 or 6-0 polyglycolic or nylon suture, or it may be left open and allowed to close secondarily.

SEGMENTAL EXCISION

Segmental excision may be used when there has been recent rupture of a early gestation, in order to conserve as much of the normal tube as possible and permit reconstructive surgery in the future. Non-absorbable (2-0 or 3-0) monofilament sutures are passed through an avascular space in the mesosalpinx and are then tied down proximal and distal to the ectopic gestation. A prior salpingostomy may be helpful. The ligated segment of the tube is then removed.

LAPAROSCOPIC EXCISION

Experienced laparoscopic surgeons have been successful in the management of unruptured ectopic pregnancy through the laparoscope alone (DeCherney, et al, 1981; Bruhat et al, 1980). The techniques described are linear salpingostomy, electrocoagulation and a snare technique. The advantages of these techniques are limitation of hospital stay and reduction of iatrogenic adhesions. However, all authors use strict criteria for the selection of patients. Failure to observe them makes complications more likely. Criteria include:

1. Extensive experience with the operating laparoscope and appropriate equipment.

2. Unruptured ectopic pregnancy in the isthmus (electrocoagulation) or in the ampullary portion of the tube (linear salpingostomy). Ectopic pregnancy near the cornu has extensive blood supply, and removal should not be attempted.

3. Ectopic gestation less than 3 cm in diameter.

4. Gestation of less than 8 weeks' duration.

5. Stable vital signs with no more than 100 to 200 ml of blood in the peritoneal cavity.

6. Normal pelvic anatomy without extensive

adhesions or limited laparoscopic view. The contralateral tube should appear normal.

7. Patients who are likely to have good follow-up.

The complications of operative laparoscopy are covered in Chapter 6. Prophylactic antibiotics are advisable. The patient should be counseled about the rare possibility of late hemorrhage.

TUBAL ABORTION

Early in the era of conservative management, tubal abortion was advocated. The technique involved expressing the products of conception out of the end of the tube. This may work well when tubal abortion has already taken place, i.e., gestation at the very distant ampulla or in the fimbria. Tubal abortion in more proximal gestations results in complications. As the ectopic pregnancy grows it invades beneath the endosalpinx and into the muscular layers. Squeezing out the tubal gestation will increase injury to the endosalpinx by stripping the mucosa from the muscle. Timonen and Neiminen (1967) showed an increased risk of repeat ectopic pregnancy in patients managed with tubal abortion.

SEGMENTAL RESECTION AND ANASTOMOSIS

Experienced tubal surgeons have advocated segmental resection and primary anastomosis in patients with unruptured isthmic ectopic pregnancies. A segmental excision is performed under microscopic control. Three sutures of 8-0 nylon on a CE-30 needle (Davis and Geckco) are placed at 8, 12 and 4 o'clock around the circumference of the tube. The sutures are placed in such a manner as to include the muscularis and the serosa but to avoid inclusion of the endosalpinx. A 6-0 nylon suture is then used to close the mesosalpinx. Tubal patency is assessed by occluding the lower uterine segment with a Buxton clamp and instilling dilute methylene blue transfundally. The distal tube is evaluated by retrograde perfusion of methylene blue from the fimbriated end. These techniques positively identify tubal patency, but should blockage be apparent the surgeon will not know whether the cause is reversible, i.e. from the decidua or edema.

Perioperative and Short-Term Complications

Table 8–14 presents the cumulative incidence of perioperative and short-term complications from selected references in the literature. Conclusions and suggested interventions are discussed.

CORNUAL OR INTERSTITIAL PREGNANCY

These pregnancies usually present later in gestation and often in a catastrophic pattern. The key to surgical management is stopping the

Table 8–14. Cumulative Morbidity of Ectopic Pregnancy in 2156 Patients*

Complications	Total No. of Patients Where Complications Assessed	No. With Complications	Percent With Complications	Range (%)
Interstitial pregnancy	1444	63	4.3	2.6–16.6
Ruptured ectopic pregnancy	1008	938	93	46.0–99
Concurrent operation				
Hysterectomy	1665	284	17.0	2.5–32
Tubal ligation	662	62	9.4	3.3–13.4
Oophorectomy	1511	484	32.0	10.7–42.7
Blood loss > 1000 ml	1199	327	27.0	18.6–43
Blood loss > 1500 ml	554	88	15.8	9.0–26
Transfusion (1 unit or more)	1760	1020	57.9	32.0–64
Antibiotic therapy	1369	619	45.2	31.0–55
Urinary tract infection	299	29	10.0	2.0–29
Pulmonary complications	998	103	10.3	3.0–13
Wound infection	944	81	8.5	3.0–9.2
Ileus	902	278	30.8	2.7–39

*Data from Weinstein L, Morris MB et al: *Obstet. Gynecol.* 61:698, 1983; Alsuleiman SA, Grimes EM: *J. Reprod. Med.* 27:101, 1982; Brenner PF, Roy S, Mishell DR: *J. Am. Med. Assoc.* 243:673, 1980; Helvacioglu A, Long EM, Yang SL: *J. Reprod. Med.* 22:87, 1979; Kitchen JD, Wein RM et al: *Am. J. Obstet. Gynecol.* 134:870, 1979; Harralson JD, Van Nagell JR, Raddick JW: *Am. J. Obstet. Gynecol.* 115:995, 1973; Halpin TF: *Am. J. Obstet. Gynecol.* 106:227, 1970; Webster HD, Barclay DL, Fischer CK: *Am. J. Obstet. Gynecol.* 92:23, 1965; Chez RA, Moore JG: *Surg. Gynecol. Obstet.* 117:589, 1963.

hemorrhage by isolation and ligation of the ascending uterine and utero-ovarian arteries. Hemorrhage and hematoma in the broad ligament will distort the normal position of the ureter; blind clamping should not be done. The bleeding may necessitate hypogastric artery ligation. This procedure is outlined in Chapter 3.

RUPTURED ECTOPIC PREGNANCY

The incidence of rupture of an ectopic pregnancy will fall with increased health care awareness, early and more sensitive pregnancy testing, early diagnosis and earlier treatment. A reasonable, modern figure is that 20 to 40% of ectopic pregnancies will be unruptured at the time of surgery and, therefore, amenable to conservative management.

CONCURRENT OPERATION

The incidence of hysterectomy is clearly falling and rightfully so. The morbidity and mortality of hysterectomy do not justify its performance. In addition, the option of in vitro fertilization emphasizes the importance of retaining the uterus.

Concurrent oophorectomy was performed more frequently in earlier studies, but does not seem to be justified (see earlier discussion). Concurrent tubal ligation is an option in surgically stable patients who provide informed consent for sterilization. Two cautions must be noted. First, the success rate is probably decreased, especially if techniques are used that do not involve burying the proximal tube. The Uchida and Irving techniques have been most successful. Second, ectopic pregnancies are associated with a 20 to 40% incidence of concurrent pelvic infection. The presence of foreign bodies (ring or clip) will increase infectious morbidity. Treatment courses of antibiotics are indicated in concurrent tubal ligation.

HEMORRHAGE

Blood loss is the greatest morbid risk of ectopic pregnancy. Except for radical operations for cancer, procedures for ectopic pregnancy have the greatest need for blood transfusion in obstetrics and gynecology. Luckily, the usual patient with an ectopic pregnancy has a healthy cardiovascular system. The surgeon must always be prepared to handle hemorrhagic shock (see Chapter 3). Transfusions should be used with discretion. There is a 7% chance of hepatitis from a one unit blood transfusion and an undefined risk of acquired immune deficiency syndrome (AIDS). Transfusion should be reserved for the hemodynamically unstable patient, the significantly symptomatic postoperative patient or the patient who will not comply with oral iron therapy postoperatively.

INFECTION

Twenty to forty percent of patients will have evidence of existing salpingitis. Usually these are multiorganism infections and may be associated with an intrauterine device or gonococcal or chlamydial infection. Because of these risks all patients with ectopic pregnancy should receive at least prophylactic antibiotics. Patients with evidence of pelvic inflammatory disease (adhesions or hydrosalpinx) should receive a full treatment course of broad spectrum antibiotics. *Chlamydia* is associated with a 20 to 40% incidence of pelvic infection and may actually cause much of the tubal and peritubal adhesions. A postoperative course of a tetracycline is indicated.

PULMONARY, URINARY, AND GASTROINTESTINAL COMPLICATIONS

These are risks seen in any surgical patient, and patients with ectopic pregnancy have a proclivity for them. The prevention and management of these complications are discussed in Chapter 4.

MORTALITY

According to data obtained by the National Center for Health Statistics, between 1970 and 1980, 523 women died from ectopic pregnancy (1.7/1000 reported pregnancies) in the United States (Rubin et al, 1983; Dorfman, 1983). An increasing death-to-case ratio is significantly associated with race. Blacks and other races have a death-to-case ratio 3.2 times higher than whites or hispanics. This may be related to differences in access to health care and patient compliance. A decreasing death-to-case ratio (fall of 75%) was noted during the 10-year period, despite a doubling of the incidence of ectopic pregnancy. This decrease has been primarily due to increasing public awareness and improved diagnosis (laparoscopy).

Schneider (1977) reviewed 102 maternal deaths from ectopic pregnancy. He observed that:

1. About 60% of patients were in shock or dead on arrival at the hospital.

2. Hemorrhage caused 81% of deaths, cardiac arrest under anesthesia 7%, postoperative complications 10% and pulmonary emboli 2%.

3. Timing of death was as follows:
   a. First symptom to medical consultation, mean of 3.5 days.
   b. First consultation to admission, mean of 3 days.
   c. From admission to death, mean of 2.2 days.

Long-Term Complications

PREVENTION

Currently there is no way to prevent ectopic pregnancy except by total sexual abstinence. Morbidity and mortality rates are most significantly altered by the location of the pregnancy (cornual or ampullary), length of amenorrhea, delay in seeking health care, delay in diagnosis and delay in therapy. Health care professionals can most readily affect the last three associations. The identification and education of a high risk population will lead to earlier and less morbid therapy. Table 8–15 depicts the incidence of ectopic pregnancy in selected populations of pregnant women. The following educational goals are appropriate for patients and health care providers.

1. Awareness of the disease entity.
2. Patient records of menstrual cycles with normal and abnormal signs or sensations.
3. Patient compliance with birth control methods.
4. Early medical follow-up on possible pregnancy.

In addition, the following are goals for high risk patients.

1. Patient awareness of signs and symptoms of ectopic pregnancy.
2. Early sensitive pregnancy testing, i.e., serum hCG, within 10 days of missed period.
3. Medical follow-up for five weeks of amenorrhea in normally ovulating women.
4. Liberal use of diagnostic testing such as ultrasonography.

FUTURE PREGNANCY

Events that lead to an ectopic pregnancy are likely to be present for future attempts at pregnancy. There is a consensus that ectopic pregnancy predicts infertility (40 to 60%) and a risk of recurrent ectopic pregnancy (6 to 22%). However, there is great variation in the literature. These differences are explained by differences in (1) methodology, such as number of patients at risk, duration of follow-up or selection of cases; (2) population under study, such as pregnancy history, age, coexisting infertility, desire for future pregnancy, contraceptive use and (3) surgical technique, salpingostomy versus salpingo-oophorectomy. The last is probably of least importance.

Sherman and co-workers (1982), in a review of fertility after ectopic pregnancy, identified four significant factors adversely affecting subsequent fertility: (1) the presence of periadnexal or peritubal disease at the index operation, (2) a history of infertility prior to the index operation, (3) the degree of damage (ruptured vs. unruptured) to the pregnant tube and (4) the mean age of the patient at index ectopic pregnancy. Additionally, they found that conservative management (salpingostomy) was only significantly helpful in the patient with either a history or operative findings suggestive of coexistent sterility factors. Further reviews of the success of surgery are given by Schenker and Evron (1983) and Cousins and Batzer (1986).

RHESUS SENSITIZATION

At the time of rupture of the pregnant tube both maternal and fetal blood cells collect in the abdominal cavity. These cells are gradually absorbed and enter the maternal blood stream. Should the mother be Rh negative and the fetal blood cells Rh positive, sensitization can occur. Katz and Marcus (1972) demonstrated significant fetal-maternal transfusion in 9 of 38 women with ruptured ectopic pregnancy. Therefore, it is recommended that a 300 mg dose of RhoGAM be given after ectopic pregnancy. Grimes and co-workers (1981) suggest that lack of utilization of RhoGAM in ectopic pregnancy is a major source of Rh-sensitized pregnancies. In their study there was only 38% utilization of RhoGAM among eligible women.

ABDOMINAL PREGNANCY

Complications of Diagnosis

Although rare (1 in 30,000 to 50,000 pregnancies), abdominal pregnancy is associated with difficult decision making, difficult surgery and significant maternal and fetal mortality and morbidity. About 80% of patients present with

Table 8–15. *Populations at High Risk for Ectopic Pregnancy*

Pregnant Population	Incidence (%)*	References
Non-white, U.S. 1978	1.2	Rubin et al (1983)
White, U.S. 1978	0.8	Rubin et al (1983)
Non-white, 35 years old	2.6	Rubin et al (1983)
Treatment with gonadotropins	2.7	Gemzell et al (1982)
Current IUD use	4.0	Tatum and Schmidt (1977)
History of DES in utero	4–6	Stillman (1982)
Laparoscopic diagnosis of PID	4.2	Westrom et al (1975)
Previous tubal sterilization	33.0	Corson and Batzer (1986)
Previous ectopic pregnancy	8–33	Corson and Batzer (1986)
Previous tubal surgery	3–20	Corson and Batzer (1986)

*Per 100 reported pregnancies.

major perinatal complications: fetal death, abdominal pain or massive intraabdominal bleeding. A preoperative diagnosis is made in about one third of gestations over 26 weeks. Failure to diagnose abdominal pregnancy preoperatively can lead the surgeon unexpectedly into one of the most complicated surgical procedures in obstetrics. In addition, accurate diagnosis will allow fetal considerations to play a part in the decision making process. Diagnosis depends on a high degree of suspicion in taking the history, the physical examination and an adequate level II ultrasonographic study. In the past, x-ray has been used to diagnose abdominal pregnancy. The major deficiencies of radiologic diagnosis are the inability to locate the placenta and to define fetal status.

Management

When to Operate?

If the diagnosis can be made, conservative management under controlled circumstances may be indicated in the stable mother with a viable pregnancy between 24 and 32 weeks' gestation. This type of management should only be considered in hospitals in which rapid, complicated surgery can be performed. Since catastrophic hemorrhage is a risk, continuous intravenous access and adequate blood banking facilities are necessary. The patient and her family must be fully informed of the risks and benefits of conservative management.

Operative management is indicated for fetal death, intraperitoneal hemorrhage, coagulopathy, diagnosis at less than 20 weeks' gestation and symptomatic abdominal organ involvement (bowel obstruction or hematuria). Pregnancies diagnosed after 32 weeks' gestation should also be managed operatively. At this point the neonatal survival in level III nurseries is essentially

equivalent to the risk of maternal death in abdominal pregnancy (5 to 10%). The neonate should be cared for by a neonatologist in the delivery room, and it is appropriate to give the mother dexamethasone 4 mg intravenously Q 8 hours for six doses preoperatively, when possible. Preoperative management should be directed at anticipating massive hemorrhage, possible bowel or bladder surgery and postoperative infection (see Chapter 2).

Surgical Technique and Intraoperative Complications

The technical problems of operation for abdominal pregnancy relate to distorted anatomy, control of hemorrhage and involvement of adjacent organs. The first principle is to obtain adequate exposure by a vertical midline incision. The bowel or the placenta may be attached to the parietal peritoneum, and careful entry is important. Fetal tissue is antigenically dissimilar to that of the mother, and spillage of amniotic fluid should be avoided if possible. After isolation of the membranes with laparotomy pads, the membranes should be entered in the least vascular space. The fetus is then removed; traction on the cord, which may dislodge placental vascular attachments, should be carefully avoided. The cord should be drained as much as possible and ligated with absorbable sutures at the base.

The biologic nature of placental tissue is to invade maternal tissue and create sinuses from the maternal blood supply. In the uterus this aggressive behavior is usually limited to the basalis of the endometrium. However, outside the uterus trophoblastic tissue is deeply invasive. Attempts at placental removal may initiate massive hemorrhage (400 to 600 ml a minute) from a wide base, making control difficult. Removal of the placenta depends on its location (preoperative ultrasound) and intraoperative complications such as placental laceration or hemorrhage. If the placenta is attached to the posterior peritoneum, bowel, bladder or vessels, it should not be removed, but left undisturbed. If there is bleeding from a laceration of the placenta, the first approach is to stop the bleeding. Attempts at removal of the placenta will initiate more uncontrolled bleeding. If local attempts at control (i.e., oversewing) are not successful, vascular embolization or a block resection must be considered. For example, if the placenta involves a loop of small bowel it may be safer to resect a portion of the small bowel rather than try to remove the placenta. If there is extensive damage, the surgical management may include salpingo-oophorectomy and hysterectomy.

As placental tissue is often left in place and this tissue is an excellent source of infection, drains should not be used. If the bowel or vagina has been entered, the prophylactic antibiotics should be continued for a full five-day course. The abdominal wound should be closed with permanent sutures using a Smead-Jones technique.

Conservative management of the placenta will lead to a decrease in operative mortality and hemorrhage, but will increase the postoperative morbidity. This includes infection, persistent fever, risk of reoperation, prolonged hospitalization and persistently elevated hCG. The retained placental tissue can be treated by methotrexate, although sepsis remains a risk (Rahman et al, 1982).

Complications

MATERNAL

The major maternal risks of abdominal pregnancy are related to intraoperative hemorrhage and postpartum infection. They are listed in Table 8–16. These risks may be reduced by early diagnosis by ultrasound, appropriate preoperative preparation and consultation, conservative management of the placenta, if possible, and meticulous attention to operative and aseptic technique.

FETAL

Most of the data on fetal risk come from large studies spanning many years. Estimates on fetal-neonatal survival usually rely on data obtained prior to the recent dramatic change in

Table 8–16. Complications of Abdominal Pregnancy*

Maternal	Percent
Death (sepsis, hemorrhage)	5–10
Morbidity	
Sepsis	25
Transfusion	75
Reoperation	5
Adjunctive surgery	
Hysterectomy	15
Salpingectomy	15
Oophorectomy	9
Omentectomy	5
Bowel surgery	1
Fetal	
Fetal death	30
Diagnosis and management <24 weeks	36
Survival after viability	65
Deformity	40
Prematurity 24–36 weeks	36
IUGR (<36 weeks and <2500 grams)	19

*Data from Beacham WD, Hunquist WC et al: *Am. J. Obstet. Gynecol.* 84:1257, 1962; Clark JF, Guy RS: *Am. J. Obstet. Gynecol.* 96:512, 1966; Hreshchyshyn MM, Bogen B et al: *Am. J. Obstet. Gynecol.* 81:302, 1961; Tan KL, Wee JH: *J. Obstet. Gynecol. Bi. Comm.* 76:1021, 1969; Rahman MS, Alsuleiman SA et al: *Obstet. Gynecol.* 59:366, 1982; Delke I, Veridiano NP, Tancer ML: Abdominal pregnancy: review of current management and addition of 10 cases. Obstet. Gynecol. 60:200, 1982; Strafford JC, Ragan WD: *Obstet. Gynecol.* 50:548, 1977.

the survival of preterm infants and the advent of antepartum fetal monitoring. A better estimate of survival would be to use survival rates at various gestational ages with modern perinatal management. The incidences of small for gestational age infants and deformities would not be expected to change. Table 8–16 depicts the frequency of these complications.

The value of the non-stress test and serial urinary estriol determinations in predicting fetal compromise with abdominal pregnancy was demonstrated by Hertz and co-workers (1977). The advent of the biophysical profile should increase the sensitivity of fetal monitoring and thus further reduce the risks of fetal death.

GESTATIONAL TROPHOBLASTIC DISEASE

Gestational trophoblastic disease, commonly referred to as gestational trophoblastic neoplasms (GTN), includes hydatidiform mole, invasive mole, choriocarcinoma and placental site tumor. Hydatidiform mole (H mole) occurs in 1:100 to 1:2000 pregnancies (Grimes, 1984).

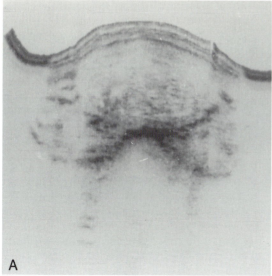

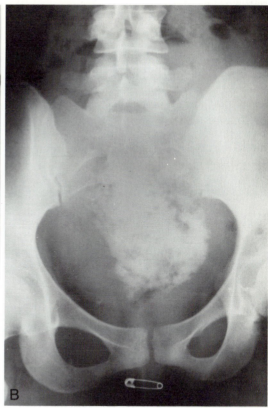

Figure 8–5. A, *Ultrasound of a hydatidiform mole.* B, *Amniogram of a hydatidiform mole.*

Twenty percent of moles develop into invasive moles and 2% of these develop into choriocarcinoma. Choriocarcinoma arises de novo in a similar number of patients. Hydatidiform mole is classically characterized by enlargement of the uterus greater than one would expect for the duration of gestation and by clinical manifestations such as hyperthyroidism, hyperemesis and lutein cysts of the ovaries, which may be related to the increased production of human chorionic gonadatropin (hCG).

Complications of Diagnosis

On examination, a large uterus that is caused by H mole may be mistaken for one caused by multiple pregnancy or leiomyomata. Since 35% of H moles occur in normal-sized uteri and 15% in uteri smaller than normal, H mole may also be confused with missed abortion or a normal intrauterine pregnancy.

Ultrasound has revolutionized the diagnosis of H mole, but the typical "honeycomb" pattern may be confused, especially by the inexperienced ultrasonographer, with normal pregnancy (especially tangential section of the placenta) leiomyomata, intrauterine fetal death or intrauterine blood clots. Injection of contrast material into the amniotic sac (amniogram) may clarify the diagnosis (Fig. 8–5). The danger of the procedure is related to the risks of midtrimester amniocentesis (see Chapter 9) rather than complications from the contrast material.

Failure to diagnose choriocarcinoma may occur in those cases in which the choriocarcinoma arises apparently without a preceding H mole and especially after abortion or term pregnancy. This may lead to unnecessary major procedures such as thoracotomy or craniotomy.

Procedure

In most instances hydatidiform moles are best evacuated by transcervical suction followed by sharp curettage with a large curette. In women over 40 and those who do not wish to preserve fertility, primary hysterectomy may be considered. Corpus lutein cysts should be managed conservatively in these instances; if they are very large, the fluid can be aspirated.

Complications

INTRAOPERATIVE COMPLICATIONS

The size of the uterus, the softness of its wall and the amount of blood and tissue to be removed present problems during the operation. Hemorrhage, perforation, and incomplete evacuation are correlated with larger uteri (greater than 16 weeks). Thus, the operation should only be undertaken in a fully equipped operating room under general anesthesia and with at least two units of blood available. The risks of severe respiratory distress and cardiovascular instability need to be anticipated. The chance of perforation can be reduced by placing the suction only in the lower part of the uterus and giving intravenous oxytocin (20 to 30 units in 1000 cc D5 1/2 NS) during the suction. Perforation of the uterus is difficult to detect because of the softness and depth of the uncontracted uterus. Contraction of the uterus from oxytocin reduces the cavity size and increases the resistance of the wall. At this point the sharp curettage may be safely performed. Should perforation occur, hysterectomy is indicated to reduce dissemination of molar tissue.

EARLY POSTOPERATIVE COMPLICATIONS

Acute Respiratory Distress. Approximately 10% of patients receiving treatment for molar pregnancy will develop acute pulmonary complications characterized by tachycardia, tachypnea and hypoxemia (Huberman et al, 1982; Twiggs et al, 1979). Generally this is a self-limited crisis occurring 1 to 12 hours after evacuation. Occasionally the complication can progress to adult respiratory distress syndrome and subsequent death (Huberman et al, 1982). There are many factors associated with its onset; trophoblastic emboli, hypervolemia, disseminated intravascular coagulation (DIC), preeclampsia or hyperthyroidism may be present. Venous thromboembolism must also be considered in the differential diagnosis. The key to the prevention of respiratory distress is the recognition of the high-risk patient and careful perioperative management. The patients at highest risk are those with uteri greater than 16 weeks' gestation in size and preexisting medical disease (DIC, preeclampsia, hyperthyroidism).

The management of the acute crisis requires an intensive care unit (see Chapter 4) with initiation of oxygen therapy, diagnostic tests such as EKG, anterial blood gases, chest x-ray

and intensive cardiac monitoring with a Swan-Ganz catheter. If elements of cardiac failure or fluid overload appear, furosemide (40 mg intravenously) should be given. If the pulmonary wedge pressure is normal, thromboembolism should be considered. Trophoblastic embolism may also cause perfusion defects, but these are likely to be smaller. The decision to heparinize a patient must be tempered with the fact that the GTN patient is at risk for hemorrhage.

Hyperthyroidism. Chemical hyperthyroidism/thyrotoxicosis can occur in as many as 40% of patients with GTN. However, clinical thyrotoxicosis occurs in only 10% of patients. Thyrotoxicosis is manifested by nervousness, hyperactivity, tremor, weight loss, sweating, temperature intolerance, muscle weakness, tachycardia and eye signs (lid lag). Occasionally the patient may have signs of thyroid storm, especially after surgery. These signs include atrial fibrillation, tachyarrhythmias, high fever, delirium, coma, severe vomiting and diarrhea. In patients with underlying cardiac disease and those over 40, congestive heart failure may also be a problem.

Hyperthyroidism is the result of direct stimulation of the thyroid gland by either hCG or a separate thyrotropin produced by the placental tissue (Hershmann, 1972; Higgins et al, 1975). The incidence of hyperthyroidism is proportional to the level of hCG, and this lends support to the theory of hCG stimulation. Regardless of the source, the therapy of hyperthyroidism associated with GTN is removal of the trophoblastic tissue. In most cases, the thyrotoxicosis will resolve in one to two weeks without further therapy. In patients with moderate to severe hyperthyroidism, preoperative iodine (2 gm over 8 hours intravenously) is warranted. Iodine, theoretically, will reduce the risk of thyroid storm precipitated by subsequent operation. Propranolol (20 mg PO Q 6 hours) should be considered to reduce the signs of adrenergic stimulation. Propranolol should be used with caution in patients with signs of congestive heart failure. The use of the thyroid blockers, propylthiouracil (100 mg PO qid) and methimazole (10 mg PO qid), may be considered, although removal of the placenta may accomplish the same end. These drugs may cause agranulocytosis (2.5%) or dermatitis (5%). Thyroid storm is a medical emergency and has been reported in GTN (Hershmann, 1972). Treatment must be started immediately (see Chapter 4). Even with the best management the syndrome may progress rapidly to coma, shock and death, with a mortality of about 20%.

LATE POSTOPERATIVE COMPLICATIONS

Approximately 20% of molar patients will have or develop persistent trophoblastic disease, invasive mole or choriocarcinoma. Adequate follow-up of all patients with evacuation of a hydatidiform mole is essential for early identification of persistent GTN. Failure to diagnose persistent GTN can lead to increased morbidity and decreased cure rates. An appropriate follow-up regime includes:

1. Weekly quantitative hCG determinations until the level is less than 4 miu/ml (levels vary with different laboratories) for three consecutive weeks. Then the hCG determinations should be repeated monthly for six months.

2. Pregnancy should be avoided for six months after the hCG has returned to normal.

3. Determination of hCG levels should be obtained six weeks after the termination of any subsequent pregnancy.

In patients with persistent GTN (steady or rising serial hCG levels), invasive mole or choriocarcinoma, treatment should be managed by specialized referral centers for GTN. Single or multiple agent chemotherapy is the cornerstone of therapy and is very successful. Regional trophoblastic centers report cure rates better than 98% for invasive mole and 50 to 90% for choriocarcinoma (Lurain et al, 1982). The complications of chemotherapy are covered in Chapter 12. Occasionally, supplementary operations and radiotherapy are needed in the management of complicated GTN. Other operations may include exploratory laparotomy, hysterectomy and extragenital operations (thoracotomy or craniotomy). The outcome of pregnancy subsequent to treatment for GTN is presented in Table 8–17 (Berkowitz and Goldstein, 1981). In general, a successful pregnancy without an increase in congenital anomalies in the infant can be expected, and the risk of recurrent GTN is less than 1%, although a woman who has had GTN once is twice as likely to have it again as one without such a history.

REFERENCES

Allibone GW, Fagan CJ, Porter SC: The sonographic features of intra-abdominal pregnancy. *JOU* 9:383, 1981.

Alsuleiman SA, Grimes EM: Ectopic pregnancy: a review of 147 cases. *J. Reprod. Med.* 27:101, 1982.

Andolsek L, Cheng M, Hern M: The safety of local anesthesia and outpatient treatment. A controlled study of induced abortion by vacuum aspiration. *Stud. Fam. Plan.* 8:118, 1977.

Atienza MF, Berkman RJ et al: Menstrual extraction. *Am. J. Obstet. Gynecol.* 121:490, 1975.

Bakketeig LS, Hoffman HJ, Harlee EY: The tendency to repeat gestational age and birthweight in successive births. *Am. J. Obstet. Gynecol.* 135:1086, 1979.

Beacham WD, Hernquist WC et al: Abdominal pregnancy at Charity Hospital in New Orleans. *Am. J. Obstet. Gynecol.* 84:1257, 1962.

Ben-Baruch G, Menczer J et al: Laparoscopy in the management of uterine perforation. *J. Reprod. Med.* 27:73, 1982.

Beral V: Reproductive mortality. *Brit. Med. J.* 2:632, 1979.

Beral V: An epidemiological study of recent trends in ectopic pregnancy. *Br. J. Obstet. Gynecol.* 82:773, 1975.

Berek JS, Stubblefield PG: Anatomic and clinical correlates of uterine perforation. *Am. J. Obstet. Gynecol.* 135:181, 1979.

Bergman P: Traumatic intrauterine lesions. *Acta Obstet. Gynecol. Scand.* 40:1, 1961.

Berkowitz RS, Goldstein DP: Pregnancy outcome after molar gestation. *Contemp. Ob/Gyn* 18:69, 1981.

Berman SM, McKay T et al: Deaths from spontaneous abortion in the United States. *J. Am. Med. Ass.* 253:3119, 1985.

Boue J, Boue A et al: Retrospective and prospective epidemiological studies of 1500 karyotyped spontaneous human abortions. *Teratology* 12:11, 1975.

Boyd EF, Holmstrom EG: Ovulation following therapeutic abortion. *Am. J. Obstet. Gynecol.* 113:469, 1972.

Bracken MB: Induced abortion as a risk factor for perinatal complications: a review. *Yale J. Biol. Med.* 51:539, 1978.

Bracken MB: Psychosomatic aspects of abortion: implications for counseling. *J. Reprod. Med.* 19:265, 1977.

Brenner PF, Roy S, Mishell DR: Ectopic pregnancy: a study of 300 consecutive surgically treated cases. *J. Am. Med. Assoc.* 243:673, 1980.

Brook I, Feingold M et al: Ultrasonography in the diagnosis of cervical incompetence in pregnancy—a new diagnostic approach. *Br. J. Obstet. Gynecol.* 88:640, 1981.

Bruhat MA, Manhes H et al: Treatment of ectopic pregnancy by means of laparoscopy. *Fertil. Steril.* 33:411, 1980.

Burkman RT, Tonasca JA et al: Untreated endocervical gonorrhea and endometritis following elective abortion. *Am. J. Obstet. Gynecol.* 126:648, 1976.

Burnhill MS: Reducing the morbidity of vacuum aspiration abortion. In Zatuchni GH, Sciarra JJ et al (Eds.): *Pregnancy Termination: Procedures, Safety and New Developments.* Hagerstown, MD, Harper and Row, 1979.

Table 8–17. Pregnancy Outcome after Molar Pregnancy*

Outcome	No.	Percent
Term deliveries	511	65.2
Preterm deliveries	76	9.7
Spontaneous abortion	157	20.0
Induced abortion	20	2.6
Ectopic pregnancy	6	0.8
Repeat moles	9	1.1
Stillbirths	4	0.5
Congenital malformations	30	5.0
Total pregnancies	783	100.0

*From Berkowitz RS, Goldstein DP: Pregnancy outcome after molar gestations. *Contemp. Ob/Gyn.* Medical Economics Company. 18:69, 1981. Reprinted with permission.

Cartwright PA, DiPietro DL: Ectopic pregnancy: changes in serum human chorionic gonadotropin concentration. *Obstet. Gynecol.* 63:76, 1984.

Cates W, Grimes DA: Deaths from second trimester abortion by dilatation and evacuation: causes, prevention, facilities. *Obstet. Gynecol.* 58:401, 1981.

Cates W, Ory HW et al: The intrauterine device and death from spontaneous abortion. *N. Eng. J. Med.* 295:1115, 1976.

Cates W, Schulz KF et al: Short-term complications of uterine evacuation techniques for abortion at 12 weeks gestation or earlier. In Zatuchni GI, Sciarra JJ et al (Eds.): *Pregnancy Termination: Procedures, Safety and New Developments.* Hagerstown, MD, Harper and Row, 1979a.

Cates W, Schulz KF et al: Complications of surgical evacuation procedures for abortions after 12 weeks gestation. In: Zatuchni GI, Sciarra JJ et al (Eds.): *Pregnancy Termination: Procedures, Safety and New Developments.* Hagerstown, MD, Harper and Row, 1979b.

Cates W, Smith JC et al: Assessment of surveillance and vital statistics data for monitoring abortion mortality in the United States 1972–1975. *Am. J. Epidemiol.* 106:200, 1978.

Cates W, Smith JC et al: Mortality from abortion and childbirth. *J. Am. Med. Assoc.* 248:192, 1984.

Chez RA, Moore JG: Diagnostic errors in the management of ectopic pregnancy. *Surg. Gynecol. Obstet.* 117:589, 1963.

Clark JF, Guy RS: Abdominal pregnancy. *Am. J. Obstet. Gynecol.* 96:512, 1966.

Corson SL, Batzer FR: Ectopic pregnancy: a review of etiologic factors. *J. Reprod. Med.* 31:78, 1986.

Cousins SL: Cervical incompetence 1980: a time for reappraisal. *Clin. Obstet. Gynecol.* 23:467, 1980.

DeCherney AH, Minkin MJ et al: Contemporary management of ectopic pregnancy. *J. Reprod. Med.* 26:519, 1981.

DeCherney AH, Romero R et al: Surgical management of unruptured ectopic pregnancy. *Fertil. Steril.* 35:21, 1981.

Delke I, Veridiano NP, Tancer ML: Abdominal pregnancy: review of current management and addition of 10 cases. *Obstet. Gynecol.* 60:200, 1982.

DeStefano F, Peterson HB et al: Risk of ectopic pregnancy following tubal sterilization. *Obstet. Gynecol.* 60:326, 1982.

Dieckmann WJ, Davis ME et al: Does the administration of diethylstilbesterol during pregnancy have therapeutic value? *Am. J. Obstet. Gynecol.* 44:1062, 1953.

Dorfman SF: Deaths from ectopic pregnancy, United States 1979–1980. *Obstet. Gynecol.* 62:334, 1983.

Duff GB: Prognosis in threatened abortion: a comparison between predictions made by sonar, urinary hormone assays and clinical judgement. *Br. J. Obstet. Gynaecol.* 82:858, 1975.

Erikson JD, Bjerkedal T: Fetal and infant mortality in Norway and the United States. *J. Am. Med. Assoc.* 247:987, 1982.

Facts of Life and Death. No. (PHS) 79-1222. *National Center for Health Statistics,* 1979.

Fielding WL, Lee SY, Friedman EA: Continued pregnancy after failed first trimester abortion. *Obstet. Gynecol.* 52:56, 1978.

Foreman H, Stadl BU et al: Intrauterine device usage and fetal loss. *Obstet. Gynecol.* 58:669, 1981.

Freda VJ, Gorman JG et al: The threat of Rh immunization from abortion. *Lancet* 2:147, 1970.

Freiman SM, Wulff GJ Jr: Management of uterine perforation following elective abortion. *Obstet. Gynecol.* 50:647, 1977.

Funderburk SJ, Guthrie D, Meldrum D: Outcome of pregnancy complicated by early vaginal bleeding. *Br. J. Obstet. Gynaecol.* 87:100, 1980.

Gemzell C, Guillome J, Wang CF: Ectopic pregnancy following treatment with human gonadotropin. *Am. J. Obstet. Gynecol.* 143:761, 1982.

Gleicher N, Giglia RV et al: Direct diagnosis of unruptured ectopic pregnancy by real time ultrasound. *Obstet. Gynecol.* 61:425, 1983.

Goldzieher JW: Double blind trial for a progestin in habitual abortion. *J. Am. Med. Assoc.* 188:651, 1964.

Goodlin RC: Cervical incompetence, hourglass membranes, and amniocentesis. *Obstet. Gynecol.* 54:748, 1979.

Grimes DA: Epidemiology of gestational trophoblastic disease. *Am. J. Obstet. Gynecol.* 150:309, 1984.

Grimes DA, Cates W: Deaths from paracervical anesthesia used for first trimester abortion 1972–1975. *N. Eng. J. Med.* 295:1397, 1976.

Grimes DA, Cates W: Complications from legally induced abortion: a review. *Obstet. Gynecol. Surv.* 34:177, 1979.

Grimes DA, Cates W et al: Fatal septic abortion in the United States 1975–1977. *Obstet. Gynecol.* 57:739, 1981.

Grimes DA, Flock ML et al: Hysterectomy as treatment for complications of legal abortion. *Obstet. Gynecol.* 63:457, 1984.

Grimes DA, Geary FH, Hatcher RA: Rh immunoglobulin utilization after ectopic pregnancy. *Am. J. Obstet. Gynecol.* 140:246, 1981.

Grimes DA, Kafrissen ME et al: Fatal hemorrhage from legal abortion in the United States. *Surg. Gynecol. Obstet.* 157:461, 1983.

Grimes DA, Ross WC et al: Rh immunoglobulin utilization after spontaneous and induced abortion. *Obstet. Gynecol.* 50:261, 1977.

Grimes DA, Schulz KF et al: Mid-trimester abortion by dilatation and evacuation. *N. Engl. J. Med.* 298:1141, 1977a.

Grimes DA, Schulz KF et al: Mid-trimester abortion by intra-amniotic prostaglandin F_2 alpha. Safer than saline? *Obstet. Gynecol.* 49:612, 1977b.

Grimes DA, Schulz KF, Cates W: Prevention of uterine perforation during curettage abortion. *J. Am. Med. Assoc.* 251:2108, 1984a.

Grimes DA, Schulz KF, Cates W: Prophylactic antibiotics for curettage abortion. *Am. J. Obstet. Gynecol.* 150:689, 1984b.

Guidotti RJ, Grimes DA, Cates W: Fetal amniotic fluid embolism during legally induced abortion: United States, 1972 to 1978. *Am. J. Obstet. Gynecol.* 141:257, 1981.

Hale RW, Kobara TY et al: Office termination of pregnancy by "menstrual aspiration." *Am. J. Obstet. Gynecol.* 134:213, 1979.

Hallatt JG: Repeat ectopic pregnancies: a study of 123 consecutive cases. *Am. J. Obstet. Gynecol.* 122:520, 1975.

Halpin TF: Ectopic pregnancy: the problem of diagnosis. *Am. J. Obstet. Gynecol.* 106:227, 1970.

Harger JH: Comparison of success and morbidity in cervical cerclage procedures. *Obstet. Gynecol.* 56:543, 1980.

Harger JH: Cervical cerclage: patient selection, morbidity and success rate. *Clin. Perinatol.* 10:321, 1983.

Harralson JD, Van Nagell JR, Roddick JW: Operative management of ruptured tubal pregnancy. *Am. J. Obstet. Gynecol.* 115:995, 1973.

Hein HA, Brown CJ: Neonatal mortality review; a basis for improving care. *Pediatrics* 68:504, 1981.

Helvacioglu A, Long EM, Yang SL: Ectopic pregnancy: an eight year review. *J. Reprod. Med.* 22:87, 1979.

Hern WM: First and second trimester abortion techniques. In Leventhal J (Ed.): *Current Problems in Obstetrics and Gynecology.* Chicago, Year Book Medical Publishers, 1983.

Hershmann JM: Hyperthyroidism induced by trophoblastic thyrotropin. *Mayo Clin. Proc.* 47:913, 1972.

Hertz JB: Diagnostic procedures in threatened abortion. *Obstet. Gynecol.* 64:223, 1984.

Hertz RH, Timor-Tritsch I et al: Diagnostic studies and fetal assessment in advanced extrauterine pregnancy. *Obstet. Gynecol.* 50(suppl):62, 1977.

Hibbard LT: Corpus luteum surgery. *Am. J. Obstet. Gynecol.* 135:666, 1979.

Higgins HP, Hershmann JM et al: The thyrotoxicosis of hydatidiform mole. *Ann. Intern. Med.* 83:307, 1975.

Hodgson JE: Major complications of 20,248 consecutive first trimester abortions. Problems of fragmented care. *Adv. Plan. Parenthood* 9:52, 1975.

Hreshchyshyn MM, Bogen B et al: What is the actual present day management of the placenta in late abdominal pregnancy? *Am. J. Obstet. Gynecol.* 81:302, 1961.

Hubbard GW: A review of the progress of psychiatric opinion regarding emotional complications of therapeutic abortion. *South. Med. J.* 70:558, 1977.

Huberman RP, Fong T, Bein ME: Benign molar pregnancies: pulmonary complications. *Am. J. Roentgenol.* 138:71, 1982.

Hulka JF, Lefler HT et al: A new electronic force monitor to measure factors influencing cervical dilatation for vacuum curettage. *Am. J. Obstet. Gynecol.* 120:166, 1974.

Irani KR, Henriques ES et al: Menstrual induction: its place in clinic practice. *Obstet. Gynecol.* 46:596, 1975.

Janis IL, Mann L: *Decision Making: A Psychological Analysis of Conflict, Choice and Commitment.* New York, New York Free Press, 1977.

Jansen RPS: Spontaneous abortion incidence in the treatment of infertility. *Am. J. Obstet. Gynecol.* 143:451, 1982.

Jeong WG, Kim CH et al: Ultrasonic sonography in the management of incomplete abortion. *J. Reprod. Med.* 26:90, 1981.

Johnson J, Lee PA et al: High risk prematurity-progestin treatment and steroid studies. *Obstet. Gynecol.* 54:412, 1979.

Johnstone FD, Beard RJ et al: Cervical diameter after suction termination of pregnancy. *Br. Med. J.* 1:68, 1976.

Kadar N, Caldwell BV, Romero R: A method of screening for ectopic pregnancy and its indications. *Obstet. Gynecol.* 58:162, 1981.

Kafrissen ME, Schulz KF et al: Midtrimester abortion: intra-amniotic instillation of hyperosmolar urea and prostaglandin F_2 alpha versus dilatation and evacuation. *J. Am. Med. Assoc.* 251:916, 1984.

Katz J, Marcus R: The risk of Rh isoimmunization in ruptured tubal pregnancy. *Br. Med. J.* 3:667, 1972.

Kaufman RH, Adam E et al: Upper genital tract changes and pregnancy outcome in offspring exposed in utero to diethylstilbestrol. *Am. J. Obstet. Gynecol.* 137:299, 1980.

Kaunitz AM, Hughes JM et al: Causes of maternal mortality in the United States. *Obstet. Gynecol.* 65:605, 1985.

Kaunitz AM, Ravira EZ et al: Abortions that fail. *Obstet. Gynecol.* 66:533, 1985.

Kelly MT, Santos-Ramos R, Dwenhoether JH: The value of sonography in suspected ectopic pregnancy. *Obstet. Gynecol.* 53:703, 1979.

Kimball AM, Hallum AU, Cates W: Deaths caused by pulmonary thromboembolism after legally induced abortion. *Am. J. Obstet. Gynecol.* 132:169,1978.

King TM, Atienza MF, Burkman RT: The incidence of abdominal procedures in a population undergoing abortion. *Am. J. Obstet. Gynecol.* 137:530, 1980.

Kitchen JD, Wein RM et al: Ectopic pregnancy: current clinical trends. *Am. J. Obstet. Gynecol.* 134:870, 1979.

Klein SM, Garcia CR: Asherman's syndrome: a critique and a current review. *Fertil. Steril.* 24:722, 1973.

Kowalski K: Managing perinatal loss. *Clin. Obstet. Gynecol.* 23:1113, 1980.

Lake M, Knuppel RA et al: The role of a grief support team following stillbirth. *Am. J. Obstet. Gynecol.* 146:877, 1983.

Läkteenmäki P: The disappearance of hCG and return of pituitary function after abortion. *Clin. Endocrinol.* 9:101, 1978.

Late consequences of abortion, editorial. *Br. Med. J.* 282:1564, 1981.

Laubach GE, Wilchins SA: Screening reveals occult pregnancies. *Contemp. Ob/Gyn* 10:51,1977.

Lauersen NH, Birnbaum S: Laparoscopy as a diagnostic and therapeutic technique in uterine perforation during first trimester abortions. *Am. J. Obstet. Gynecol.* 117:522, 1973.

Lauersen NH, Dent T et al: Cervical priming prior to dilatation and evacuation: a comparison of methods. *Am. J. Obstet. Gynecol.* 144:890, 1982.

Lawson TL: Ectopic pregnancy: criteria and accuracy of ultrasonic diagnosis. *Am. J. Radiol.* 131:153, 1978.

Lazar P, Gueguen S et al: Multicentered controlled trial of cervical cerclage in women at moderate risk of preterm delivery. *Br. J. Obstet. Gynaecol.* 91:731, 1984.

Lee KS, Paneth N et al: Neonatal mortality: an analysis of the recent improvement in the United States. *Am. J. Publ. Health* 70:15, 1980.

Levi S, Leblicq P: The diagnostic value of ultrasonography in 342 suspected cases of ectopic pregnancy. *Acta Obstet. Gynecol. Scand.* 59:29, 1980.

Lewis E: The management of stillbirth: coping with an unreality. *Lancet* 2:619, 1976.

Lindahl B, Ahlgren M: Identification of chorionic villi in abortion specimens. *Obstet. Gynecol.* 67:79, 1986.

Lurain JR, Brewer JI et al: Gestational trophoblastic disease: treatment results at the Brewer Trophoblastic Disease Center. *Obstet. Gynecol.* 60:354, 1982.

Mantoni M: Ultrasound signs in threatened abortion and their prognostic significance. *Obstet. Gynecol.* 65:471, 1985.

Marrs RP, Kletzky DA et al: Disappearance of human chorionic gonadotropin and the resumption of ovulation following abortion. *Am. J. Obstet. Gynecol.* 135:731, 1979.

McCarthy BJ, Terry J et al: The under-registration of neonatal deaths: Georgia 1974–1977. *Am. J. Publ. Health* 70:977, 1980.

Mikano K: Anatomic and chromosomal anomalies in spontaneous abortion. *Am. J. Obstet. Gynecol.* 106:243, 1970.

Munsick RA: Clinical test for placenta in 300 consecutive menstrual aspirations. *Obstet. Gynecol.* 60:738, 1982.

Nathanson BN: Ambulatory abortion: experience with 26,000 cases. *N. Engl. J. Med.* 286:403, 1972a.

Nathanson BN: Management of uterine perforation suffered at elective abortion. *Am. J. Obstet. Gynecol.* 119:1054, 1972b.

National Center for Health Statistics: Birth, marriage, divorce, death. Monthly Vital Statisics Report, 33(12) March 26, 1985.

Newton ER, Kennedy JL et al: Obstetric diagnosis and perinatal mortality. *Am. J. Perinatol.* In Press.

Niswander KR, Gordon M et al. *The Women and Their Pregnancies: The Collaborative Perinatal Study of the National Institute of Neurological Diseases and Stroke.* DHEW Publication No (NIH) 73–379, 1972.

Obel EB, Madsen M: Urinary estrogen excretion and concentration of serum human placental lactogen in pregnancies following legally induced abortions. *Acta Obstet. Gynecol. Scand.* 59:37, 1980.

Olatunbosun OA, Dyck F: Cervical cerclage operation for a dilated cervix. *Obstet. Gynecol.* 57:166, 1981.

Ornoy A, Benedy S et al: Association between maternal bleeding during gestation and congenital anomalies in the offspring. *Am. J. Obstet. Gynecol.* 124:474, 1976.

Osser S, Persson K: Postabortal pelvic infection with chlamydia trachomatis and the influence of humoral immunity. *Am. J. Obstet. Gynecol.* 150:699, 1984.

Peterson HB, Grimes DA et al: Comparative risk of death from induced abortion at less than 12 weeks gestation performed with local versus general anesthesia. *Am. J. Obstet. Gynecol.* 141:763, 1981.

Peterson WF, Berry FN et al: Second trimester abortion by dilatation and evacuation: an analysis of 11,747 cases. *Obstet. Gynecol.* 62:185, 1983.

Rahman MS, Alsuleiman SA et al: Advanced abdominal pregnancy: observation in 10 cases. *Obstet. Gynecol.* 59:366, 1982.

Romero R, Kada N et al: Diagnosis of ectopic pregnancy: Value of the discriminatory human chorionic gonadotropin zone. *Obstet. Gynecol.* 66:357, 1985.

Rubin GL, Cates W et al: Fatal ectopic pregnancy after attempted legally induced abortion. *J. Am. Med. Assoc.* 244:1705, 1980.

Rubin GL, McCarthy B et al: The risk of childbearing reevaluated. *Am. J. Publ. Health* 71:712, 1981.

Rubin GL, Peterson HB et al: Ectopic pregnancy in the United States 1970 through 1978. *J. Am. Med. Assoc.* 249:1725, 1983.

Rush RW, Isaacs S et al: A randomized controlled trial of cervical cerclage in women at high risk of spontaneous preterm delivery. *Br. J. Obstet. Gynaecol.* 91:724, 1984.

Sachs BP, Lande PM et al: Reproductive mortality in the United States. *J. Am. Med. Assoc.* 247:2789, 1982.

Samuelson S, Sjovall A: Laparoscopy in suspected ectopic pregnancy. *Acta Obstet. Gynecol. Scand.* 51:31, 1972.

Schenker JG, Evron S: New concepts in the surgical management of tubal pregnancy and consequent postoperative results. *Fertil. Steril.* 40:709, 1983.

Schinfeld JS, Reedy G: Mesosalpingeal vessel ligation for conservative treatment of ectopic pregnancy. *J. Reprod. Med.* 28:823, 1983.

Schneider J, Berger CJ, Cattell C: Maternal mortality due to ectopic pregnancy; a review of 102 cases. *Obstet. Gynecol.* 49:557, 1977.

Schulz KF, Grimes DA, Cates W: Measures to prevent cervical injury during suction abortion. *Lancet* 1:1182, 1982.

Selik RM, Cates W, Tyler CW Jr: Behavioral factors contributing to abortion death: a new approach to mortality studies. *Obstet. Gynecol.* 58:63, 1981.

Shearman RP, Garrett WJ: Double blind study of the effect of 17-hydroxyprogesterone caproate on abortion rate. *Br. Med. J.* 1:292, 1963.

Sherman D, Langer R et al: Improved fertility following ectopic pregnancy. *Fertil. Steril.* 37:497, 1982.

Steier JA, Bergsjo P, Myking OL: Human chorionic gonadotropin in maternal plasma after induced abortion, spontaneous abortion and removed ectopic pregnancy. *Obstet. Gynecol.* 64:391, 1984.

Stillman RJ: In utero exposure to diethylstilbestrol: adverse effects on the reproductive tract and reproductive performance in male and female offspring. *Am. J. Obstet. Gynecol.* 142:905, 1982.

Strafford JC, Ragan WD: Abdominal pregnancy: review of current management. *Obstet. Gynecol.* 50:548, 1977.

Stroh G, Hinman AR: Reported live births following induced abortion: two and one-half years experience in upstate New York. *Am. J. Obstet. Gynecol.* 126:83, 1976.

Tan KL, Wee JH: The pediatric aspects of advanced abdominal pregnancy. *J. Obstet. Gynaecol. Brit. Comm.* 76:1021, 1969.

Tatum HJ, Schmidt FH: Contraception and sterilization practices and extrauterine pregnancy: a realistic perspective. *Fertil. Steril.* 28:407, 1977.

Tho PT, Byrd JR et al: Etiologies and subsequent reproductive performance of 100 couples with recurrent abortion. *Fertil. Steril.* 32:389, 1979.

Tietze C, Lewit S: Joint program for the study of abortion (JPSA): early medical complications of legal abortion. *Stud. Fam. Plann.* 3:97, 1972.

Timonen S, Nieminen U: Tubal pregnancy: choice of operative method of treatment. *Acta Obstet. Gynecol. Scand.* 46:327, 1967.

Twiggs LB, Morrow CP et al: Acute pulmonary complication of molar pregnancy. *Am. J. Obstet. Gynecol.* 135:189, 1979.

U. S. Department of Commerce: *Bureau of Census, Statistical Abstracts of U. S. 1986.* 106:72, 1986.

Valle RF, Sabbagha RE: Management of first trimester pregnancy termination failure. *Obstet. Gynecol.* 55:625, 1980.

Vitsky M: Pessary treatment of the incompetent cervical os. *Obstet. Gynecol.* 87:144, 1968.

Warburton D, Fraser FC: Spontaneous abortion risks in man: data from reproductive histories collected in a medical genetics unit. *Am. J. Hum. Genet.* 16:1, 1964.

Webster HD, Barclay DL, Fischer CK: Ectopic pregnancy: a seventeen year review. *Am. J. Obstet. Gynecol.* 92:23, 1965.

Wegman ME: Annual summary of vital statistics. *Pediatrics.* 76:861, 1985.

Weinstein L, Morris MB et al: Ectopic pregnancy—a new surgical epidemic. *Obstet. Gynecol.* 61:698, 1983.

Westrom L: Effect of acute pelvic inflammatory disease on fertility. *Am. J. Obstet. Gynecol.* 121:707, 1975.

Westrom L, Bengtsson LP, Mordh PA: Incidence, trends and risks of ectopic pregnancy in a population of women. *Br. Med. J.* 282:3, 1981.

Wheeler RG, Schneider K: Properties and safety of cervical dilators. *Am. J. Obstet. Gynecol.* 146:597, 1983.

Williams RL, Chen PM: Identifying the sources of the recent decline in perinatal mortality rates in California. *N. Eng. J. Med.* 306:207, 1982.

Williams RL, Hawes WE: Cesarean section, fetal monitoring and perinatal mortality in California. *Am. J. Publ. Health* 69:864, 1979.

Wilson JG, Brent RL: Are female sex hormones teratogenic? *Am. J. Obstet. Gynecol.* 141:567, 1981.

Woodward G: Estimation of blood loss in second trimester dilatation and curettage. *Obstet. Gynecol.* 63:230, 1984.

COMPLICATIONS OF DIAGNOSTIC AND THERAPEUTIC PROCEDURES

9

EDWARD R. NEWTON

BIOSTATISTICS

Until about 20 years ago the obstetrician had very little information about the health of the feto-placental unit until the time of delivery. Modern technology has allowed the prenatal diagnosis of chromosomal and developmental defects, abnormalities in placental position, disorders of fetal growth, antepartum fetal hypoxia and the antenatal prediction of infants at risk for respiratory distress. These techniques are rightfully credited with reducing mortality and morbidity in many infants. However, modern diagnostic technology is not without its cost. The risks of diagnosis are not just the physical risks of the procedure, for example, the incidence of rupture of membranes with amniocentesis. A major risk of an indirect assessment of the fetus during pregnancy is intervention based on the accuracy of the test. The risk of inappropriate intervention can only be assessed with a knowledge of testing statistics and their usage.

The basic requirements of any test are measures of (1) validity, (2) reliability, (3) sensitivity, (4) specificity, (5) the predictive value of a positive or negative test and (6) the practicality in terms of compliance or cost.

Validity is a measure of how closely the test measures a disease state. The incidence or prevalence of a disease can have profound effects on the practical testing of validity. For example, the focus of electronic fetal monitoring is the prediction of asphyxial neonatal death or subsequent long-term neurologic handicap. The incidences of neonatal death and cerebral palsy in term infants are 0.8% and 0.2% respectively. In order to test the validity of fetal monitoring 200 to 300 patients must be monitored to identify just one disease state. As a result, most studies focus on a more frequent but less accurate outcome parameter—Apgar score less than 7. This seriously weakens the validity of predicting long-term neurologic handicap; very few infants (1:1000) develop cerebral palsy after an Apgar score of less than 7.

Reliability is a measure of the exactness of a test. In other words, reliability is the variation of the results, given the same disease state. Reliability can have intra-observer or inter-observer variation. For example, different laboratories may give very different results from the same serum (inter-observer reliability), or the same serum run several times at the same laboratory may give different results (intra-observer reliability). The measurements of validity and reliability are demonstrated schematically in Figure 9–1. Test I is a very reliable test but with little validity, whereas Test II is a more valid test but with less reliability.

The sensitivity and specificity are essential facts to know. Sensitivity is the ability of an abnormal test to predict the disease state. Specificity is the ability of a normal test to predict the normal state. These measurements are demonstrated in Figure 9–2. Sensitivity is more affected by differences in outcome parameters. For example, the goal of fetal monitoring is to test for hypoxia that leads to neonatal death or cerebral palsy. However, the incidence of this disease state (hypoxia) is so small that fetal monitoring studies evaluate the sensitivity against abnormal fetal scalp pH or low Apgar scores. Yet, these parameters are not valid predictors of infant outcome. Abnormal fetal monitoring plus a scalp pH of less than 7.20 predicts about 60% incidence of an Apgar score of 0 to 3 at one minute. This Apgar score only predicts a 1.5% incidence of cerebral palsy in term infants. In this case the actual sensitivity of fetal monitoring falls from 60% to 0.9%.

The clinician attempting to make a diagnosis is not really interested in the academic question: if my patient has the disease, how likely is she to have a positive test (sensitivity)? A more practical question is: if my patient's test is positive, how likely is the disease to be actually present? Using Figure 9–2, of those patients with a positive test (A + B), the proportion with actual disease is A/A + B. This is called the predictive value of a positive test. Many articles will refer to a false positive test. Usually this is the proportion between the number of positive tests in which the disease is absent (B) and the total positive tests (B/A + B).

The converse question is: if my patient's test is negative, how likely is the disease not to be present? This is the predictive value of a negative test (D/C + D). Many articles will refer to a false negative test, which is the proportion of negative tests with disease present to total patients with negative tests (C/C + D). The accuracy of a test is the ability of the test to discriminate both the disease state and the healthy state (A + D)(A + B + C + D).

The prevalence of a disease state within a population can cause wide variation in the predictive values of a positive test. This variation is illustrated in Table 9–1. The rapid deterioration of the predictive value of a positive test with decreasing prevalence is of crucial concern. If one intervenes in the face of a positive

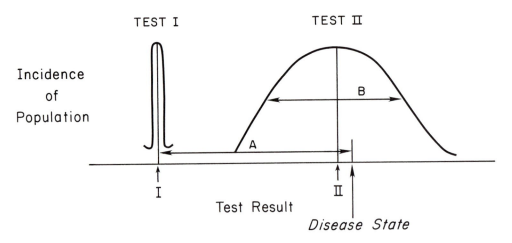

A – Distance between Test Value
     and Real Value = Validity

B – Variance of Samples = Reliability

Figure 9–1. Validity and reliability.

DISEASE

	Present	Absent	Total
Test Result Positive	A	B	A + B
Negative	C	D	C + D
Total	A + C	B + D	A + B + C + D

$$\text{Sensitivity} = \frac{A}{A + C}$$

$$\text{Specificity} = \frac{D}{B + D}$$

$$\text{Predictive Value of Positive Test} = \frac{A}{A + B}$$

$$\text{Predictive Value of Negative Test} = \frac{D}{C + D}$$

$$\text{Accuracy} = \frac{A + D}{A + B + C + D}$$

$$\text{Prevalence} = \frac{A + C}{A + B + C + D}$$

Figure 9–2. Sensitivity and specificity.

test, for example, abnormal fetal monitoring, a low risk population (prevalence 1%) faces many more unnecessary interventions.

ULTRASOUND

Most American fetuses are exposed to ultrasound radiation through the use of one or more modalities: office Doppler detection of the fetal heart beat, diagnostic ultrasound and fetal monitoring by ultrasound during the antepartum and intrapartum periods. A recent consensus conference prompted by the National Institutes of Health and the Food and Drug Administration (Consensus Conference, 1984) reviewed the indications for, use of and safety of diagnos-

tic ultrasound in pregnancy. Ultrasound is an extremely versatile and efficacious diagnostic technique, which has largely replaced x-ray diagnosis. High intensity, whole body ultrasound radiation can have adverse biologic ef-

Table 9–1. Effect of the Prevalence of a Disease/Condition on Positive Predictive Values and Frequency of False Positive Tests*

Prevalence (%)	Positive Predictive Value (%)	False Positive Tests (%)
20	53	47
10	33	67
5	19	81
1	4	96

*Assumption: Test is 90% sensitive and 80% specific.

fects, but these doses are 30 to 50 times more than those used in current techniques (O'Brien, 1984; Mole, 1986). There is a lack of adequate scientific study of the biologic effects of currently used intensities and duration in clinical ultrasound. This has been largely due to the inability to determine objectively biologic effects with clinical ultrasound. The adverse effects of high intensity and long duration of ultrasound radiation seen in whole laboratory animals or cell cultures may not be produced in humans. Nevertheless, several epidemiologic studies tend to support the safety of clinical ultrasound (Petitti, 1984). In fact, maternal bonding resulting from ultrasound seems to have a significant beneficial effect on obstetric and neonatal outcome (Fletcher and Evans, 1983; Field et al, 1985). However, a recent review of the controlled trials of routine ultrasound screening revealed significant methodologic weaknesses, with no clear statement of benefit or lack of benefit (Grant, 1986).

Despite the widespread agreement among experts that ultrasound is safe, ultrasound remains a focus of individuals and groups opposed to the technologic approach to obstetrics (Haire, 1984). A review of the biomechanics of ultrasound will allow improved interpretation of the arguments against ultrasound (Baker and Dalrymple, 1978).

Diagnostic ultrasound is based on the transmission of high-frequency sound waves at a rate of 1000 times/second and the reception and interpretation of the echopattern produced from the interfaces of tissues of different acoustic impedance or densities. During diagnostic ultrasound, the machine is receiving and interpreting the echopattern for 99.9% of the time, during which time the target tissue is not being impacted by ultrasound radiation. This ratio between emitting and receiving time is the duty cycle and varies with the ultrasound modality; continuous Doppler is 1:1, diagnostic ultrasound 1:1000. For example, in a 24-hour period of use with continuous Doppler (fetal monitoring) the target tissue receives 12 hours of energy. However, in 24 hours of use with a linear array realtime ultrasound the total exposure is less than 30 seconds.

The distance to the target tissue (the fetus) will also affect the amount of energy the target tissue receives. The rate at which energy is lost is a function of the square of half the distance: energy loss = $Km \left(\frac{d}{2}\right)^2$, when Km is the constant for a given medium and d is the

distance to the target tissue. Most commercial ultrasound instruments operate at energies between 10 and 20 mW/cm² at 2.5 to 7.5 mHz. Thus, a fetal target 8 cm distant from the source receives on the average 0.01 to 0.03 mW/cm².

Duty cycle and distance greatly reduce the energy received by the target tissue. In addition, the biologic effect of ultrasound radiation is different from that of ionizing radiation (x-rays). X-ray radiation forms free radicals that in turn disrupt biologic systems by chemical reactions. Ultrasound does not have the energy required to produce free radicals. The biologic mechanisms by which ultrasound produces effects include absorption heating, cavitation and microstreaming. Absorption heating probably occurs as the electromagnetic energy (sound) is changed to mechanical energy and heat by molecular vibration. This absorption phenomenon is approximately proportional to the frequency (mHz). The higher the frequency, the higher the temperature rise, but over a shorter distance. The thermal conductivity of the target tissue and the ability of the blood circulation to extract the heat greatly affect the temperature rise in the target tissue. Whole body radiation of laboratory animals or irradiation of a cell culture eliminates this important protective mechanism and seriously weakens the application of these experiments to human diagnostic ultrasound. Theoretic calculations suggest that diagnostic ultrasound does not produce biologically significant temperature rises.

Cavitation is the formation and dynamics of microbubbles and bubbles in media through which sound is propagated. Most ordinary liquids contain stable microbubbles that are found to grow in size during the negative pressure phase of a sound wave. At a critical size determined by the sound frequency, the bubbles exhibit mechanical resonance. The mechanical resonance and the uniform fluid patterns that it induces (microstreaming) can lead to localized regions of high shear and stress in the liquid (intracellular) sufficient to disrupt subcellular structures. This is called stable cavitation. In the 1 to 4 mHz frequency range stable cavitation may occur in the liquid state when the intensity exceeds 0.2 to 5.0 W/cm². Diagnostic ultrasound uses a 1 to 4 mHz range, but the tissue intensity is 0.01 to 0.03 mW/cm². At extreme intensities (greater than 300 W/cm²) more violent disruption occurs, with collapse of the bubbles during the early compression phase of the sound wave (collapse cavitation). The in-

Table 9–2. Accuracy of Ultrasound

Condition	Measurement	Sensitivity	Specificity	Predictive Value of Positive Tests	Author
Birthweight <5th percentile	Serial biometry	75.0	85.0	53.0	Pavelka et al, 1982
	BPD + NST	75.0	100.0	98.0	Pavelka et al, 1982
	Estimated fetal weight	60.0	99.0	65.0	Persson & Kullander, 1983
Birthweight >4000 gm	BPD − chest diameter >1.4 cm	61.0	92.0	87.0	Elliot & Garite, 1982
Multiple gestation	2 or more fetuses	98.0	100.0	98.0	Persson & Kullander, 1983
Placenta previa	Present	93.0	92.0	55.0	Bowie et al, 1978
Fetal sex	Accuracy	93.0	—	—	Plattner et al, 1983
Biophysical outcome	Abnormal outcome	31.8	99.5	87.5	Platt et al, 1985
Fetal lung maturity LS >2	BPD >9.2	92.0	—	—	Newton et al, 1983
Fetal lung maturity no RDS	BPD >9.2	100.0	—	—	Golde et al, 1982
Major congenital abnormality	Presence	68.4	—	—	Manning & Baskett, 1981
	Presence	16.7	—	—	Platt et al, 1985
	Presence	95.0	99.0	95.0	Sabbagha et al, 1985
	Presence	45.7	—	—	Hill et al, 1985
Spina bifida	Presence	83.0	97.0	83.0	Sabbagha et al, 1985

tensities needed to produce either stable or collapse cavitation are more than 1000 times greater than those used in clinical ultrasound.

In summary, widespread clinical experience has supported the safety of ultrasound in pregnancy. Physics and biomedical principles predict a very large margin of safety. However, good studies of long-term handicaps and disease following prenatal ultrasound have not been performed. Ultrasound may not have a biologic risk, but complications from its use may be important. The single greatest risk or complication of diagnostic ultrasound is obstetric intervention or lack of intervention based on an inaccurate ultrasound diagnosis. For example, an elective repeat cesarean section based on ultrasound dating alone may result in a small baby with respiratory distress syndrome. Tables

9–2, 9–3 and 9–4 give a representative incidence of the sensitivity, specificity and accuracy of common ultrasound measurements. Clinical judgment depends on an understanding of the limitations of the test and a knowledge of alternative tests that may support the results of ultrasound. An example is the collaborative use of ultrasound and the measurement of alpha-fetoprotein in the diagnosis of neural tube defects.

DIAGNOSTIC X-RAYS

In the United States until the early 1970's about 20% of women received x-ray radiation during pregnancy. Since then the use of ultra-

Table 9–3. The Sensitivity of Ultrasound in the Diagnosis of Selected Congenital Abnormalities

Organ System	Authors		Sensitivity (%)
	Hill et al, 1985	Sabbagha et al, 1985	
Central nervous system	9/11	30/32	39/43 (91)
Gastrointestinal system	3/15	16/16	19/31 (61)
Cardiothoracic systems	4/21	—	4/21 (19)
Skeletal system	4/10	6/6	10/16 (62)
Urinary tract system	12/13	12/13	24/26 (92)

Table 9–4. Accuracy of Ultrasonographically Determined Fetal Weight

Birthweight	Mean Percent Error	
	Ott (1981)	Hadlock et al (1985)
<1500 grams	+ 9.4	+ 5.4
1501–4000 grams	+ 7.0 to + 8.2	– 2.6 to + 0.9
>4000 grams	+ 11.7	– 4.0

sound has dramatically reduced the frequency. Currently, between 5 and 10% of women are exposed to x-ray radiation during pregnancy. There will always be an irreducible percentage in which x-ray diagnosis is superior to that obtainable with ultrasound. Examples are medical conditions requiring diagnostic x-ray, pelvimetry for trial of labor in breech presentation, amniography, or delineation of fetal positions in multiple gestation. Nor does the neonate escape irradiation, especially if she is admitted to the intensive care unit. The median number of films was five and the median exposure was 28 mR to neonates in the intensive care unit at Baltimore City Hospital (Mazzi et al, 1978).

The fear of radiation and lack of understanding about it have led the public to blame x-rays for bad pregnancy outcomes (malpractice cases) and have encouraged physicians to over-intervene (abortion) when early exposure has occurred (Brent, 1980). In very large doses (greater than 100 R) there is definite fetal damage—intrauterine growth retardation, microcephaly, mental retardation, microphthalmia, genital and skeletal malformations and cataracts (Dekaban, 1968). However, the doses in this study and the doses after the nuclear explosions at Hiroshima and Nagasaki far exceeded the doses received in diagnostic x-ray. Table 9–5 depicts an average dose to the fetus during common diagnostic x-rays. Fluoroscopy has an exposure rate of 15 to 150 mrads/min. In general, the usual exposure in diagnostic x-ray is less than 5 rads. This dose is much below the threshold dose (>20 rads) needed to demonstrate statistical increases in adverse outcomes. However, should exposure occur, the physician should more accurately estimate the doses and risk. Brent (1980) recommends documentation of the following as a minimal systematic approach:

1. Gestational age at exposure.
2. Menstrual history.
3. Previous pregnancy history.

4. Familial genetic or developmental risk, i.e., family history of birth defects.
5. Other concurrent environmental risks: smoking, alcohol use, drug abuse, toxic chemical exposure.
6. Age of mother and father.
7. Type of radiation study. Dates and number of films performed.
8. Calculation of the embryonic exposure by a medical physicist or competent radiologist.
9. Status of the pregnancy: wanted or unwanted.
10. Documentation in the chart of the workup and the counseling of the patient: bad outcomes can occur with or without irradiation, and, in most cases, diagnostic x-rays do not increase the risk.

The damage from x-ray exposure can be manifested in genetic defects, malformations, maldevelopment (growth retardation), loss of pregnancy or carcinogenesis. The periods of greatest risk for genetic disease are the first five months of fetal life and at ovulation. Pregnancy loss is most likely to occur with exposure in the first 17 days after conception. Malformation in most organ systems results when an insult occurs between 17 and 56 days. However, the development of the reproductive system (20 weeks), immune system (3 to 6 months postnatal) and the neurologic system (several years postnatal) takes considerably longer. The neurologic system is a major focus of the studies on irradiation in pregnancy, i.e., mental retardation and microcephaly. Mole (1982) has reviewed the development of the fetal brain and its relationship

Table 9–5. Fetal Irradiation from Diagnostic X-ray

Diagnostic X-ray	Fetal Absorbed Dose (rads)
Exchange transfusion	10.0
Barium enema	5.0
Hysterosalpingogram	3.27
Pelvimetry	2.0
Intravenous pyelogram	1.75
"Two shot" pyelogram	0.35
Amniogram	1.4
Lumbar spine	0.54
Upper gastrointestinal examination	0.29
Abdomen for fetal skeletal abnormalities	0.28
Pelvis	0.113
Femur	0.005
Gallbladder	0.003
Chest	0.001
Dental x-rays	0.001
Mammogram	0.001

to fetal damage. Cellular division marks the time of greatest vulnerability. Neuroblast division into neurons occurs at an exponential rate between 12 and 20 weeks' menstrual age. This is shown by an increase in DNA. Glial cells hallmark the second phase of cellular division, 20 weeks' to the postnatal period. The location and number of synapses are developed at this time.

Several large epidemiologic studies have suggested a small risk of carcinogenesis from exposure in utero to x-ray radiation (0.5 to 5 rads), especially from pelvimetry. Several authors have described a 40 to 60% increase in the frequency of childhood cancers (leukemia, neuroblastoma) in children exposed to irradiation in utero (Brent, 1980). Although this is statistically significant, the practical risk is remote (Brent, 1980). For example, in the United States, white children less than 15 years of age have a risk of leukemia of 1:2800, children exposed to pelvimetry in utero have a risk of 1:2000 and siblings of a child with leukemia have a 1:720 risk of childhood leukemia. In addition, until we know more about the induction of malignancy, one cannot say that irradiation causes childhood leukemia; it may only be a co-variant.

During their meiotic and mitotic divisions the germ cells are at risk for insult. These insults may be manifested as gross genetic disease such as trisomies or autosomal dominant or recessive disease. It may take several generations of an exposed population to exhibit the disease state. X-ray radiation has been discussed as a possible mechanism in the induction of genetic disease. The response of the oocyte to irradiation varies considerably, according to age, species, strain, physical factors (dose, dose rate, etc.) and according to the criteria used to assess the effect (Amatuzzi, 1980; Brent and Gorson, 1972). Although cytogenetic abnormalities are reported in peripheral lymphocytes in many of the victims exposed to greater than 100 rads (Bloom and Tijio, 1964), the risk of genetic disease in the offspring of radiation-exposed women is remote (less than 1%). The genetic risk of diagnostic x-ray is more difficult to ascertain. One must recognize that the average pregnant woman in the United States absorbs about 80 to 100 millirads background radiation during the nine months of pregnancy. This and other factors contribute to the 1% spontaneous mutation rate in the United States (Brent and Gorson, 1972).

In summary, malformation or maldevelopment cannot be ascribed to radiation exposure alone. There is a very small association between in utero radiation exposure and childhood cancers, but a cause and effect relationship has not been established in humans. The genetic risks are probably remote, but animal studies are limited in their application to human experience. The American College of Obstetricians and Gynecologists' guidelines for diagnostic x-ray examinations in fertile women (1977) are outlined in Table 9–6.

Specific Procedures

AMNIOGRAPHY

Amniography is used to outline either the surface topography of the fetus or the fetal gastrointestinal tract. Amniography is performed using the usual amniocentesis technique, after which water-soluble contrast material is injected. The volume is 1.5 ml per week of gestation but not to exceed 50 ml. This is followed by injection of 1 or 2 ml of lipid-soluble material for better contrast. Anteroposterior and lateral radiographs of the abdomen are obtained 30 minutes and 2 hours after the injection. The fetal gastrointestinal tract will be visualized within two hours; if it is not, another film is taken 24 hours later. The risks of the procedure are similar to those of amniocentesis—premature rupture of membranes, preterm labor, uterine bleeding and fetal injury. The cumulative risk is about 1%. Grech and Spitz (1977) reported two cases of tissue necrosis in 241 amniographs. The use of iodine solutions

Table 9–6. Guidelines for Diagnostic X-ray in Pregnancy*

1. The use of x-ray examinations should be considered on an individual basis. Concern over harmful effects should not prevent the proper use of radiation exposure when significant diagnostic information can be obtained. Pre-examination consultation with a radiologist may be useful in obtaining optimal information from the x-ray exposure.
2. There is no measurable advantage to scheduling diagnostic x-ray examinations at any particular time during a normal menstrual cycle.
3. The degree of risk involved in an x-ray examination if the person is pregnant, or should become pregnant, should be explained to the patient and documented in her record.

*From American College of Obstetricians and Gynecologists: Guidelines for diagnostic x-ray examination of fertile women. ACOG Statement of Policy, May, 1977. Reprinted with permission.

can result in transient impairment of fetal thyroid function (Rodesch et al, 1976). This appears to resolve spontaneously without lasting fetal effect.

PELVIMETRY

Early studies of pelvimetry demonstrated strong associations between decreased pelvic diameter and poor obstetric outcome, especially operative delivery (Steer, 1958). However, methodologic problems complicate the investigation of pelvimetry: lack of a uniform set of indications for performing pelvimetry, not all patients meeting clinical criteria have pelvimetry, wide variation in clinical management after the results of pelvimetry are known, inability to measure fetal biparietal diameter and failure to adjust for the normal changes in pelvic and fetal size during labor, i.e., molding. The recognition of these weaknesses and the more recent data suggesting a carcinogenic effect of in utero irradiation have led to a dramatic reduction in the frequency of x-ray pelvimetry. In most teaching institutions it has fallen from use in 10 to 15% of patients in the early 1970's to use in less than 1% more recently. The management of labor currently rests on the progress determined by dilatation of the cervix, descent of the fetal head and manual evaluation of the pelvic size. In fact, in one study (Fine et al, 1980) manual pelvimetry predicted cephalopelvic disproportion as well as two different x-ray techniques of pelvic measurement, Thoms's method and the modified Ball method. In this study, the incidence of cesarean section with the diagnosis of an inadequate or borderline pelvis was 29% by manual evaluation, 32% by the modified Ball method and 25% by Thoms's method. Absolute cephalopelvic disproportion increased the incidence of cesarean section to 70 to 90%. These data show that the use of pelvimetry alone to determine management by cesarean section would result in 30 to 50% of women having an unnecessary cesarean section. Nor is pelvimetry helpful clinically. Parsons and Spellacy (1986) performed a prospective randomized trial of x-ray pelvimetry or no pelvimetry prior to oxytocin augmentation of labor. No differences in maternal or neonatal outcomes were found.

Current clinical situations in which pelvimetry may be valuable are in patients with breech presentation when a vaginal delivery is anticipated, with multiple gestation in labor or with known distortion of the pelvis. As an adjunct,

the fetal biparietal measurements can be obtained by ultrasound. In these cases the benefits of the information obtained may outweigh the remote risks of diagnostic irradiation.

FETOSCOPY

Fetoscopy can be an adjunct to the diagnosis of fetal disease in at least three ways, visualization of anatomic defects, intrauterine fetal therapy and the diagnostic biopsy of fetal tissue (blood, skin or liver). The transuterine insertion of fetoscopes has its roots in the early 1950's. With increased motivation and improved optic technology an increasing number of investigators are using the technique for prenatal diagnosis and therapy. The fetoscopes currently used have a diameter of 2.0 to 2.7 mm with a field of vision ranging from 50 to 70 degrees. For diagnosis or treatment other than visualization, accessory instrumentation is needed. Blood or skin samples are taken by instruments introduced next to the fetoscope. The actual equipment and technique are both complex and costly. These are described by Goldberg and Golbus (1984), and the technique is best performed by individuals and centers equipped and motivated to handle the complexities of this procedure.

The major risks of fetoscopy include loss of pregnancy, maternal bleeding, fetal injury, placental injury, maternal bowel or bladder injury, premature rupture of membranes, preterm labor or third trimester bleeding. The risk of fetal loss is about 5%, and the risk of prematurity about 10% (Elias and Esterly, 1981). All investigators report a decrease in the complication rate and an increase in the success rate with increasing technical experience. Skill in fetoscopy should be obtained from the performance of 30 to 40 procedures in patients undergoing elective midtrimester abortions.

The need for fetoscopy may be greatly reduced in the future. Ultrasonographically directed needle aspiration of the umbilical cord has proved safer and more accurate in the diagnosis of fetal disease. The range of diagnosable conditions includes: karyotype abnormalities, blood component deficiencies, acid-base inequalities and hemoglobin abnormalities. Daffos and co-workers (1985) reported a series of 606 consecutive needle aspirations of the umbilical cord. Using an ultrasonographically guided 20-gauge needle, fetal blood was aspirated in 99.5% of cases. In 2.9% of cases, two attempts were required, and 2.4% of samples were contaminated. In 2% of cases bleeding from the cord lasted more than two minutes. Nine percent of fetuses had bradycardia. However, only two patients had major complications related to the procedure, one premature rupture of membranes and one fetal death.

CHORIONIC VILLUS SAMPLING

Hahnemann and Mohr (1969) and Kullander and Sandahl (1973) were among the first investigators to describe the sampling of chorionic villi for the diagnosis of genetic disease. In theory, the numbers of cells and their high mitotic rate make trophoblastic cells superior to amniotic fluid cells. Sampling in the first trimester would allow termination of the pregnancy at a much safer gestational age. However, early attempts were hampered by the difficulty of the procedure and the increased rate of complications. The recent development of high resolution realtime ultrasound and new diagnostic techniques for cytogenetic and molecular analysis have led to a renewed interest in chorionic villus biopsy.

Procedure

Chorionic villus sampling is the transcervical biopsy of the placenta between 7 and 11 weeks' gestation. The biopsy procedure requires an experienced ultrasonographer and obstetrician-gynecologist. The preoperative preparation involves a Pap smear and cervical cultures for gonococcus and chlamydia. The procedure itself is done under sterile conditions. The ultrasonographer scans the uterus to determine placental location, fetal life and gestational age. Under ultrasound guidance, the sampling device is directed into the placental bed and a sample is taken from the amniotic membrane side. Samples from the maternal side contain more maternal tissue. The actual sampling is done by one of two techniques, direct vision using a fetoscope or a contact hysteroscope or with a small suction cannula directed by ultrasound. More recently a transabdominal approach has been used with ultrasonic guidance. This approach avoids the relatively unsterile vaginal environment.

Complications

Instrumentation of the cervix with trauma to the villi has a predictable risk of complications. Infection, hemorrhage and rupture of membranes with subsequent pregnancy loss are immediate. The morbid risks to the fetus stem from the proportional reduction of viable placental tissue caused by the sampling and operative site bleeding. The late risks include intrauterine growth retardation and placental site bleeding late in pregnancy. Injury at 7 to 10 weeks also has an undefined teratogenic risk. There is also the potential for an adherent placenta at the time of delivery because of scarring at the operative site.

The fetal loss rate up to eight weeks after the procedure is between 2 and 5% (Jackson, 1984; Lilford, 1985; Brambati and Oldrini, 1985). Infection, bleeding and rupture of membranes seem to be associated with acute loss in the first two weeks. However, 30 to 40% of the losses occur between 15 and 20 weeks, and these fetal deaths are often unexplained. Greater operator experience seems to reduce losses. Of the two techniques, sampling under direct vision has the potential advantages of a purer sample and decreased incidence of rupture of membranes. However, the use of a disposable plastic suction cannula, under ultrasound guidance, has more practical appeal. The acute complication rate and the success rate (90%) are comparable with the two techniques. Fetal-maternal bleeding is also a risk, and unsensitized Rh negative women should receive RhoGAM after chorionic villus sampling.

The trophoblast is perhaps the most aggressive cell in the human body. In many senses it behaves like a malignant cell. It is pleomorphic and multinucleated with a high mitotic index. It rapidly invades normal tissue. With this activity, the DNA within the trophoblastic cell replicates much more quickly than usual. One would expect a discordancy between the analysis of trophoblastic tissue and fetal tissue. This is a real problem with chorionic villus sampling (Kalousek and Dill, 1983). In about 2 to 5% of cases the cell culture from the chorion will show an abnormality and the fetal cells will be normal. Action based on chorionic villus sampling abnormality may lead to some unnecessary pregnancy terminations.

In summary, chorionic villus sampling is an exciting new technique. However, it must still be considered experimental until the risks are better defined, including long-term fetal complications, maternal complications and discordancy with amniocentesis data. The technique will probably not replace amniocentesis but supplement it. Newer techniques of harvesting trophoblasts from maternal blood in the first trimester may significantly change the picture of prenatal genetic diagnosis, as phlebotomy is much safer than chorionic villus sampling or amniocentesis.

AMNIOCENTESIS

The major indication for midtrimester amniocentesis is prenatal diagnosis by the cytogenetic study of cultured amniotic fluid cells (fetal squames). The late second trimester amniotic fluid studies of optical density at 450 nm have been valuable in the management of isoimmunization. The current recommendations for midtrimester genetic amniocentesis are listed in Table 9–7, with an estimate of the incidence of abnormal results. In general, the most frequent indication (85%) will be advanced maternal age (greater than 35) or a low serum alphafetoprotein level. The incidence of abnormal results is about 1%. Cytogenetic analysis of amniocytes will not provide useful information on the effect of trauma, either physical or chemical, to the genetic material of the developing fetus.

The major indication for late third trimester amniocentesis is to evaluate fetal lung maturity. Respiratory distress is a major factor in neonatal morbidity and mortality. Only term spontaneous labor assures the lowest incidence of neonatal respiratory distress. In any other situation the risk of respiratory distress syndrome (RDS) must be recognized. Amniocentesis for fetal lung maturity studies should be performed in any case in which the risk of neonatal respiratory morbidity or mortality exceeds that of continued in utero management, i.e., prior to elective repeat cesarean. In cases in which there are good menstrual dates (Frigoletto and Phillippe, 1980) an amniocentesis can be avoided. Acceptable criteria would be (1) 33 weeks after a positive urine pregnancy test, (2) 35 weeks after a positive hCG test or (3) 20 weeks after the fetal heart tones are heard by stethoscope. In cases in which amniocentesis is impossible, a fetal biparietal diameter (BPD) greater than 9.3 and a negative maternal glucose challenge test will predict fetal lung maturity and a lack of neonatal RDS (Newton et al, 1983).

Procedure

The technique is the same for both midtrimester and third trimester amniocentesis. All amniocenteses should be preceded by a thorough ultrasonographic examination, including dating measurements, determination of fetal position and cord position, screening for fetal abnormalities and placental localization. At the time of amniocentesis and after the bladder has been emptied, a pocket of free fluid is visualized. A site away from the fetal face and umbilical cord is best. A site high on the fundus has the risk of maternal bowel perforation and a site far lateral on either side has the risk of uterine artery injury. Special caution should be used when the patient has had abdominal surgery because of fixation of the bowel to the anterior abdominal wall or uterus. The depth of the pocket should also be noted. The insertion site should be marked by pressing a small round object against the maternal skin for 10 to 15 seconds so that an impression remains.

The skin is then prepared with an antiseptic solution and a sterile drape is applied. Lidocaine can be used to anesthetize the skin, fascia and peritoneum. A 22-gauge spinal needle is sharply inserted to the angle and depth demonstrated on ultrasound. Insertion of the needle can be observed on lateral scan by the ultrasound or through an ultrasound aspiration transducer. The author finds lateral visualization helpful in the more difficult cases, and in these situations the free movement of the needle is important. The aspiration transducer can limit mobility.

When the needle enters the amniotic cavity, the loss of resistance is felt. The stylet is removed and 2 to 3 ml of fluid are aspirated in a 5-ml syringe. This is discarded, since it may be blood tinged. Fluid is aspirated (up to 20 ml) until the fluid clears. Then a fresh plastic syringe is used to withdraw 20 ml of fluid. The plastic syringes and transport containers must be checked beforehand for cytotoxic substances. The stylet is then reinserted and the needle is quickly withdrawn. After the procedure the fetal heart movement is documented and the placental surface is inspected for hematoma formation. The fluid is properly labeled and sent to the appropriate laboratory at room temperature.

If the scan reveals an anterior placenta with no "clear" window, the situation needs to be discussed with the patient. Insertion through the placenta in the midtrimester increases the

Table 9–7. Indications for Midtrimester Amniocentesis

Indication	Incidence of Abnormal Karyotype per 1000 Population
Advanced maternal age	
Trisomy 21 <30 years old	1.2
Trisomy 21 35 years old	2.5– 3.9
Trisomy 21 42 years old	13.8–23.4
Advanced paternal age >55	3.3
Abnormal parental karyotype	
Father with balanced translocation	30
Mother with balanced translocation	100
21/21 and 22/22	100
21/22	50
13/21 Mother	20
13/21 Father	0
Inversion	
no previous aneuploid children	10
previous aneuploidy male	50
previous aneuploidy female	100
Mosaicism	Risk proportional to frequency of abnormal cells
Previous child with Down's syndrome and mother <29 years old	10
Serum alpha-fetoprotein <0.5 multiples of the mean	10–15
Carrier of X linked recessive	XY karyotype
Sex limited autosomal dominant	Variable
Carrier of diagnostic biochemical abnormality	Variable

incidence of bloody taps, fetal-maternal blood transfusion and a possible increase in the pregnancy loss rate. The major complication rate probably does not exceed 1 to 2% (Crane and Kopta, 1984). The best plan is to delay one week in the hope that further uterine growth will permit a safer tap. If delay is not possible, the risks and benefits need to be assessed. If amniocentesis is performed, a site through the thinnest part of the placenta and away from the insertion of the cord is selected.

If twins are identified, another decision point is reached. The greater the number of taps, the greater is the likelihood for an iatrogenic fetal loss to occur. In addition, the results of genetic amniocentesis may be confusing. Since two thirds of twins are dizygotic and most dizygotic twins have discordant karyotypes, the patient may be faced with the dilemma of one healthy infant and one abnormal infant. If multiple taps are elected, it is important that the ultrasonographer identify the location of the dividing membrane and the relative positions of the two sacs. After the fluid is removed from one sac, 0.5 ml of indigo carmine (0.8%) diluted in 10 ml of normal saline is injected into the first sac. The second sac is then tapped. Clear fluid shows that the second sac has been sampled. The two samples must be clearly labeled to avoid confusion if abnormal results are obtained. If the

amniotic membrane cannot be identified on the scan, the needles are inserted as close to the small parts of each fetus as possible.

All Rh negative unsensitized gravidas should receive RhoGAM after amniocentesis. After third trimester amniocentesis a non-stress test should be obtained. A spontaneous contraction stress test is often present. The patient is then sent home, after having been instructed to limit activity until the next morning. She should report contractions, bleeding, leakage of fluid, decreased fetal activity or signs of chorioamnionitis.

Complications

RELIABILITY OF THE DATA

Midtrimester Amniocentesis. Cytogenetic analysis of amniocytes is an extremely accurate procedure (Roberts et al, 1983). Repeat amniocenteses were required in only 1.7 to 4.9% of cases and failure to report results (loss of culture) occurred in only 0.5 to 2.1%. Errors in diagnosis occurred in only 7 of 9,352 cases. The largest single source of error was maternal cell contamination. The accuracy of biochemical measurements depends on the clinical situation. The most common determination is alpha-fetoprotein, used in ascertaining the risk of neural tube defects. The sensitivity of amniotic fluid alpha-fetoprotein in the detection of open neural tube defects is 98%. Amniotic fluid acetycholinesterase, which is relatively specific for neural tube disease, helps separate neural tube defects from other sources of elevated amniotic fluid alpha-fetoprotein levels (abdominal wall defects, tracheal abnormalities, etc.). However, closed neural tube defects will not be detected, and these comprise between 5 and 10% of defects in affected infants.

Late Third Trimester Amniocentesis. Many tests have been used to predict fetal lung maturity and the lack of respiratory distress. The more common criteria are the lecithin/sphingomyelin (L/S) ratio (greater than 2.0), the presence of phosphatidylglycerol and optical density at 650 nm (OD 650) greater than 0.15. The presence of glucose intolerance, polyhydramnios, blood or meconium can affect the reliability of these tests. However, in the absence of these complications, fetal lung maturity studies are very specific tests. When the L/S ratio is greater than 2.0 the incidence of RDS is 1 to 2%. On the other hand, fetal lung maturity studies are not sensitive. With an L/S ratio between 1.5 and 2.0 the incidence of RDS is 20% and between 1.0 and 1.5 it is only 50%.

PREGNANCY LOSS

The worst complication is the loss of a healthy fetus after a diagnostic midtrimester amniocentesis. The recommendation to perform a genetic amniocentesis must weigh the chance of pregnancy loss against the benefit of clinically useful information. O'Brien (1984) has reviewed the major studies and their research designs in the examination of the risk of midtrimester amniocentesis. Table 9–8 depicts the cumulative statistics for prospective controlled studies of pregnancy loss following mid-trimester amniocentesis (O'Brien, 1984). These showed an

iatrogenic pregnancy loss rate of 0.5 to 1.0% above the expected loss rate of between 2 to 3%.

The factors associated with increased fetal loss are a transplacental tap, multiple taps, bloody taps, multiple gestation, oligohydramnios and operator experience. The largest single factor may be operator experience; the risk of pregnancy loss may be reduced to one tenth among physicians with experience in 50 or more cases (Hecht, 1982). With a cumulative experience of less than 10 midtrimester taps the loss was 3.7%, between 11 and 50 taps it was 1.8% and with greater than 50 taps the loss was 0.3%.

Intuitively, ultrasound guidance would seem to reduce the risk of complications. However, the evidence to support this is confusing. Many non-randomized studies have supported ultrasound's efficacy in reducing the frequency of failed taps, bloody taps and pregnancy loss (Carpenter et al, 1983). In fact, Farahani and co-workers (1984) reported an extremely low incidence of complications in 2100 patients using an ultrasound aspiration transducer in midtrimester amniocentesis. They reported 99.2% successful taps, 2.37% bloody taps and 0.38% iatrogenic fetal loss. In contrast, two randomly assigned prospective studies (Nolan et al, 1981; Levine et al, 1978) failed to report a significant difference whether ultrasound was used or not. Large collaborative studies have showed mixed results. The NICHD study showed no benefit (NICHD, 1976). The Canadian study (Simpson et al, 1976) showed that ultrasound improved the success rate but did not change the risk of pregnancy loss. The discrepancy in these studies may be explained by the varied experience of the physician in performing the amniocentesis and in using ultrasound guidance. It is without question that an ultrasound scan for structural abnormalities performed at the time of amniocentesis greatly assists counseling the patient.

Table 9–8. Pregnancy Loss and Midtrimester Amniocentesis*

	Amniocentesis			Control		
	No.	Loss	Percent	No.	Loss	Percent
Spontaneous abortion	2,027	56	2.76	2,018	37	1.83†
Total fetal and neonatal loss	3,423	111	3.26	3,405	96	2.82‡

*Data from National Institute of Child Health and Human Development, *J. Am. Med. Assoc.* 236:1471, 1978; Turnbull AC, Fairweather DV et al: *Br. J. Obstet. Gynaecol.* 85:1, 1978.
†P <0.01 (X²)
‡P <0.001 (X²)

BLOODY TAP

The aspiration of blood signifies either maternal or fetal trauma. The major complications of maternal trauma are hematoma or abruptio placentae. Hematoma of the abdominal wall, peritoneum, broad ligament or uterus occurs rarely. Galle and Meis (1982) found seven case reports of significant maternal trauma associated with amniocentesis. The incidence of abruptio placentae in midtrimester amniocentesis is hard to separate from the data on pregnancy loss. In third trimester amniocentesis two studies report an 0.3% (Sabbagha, 1979) and 0.38% (Young, 1979) incidence of abruptio placentae.

Fetal trauma includes injury to the fetus and the placental vessels, including the umbilical cord (Tables 9–9 and 9–10). In most cases fetal injury is relatively benign and is manifested only by cutaneous injury. However, major injury has been reported, including pneumothorax, hemopericardium, spinal tap, renal trauma, gastrointestinal atresia, arteriovenous fistula, brain injury, spinal cord injury and ocular injury (Galle and Meis, 1982). The incidence of fetal injury varies according to the type of study and the care with which the neonates are examined. The collaborative studies reveal rates of less than 1%, but other studies show rates between 2 and 3% (Galle and Meis, 1982).

The amount of fetal blood mixing with maternal blood and amniotic fluid marks the severity of fetal injury. Young and co-workers (1977) examined the ratio of fetal to maternal red cells obtained by amniocentesis for genetic study from 242 consecutive patients. The study material included both clear and bloody taps. They noted that 38% of the samples contained at least microscopic red blood cells and 14% were grossly bloody on inspection. In grossly bloody taps, 57% contained more than 75%

Table 9–9. Complications of Midtrimester Amniocentesis

Complication	Incidence (%)
Failure to obtain fluid	5–10
Bloody amniotic fluid	10–15
Two or more needle insertions	10–15
Fetal injury	
Cutaneous scars	1–5
Exsanguination	Rare
Fetal to maternal bleed	1.0
Abruptio placentae at the time of amniocentesis	Unknown
Rupture of membranes	0.1–1.3
Pregnancy loss	0.5–1.0
Musculoskeletal abnormalities	1.0

Table 9–10. Complications of Third Trimester Amniocentesis

Complication	Incidence (%)
Failed attempt	5–10
Rupture of membranes	
<24 hours	2–3
Between 24–48 hours	2–3
Fetal injury	1–2
Infection	0.5–1
Preterm labor	0.5–1
Injury to fetal vessels	1–2
Bloody tap	5–10

fetal red cells. One case of fetal exsanguination was reported, and the incidence of fetal bleeding was correlated with an anterior placenta. Except for the management of fetal-maternal bleeding, the presence of fetal blood after a midtrimester amniocentesis is treated conservatively.

Fetal trauma, including injury to the umbilical cord, occurs at similar rates in third trimester amniocentesis (see Table 9–10) but has very different management goals. First, a clear tap does not absolutely guarantee that significant fetal trauma has not occurred. Klein and Young (1981) have supported the recommendation that a post-amniocentesis fetal monitoring strip should show a reactive fetus and a negative contraction stress test. Any bloody fluid should be evaluated for the presence of fetal cells. A hematocrit is obtained on the fluid and then the fluid is spun down (1000 g for 10 minutes) to a "pellet." The cells are examined by the Kleihauer-Betke technique and the percentage of fetal cells is determined. The Apt test is another method to identify fetal cells, but the technique will miss small amounts of fetal blood in a mixture with maternal blood (less than 50% fetal cells). Hemoglobin electrophoresis (Richards and Miller, 1983) can also be used, but the technique is long and complicated and may not be available in smaller laboratories. The presence of fetal blood signifies a potentially dangerous situation. If there are fetal heart abnormalities, delivery is mandatory, and in most cases this is by cesarean section. In cases in which the post-amniocentesis strip is normal, the knowledge of fetal lung maturity is critical. The presence of blood or meconium will reduce the reliability of the L/S ratio and OD 650, but the phosphatidylglycerol determination is less affected. Good dating or a fetal biparietal diameter greater than 9.4 cm also assures fetal lung maturity unless there is maternal glucose intolerance. If fetal lung maturity is assured, delivery is recommended. If the fetal lungs are immature, the mother should be given steroids (dexamethasone 4 mg Q 8 hours for 6 doses), and the fetus should be continuously monitored. In most cases delivery is indicated after 24 to 48 hours. Another option is to repeat the amniocentesis to evaluate the amount of intra-amniotic bleeding.

Fetal-Maternal Bleeding

Fetal to maternal transfusion can occur with any diagnostic amniocentesis, midtrimester or third trimester, and is positively correlated with anterior placenta, multiple taps and the presence of bloody tap. About one quarter of these transfusions exceed 0.1 ml fetal blood (Thomsen et al, 1983). Three quarters of the fetal-maternal bleeds in amniocentesis occur in women with grossly clear amniotic fluid. By examining the pre- and post-amniocentesis maternal serum alpha-fetoprotein levels or the Kleihauer-Betke test, approximately 5 to 15% of patients will have evidence of a bleed (Lele et al, 1982). The determination of serum alpha-fetoprotein is a more sensitive test. An accurate Kleihauer-Betke test requires the examination of at least 2000 red cells to reach the desired level of sensitivity (0.1 ml fetal blood transfusion). This is a lengthy and inaccurate procedure.

The diagnosis of fetal-maternal bleeding has important perinatal implications. There is a significant risk of fetal death (Lele et al, 1982), lower birth weight (Thomsen et al, 1983) and Rh sensitization (Hill et al, 1980). In view of these complications the remaining part of the pregnancy should be considered at high risk and prophylactic RhoGAM (150 mcgm) should be given after any amniocentesis in an unsensitized Rh negative woman.

Premature Rupture of Membranes and Preterm Labor

About 2 to 3% of women will complain of cramping or the leakage of fluid after diagnostic midtrimester amniocentesis (see Table 9–9). These complications are generally treated conservatively. In the case of early premature rupture of membranes, the leakage may cease in three to four days. Since infection is a risk in these cases, close observation and prohibition of coitus or other vaginal insertions are warranted. Any signs of infection should initiate termination of pregnancy. Cramping should be managed with reduced activity for 48 to 72 hours.

Premature rupture of membranes and preterm labor occur at a somewhat higher frequency in late third trimester amniocentesis (see Table 9–10). Between 2 and 5% of women will have rupture of membranes within 48 hours of amniocentesis (Teramo and Sipinen, 1978). Rupture of membranes seems to be related to the number of attempts and the site of amniocentesis. Teramo and Sipinen (1978) found that amniocentesis behind the fetal neck was associated with a greater incidence of multiple taps and a higher incidence of ruptured membranes.

Premature labor is stimulated in 3 to 5% of patients after amniocentesis in the third trimester (Young, 1979). Prior to 38 weeks the risk is reported to be 1 to 2% (Rome et al, 1975). The maturity of the fetal lung determines the management of this preterm labor. In most cases labor can continue. The risk of RDS with a mature L/S ratio is 0.19% in this situation (Young, 1979). Preterm labor in the presence of immature fetal lung studies should be treated aggressively with a tocolytic agent.

The risk of respiratory distress from third trimester amniocentesis depends in part on the population studied. Among patients undergoing repeat cesarean sections the risk may be lower. However, in a high risk population in which the amniocentesis is done earlier the risk may be higher. Young (1979) reported a 0.77% incidence of respiratory distress as a result of third trimester amniocentesis.

Miscellaneous Complications

A number of studies have considered the incidence of antepartum hemorrhage later in pregnancy after a midtrimester amniocentesis. There seems to be a small but significant risk of about 1.1%, or about 40% over the usual incidence (0.69%) (O'Brien, 1984). The cause and effect relationship is not clear because risk factors for antepartum bleeding such as smoking have not been controlled.

Cesarean section seems to be more common in women undergoing midtrimester amniocentesis (O'Brien, 1984). The estimate of the increase in cesarean births is 2.2%, or about a 10% increase. The increased risk of antepartum hemorrhage and cesarean birth may help to explain the consistent increase in RDS noted in patients who have undergone midtrimester amniocentesis (O'Brien, 1984). This is about 1.44%, or a 60% increase over the usual incidence (0.80%).

The risk of orthopedic deformity in neonates following midtrimester amniocentesis was raised by the British Collaborative Study (Turnbull et al, 1978). The significant findings were severe talipes equinovarus and congenital dislocation and subluxation of the hip. An explanation of the abnormalities may be chronic low amniotic fluid volume. However, other large studies have failed to find significant orthopedic problems, and pooled data suggest no significant increase in orthopedic problems among neonates (O'Brien, 1984).

Long-term follow-up studies of fetuses exposed to midtrimester genetic amniocentesis have shown no abnormalities of neurobehavioral status compared to fetuses not so exposed (Finegan et al, 1984; Gillberg et al, 1982). These small controlled studies require continued follow-up and larger numbers for confirmation.

EXTERNAL VERSION

The external manipulation of a fetus from a non-vertex to a vertex presentation (external cephalic version) has been reported for many years, and there have been rises and falls in its popularity. Randomly assigned prospective trials under controlled conditions (Van Dorsten et al, 1981; Hofmeyer, 1983) have demonstrated the efficacy and safety of the technique. The incidence of breech presentation at the onset of labor can be reduced by 75 to 80%, and the incidence of cesarean section for breech presentation is reduced according to the particular institutional policy on vaginal breech delivery. This reduction can be as high as 80 to 90% for institutions in which all breeches are delivered by cesarean section.

Current protocols call for external cephalic version under tocolysis and ultrasound evaluation after 37 weeks' gestation. Delay until after 37 weeks' has obvious advantages; fewer procedures are needed, since 10 to 20% of breech presentations will convert to vertex between 35 and 37 weeks, and complications of external cephalic version can be managed by timely delivery of a mature infant. The disadvantage of late external cephalic version is that 20 to 30% of breech deliveries occur prior to 37 weeks. Tocolysis has been felt to aid external version and reduce the risk of uterine contraction during the procedure (Saling and Muller-Holve, 1975).

The absolute contraindications to the procedure are multiple pregnancy (except for version of the second twin after delivery of the first), antepartum hemorrhage, low lying placenta, ruptured membranes, fetal anomalies, uteroplacental insufficiency (intrauterine growth retardation or abnormal fetal testing) and cases in which cesarean section is required regardless of presentation. Relative contraindications are a uterine scar (cesarean section), uterine anomalies (leiomyomata, mullerian duct abnormalities) or a contraindication to tocolysis. The prerequisites for external cephalic version include assurance of mature fetal lungs, a reactive non-stress test or a negative contraction stress test and informed consent.

Procedure

Immediately prior to the procedure a blood sample is taken for a blood count and a tube of blood for type and antibody screen. Patients who are Rh negative should have a sample drawn prior to and 30 minutes after the procedure for comparison of serum alpha-fetoprotein level and a Kleihauer-Betke test for demonstration of fetal-maternal bleeding. All Rh negative unsensitized women should receive 300 mcgm of RhoGAM. Vital signs are taken prior to the start of tocolysis. Tocolysis may be accomplished by a variety of techniques: intravenous ritodrine or magnesium sulfate or terbutaline subcutaneously. A suggested protocol is to give terbutaline 0.25 mg subcutaneously 20 minutes prior to the procedure. If needed, a second dose is given 40 minutes later. During the procedure maternal heart rate and blood pressure are taken every five minutes. No anesthesia is needed.

The patient is placed supine with a lateral tilt to prevent supine hypotension. Hofmeyer (1983) describes the maneuver with steep lateral positioning and back support. Both are equally effective. Realtime ultrasound is used to locate the fetal position, to demonstrate a BPD greater than 9.3 cm and to document the presence of an amniotic fluid pocket greater than 3 cm in the vertical plane. The fetal heart rate is recorded by Doppler monitoring every two minutes during the procedure. Version is accomplished by either the classic forward roll or by a back flip. If the fetal spine and head are on the same side of the maternal spine, a back flip is attempted; if the fetal head and spine are on opposite sides of the midline, a forward roll is chosen. If the initial attempt fails, the opposite method is attempted. The procedure is interrupted for intolerable maternal discomfort, fetal heart rate decelerations or uterine contractions. Most successful versions occur within five min-

Table 9–11. Efficacy of External Cephalic Version

Author	No. of Versions	Gestational Age (weeks)	Success (%)	Spontaneous Version (%)	Reversion (%)
Ylikorkala & Hartikainen-Sorri (1977)	649	32–36	76.2	5.3	9.2
Fall & Nilsson (1979)	53	>36	70.0	—	0
Van Dorsten et al (1981)	51	>37	68.0	18.0	0
Hofmeyr (1983)	30	>37	97.0	33	3.0

utes and should be followed by ultrasound confirmation of presentation and fetal heart activity. The fetus is maintained in the new attitude for several minutes and a fetal monitor is applied. A reactive non-stress test or a negative contraction-stress test is obtained prior to discharge. A repeat Kleihauer-Betke test and alpha-fetoprotein measurements are obtained 30 minutes after the version, and RhoGAM is given to all eligible gravidas. Some authors have argued for immediate induction of labor, but most institutions have allowed the patients to go home.

Complications

FAILED VERSION

The rates of success, spontaneous version and reversion are depicted in Table 9–11. Factors associated with failed external cephalic version are multiparity, maternal weight greater than 175 lbs, engagement of the breech and advanced gestational age. Ranney (1973) in 860 patients showed a doubling of the failure rate between 36 and 40 weeks (25 vs. 50%). Placental position has only a limited role in failed version. Ylikorkala and Hartikainen-Sorri (1977) showed no differences between anterior, posterior or lateral wall placental position. The author has found decreased success when the fetus is in a frank breech sacrum anterior presentation. In this case, the extended legs on either side of the maternal spine make rotation difficult. A deeply engaged breech may prevent rotation, although elevation of the vagina by a second operator will occasionally allow success. In general, if the attempt takes longer than five minutes and the mother is uncomfortable the success rate drops significantly.

UTERINE BLEEDING OR ABRUPTIO PLACENTAE

Table 9–12 depicts the complication rates in a large group of external cephalic versions under tocolysis and ultrasound guidance (Ylikorkala

and Hartikainen-Sorri, 1977). Uterine bleeding with or without contractions occurred in 5 of 649 procedures (0.8%). All placentas were examined for retroplacental clot; in two cases a small clot was found. Bradley-Watson (1975) reported a series of 1308 attempted external cephalic versions. These were not performed under tocolysis or with ultrasound guidance. Non-stress testing was not performed. Anesthesia and analgesia were used in many cases. He reported a 0.9% fetal mortality rate and a 0.4% emergency cesarean section rate. He related three of eight fetal deaths due to abruptio placentae. This experience illustrates the importance of control over the procedure. The assurance of fetal lung maturity decreases the fetal risk of emergency cesarean section precipitated by external version. A reactive non-stress test will identify a healthy infant prior to the procedure. Maternal discomfort is an important guide to the gentle manipulation of the fetus. Analgesia and anesthesia allow greater and perhaps more dangerous manipulation and thus increases the risk to the fetus and placenta.

FETAL HEART RATE VARIATION

Ylikorkala and Hartikainen-Sorri (1977) reported a 0.5% incidence of fetal bradycardia (less than 100 BPM) or tachycardia (greater than 160 BPM). Van Dorsten and co-workers (1981)

Table 9–12. Complications of External Cephalic Version (649 Versions)*

Complication	No.	%
Uterine contraction	27	4.2
Uterine bleeding	3	0.5
Uterine bleeding and contractions	2	0.3
Variation in fetal heart rate	3	0.5
Rupture of membranes	1	0.2
Abruptio placentae	0	0
Fetal death	0	0
Total	36	5.5

*From Ylikorkala O, Hartikainen-Sorri A: Value of external version in fetal malpresentation in combination with use of ultrasound. *Acta Obstet. Gynecol. Scand.* 56:63, 1977. Reprinted with permission.

and Phelan and co-workers (1984) reported about a 40% incidence of bradycardia (a fall greater than 40 BPM from baseline). In most cases these are variable decelerations probably occurring because of compression of the cord. A healthy infant (reactive non-stress test) should tolerate this stress without injury. The fetal heart is monitored by ultrasound and Doppler throughout the procedure. If a deceleration occurs, the version is stopped and the fetal heart is allowed to recover for 60 seconds. If a bradycardia recurs on further attempts with that version technique, for example a back flip, the fetal heart should be allowed to recover and the alternate method (forward roll) should be tried. Recurrent bradycardia is an indication for discontinuing version.

FETAL-MATERNAL HEMORRAGE

Fetal-maternal hemorrhage is a consistent risk of external cephalic version. The incidence varies between 5 and 28% (Van Dorsten et al, 1981; Gjode et al, 1980; Marcus et al, 1975). The volume transfused is usually small, 0.1 to 6.0 ml, although life-threatening transfusion has been reported (Loyet et al, 1976). The risk of Rh sensitization when patients are not treated with RhoGAM is around 8% (Vos, 1967). The risk seems to be increased when there is a failed attempt at external version. The lowest incidences are reported in trials in which tocolysis and ultrasound are used and in which no anesthesia is used.

A dangerous transfusion is identified by post-procedure non-stress testing and Kleihauer-Betke tests. Small transfusions are treated expectantly except in Rh negative unsensitized patients. These patients should receive 300 mcgm of RhoGAM.

INTRAUTERINE TRANSFUSION

The etiology of isoimmunization syndromes is well established, involving exposure of the maternal host to foreign red cell antigens, maternal antibody production, transplacental antibody passage and destruction of fetal red cells. The most common and significant red cell antigens are A, B, O, Rhesus, Kell, C, c, E, e. Other antigens are rare, but some can cause severe disease. The reader is referred to standard obstetric and perinatal medicine textbooks for further details. The destruction of fetal red cells produces the amniotic bilirubin that is used as a guide for the management of isoimmunization. Fetal over-compensation for the anemia results in hydrops and intrauterine fetal death. Extramedullary hematopoiesis leads to extensive displacement of liver parenchyma by erythropoietic tissue and fibroblasts, decreasing the synthesizing capacity of the liver cells and leading to hypoproteinemia and consequent edema. Obstruction of the portal and umbilical veins by the abnormal liver parenchyma leads to ascites and placental villous edema. The resultant decrease in fetal O_2 uptake and the anemia lead to fetal cardiac failure, but this is a late event.

The purpose of intrauterine transfusion is to keep the fetus alive until delivery can be reasonably be expected to result in an infant with less mortality or morbidity than the intrauterine treatment itself produces. Intrauterine transfusion replaces antigen-present red cells (Rh positive) with antigen-absent red cells (Rh negative). This partially corrects the fetal anemia and turns off the stimulus for extramedullary hematopoiesis.

A positive antibody titer indicates that a mother has been sensitized to that antigen. Considerable experience with isoimmunization is needed to predict the absence of significant fetal disease with titers below a critical level. Relatively few centers now encounter adequate numbers of sensitized patients. Unless the titer is done at a center with sufficient experience, all patients with positive titers should have amniocentesis. In all cases in which the critical titer is not known, amniocentesis is performed at 26 weeks for the first sensitized pregnancy. In cases in which the critical titer is known, amniocentesis is performed at 20.5 weeks for a history of an affected infant or a titer greater than the critical level. If the critical titer is known and the titers are less than the critical level, they are repeated at two week intervals. Once the critical titer has been reached amniocentesis is performed within three to five days. Through amniocentesis the excess bilirubin is measured in the amniotic fluid (delta 450 nm) and plotted on a graph relating the delta 450 nm reading to gestational age (Liley curve). From this curve an individual plan of diagnosis and treatment can be made. In a case with a history of late second trimester loss, fetal transfusion can be performed at 22 to 23 weeks. Blood, meconium, renografin, maternal liver disease or steroid usage will make the measurement of amniotic fluid bilirubin unreliable.

Procedure

Intraperitoneal transfusion has been the standard procedure for many years. The techniques and their complications have been well established. This procedure is described in the following paragraphs. However, techniques for direct intravascular transfusion are being developed. Once the technique has been refined and its complications have been determined, direct intravascular transfusion will become the standard procedure.

The use of continuous realtime ultrasound has dramatically reduced the need for radiography in intrauterine transfusion (IUT). A realtime ultrasound will show the placental position and status of the fetus, including the presence of edema and ascites. The ultrasound allows continuous tracking of the moving target, the fetal peritoneum, and can accurately measure the depth of penetration for the needle. However, x-rays are needed for confirmation of catheter placement. Thus, the procedure needs to be performed in the radiology department with a high quality portable realtime ultrasound unit.

Heavy maternal sedation (diazapam and an opiate) is important in reducing fetal morbidity by reducing fetal activity. Ideally the fetus should be lying in a lateral position. This allows paracentesis below the umbilicus, cephalad to the fetal bladder and halfway between the midline and the lateral abdominal wall. Midline penetration should be avoided because of possible laceration of umbilical vessels. Penetration superiorly risks hepatic or splenic injury. In cases in which the fetal back is anterior, an effort should be made to change it to a lateral position, because entry through the retroperitoneum risks kidney or large vessel injury. If intrauterine transfusion cannot be delayed, an oblique insertion of the needle may be attempted.

The risk of IUT increases when the placenta is placed anteriorly. The placenta should be avoided; if it cannot be avoided, it should be traversed away from the insertion of the cord and near the periphery. External manipulation may be necessary to improve the fetal lie.

The maternal abdomen is prepared and anesthesized with 1% lidocaine. The needle insertion is observed with the ultrasound transducer covered with a sterile glove. A small 5-mm skin incision is made, and an 18-cm, 16-gauge Touhy needle is inserted to the predetermined depth. Loss of resistance is felt successively as the needle enters the maternal peritoneal cavity, the amniotic sac and the fetal peritoneal cavity. The stylet is removed and a size 16 epidural catheter is threaded down the needle. The tip and side hole of the catheter are removed beforehand, since red blood cells can be lysed by the side holes. Free passage of the catheter past the needle tip indicates its placement in a cavity. Approximately 30 cm are threaded down the needle. The needle is then withdrawn and 2 to 3 ml of radiopaque medium is injected. Often realtime ultrasound will demonstrate the passage of small air bubbles and contrast. A single A-P radiograph is taken. If the catheter is in the peritoneal cavity and is unobstructed, the characteristic half moons of contrast outline the fetal intestine.

If the catheter cannot be threaded past the tip of the needle, the needle is usually embedded in fetal soft tissue. No attempt should be made to force the catheter, and the needle is removed and redirected under ultrasound guidance. The appearance of fluid in the needle alerts the perinatologist to its location. Rarely does amniotic fluid come up the needle under pressure. Fetal urine is colorless. Contrast material may be injected down the needle to confirm its position. If the needle is in the bladder, the bladder is emptied and the needle is withdrawn and reinserted. Ascitic fluid coming from the needle is recognized by its clear, bright yellow appearance and viscosity. Blood-stained ascitic fluid may be obtained on repeat IUT.

When free peritoneal placement is demonstrated, fresh Group O negative red cells that have been tightly packed with all plasma and buffy coat removed and cross-matched with the maternal serum are prepared for transfusion. The total volume to be transfused is calculated from the formula: IUT volume = (weeks gestation − 20) × 10 ml. This volume is diluted with 15 ml isotonic saline to reduce the viscosity of the blood. If the unit has been prepared properly, the hemoglobin of the mixture is about 29 gm/dl with a hematocrit of 90%.

The blood is filtered and transfused in 10 ml aliquots, each 10 ml taking about five minutes. A Harvard pump may be useful in maintaining an even flow. The fetal heart rate is monitored continuously throughout the transfusion. Fetal tachycardia of 160 to 190 BPM is common in a fetus with an intact autonomic nervous system. Bradycardia early in the procedure is a poor prognostic sign. Late bradycardia is an indication to stop the transfusion immediately because the intraperitoneal pressure may be approaching umbilical venous pressure.

After termination of the IUT the fetal heart rate is monitored continuously for four to six hours. Tachycardia and a gradual return to good long-term variability is the expected response. The presence of a sustained sinusoidal heart rate, persistent late decelerations or a baseline bradycardia is an indication for corrective measures including delivery if the fetus is viable. In order to evaluate the status of the transfused blood and to confirm fetal well-being, a biophysical profile and ultrasound should be performed twice a week in the non-hydropic fetus and daily in the hydropic fetus.

When gross fetal ascites is present at IUT, some of the ascitic fluid is aspirated prior to threading the catheter. A volume of ascitic fluid 20 to 30 ml in excess of the planned volume of red cells to be transfused should be aspirated. Up to 150 ml of ascitic fluid can be removed. If more ascitic fluid is removed than the planned volume of red cells to be infused, the total volume of the transfusion should be increased 20 to 30%. Some authors advocate the use of intraperitoneal digitalis (digoxin 0.035 to 0.040 mg/kg of estimated non-hydropic fetal weight), infused into the fetal peritoneal cavity at the time of IUT (Bowman, 1984).

The timing of a subsequent transfusion is dependent on gestational age and the estimated concentration of donor cells within the fetus. The gestational age is important, since delivery should be performed when the risks of transfusion exceed the risk of neonatal death from prematurity. Intrauterine transfusions are performed to maintain the estimated concentration of donor (O negative) hemoglobin above 10 to 11 gm/100 ml. This estimation is based on the following formula.

$$\text{Hb concentration (grams/100 ml)} = \frac{0.55(a) \times 120 - (c)}{85(b) \times 120}$$

The fraction 0.55 is the proportion of intraperitoneal red cells that appears in the fetal circulation, (a) is the amount (ml) of donor cells transfused, (b) is the estimated fetal weight (Kg) at the time of the calculation, (c) is the interval in days from the time of transfusion to the time of calculation, 120 is the life span of the donor cells, and 85 ml/Kg is the estimated blood volume of the fetus.

One intrauterine transfusion cannot raise the donor (O negative) hemoglobin to above 10 gm/ 100 ml. Therefore, a second transfusion is performed in 8 to 10 days. Subsequent transfusions are given at four-week intervals, with the last being performed at around 28 to 30 weeks.

Complications

RISKS OF DIAGNOSIS

As reviewed earlier in this chapter, amniocentesis has its own risks; approximately 1% of pregnancies will have serious complications resulting from each amniocentesis done to determine optical density. Operator experience and ultrasound guidance will reduce the complications to a bare minimum. Contamination of the amniotic fluid with blood or meconium will abolish the value of the OD 450 measurement. In these cases ultrasound is the only method of determining the timing of transfusion; it is performed at three- to four-day intervals. Ultrasound can also evaluate the fetus for progressive changes leading to hydrops. Useful signs are increasing liver or placental size and sonolucency, dilatation of hepatic veins and right atrium, or the appearance of peritoneal, pericardial or pleural fluid. Edema of the subcutaneous tissue is a late sign.

The accuracy of the Liley curve is very high, but life-threatening inaccuracies can occur. Bowman (1984) reviewed a series of 3,177 samples and noted a overall inaccuracy rate of 5.3%. The rate of life-threatening inaccuracy for the zone of the last sample was 1.2% for zone I, 3.6% for zone II and 0.6% for zone III. In a patient without increasing titer and with a poor obstetric history, a falling OD 450 curve is suggestive of inaccurate testing.

TRAUMA

Intrauterine transfusion is an invasive procedure with a major risk of trauma to the mother and fetus (Table 9–13). Maternal trauma includes abdominal wall or uterine hematoma. Trauma to the placenta or membranes may lead to premature labor or abruptio placentae. Amniotic fluid embolism from catheterization of a maternal uterine venous sinus has been reported. The incidence of significant maternal trauma is 1 to 3%. Penetration of the moving fetal abdomen runs a major risk of fetal trauma. Lacerations of fetal vessels and intra-abdominal organs are possible. Insertion of the needle and catheter into the thorax, retroperitoneum, bladder, bowel or stomach is relatively inconse-

Table 9–13. Hazards of Intrauterine Transfusion

Maternal
Infection
Maternal tissue trauma
Abruptio placentae
Amniotic fluid embolism
Fetal
Early
   Over-transfusion
   Trauma
   Infection
   Premature labor
   Premature rupture of membranes
Late
   Graft-versus-host disease
   Radiation exposure
   Transient susceptibility to neonatal infection

quential unless there is vascular injury. The error must be recognized; blood is not injected, and the needle and catheter are removed and replaced properly. Approximately 10 to 20% of perinatal mortality due to IUT is secondary to fetal trauma (Bowman, 1984). The use of direct ultrasonographic guidance, avoiding the placenta when possible and taking care not to insert the needle too deeply, will reduce the risk of trauma.

PREMATURE LABOR

Precipitation of labor after fetal transfusion is a major risk. Bowman (1984) reports a 20% incidence after IUT. Preterm labor tends to occur more commonly at later gestational ages. Preterm labor prior to viability (less than 26 weeks) should be treated aggressively with a tocolytic agent, as continued pregnancy is the only chance for survival. Frank evidence of abruptio placentae or infection is the only contraindication to the use of intravenous ritodrine, assuming no maternal allergy or cardiac disease. Between 26 and 30 weeks the question is more difficult. Abruptio placentae may add significant stress to the already stressed infant, and delivery may be indicated. Preterm labor at this stage without bleeding can be treated with intravenous ritodrine.

PERINATAL MORTALITY

The severity of the disease, premature delivery and trauma are the commonest causes for perinatal mortality in IUT (Bowman, 1984). The severity of the disease causes 40% of deaths in the IUT population. The remaining 60% result from the IUT's. Twenty percent of the deaths associated with the IUT procedure are caused by trauma. Low gestational ages and the presence of hydrops at the first IUT significantly lower survival. The first transfusion prior to 26 weeks increases perinatal mortality by 15 to 20% and the risk of traumatic death by 50 to 60%. The survival for hydropic infants at first IUT is about 30% less than for non-hydropic infants.

Fetal mortality within the first 48 hours of the procedure is usually the direct result of the IUT. The fetal risk per IUT is between 3 and 10%, with an average figure of 5% (Larkin et al, 1982). Ultrasound guidance and experience with the procedure minimize the risk of IUT. Adequate experience is indicated by the management of four or five severely affected pregnancies, requiring 12 to 16 transfusions a year. To reach this volume of patients the IUT team must have all the transfusion candidate referrals from a population base of 25,000 to 30,000 deliveries.

LONG-TERM COMPLICATIONS

The major long-term complication is handicapping neurologic disease, and this complication is related more to prematurity and the disease process than to IUT. Two case-controlled studies (White et al, 1978; Knobbe et al, 1979) demonstrated no increased risk from IUT over the disease process itself. In a review of 15 published reports that included 450 IUT patients, Hardyment and co-workers (1979) noted that 80% of the infants were normal and only 5% had major handicaps.

Transient susceptibility to infection in the first few months of life has been reported (Bowman, 1984). Premature delivery and respiratory distress are also associated with an increased susceptibility to respiratory infection over the same period. The reality of this risk must await adequately controlled studies.

Graft-versus-host disease and the risk of in utero irradiation are remote theoretical risks. Donor lymphocyte grafting has been reported. Specific steps to reduce this risk are removal of the buffy coat from and irradiation of donor cells. However, this complication is exceedingly rare, and irradiation of donor cells may be unnecessary. The use of dynamic ultrasound has reduced the fetal x-ray exposure, and only one or two plain A-P films are required for confirmation of catheter placement. In most cases the fetal exposure is probably less than 1 rad. The safety of in utero exposure to radiation has been reviewed earlier in this chapter.

The advent of umbilical blood sampling and transfusion may significantly change the management of isoimmunization and intrauterine transfusion. Direct measurement of the fetal hematocrit will allow a more precise gauge of fetal disease. Direct fetal transfusion through the umbilical cord will avoid the variability of absorption from the peritoneal cavity, especially in hydropic fetuses. Preliminary reports by Daffos and co-workers (1985) suggest a degree of safety greater than that of intrauterine transfusion. However, larger series and greater experience with isoimmunization are needed.

FETAL MONITORING

The evaluation of the fetus during pregnancy, labor and delivery has radically changed the practice of obstetrics over the last 30 years. Obstetric evaluation of the fetus has matured from palpation and auscultation to highly sophisticated ultrasound diagnosis and electronic fetal monitoring. Biochemical testing and evaluation of fetal behavioral states are new dimensions in the diagnosis of fetal health and disease. Modern fetal monitoring methods are much superior to older techniques. However, they remain insensitive and may lead to over-diagnosis and over-intervention. A distorted sense of validity and reliability in fetal heart rate monitoring has contributed significantly to the current medicolegal crisis.

Fetal monitoring has several interrelated goals: to distinguish the healthy from the diseased fetus (heart rate monitoring), to predict the progression or development of a diseased state within an arbitrary time frame (non-stress testing) and to evaluate the physical strength and stress of uterine contractions (uterine contraction monitoring). The ideal result of monitoring would be a reduction in perinatal mortality and long-term neurologic handicap. The evaluation of fetal monitoring in reaching these goals raises several questions. First, what is the relationship of hypoxia/asphyxia to mortality and morbidity? Second, does hypoxic/asphyxic insult occur antepartum, intrapartum or neonatally? Third, are the currently available techniques, i.e., electronic fetal heart rate monitoring, sensitive and specific? Four, does intervention based on the diagnostic test results affect the outcome? Fifth, is there a direct or indirect effect of monitoring on the normal course of labor?

Pathophysiology of Hypoxia/Asphyxia

Hypoxic damage to organ systems, especially the central nervous system, is dependent on the degree of oxygen deprivation and circulatory collapse. Hypotension impedes the removal of the acidotic end-products of anaerobic metabolism (lactic acid). The organic acids disrupt intracellular function and encourage tissue swelling. Tissue swelling within the cranium increases intracranial pressure and further compromises the circulation. The combination of hypoxia and hypotension is termed asphyxia.

Two patterns of anoxic brain lesions occur. Acute total hypoxia (umbilical cord clamping) causes damage in tissues with the highest metabolic rate and, therefore, the highest blood flow—the myocardium and brainstem. Permanent brainstem lesions and congestive heart failure begin to occur after total acute hypoxia for 10 to 13 minutes. These lesions are rarely seen in the surviving infant because few fetuses are able to withstand multiorgan system failure. The effects of partial asphyxia are the diseases most often seen in human neonates. The pattern of disease suggests a strong gestational age factor (Niswander, 1983). In the preterm infant partial asphyxia may precede the development of periventricular leukomalacia, a lesion associated with spastic dysplagia. In the mature infant (greater than 34 weeks) partial asphyxia most frequently causes generalized cerebral edema with flattening of the cerebral convolutions and subsequent necrosis and atrophy of cerebral tissue. This may result in a decrease in intelligence test scores as well as cerebral palsy. However, prolonged and severe partial asphyxia usually results in fetal or neonatal death with multiorgan system failure from asphyxia.

The variation of the fetal heart rate over time is used to predict the status of the fetus. It reflects an intricate balance between many regulatory influences (Fig. 9–3). Fetal cardiac output varies to a large extent with increases and decreases in heart rate. An increase in cardiac output through changes in stroke volume is blunted by a limited ventricular compliance, as compared with compliance in the adult cardiac ventricle. Fetal heart rate variation reflects the balance between sympathetic and parasympathetic influences. The parasympathetic nervous system seems to play the largest role in the

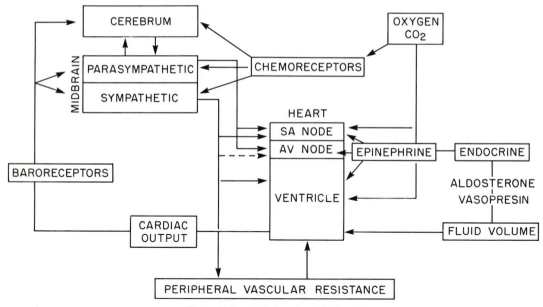

Figure 9–3. Control of the fetal heart.

rapid response to acute cord compresion and heart rate variability. The parasympathetic system matures more slowly than the sympathetic system, and a mature fetal heart rate shows a slower rate, increased reactivity and increased variability. Beat-to-beat variability is thought to reflect cerebral control over the parasympathetic system.

The fetus responds to acute stress, i.e., decreased uteroplacental perfusion during a contraction, by a series of responses: (1) redistribution of blood to vital organs (brain and heart), (2) decreased total O_2 consumption, (3) anaerobic glycolysis. In studies of hypoxic sheep, cerebral oxygen consumption is maintained at 4 ml/min/Kg of tissue over a wide range of arterial oxygen contents because the decrease in arteriovenous oxygen content is compensated by an increase in cerebral blood flow (Jones et al, 1977). Compensatory mechanisms enable the fetus to tolerate moderately long periods (up to 60 minutes) of limited O_2 supply without decompensation of the heart and brain. Decompensation of the heart is manifested as a fall in cardiac output and heart rate after the stress of a contraction. Decreasing variability and reactivity are thought to represent decompensation of the higher cortical areas. This decompensation occurs somewhere below an arterial O_2 level of 2 ml/100 ml in fetal sheep. These early changes are usually reversible without long-term neurologic deficiency. With increasing severity and duration of the insult cardiac decom-

pensation and subsequent cerebral hypotension exacerbate the damage. The acidotic end-products of anaerobic metabolism accumulate, and cellular damage, tissue swelling and intracranial hypertension ensue. A poor prognostic sign is evidence of parasympathetic paralysis. This damage is shown by a rising baseline rate and an overshoot pattern with absent variability (Fig. 9–4). In most cases in which this pattern appears, the damage is chronic, and delivery may not change the prognosis.

Procedures

FETAL HEART RATE

Auscultation. The fetal heart rate is assessed by stethoscope auscultation or doptone localization. A standard protocol (MacDonald and Grant, 1985) describes the auscultation of the fetal heart for 60 seconds after a uterine contraction at least every 15 minutes during the first stage of labor and during every interval between contractions in the second stage. If the fetal heart rate is greater than 160 beats per minute or less than 100 beats per minute and the abnormality fails to respond to conservative measures, then a scalp pH is estimated and electronic fetal heart rate monitoring is commenced. This level of care requires one nurse to one patient nursing care.

Electronic Fetal Heart Rate Monitoring. The fetal heart rate is determined by fixing a point

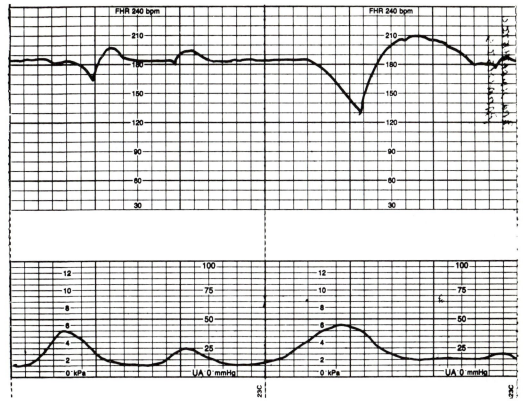

Figure 9–4. Fetal heart rate patterns: Chronic hypoxic changes.

in the fetal cardiac cycle and measuring the time lapse between that point and a similar point in the next cardiac cycle. This can be done by an external or an internal monitor. The most commonly used external technique is the Doppler ultrasound transducer. This device transmits a high frequency sound of 2.0 to 3.0 megahertz. The sound pulse is reflected from a moving structure, i.e., the ventricular wall. The reflected beam has a different frequency because of the object's motion. This frequency change is the fixed point in the fetal cardiac cycle by which Doppler ultrasound measures heart rate.

Internal monitoring is obtained from a direct electrode, which consists of a small disposable stainless steel spiral device that is screwed into the fetal scalp to a maximum depth of 2 mm. This device gives a direct fetal electrocardiogram. The fetal heart rate is determined by measuring the R-R wave time interval. The beats per minute (BPM) corresponding to each interval between beats (t) is computed as follows: rate (BPM) = 60/t (seconds). A new rate is calculated with each successive beat, and the recording pen moves to a new rate only after

the latest impulse is received. Instantaneous beat-to-beat variations of less than 0.5 beats per minute are detectable using the direct electrode. If no new impulse is recognized, the pen will remain at its previous level until machine logic determines that no signal is present or that an artifact is being recorded.

In either the Doppler method or the direct electrode method the computed rates are screened for variations likely to be artifacts. The screening criteria are the property of the individual machine. This screening may reject true rates that change rapidly or are extremely fast or slow. This may result in a doubling of slow rates or a halving of fast rates (Fig. 9–5).

The reliability of the fetal heart rate pattern is most affected by signal quality when Doppler ultrasound is used. The transducer must isolate cardiac ventricular wall motion from many other moving targets, such as maternal blood vessels. Increased activity by the mother or fetus will decrease the reliability of the signal. The most important effect on signal quality is that of short-term variability. The machine is not always able to select with accuracy and consistency the same fixed point in the cardiac cycle, and the signal

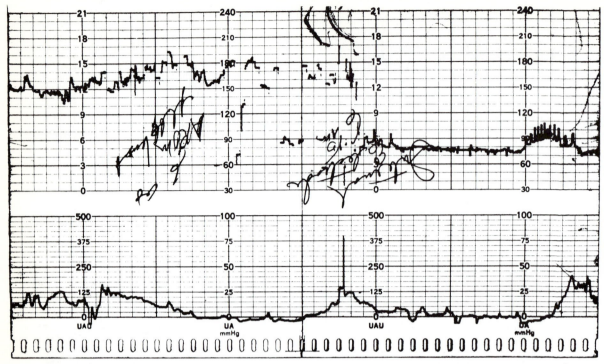

Figure 9–5. Fetal heart rate patterns: Mechanical complications. Internal fetal electrode (right) demonstrates a congenital heart block. External fetal heart monitor (left) depicts a doubling of the low rate.

is slurred. Hence an artificial short-term variability is introduced. Attempts to limit maternal movement to improve signal quality may artificially restrict the normal movement of the mother and this will affect the normal course of labor (Chapter 11).

The two major concerns in evaluating the fetal heart rate pattern are baseline characteristics and periodic changes. Baseline markers are heart rate, variability and reactivity. The normal fetal heart rate varies from 120 to 160 BPM. In more mature fetuses, heart rates between 100 and 120 BPM may be normal when associated with good variability. Prolonged bradycardia (rate less than 120 BPM) with good variability implies a strong parasympathetic influence, i.e., vagal stimulation from head compression in an occiput posterior position. Bradycardia without variability can be associated with a severely hypoxic fetus. Scalp stimulation and scalp sampling for fetal pH and base excess are indicated in fetal bradycardia without variability. However, most often bradycardia is associated with other causes such as congenital defects, hypothermia and drugs such as beta blockers and local anesthetics.

An increase in fetal heart rate is the mechanism by which the infant increases its cardiac output. Changes in stroke volume are minimal and secondary to decreased contractability and compliance of the immature myocardium. Thus, tachycardia can be a normal response to stress. Any stress can increase the baseline heart rate. These stresses may be maternal or fetal infection (chorioamnionitis), drugs (betamimetics or parasympathetic blockers), birth defects or fetal anemia. Hypoxia is not the most common cause of tachycardia but may be the most important. An increasing baseline heart rate, especially with decreasing variability, should initiate corrective action (see later section) and evaluation of the fetal acid-base status (fetal scalp sampling or scalp stimulation).

Variability in the fetal heart rate is the second important parameter to evaluate. Despite the presence of other abnormal patterns, the presence of normal short-term and long-term variability assures that the fetus is not suffering cerebral tissue asphyxia. The variability implies a normal compensatory response to the stresses—redistribution of available oxygen and blood flow to the cerebrum and myocardium. Variability is divided into two types: short-term and long-term. Short-term variability is the beat-to-beat variation of rate. This requires an accurate measurement of a fixed point in a cardiac cycle, i.e., the R wave on a fetal electrocardiogram. Doppler ultrasound is not suitable for beat-to-beat evaluation because of the inability to locate the same fixed point in the cycle. Figure 9–6 depicts the difference in perceived variability from simultaneous measurements of Doppler and direct fetal electrocardiogram data. Short-term variability is described as present when the beat-to-beat variability is greater than 2 beats per minute. Long-term variability consists of waves of variation with a cycle of 3 to 6 per minute. Long-term variability describes the range of fetal heart rates over a one-minute period. There are four categories: (1) normal variability in which the range of variation is 6 BPM or greater, (2) decreased variability in which the range of variation is 3 to 5 BPM, (3) absence of variability in which the range of variation is less than 2 BPM and (4) saltatory variability when the range is greater than 25 BPM. On a practical basis the evaluation of variability involves a quantitative estimate of long-term variability and a qualitative estimate of superimposed short-term variability (Fig. 9–7).

Although hypoxia is the most important cause of decreased variability, other causes include (1) central nervous system or cardiac abnormalities, (2) depressant drugs (narcotics), (3) cardiolytic drugs such as atropine, scopolamine, antiarrhythmia drugs and antihypertensive drugs, (4) fetal sleep cycles, (5) tachycardia.

Decreased long-term variability or absent short-term variability is an indication for determination of fetal reactivity by scalp stimulation. Lack of reactivity should then lead to investigation of acid-base status by fetal scalp sampling.

Closely related to long-term variability is fetal reactivity. This refers to the acceleration of the fetal heart rate for greater than 15 seconds by more than 15 BPM in association with fetal movement (Fig. 9–8). Accelerations imply intact function of the higher cortical centers, which control the heart rate. By inference the oxygenation of the fetal cerebrum can be assumed to be normal. Accelerations are widely used in antepartum testing and in general are highly predictive of a healthy infant at that moment. A commonly used protocol, the nonstress test, is called reactive if two accelerations occur with two fetal movements within 10 minutes. Reactivity is present throughout labor, although it is somewhat decreased in the second stage.

Periodic changes in the fetal heart rate such as early, late and variable decelerations have been the focus of evaluation for many years. The classic patterns are depicted in Figure 9–9. Periodic changes are markers of the acute stresses of labor. In general, the normal fetus tolerates these stresses well. The fetal heart rate pattern depicts the type and severity of the stress. Myocardial dysfunction and paralysis of the vagus can be demonstrated in the most pathologic fetal response to the acute stress.

Early decelerations indicate a parasympa-

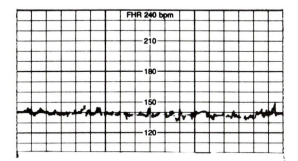

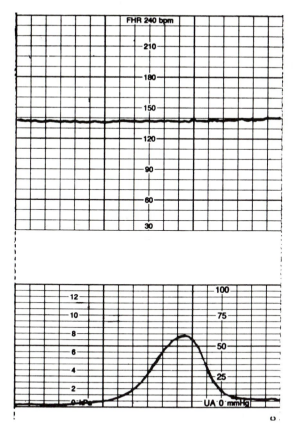

Figure 9–6. Fetal heart rate patterns: Mechanical complications. External monitor (upper tracing) demonstrates mechanical variability not shown on simultaneous internal fetal electrode (lower tracing).

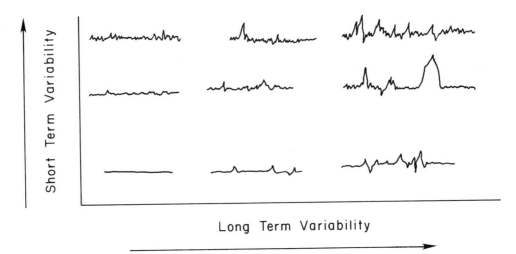

Figure 9–7. The evaluation of variability.

thetic response to head compression and are not considered to be of major significance. Because of the similarities of pattern, shape and consistency, differentiation from late decelerations is important.

The increased severity of the stress is marked by the presence of late decelerations (type II) or severe variable decelerations (type III). Late decelerations are repetitive, uniform decelerations that reach their greatest depth at more than 15 seconds after the peak of the contraction. The depth of the deceleration is proportional to the strength of the contraction. Late decelerations are of two types. Reflex late decelerations are seen when an acute, sudden insult affects a previously well-oxygenated fetus. The deceleration results from the effect of low oxygen tension on the fetal chemoreceptors and a subsequent vagal discharge. Between contractions, normal oxygen delivery is maintained and the variability and heart rate are normal. Maternal hypotension from conduction anesthesia is a common source of this type of stress.

The second type of late decelerations due to myocardial hypoxia has the same initial mechanism. A bolus of hypoxic blood from the placental circulation is transported to the coronary arteries and the fetal chemoreceptors. In this case the myocardium cannot tolerate the transient stress, and bradycardia and a fall in cardiac output ensue. The bradycardia is further amplified by the vagal response. The lag time (late appearance of the deceleration) is a reflection of placenta to myocardium circulation time and thus an indirect measurement of cardiac output. An increasing lag time is a very ominous sign.

The fetal cerebrum, like the myocardium, reflects the decreased oxygenation and hypotension; tachycardia and absent variability are present (Fig. 9–10). At this point further labor will continue to stress the cerebrum and myocardium. Documentation of fetal acid-base status and delivery are the next steps.

Variable decelerations (type III) (see Fig. 9–9) represent a healthy response to cord compression. The mechanism in these cases is a sudden increase in fetal peripheral resistance when the cord is compressed. An acute increase in fetal blood pressure initiates a strong vagal response through baroreceptor stimulation. The depth and duration of the vagal response reflect the severity of the stress. Variable decelerations are not pathologic. However, the stress they reflect may cause fetal decompensation. In cases in which there are repetitive variable decelerations falling to less than 60 BPM from the baseline and lasting longer than 60 seconds, cerebral asphyxia and acidosis may ensue. The development of acidosis may be prevented by conservative management (see later section).

The length of time a fetus can tolerate reflex late or severe variable decelerations depends on fetal-placental reserve (presence of antepartum insults), uterine blood flow and recovery time between contractions. Fleischer and coworkers (1982) studied the development of fetal acidosis after the diagnosis of an abnormal fetal heart rate tracing. In normally grown infants there was a dramatic increase in the incidence of fetal acidosis after 115 minutes of late decelerations and 145 minutes of variable decelerations. When no decelerations were present but

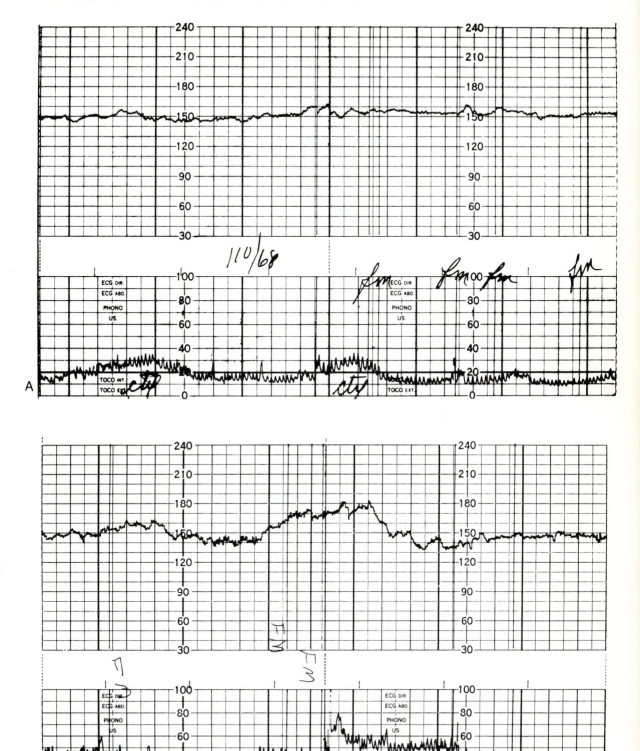

Figure 9–8. Fetal heart rate patterns: Evaluation of reactivity. A, Nonreactive nonstress test in a normal fetus at 30 weeks. B, Reactive nonstress test in the same fetus at 35 weeks.

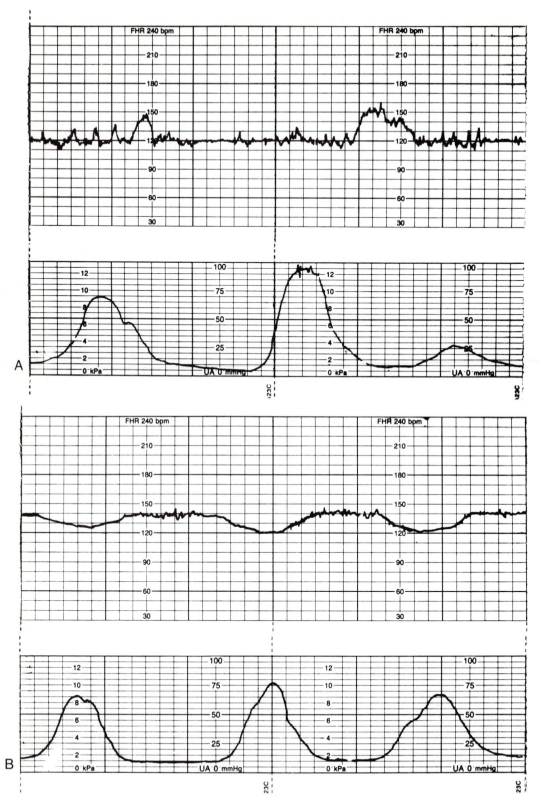

Figure 9–9. Fetal heart rate patterns: Decelerations. A, Normal heart rate with accelerations. B, Type I or early decelerations.

Illustration continued on opposite page

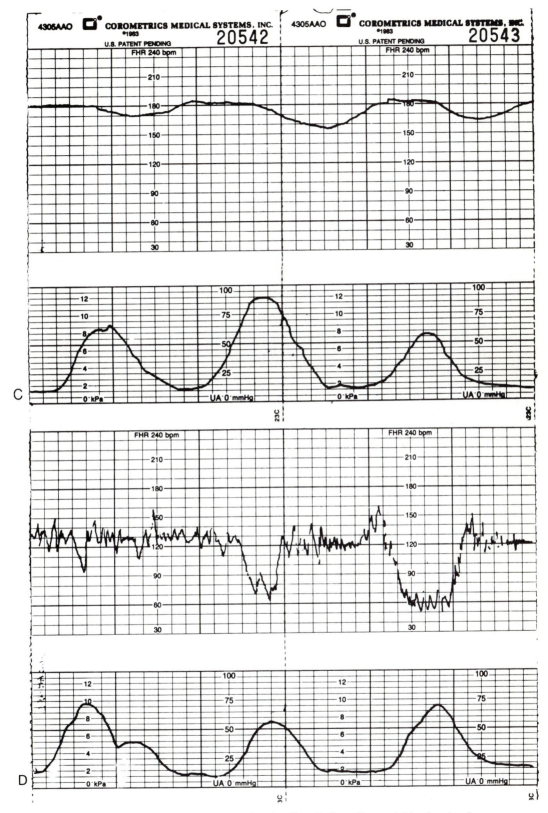

Figure 9–9 Continued C, *Type II or late decelerations.* D, *Type III or variable decelerations.*

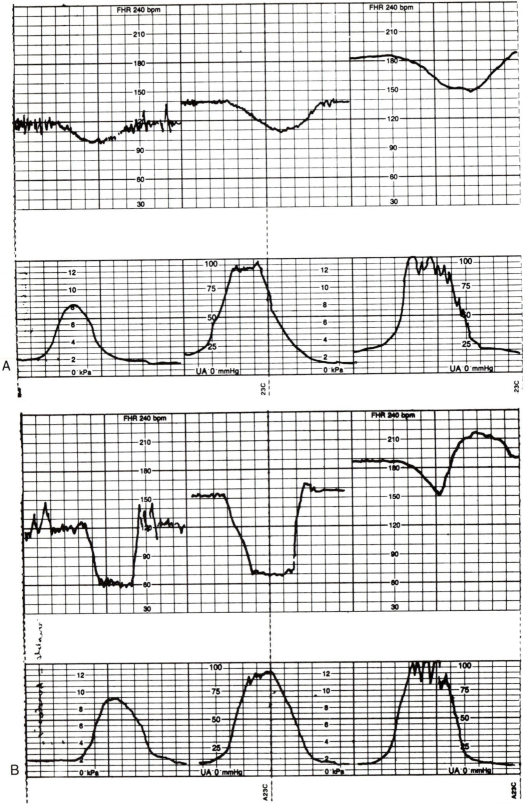

Figure 9–10. Fetal heart rate patterns. Evidence of progressive fetal decompensation: Loss of variability and tachycardia after prolonged acute stress. A, Late decelerations; B, variable decelerations.

tachycardia and decreased variability developed, the incidence of peripheral fetal acidosis increased after 185 minutes. The importance of preexisting antepartum insult must not be underestimated. For example, Lin (1980) showed a greater incidence of acidosis in the poorly grown fetus. The recovery time between contractions and baseline uterine tone can affect the ability of the fetus to tolerate stress. Uteroplacental perfusion is restored between contractions. High uterine tone and increased frequency and duration of contractions will hasten the onset of acidosis with intermittent stress. Conservative management of acute stress manifested by an abnormal tracing is directed at increasing uterine blood flow by placing the patient on her left side to decrease compression of the vena cava and aorta and increasing circulating blood volume by a bolus of balanced salt solution. Oxygen delivery to the fetus is increased by giving the mother 5 L/m of oxygen by mask. The stress caused by contractions can be reduced by halting any oxytocin infusion. If there is no oxytocin augmentation, contractions are harder to eliminate. Betamimetic agents such as infusion of ritodrine at 150 microgram/liter or terbutaline 0.25 mg intravenously can be used to stop the contractions and allow placental resuscitation.

UTERINE CONTRACTION MONITORING

The four important aspects of uterine contraction monitoring are baseline tone, frequency, intensity and duration. Uterine contraction monitoring has two objectives. The first is to measure the amount and duration of stress for the fetus. While the uterine wall tension exceeds the maternal arteriolar pressure (20 to 30 mmHg) the fetus must rely on placental and respiratory reserve to compensate for the transient stress. Second, a recording of uterine activity allows a measurement of uterine work in relationship to the progress of labor. Most often failure to progress in labor is a function of inadequate or ineffective uterine work.

The oldest method of uterine contraction monitoring is palpation and self-report. Many mothers can accurately perceive the frequency of contractions. Palpation of a contraction allows a rough estimation of its strength. A uterus that can be indented at the peak of a contraction usually has an intrauterine pressure of less than 50 mmHg. The duration of a contraction estimated by self-reporting or palpation is 20 to 30% shorter than the actual duration. Tone can

only be estimated by this technique. These weaknesses make palpation and self-report unreliable when uterine work or fetal stress need to be quantified.

The most commonly used external monitor of uterine contractions is the tokodynamometer. In this technique a strain gauge is placed on a fixed length of strap around the maternal abdomen. Pressure on this transducer is produced by changes in the maternal abdominal circumference as the uterus contracts. However, changes in maternal position or fetal movement may produce a monitor artifact. This method provides a fairly accurate description of the frequency and is an improvement in the measurement of the duration of contractions. However, intensity and tone are inadequately measured.

Intra-amniotic pressures can be measured by a saline-filled catheter introduced through the cervix posteriorly and away from the fetal face. A rigid plastic sleeve is used as an initial guide by placement no more than 1 cm into the cervix. Intrauterine pressure is commonly felt to be directly proportional to myometrial wall tension, i.e., LaPlace's law ($WT = IUP \times R/2$; where WT = wall tension, IUP = intrauterine pressure and R = radius of the spherical uterus). However, Anderson and co-workers (1967) have shown that IUP is rarely a proportional measurement. Deviation of the uterus from the shape of a sphere and rupture of membranes will introduce error into the calculation.

Despite these theoretical weaknesses, the intrauterine pressure catheter remains the best method to approximate uterine work. Various measurements have been used to quantify uterine work (Fig. 9–11). From a practical point of view, only about 5% of the time is normal progress in labor associated with a three contraction average amplitude under 25 mmHg, periods greater than 240 seconds, and Montevideo units less than 100.

FETAL SCALP SAMPLING

Fetal scalp blood is collected anaerobically using an endoscope, a light source, a knife blade and holder, sponges, preheparinized capillary tubing and silicone grease. The pH and pCO_2 are measured in anaerobic blood samples by separate glass electrodes at a standard 37 degrees C. The variation within samples between well-calibrated machines is at least 0.03 pH units. pH values of greater than 7.25, between

MONTEVIDEO UNITS
Average Intensity x Frequency / 10 Minutes

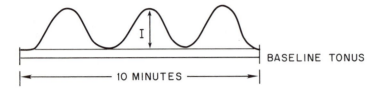

ALEXANDRIA UNITS
Montevideo Units x Average Duration (minutes)

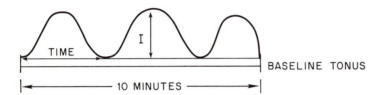

Figure 9–11. Quantification of uterine work.

7.20 and 7.25 and below 7.20 are considered normal, intermediate and abnormal, respectively.

The usual indications for fetal blood sampling include identification of fetal acid-base status or evaluation of fetal blood constituents (platelet count). The contraindications to sampling include known or suspected fetal coagulopathy; active viral (herpes) infections of the vagina, cervix or vulva; placenta previa or a sampling site on brow, face or genitals. Suture lines and fontanelles are best avoided. The site for fetal blood sampling is isolated by the endoscope to exclude amniotic fluid and maternal blood. The site is wiped clean with sponges. A reactive hyperemia may be created by spraying the site with ethyl chloride. The site is then smeared with silicone grease to facilitate beading of the blood. In general, a single stab will suffice to produce free flowing blood; occasionally a cruciate incision is needed. The capillary tube is placed in the center of the droplet. The advantage of gravity and a slight to-and-fro movement of the tip will facilitate the collection of 0.25 ml of blood. Two or three samples are taken from the same place. After the collection of blood, a sponge is pressed against the sampling site until hemostasis is evident during a contraction.

The reliability of fetal scalp sampling has been tested in monkeys. Simultaneous sampling of the carotid artery and jugular vein shows that the scalp pH is generally between the two values. In 5% of cases, the capillary blood was 0.01 pH units lower than the carotid artery sample. Other factors that may affect reliability

are scalp edema (lower pH), meconium or amniotic fluid contamination (higher pH), maternal acid-base status and air contamination. The maternal acid-base status can have a dramatic effect on scalp sample validity. Prolonged stressful labor with mild starvation ketosis can cause a maternal metabolic acidosis, and an equilibrium of fixed acids develops across the placenta. In these cases, maternal arterial pH may be 7.30 with a base deficit of 9 mEq/liter. This is generally asymptomatic, but a fetal acidosis (pH less than 7.20) may be found which in fact is just a reflection of maternal status and not an indication of fetal anaerobic metabolism. Maternal acid-base status can be determined by collecting a venous specimen from a large vein in a heparinized syringe without blood stasis (no tourniquet). A maternal arterial sample can further confirm maternal metabolic acidosis. In general, a base deficit difference between the maternal and fetal blood of greater than 6 mEq/liter should suggest fetal reliance on anaerobic metabolism. A fetal pH of 0.15 to 0.19 less than the maternal pH is preacidotic and less than 0.20 is acidotic.

The temporal relationship between a scalp sample and a uterine contraction can affect the validity of a scalp pH determination. At the end of a contraction there is a respiratory acidosis. The pH may be significantly depressed secondary to CO_2 retention. Hence, it is preferable to obtain the fetal blood sample just before the next contraction because it will best reflect the fetal acid-base status.

One major objection to the use of scalp

sampling is the complicated nature of the procedure and the discomfort to the patient. In fact, there is strong sentiment to reduce the frequency of scalp sampling (Perkins, 1984). Improved skill at fetal heart rate monitoring will help to do this. However, fetal scalp sampling can clarify fetal tolerance of labor and reduce cesarean section rates by as much as 50%. The development of better and more acceptable techniques will further improve this diagnostic modality. The frequency of scalp sampling may also be reduced by a scalp stimulation test (Clark et al, 1984). Scalp stimulation by a finger or an atraumatic clamp with a fetal heart rate acceleration of greater than 15 BPM for 15 seconds is usually associated with scalp pH greater than 7.19.

Complications

RELIABILITY

Much has been written about the "correct" interpretation and intervention based on fetal heart rate monitoring. However, even researchers and educators experienced in fetal heart rate pattern interpretation cannot agree on the interpretation and management of individual monitor patterns. Cohen and co-workers (1982) presented 14 fetal heart patterns to 12 perinatal obstetricians. The average pairwise agreement was 68% in classifying the patterns as ominous, non-reassuring or innocuous. The option of using fetal scalp sampling reduced the average agreement to 59%. Peck (1980) had five Board certified obstetricians blindly review 50 contraction stress tests that had been read as positive or negative and had been acted upon. In only 18% of the cases did four of five specialists agree with the original positive reading. Likewise in only 62% did four of five specialists agree that the original negative tests were negative. Lotgering and co-workers (1982) and Hage (1985), in the evaluation of non-stress tests by qualified obstetricians, found an inter-observer agreement of 40 to 50%. There were highly significant intra-observer correlations. Auscultation has not been studied in the same fashion. However, Miller and co-workers (1984) studied the auscultatory recognition of fetal heart rate patterns. They found that late decelerations with and without good baseline variability were misdiagnosed in 18.4 and 33% of cases respectively.

In a different approach to reliability testing, Sykes (1983) performed a prospective audit of obstetric management, operative delivery for fetal distress and the acid-base status of the newborn. An acidotic infant was defined as an infant with an umbilical artery pH less than 7.12, a base deficit greater than 12 millimols and a one minute Apgar score of less than 7. Continuous fetal monitoring with scalp sampling led to operative delivery for fetal distress in only 23% of these acidotic infants.

VALIDITY OF FETAL HEART RATE MONITORING

Validity is the measure of how well the test reflects the true disease state. In perinatal medicine the true disease state caused by hypoxia/asphyxia is perinatal mortality and long-term neurologic defects. The incidence of perinatal mortality, severe mental retardation and cerebral palsy caused by hypoxic insult is 4/1000 births, 0.6/1000 population and 0.4/1000 population, respectively. For diseases so rare enormous numbers of patients would be needed for scientific evaluation of electronic fetal monitoring validity. As a consequence, validity studies of fetal monitoring have used more common outcome parameters such as Apgar scores, cord acid-base status and neonatal seizures. These outcomes occur in 0.5 to 5% of live births. They are very poor predictors of long-term abnormal neurologic findings. Apgar scores of 0 to 3 at one minute will predict only a 16% incidence of neonatal mortality and a 1 to 2% incidence of cerebral palsy or severe mental retardation in infants weighing over 2500 gm (Nelson and Ellenberg, 1981). A cord pH of less than 7.10 cannot separate a population of infants at greater risk of long-term neurologic defects (Low et al, 1983). A prospective study of neonatal seizures only showed a 19% incidence of cerebral palsy on later follow-up (Nelson and Ellenberg, 1981).

Two studies have compared specific abnormal fetal heart rate patterns with abnormal neurologic findings. Painter and co-workers (1978) performed serial neurologic examinations after an abnormal heart rate pattern. The sensitivity of the abnormal patterns was about 50%. However, an abnormal neurologic examination did not imply persistent disease or major handicap. By five years of age all abnormal infants were normal except for one with genetically caused disability. Keegan and co-workers (1985) examined heart rate patterns in regard to early neonatal seizures. They found a clear relationship between neonatal seizures and abnormal heart rate with absent variability (30/66 vs. 8/66 in controls). However, only 45% of infants with seizures had long-term defects. More importantly, in a subgroup with the diagnosis of fetal distress and delivery within one half hour of diagnosis, seizure activity was present in all infants and long-term neurologic disease was present in 45%. In other words, rapid intervention based on fetal heart rate patterns may not change ultimate neurologic outcome. However, the numbers of patients were small and further study is needed.

The role of antepartum insult cannot be underestimated and can explain the discouraging findings of Keegan and co-workers (1985). Most reviews suggest that the majority (70 to 80%) of insults occur prior to the onset of labor (Illingsworth, 1981; Niswander 1983; Freeman, 1985). These estimates come from retrospective reviews of obstetric history in children with cerebral palsy (Holm, 1982), prospective evaluations of infants up to the time they are seven years old (Nelson and Ellenberg, 1984, 1985, 1986) and the examination of other fetal tissues that are oxygen sensitive (Emery et al, 1967; Cohen and Diner, 1970). Alberman and Stanley (1984) have outlined the specific pitfalls of the epidemiologic study of cerebral palsy. Most studies have major methodologic weaknesses that tend to over-estimate the obstetric contributions to long-term defect.

Studies of other oxygen-sensitive tissues in the fetus have found evidence of hypoxic damage on dental enamel and cartilage structure (Emery et al, 1967; Cohen and Diner, 1970). The abnormal growth of cartilage requires exposure to an abnormal environment over days not just the 10 to 20 hours of labor. Emery and co-workers (1967) examined abnormal cartilage growth in an extensive study of 574 autopsies of infants who died in utero or within 48 hours of birth. The incidence of antepartum insult (i.e., abnormal cartilage growth), was 59% at 19 to 30 weeks, 58% at 31 to 33 weeks, 73% at 33 to 38 weeks, 71% at 39 to 41 weeks and 92% at greater than 41 weeks.

SENSITIVITY AND SPECIFICITY OF ELECTRONIC FETAL MONITORING (EFM)

Until recently most studies have relied on retrospective reviews of population statistics before and after the introduction of electronic fetal monitoring in order to evaluate the efficacy of electronic fetal monitoring. The most consistent effect noted has been a reduction in the incidence of intrapartum death by 60 to 70% (Kiely et al, 1985). The effects on antepartum fetal death and neonatal death from asphyxia have not been well defined. The other approach

to evaluating electronic fetal monitoring efficacy has been to examine early neonatal outcome parameters, Apgar scores and neonatal seizures. Banta and Thacker (1979) reviewed the sensitivity and specificity of electronic fetal monitoring using an outcome parameter of one minute Apgar scores less than 7. The combination of electronic fetal monitoring and fetal scalp blood sampling had a sensitivity of 32%, specificity of 91.6%, false positive incidence of 43.6% and false negative incidence of 19.9%. When the maternal-fetal pH difference is used in addition to EFM, the sensitivity is 69.2%, specificity 88.4%, false positives 10.9% and false negatives 1.9%, according to Bowen and co-workers (1986).

Neonatal seizures within 48 hours of birth have been used as a predictor of quality of prenatal care and long-term prognosis (Dennis and Chalmers, 1982). MacDonald and co-workers (1985) described a large prospective randomized trial of electronic versus auscultatory fetal monitoring. Electronic fetal monitoring was associated with one third the risk of neonatal seizures compared with auscultatory fetal monitoring. Other smaller randomized studies have failed to show significant benefit to electronic fetal monitoring (Haverkamp and Orleans, 1983). However, the numbers of patients in these studies were inadequate to evaluate for early neonatal seizures.

MATERNAL COMPLICATIONS

Increased Cesarean Section Rate. The two principal mechanisms by which electronic fetal monitoring may increase cesarean delivery rates (CDRs) are increases in the diagnosis of fetal distress and dystocia. Ten to fifteen percent of the recent tripling of the national CDR is due to the increase in diagnosis of fetal distress. Most retrospective studies suggest an increase in CDR after the introduction of electronic fetal monitoring (EFM). These studies have been supported by a few randomized trials (Haverkamp and Orleans, 1983). These showed a doubling of the CDR rate in the EFM groups. Haverkamp and co-workers (1979) and Zalar and Quilligan (1979) reported a 50% drop in the CDR for the diagnosis of fetal distress when fetal acid-base status was used in conjunction with heart rate pattern interpretation. Perkins (1984) has argued that more sophisticated pattern reading without fetal scalp sampling will also prevent the over-diagnosis of fetal distress. In a large randomized study EFM did not increase the CDR, although the use of fetal scalp sampling was increased in the EFM group (McDonald et al, 1985).

The restriction of maternal movement with continuous fetal monitoring and maternal anxiety combine to increase the risk of cesarean delivery for the diagnosis of dystocia. The negative impact of maternal anxiety on the duration of labor and fetal heart rate patterns has been supported by animal studies (Rosenfeld et al, 1976), fetal heart rate studies (Lederman et al, 1981) and human epinephrine studies (Lederman et al, 1985). The negative impact of maternal position has been reviewed by McKay and Mahan (1984).

Maternal Anxiety. The effect of electronic fetal monitoring on maternal anxiety has received very little scientific interest. Anxiety and its source are notoriously hard to isolate. Many factors may create or modify maternal anxiety independent of the fetal monitor. Such factors might be basic psychologic make-up, support personnel, previous birth experience, concurrent discomforts (i.e., intravenous line placement) and the patient's knowledge of fetal monitoring. Starkmann (1977) performed structured interviews on 35 postpartum women and found a mixed reaction to the monitor. The patients often viewed the monitor as a protector but were uncomfortable. Anxiety was not a major response except when the patient worried about the variations displayed by the monitor. Garcia and co-workers (1985) studied randomly selected women from a large prospective trial comparing EFM to auscultation. They found no evidence that the method of monitoring provided significant reassurance and neither method influenced the support that they said they experienced nor made them feel more or less in control. In summary, electronic fetal monitoring by itself does not increase maternal anxiety. The potential for anxiety can be reduced by adequate prenatal education and adequate explanation and support during labor.

Increase in Maternal Infection. The incidence of puerperal infection is related to many factors. These include host factors, presence of virulent organisms, rupture of membranes, number of examinations, length of labor, invasive fetal monitoring and method of delivery. Of these, cesarean delivery is associated with the highest incidence of infection. An increase in maternal infection attributed to invasive fetal monitoring must be separated from other factors known to increase infection rates. Neither of two major prospective trials of intermittent aus-

cultation versus EFM showed statistical differences in the rates of infectious morbidity (Haverkamp et al, 1979; MacDonald et al, 1985). Despite the reassurance from these studies, the placement of invasive monitoring equipment should be done in the most aseptic manner possible. In patients in whom a fetal scalp electrode or a pressure catheter has been used, prophylactic antibiotics should be used in the event of cesarean delivery.

FETAL COMPLICATIONS

Fetal complications are either indirect or direct. Indirect fetal risks rarely receive attention, but can be significant. They result from intervention based on faulty diagnostic data. An example would be a cesarean section performed at 32 weeks' gestation based on abnormal antepartum testing that produces a vigorous, normally grown infant with a normal acid-base status. The risks of prematurity (respiratory distress, intraventricular hemorrhage and necrotizing enterocolitis) are major and should be considered indirect complications of fetal monitoring. Unfortunately, the incidence of false positive antepartum tests can be as high as 40%. Any decision to deliver a preterm infant on the basis of abnormal fetal monitoring must be undertaken with as much information as possible. The battery of tests includes a non-stress test, biophysical profile, contraction stress test and an ultrasonographic examination for fetal abnormalities. Amniocentesis for fetal lung maturity studies can also be helpful. The decision for cesarean section should be made in conjunction with an obstetrician who has a special interest in and knowledge of high-risk obstetrics.

Scalp Abscess. The incidence of scalp abscess after invasive fetal monitoring varies between 0.1 and 4% (Parer, 1980; Cordero and Anderson, 1983). It seems to be increased with high-risk pregnancies, long periods of fetal monitoring and the presence of prolonged rupture of membranes. The abscesses usually appear between the second and tenth postnatal day as a single localized induration 1 to 3 cm in diameter. The lesion may fluctuate, suppurate and cause regional lymphadenopathy. The organisms most commonly recovered are those of the normal vaginal flora in the third trimester. Systemic invasion by virulent organisms including gonococcus, group B streptococcus and herpes simplex virus have been associated with invasive fetal monitoring. Active herpetic lesions contraindicate the use of internal fetal electrodes or fetal scalp sampling. Invasive monitoring in the face of other virulent organisms should be used with caution, and prophylactic antibiotics should be used when appropriate. The initial management of a scalp abscess is similar to that of any other superficial soft tissue infection. The lesion is initially cleaned and drained. Topical antibiotics are used. The lesion is then cleaned and dressed four times a day using a dilute solution of hydrogen peroxide. About 5% of reported abscesses have been associated with major and potentially life-threatening bacterial complications such as septicemia, osteomyelitis, cellulitis and infected cephalohematoma.

Trauma. Persistent scalp bleeding has been associated with fetal scalp sampling and internal scalp electrode placement. Occasionally bleeding can occur in the nursery owing to the disappearance of vasoconstriction that previously prevented bleeding. Neonatal death is extremely rare unless there is an underlying fetal coagulopathy. In cases in which fetal coagulopathy is suspected, fetal scalp sampling for acid-base status should be used with caution. Persistent scalp bleeding should be first controlled with pressure. Occasionally an Allis clamp can be used. If these measures fail, a suture ligature is needed. Persistent bleeding should initiate workup of the neonate's coagulation system.

Other traumatic injury from invasive monitoring has been described in single case reports. These include injury to the face, genitals and subarachnoid space. These injuries are extremely rare and can be avoided by careful selection of monitoring areas and attention to technique.

References

Alberman E, Stanley F: Guidelines to the epidemiological approach. In Stanley F, Alberman F (Eds.): *The Epidemiology of the Cerebral Palsies*. Philadelphia, JB Lippincott, 1984.

Amatuzzi R: Hazards to the human fetus from ionizing radiation at diagnostic dose levels: review of the literature. *Perinatal Neonatol.* Dec. 23, 1980.

American College of Obstetricians and Gynecologists: Guidelines for diagnostic x-ray examination of fertile women. ACOG Statement of Policy, May, 1977.

Anderson ABM, Turnbull AC, Murrey AM: The relationship between amniotic fluid pressure and uterine wall tension in pregnancy. *Am. J. Obstet. Gynecol.* 97:992, 1967.

Baker ML, Dalrymple GV: Biological effects of diagnostic ultrasound—a review. *Radiology* 126:479, 1979.

Banta HD, Thacker SB: Assessing the costs and benefits of electronic fetal monitoring. *Obstet. Gynecol. Surv.* 35:627, 1979.

Bloom A, Tijio JH: In vivo effects of diagnostic x-irradiation on human chromosomes. *N. Engl. J. Med.* 270:1341, 1964.

Bowen LW, Kochenour NK et al: Maternal-fetal pH difference and fetal scalp pH as predictors of neonatal outcome. *Obstet. Gynecol.* 67:487, 1986.

Bowie JD, Rochester D et al: Accuracy of placental localization by ultrasound. *Radiology* 128:177, 1978.

Bowman JM: Rh hemolytic disease. In Creasy RK, Resnick R (Eds.): *Maternal Fetal Medicine: Principles and Practice*. Philadelphia, W.B. Saunders Company, 1984.

Bradley-Watson PJ: The decreasing value of external cephalic version in modern practice. *Am. J. Obstet. Gynecol.* 123:237, 1975.

Brambati B, Oldrini A: CVS for first-trimester fetal diagnosis. *Contemp. Ob/Gyn* 25:94, 1985.

Brent RL: Radiation teratogenesis. *Teratology* 21:281, 1980.

Brent RL, Gorson RO: Radiation exposure in pregnancy. *Curr. Probl. Radiol.* 2:3, 1972.

Carpenter RJ, Hinkley CM, Carpenter AI: Midtrimester genetic amniocentesis: use of ultrasound direction versus blind needle insertion. *J. Reprod. Med.* 28:35, 1983.

Clark SL, Gimovsky ML, Miller FC: The scalp stimulation test: a clinical alternative to fetal scalp blood sampling. *Am. J. Obstet. Gynecol.* 148:274, 1984.

Cohen AB, Klapholz H, Thompson MS: Electronic fetal monitoring and clinical practice: a survey of obstetric opinion. *Med. Decis. Making* 2:79, 1982.

Cohen HJ, Diner H: The significance of developmental dental enamel defects in neurological diagnosis. *Pediatrics* 46:737, 1970.

Consensus Conference: The use of diagnostic ultrasound imaging during pregnancy. *J. Am. Med. Assoc.* 252:669, 1984.

Cordero L, Anderson CW: Coping with complications from fetal scalp electrode. *Contemp. Ob/Gyn* 22:28, 1983.

Crane JP, Kopta MM: Genetic amniocentesis: impact of placental position upon the risk of pregnancy loss. *Am. J. Obstet. Gynecol.* 150:813, 1984.

Daffos F, Capella-Paulousky M, Forestier F: Fetal blood sampling during pregnancy with use of a needle guided by ultrasound: a study of 606 consecutive cases. *Am. J. Obstet. Gynecol.* 153:655, 1985.

Dekaban AS: Abnormalities in children exposed to x-radiation during various stages of gestation: tentative time table of radiation injury to the human fetus. *J. Nucl. Med.* 9:471, 1968.

Dennis J, Chalmers I: Very early neonatal seizure rate: a possible epidemiological indication of the quality of perinatal care. *Br. J. Obstet. Gynecol.* 89:418, 1982.

Dyson DC, Ferguson JE, Hensleigh P: Antepartum external cephalic version under tocolysis. *Obstet. Gynecol.* 67:63, 1986.

Elias S, Esterly NB: Prenatal diagnosis of hereditary skin disorders. *Clin. Obstet. Gynecol.* 24:1069, 1981.

Elliott JP, Garite TJ: Ultrasonic prediction of fetal macrosomia in diabetic patients. *Obstet. Gynecol.* 60:159, 1982.

Emery JL, Kalpaktsoglou PK, Soglov PK: The costochondral junction during later stages of intrauterine life and abnormal growth patterns found in association with perinatal death. *Arch. Dis. Child.* 42:1, 1967.

Fall O, Nilsson BA: External cephalic version in breech presentation under tocolysis. *Obstet. Gynecol.* 53:712, 1979.

Farahani G, Goldman MA et al: Use of the ultrasound aspiration transducer in midtrimester amniocentesis. *J. Reprod. Med.* 29:227, 1984.

Field T, Sandberg D et al: Effects of ultrasound feedback on pregnancy anxiety, fetal activity and neonatal outcome. *Obstet. Gynecol.* 66:525, 1985.

Fine EA, Bracken M, Berkowitz RL: An evaluation of the usefulness of x-ray pelvimetry: comparison of the Thoms and modified Ball methods with manual pelvimetry. *Am. J. Obstet. Gynecol.* 137:15, 1980.

Finegan JK, Quarrington BJ et al: Midtrimester amniocentesis: obstetric outcome and neonatal neurobehavioral status. *Am. J. Obstet. Gynecol.* 150:989, 1984.

Fleischer A, Schulman H et al: The development of fetal acidosis in the presence of an abnormal fetal heart rate tracing. *Am. J. Obstet. Gynecol.* 144:55, 1982.

Fletcher JC, Evans MI: Maternal bonding in early fetal ultrasound examination. *N. Engl. J. Med.* 308:392, 1983.

Freeman JM (Ed.): Prenatal and perinatal factors associated with brain disorders. US Dept. of Health and Human Services, NIH No. 85-1149, 1985.

Frigoletto FD, Phillippe M: Avoiding iatrogenic prematurity with elective repeat cesarean section without the routine use of amniocentesis. *Am. J. Obstet. Gynecol.* 137:521, 1980.

Galle PC, Meis PJ: Complications of amniocentesis. *J. Reprod. Med.* 27:149, 1982.

Garcia J, Corry M et al: Mother's view of continuous electronic fetal heart monitoring and intermittent auscultation in a randomized controlled trial. *Birth* 12:2, 1985.

Gillberg C, Rasmussen P, Wahlstrom J: Long-term follow-up of children born after amniocentesis. *Clin. Genet.* 21:69, 1982.

Gjode P, Rasmussen TB, Jorgensen J: Fetomaternal bleeding during attempts at external version. *Br. J. Obstet. Gynaecol.* 87:571, 1980.

Goldberg JD, Golbus MS: Fetoscopy. In Iffy L, Charles D (Eds.): *Operative Perinatology: Invasive Obstetric Techniques.* New York, Macmillan Publishing Co., 1984.

Golde SH, Petrucha R et al: Fetal lung maturity: the adjunctive use of ultrasound. *Am. J. Obstet. Gynecol.* 142:445, 1982.

Grant A: Controlled trials of routine ultrasound in pregnancy. *Birth* 13:22, 1986.

Grech P, Spitz L: Fetal complications of amniography. *Br. J. Radiol.* 50:110, 1977.

Hadlock FP, Harrist RB et al: Estimation of fetal weight with the use of head, body and femur measurements—a prospective study. *Am. J. Obstet. Gynecol.* 151:333, 1985.

Hage ML: Interpretation of non-stress tests. *Am. J. Obstet. Gynecol.* 153:490, 1985.

Hahnemann N, Mohr J: Antenatal fetal diagnosis in genetic disease. *Bull. Eur. Soc. Hum. Genet.* 3:47, 1969.

Haire D: Fetal effects of ultrasound: a growing controversy. *J. Nurse Midwifery* 29:241, 1984.

Hardyment AF, Salvador HS et al: Follow-up of intrauterine transfused surviving children. *Am. J. Obstet. Gynecol.* 133:235, 1979.

Haverkamp AD, Orleans N: An assessment of electronic fetal monitoring. In Young D (Ed.): *Obstetrical Intervention and Technology in the 1980's.* New York, Haworth Press, 1983.

Haverkamp AD, Thompson HE et al: A controlled trial of the differential effects of intrapartum fetal monitoring. *Am. J. Obstet. Gynecol.* 134:399, 1979.

Hecht F: The physician as a risk factor in midtrimester amniocentesis. *N. Engl. J. Med.* 306:1553, 1982.

Hill LM, Breckle R, Gehrking WC: Prenatal detection of congenital malformation by ultrasonography. *Am. J. Obstet. Gynecol.* 151:44, 1985.

Hill LM, Platt LD, Kellog B: Rh sensitization after genetic amniocentesis. *Obstet. Gynecol.* 56:459, 1980.

Hofmeyr GJ: Effect of external cephalic version in late pregnancy on breech presentation and cesarean section rate: a controlled trial. *Br. J. Obstet. Gynaecol.* 90:392, 1983.

Holm VA: The causes of cerebral palsy, a contemporary perspective. *J. Am. Med. Assoc.* 247:1473, 1982.

Illingsworth RS: Why blame the obstetrician? A review. *Br. Med. J.* 1:797, 1981.

Jackson L: Chorionic villus sampling newsletter. Aug. 16, (6), 1984.

Jones MD, Sheldon RE et al: Fetal cerebral oxygen consumption at different levels of oxygenation. *J. Appl. Physiol.* 43:1080, 1977.

Kalousek DK, Dill FJ: Chromosomal mosaicism confined to the placenta in human conception. *Science* 221:665, 1983.

Keegan KA, Waffarn F, Quilligan EJ: Obstetric characteristics and fetal heart rate patterns of infants who convulse during the newborn period. *Am. J. Obstet. Gynecol.* 153:732, 1985.

Kiely JL, Paneth N, Sasser M: Fetal death during labor: an epidemiologic indicator of level of obstetric care. *Am. J. Obstet. Gynecol.* 153:721, 1985.

Klein SA, Young BK: Continuous fetal monitoring following third trimester amniocentesis. *Obstet. Gynecol.* 58:444, 1981.

Knobbe T, Beier P et al: Psychological development of children who received intrauterine transfusions. *Am. J. Obstet. Gynecol.* 133:235, 1979.

Kullander S, Sandahl B: Fetal chromosome analysis after transcervical placenta biopsy during early pregnancy. *Acta Obstet. Gynecol. Scand.* 52:355, 1973.

Larkin RM, Knochel JQ, Lee TG: Intrauterine transfusion: new technology and results. *Clin. Obstet. Gynecol.* 25:303, 1982.

Lederman E, Lederman RP et al: Maternal psychological and physiologic correlates of fetal-newborn health status. *Am. J. Obstet. Gynecol.* 139:956, 1981.

Lederman RP, Lederman E et al: Anxiety and epinephrine in multiparous women in labor: relation to duration of labor and fetal heart rate pattern. *Am. J. Obstet. Gynecol.* 153:870, 1985.

Lele A, Carmody P et al: Fetomaternal bleeding following diagnostic amniocentesis. *Obstet. Gynecol.* 60:60, 1982.

Levine SC, Filly RA, Golbus MS: Ultrasonography for guidance of amniocentesis in genetic counseling. *Clin. Genet.* 14:133, 1978.

Lilford RJ: Chorionic villus biopsy. *Arch. Dis. Child.* 60:897, 1985.

Lin CC, Moawad AH et al: Acid-base characteristics of fetuses with intrauterine growth retardation during labor and delivery. *Am. J. Obstet. Gynecol.* 137:553, 1980.

Lotgering FK, Wallenburg HCS, Schouten HJA: Interobserver and intraobserver variation in the assessment of antepartum cardiotocograms. *Am. J. Obstet. Gynecol.* 144:701, 1982.

Low JA, Galbraith RS et al: Intrapartum fetal hypoxia: a study of long term morbidity. *Am. J. Obstet. Gynecol.* 145:129, 1983.

Loyet F, Schmid J et al: Massive fetomaternal transfusion

during external cephalic version with fatal outcome. *Arch. Gynaekol.* 221:273, 1976.

MacDonald D, Grant A et al: The Dublin randomized controlled trial of intrapartum fetal heart rate monitoring. *Am. J. Obstet. Gynecol.* 152:524, 1985.

Manning FA, Baskett TF: Fetal biophysical profile scoring: a prospective study in 1,184 high risk patients. *Am. J. Obstet. Gynecol.* 140:289, 1981.

Marcus RG, Crewe-Brown H et al: Fetomaternal hemorrhage following successful and unsuccessful attempts at external cephalic version. *Br. J. Obstet. Gynaecol.* 82:578, 1975.

Mazzi E, Herrera AJ, Hebert L: Neonatal intensive care and radiation. *Johns Hopkins Med. J.* 142:15, 1978.

McKay S, Mahan CS: Laboring patients need more freedom to move. *Contemp. Ob/Gyn* 24:90, 1984.

Miller FC, Pearse KE, Paul RH: Fetal heart rate pattern recognition by the method of auscultation. *Obstet. Gynecol.* 64:332, 1984.

Mole RH: Consequences of prenatal exposure for postnatal development. A review. *Int. J. Radiat. Biol.* 4:1, 1982.

Mole RH: Possible hazards of imaging and doppler ultrasound in obstetrics. *Birth* 13:29, 1986.

National Institute of Child Health and Human Development: National Registry for Amniocentesis Study Group: midtrimester amniocentesis for prenatal diagnosis, safety and accuracy. *J. Am. Med. Assoc.* 236:1471, 1976.

Nelson KB, Ellenberg JH: Neonatal signs as predictors of cerebral palsy. *Pediatrics.* 64:225, 1979.

Nelson KB, Ellenberg JH: Apgar scores as predictors of chronic neurologic disability. *Pediatrics.* 68:36, 1981.

Nelson KB, Ellenberg JH: Obstetric complications as risk factors for cerebral palsy or seizure disorder. *J. Am. Med. Assoc.* 251:1843, 1984.

Nelson KB, Ellenberg JH: Antecedents of cerebral palsy I. Univariate analysis of risk. *Am. J. Dis. Child.* 139:1031, 1985.

Nelson KB, Ellenburg JH: Antecedents of cerebral palsy. Multivarate analysis of risk. *N. Engl. J. Med.* 315:81, 1986.

Newton ER, Cetrulo CL, Kosa DJ: Biparietal diameter as a predictor of fetal lung maturity. *J. Reprod. Med.* 28:480, 1983.

Niswander KR: Asphyxia in the fetus and cerebral palsy. In Pitkin RM, Zlatnik FJ (Eds.): *Yearbook of Obstetrics and Gynecology.* Chicago, Yearbook Medical Publishers, 1983.

Nolan GH, Schmickel RD et al: The effect of ultrasonography on midtrimester genetic amniocentesis complications. *Am. J. Obstet. Gynecol.* 140:531, 1981.

O'Brien WD: Ultrasonic bioeffects: a review of experimental studies. *Birth* 11:149, 1984.

O'Brien WF: Midtrimester genetic amniocentesis: a review of fetal effects. *J. Reprod. Med.* 29:59, 1984.

Ott WJ: Clinical application of fetal weight determinations by real-time ultrasound measurements. *Obstet. Gynecol.* 57:758, 1981.

Painter MJ, Depp R, O'Donoghue PD: First heart rate patterns and development in the first year of life. *Am. J. Obstet. Gynecol.* 132:271, 1978.

Parer JT: The current role of intrapartum fetal scalp blood sampling. *Clin. Obstet. Gynecol.* 23:565, 1980.

Parsons MT, Spellacy WN: Prospective randomized study of x-ray pelvimetry in the primigravida. *Obstet. Gynecol.* 66:76, 1986.

Pavelka R, Schmid R, Reinhold E: Evaluation of monitoring techniques in late pregnancy to detect poor intrauterine fetal growth. *Gynecol. Obstet. Invest.* 13:65, 1982.

Peck TM: Physicians' subjectivity in evaluating oxytocin challenge tests. *Obstet. Gynecol.* 56:13, 1980.

Perkins RP: Perinatal observation in a high-risk population managed without intrapartum fetal pH studies. *Am. J. Obstet. Gynecol.* 149:327, 1984.

Persson PH, Kullander S: Long-term experience of general ultrasound screening in pregnancy. *Am. J. Obstet. Gynecol.* 146:942, 1983.

Petitti DB: Effects of in utero ultrasound exposure in humans. *Birth* 11:159, 1984.

Phelan JP, Stine LE et al: Observations of fetal heart rate—characteristics related to external version and tocolysis. *Am. J. Obstet. Gynecol.* 149:658, 1984.

Platt LD, Walker CA et al: A prospective trial of the biophysical profile versus the non-stress test in the management of high risk pregnancies. *Am. J. Obstet. Gynecol.* 153:624, 1985.

Plattner G, Renner W et al: Fetal sex determination by ultrasound seen in the second and third trimesters. *Obstet. Gynecol.* 61:454, 1983.

Ranney B: The gentle art of external cephalic version. *Am. J. Obstet. Gynecol.* 116:239, 1973.

Richards SR, Miller MM: Bloody tap amniocentesis: discrimination between fetal and maternal blood by means of hemoglobulin electrophoresis. *Am. J. Obstet. Gynecol.* 145:837, 1983.

Roberts NS, Dunn LK et al: Midtrimester amniocentesis, indications, technique, risks and potential for prenatal diagnosis. *J. Reprod. Med.* 28:167, 1983.

Rodesch F, Camus M et al: Adverse effect of amniofetography on fetal thyroid function. *Am. J. Obstet. Gynecol.* 126:723, 1976.

Rome RM, Glover JT, Simmons SC: The benefits and risks of amniocentesis for the assessment of fetal lung maturity. *Br. J. Obstet. Gynaecol.* 82:662, 1975.

Rosenfeld CR, Barton MD, Meschia G: Effects of epinephrine on the distribution of blood flow in the pregnant ewe. *Am. J. Obstet. Gynecol.* 113:156, 1976.

Sabbagha R: Report on third trimester amniocentesis at Prentice Women's Hospital of Northwestern University Medical School. *Antenatal Diagnosis*, NIH 79-1973, April, 1979, p. 61.

Sabbagha RE, Sheikh Z et al: Predictive value, sensitivity, and specificity of ultrasonographic targeted imaging for fetal anomalies in gravid women at high risk for birth defects. *Am. J. Obstet. Gynecol.* 152:822, 1985.

Saling E, Muller-Holve W: External cephalic version under tocolysis. *J. Perinat. Med.* 3:115, 1975.

Scheidt PC, Stanley F, Bryla DA: One year follow-up of infants exposed to ultrasound in utero. *Am. J. Obstet. Gynecol.* 131:743, 1978.

Simpson NE, Dallaire L et al: Prenatal diagnosis of genetic disease in Canada: report of a collaborative study. *Can. Med. Assoc. J.* 115:739, 1976.

Stark CR, Orleans M et al: Short and long-term risks after exposure to diagnostic ultrasound in utero. *Obstet. Gynecol.* 63:194, 1984.

Starkmann MN: Fetal monitoring: psychological consequences and management recommendations. *Obstet. Gynecol.* 50:500, 1977.

Steer CM: X-ray pelvimetry and the outcome of labor. *Am. J. Obstet. Gynecol.* 76:118, 1958.

Stine LE, Phelan JP et al: Update on external cephalic version performed at term. *Obstet. Gynecol.* 65:642, 1985.

Swartz HM, Reichling BA: Hazards of radiation exposure for pregnant women. *J. Am. Med. Assoc.* 239:1907, 1978.

Sykes GS, Molloy PM et al: Fetal distress and the condition of newborn infants. *Br. Med. J.* 287:943, 1983.

Teramo K, Sipinen S: Spontaneous rupture of membranes after amniocentesis. *Obstet. Gynecol.* 52:272, 1978.

Thomsen SG, Isager-Sall L et al: Elevated maternal serum alpha-fetoprotein caused by midtrimester amniocentesis: a prognostic factor. *Obstet. Gynecol.* 62:297, 1983.

Turnbull AC, Fairweather DV et al: An assessment of the hazards of amniocentesis. *Br. J. Obstet. Gynaecol.* 85(S):1, 1978.

Van Dorsten JP, Schifrin BS, Wallace RL: Randomized control trial of external cephalic version with tocolysis in late pregnancy. *Am. J. Obstet. Gynecol.* 141:417, 1981.

Vos GH: The effect of external version on antenatal immunization by the Rh factor. *Vox Sang.* 12:390, 1967.

White CA, Goplerud CP et al: Intrauterine fetal transfusion, 1965–1976, with an assessment of the surviving children. *Am. J. Obstet. Gynecol.* 130:933, 1978.

Ylikorkala O, Hartikainen-Sorri A: Value of external version in fetal malpresentation in combination with use of ultrasound. *Acta Obstet. Gynecol. Scand.* 56:63, 1977.

Young BK: Report on third trimester amniocentesis at Bellevue Hospital of New York University Medical Center. *Antenatal Diagnosis*, NIH 79-1973, April, 1979, p. 65.

Young PE, Matson MR, Jones OW: Fetal exsanguination and other vascular injuries from midtrimester genetic amniocentesis. *Am. J. Obstet. Gynecol.* 129:21, 1977.

Zalar RW, Quilligan EJ: The influence of scalp sampling on the cesarean section rate for fetal distress. *Am. J. Obstet. Gynecol.* 135:239, 1979.

COMPLICATIONS OF NON-OBSTETRIC OPERATIONS AND INTERVENTIONS

10

EDWARD R. NEWTON

About one in 200 pregnant women will undergo non-obstetric surgery during pregnancy (Table 10–1). Pregnancy adaptation complicates surgery. One unique feature of pregnancy is the fetus, and recognition of the risks to it is mandatory. The fetus is a passive participant in non-obstetric surgery, yet complications can seriously affect its well-being. Caretaker ignorance may be its greatest risk. Perinatal morbidity and mortality statistics have changed radically over the last 10 to 15 years, and many non-obstetric specialists do not realize the good prognosis for the tiny neonate. All too often the perinatal specialist hears non-specialists discount the 28-week fetus: "It probably will not survive, and if it does it will be handicapped." In reality, neonatal survival is 40 to 60% at 26 weeks and 70 to 90% at 28 weeks, with a 70 to 90% chance of survival without major handicap. Representative statistics for most tertiary care perinatal centers are illustrated in Table 10–2.

The four major factors associated with fetal risk in maternal surgery during gestation are hypoxia, infection, preterm labor and drug effects on the fetus. The growing fetus, especially its central nervous system, is sensitive to oxygen deprivation. There is a constant danger, for example, of a hypotensive episode related to the supine position of the mother in the third trimester. Infection may injure the fetus by direct extension (chorioamnionitis) or by endotoxin transfusion. The source of an intra-abdominal infection is one of the most difficult surgical issues. Genital tract manipulation may disrupt hormonal support (corpus luteum resection) or directly stimulate uterine contractions. The risks to the fetus of drugs are teratogenic (thalidomide), carcinogenic (diethylstilbestrol) and physiologic. The major risk of maternal drug use is often adverse changes in fetal physiology or in maternal physiology, for example, decreased uterine blood flow from alpha adrenergic agents.

The surgeon and anesthesiologist must be knowledgeable of both the normal maternal adaptation to pregnancy and the risks to the fetus of surgery and anesthesia. Failure to recognize these may result in congenital injury or premature delivery. Any surgeon

Table 10–1. Concurrent Non-Obstetric Surgery During Pregnancy per 1000 Pregnancies*

Head and neck, including dental	3.6
Cystoscopy	2.3
Reduction of fracture	1.0
Breast biopsy	0.8
Non-abdominal—major	0.8
Appendectomy	0.5
Myomectomy	0.5
Ovarian cystectomy	0.3
Laparotomy	0.3
Cholecystectomy	0.3

*From Peckham CH, King RW: A study of intercurrent conditions observed during pregnancy. *Am. J. Obstet. Gynecol.* 87:609, 1963. Reprinted with permission.

operating on a pregnant patient must be able to recognize and manage alone or in consultation with an obstetrician the obstetric complications of surgery.

MATERNAL PHYSIOLOGIC CHANGES IN PREGNANCY

Respiratory System

Hormonal and mechanical changes (enlarging uterus) combine to produce hyperventilation and earlier onset of respiratory hypoxia. Progesterone acts early to increase respiratory rate by 15%. Minute ventilation and tidal volume are increased 50% and 40% respectively. The relative hyperventilation is reflected by a hypocapnia ($PaCO_2$ = 28 to 32 mmHg). Thus, inhalation anesthesia has a more rapid onset in the pregnant patient. After the first trimester, progressive anatomic changes reduce the functional residual capacity and residual volume by 20%. When these changes are coupled with an increase in oxygen consumption (15%), hypoventilation or apnea results in a more rapid onset of hypoxia. During pregnancy the closing capacity is elevated in the first 48 to 72 hours after abdominal or thoracic surgery. The resultant arteriovenous shunting further shortens the onset of hypoxia in the pregnant woman.

Cardiovascular System

Hypervolemia, increased cardiac output and positional hypotension are the major changes and risks of the pregnancy-induced adapations of the cardiovascular system. A combination of increasing fetal metabolic requirements, maternal vasodilatation and arteriovenous shunting through the placenta initiates a 50% increase in circulating blood volume. The plasma volume is increased prior to the red cell volume increase. Hence, it is common for the hematocrit to fall in the midtrimester. A hematocrit of less than 30% is considered significant in pregnancy. The full effects of vasodilatation and arteriovenous shunting reach their maximum between 24 and 30 weeks, and a 20% fall in both systolic and diastolic blood pressures is expected. Cardiac output also rises rapidly until 24 to 28 weeks' gestation. This is accomplished by an increase in heart rate to 80 to 90 beats per minute and a lesser increase in stroke volume. In the third trimester maternal position has a great impact on intravascular pressures and cardiac output. In the supine position the uterus obstructs both the inferior vena cava and the aorta. Venous pressures in the lower leg can be as high as 20 to 25 mmHg, and the caliber of the aortic lumen is reduced by 35 to 40%. Subsequently, cardiac output in the supine position may be reduced as much as 20 to 30% when compared to that in the left recumbent position. About 10% of pregnant women in the third trimester will have the supine hypotensive syndrome. This is manifested by profound maternal hypotension and fetal hypoxia.

Gastrointestinal System

Physiologic changes in the gastrointestinal tract during pregnancy increase the risk of aspiration during surgery and anesthesia. Progesterone is a smooth muscle relaxant. Thus, lower esophageal sphincter tone is decreased.

Table 10–2. Current Perinatal Mortality and Morbidity Statistics*

Gestational Age (Weeks)	Survival (%)	Survival Free of Major Morbidity (%)	Survival Free of Long-Term Handicap (%)
24	17	50	9
26	51	80	41
28	75	89	67
30	87	93	81
32	95	95	90
34	98	97	95
36	99+	98	97

*From Goldenberg RL, Nelson KG et al: Delay in delivery: influence of gestational age and the duration of delay on perinatal outcome. *Obstet. Gynecol.* 64:480, 1984. Reprinted with permission from the American College of Obstetricians and Gynecologists.

One fourth of pregnant women have symptomatic lower esophogeal reflux. Gastrin, the hormone that increases the volume of gastric secretion and lowers the pH of the stomach contents, increases considerably during pregnancy. In addition, intragastric pressure is increased by the large uterus, supine/lithotomy position, fundal pressure and light anesthesia. Thus, approximately one fourth of gravidas undergoing abdominal surgery after an overnight fast will have gastric contents of sufficient volume and of sufficiently low pH to classify them as being at high risk of aspiration.

Renal System

Pregnancy-induced changes of the renal system include ureteral obstruction in the third trimester and increased glomerular clearance. A combination of smooth muscle relaxation by progesterone and compression by the enlarging uterus creates a "physiologic hydronephrosis of pregnancy." Changes can occur prior to 12 weeks, and the obstruction is more pronouced on the right. The anatomic changes revert to normal by six weeks postpartum. Changes in the cardiovascular system are reflected in changes in the renal sytem. The 50% increase in blood volume during pregnancy results in an increased renal plasma flow and an increased glomerular filtration rate. As a result, there is an increase in the excretion of metabolic products, proteins and glucose. Often the excretion of protein and glucose will exceed tubular reabsorption. Normal pregnancy blood urea nitrogen (BUN) and creatinine levels are 10 mg/dl and 0.7 mg/dl respectively. Glucosuria on two or more occasions occurs in 5 to 10% of women as a result of a reduction in the renal threshold to 140 to 160 mg/dl. Proteinuria up to 300 mg/day is considered normal.

Hematologic System

A unique surgical risk in pregnancy is the risk of thrombosis. The pregnant woman has two of Virchow's triad: venous stasis and hypercoagulability. The enlarged uterus compresses the vena cava and triples the venous pressures (24 mmHg) in the lower extremities. Estrogen increases the hepatic production of coagulation factors, with a 30 to 50% rise in fibrinogen and factors VII, VIII, IX and X. Fibrinolysis is decreased in the second and third trimesters. These changes increase the risk of thrombo-

phlebitis to 1:70. General anesthesia and surgery will further exaggerate the risk when the third of Virchow's triad, vascular injury, is added. Postoperative bed rest further increases the risk of stasis. Prevention is the cornerstone of management; identification of high risk patients, prophylactic heparin (5,000 units Q 12 hrs), pressure stockings and early ambulation are necessary.

Central Nervous System

Pregnancy critically changes the needs for several anesthetic drugs. The requirement for halogenated anesthetics (halothane) is reduced by 40% because of the increased minute volume. Serum pseudocholinesterase is decreased by 20% in late pregnancy. However, clinically significant increases in the duration of succinylcholine neuromuscular block are rarely reported. Venous distension will increase the caliber of epidural veins. Thus, the dose of epidural anesthetic agents is reduced by 50%. The uterine vasculature is very sensitive to alpha adrenergic stimulation. Shock, anxiety or alpha-adrenergic vasopressors can result in fetal hypoxia and acidosis.

OPERATIONS FOR THE MANAGEMENT OF CERVICAL NEOPLASIA

Papanicolaou's smears during pregnancy have become routine in the United States. As a consequence, the pregnant woman is in the best-screened population for cervical dysplasia. Over the last 20 years the incidence of cervical intraepithelial neoplasia (CIN) has risen from 0.2 to 0.5% in the 1960's to 1 to 2% in the early 1980's. This may be explained by either an increasing screening rate or a real change in incidence. The incidence of carcinoma in situ reflects a similar increase from 1:1670 in 1966 to 1:600 in 1977 (Hacker et al, 1982). The incidence of invasive cervical carcinoma in pregnancy has stayed relatively constant at 1:2,200 (Hacker et al, 1982).

Intraepithelial Neoplasia

CERVICAL BIOPSY + Colposcopy

Colposcopy has been an extremely important adjunct to the management of cervical lesions. In both pregnant and non-pregnant patients the need for cone biopsy has been reduced dramatically. The pregnant patient and her fetus have benefited the most. However, colposcopy and subsequent directed biopsy are somewhat more difficult. The squamocolumnar junction is generally more visible in pregnancy, but the increased metaplasia and vascularity raise the likelihood of misinterpretation. Hacker and coworkers (1982) reviewed nine studies of colposcopy in pregnancy, which involved 1,064 patients. The diagnostic accuracy was 99.5% and no cases of invasive carcinoma were missed. The complication rate was 0.6% and consisted almost entirely of excessive bleeding at the biopsy site. Bleeding can be controlled by pressure or chemical cautery with such agents as silver nitrate or ferrous subsulfate (Monsel's solution). It must be noted that endocervical curettage is not recommended during pregnancy because of the possibility of damage to the conceptus. Random biopsies should not be used in place of a colposcopically directed biopsy; false negative rates are between 8 and 40% (Hacker et al, 1982). Cervical intraepithelial neoplasia, including carcinoma in situ, should be managed conservatively (Fig. 10–1). The pregnancy can be allowed to proceed to term, and delivery can occur vaginally. Cytologic and, if necessary, colposopic examination should be repeated every three months.

CONE BIOPSY

Conization in pregnancy is reserved for situations in which there is (1) no lesion visible colposcopically and a confirmed abnormal Pap smear; (2) incomplete visualization of the lesion; (3) a confluent lesion involving more than 50% of the ectocervix; (4) marked discrepancy (more than one grade) between the results of the Pap smear and those of the biopsy or (5) suspicion of invasive carcinoma.

In addition to reducing the frequency of cone biopsy during pregnancy, preoperative colposcopy can reduce its morbidity. The entire extent of abnormal tissue can be seen, and excision can be limited to that area. With the reduction in the size of the biopsy area, there is considerable reduction in blood loss and the need for anesthesia. Although most patients will need spinal or general anesthesia, a small lesion may be excised under paracervical block.

Preoperative and Intraoperative Complications. Preoperative management is essentially the same as in the non-pregnant patient. Excessive preoperative vaginal preparation will result in loss of abnormal tissue. Schiller's stain

may be used without significant risk to the growing fetus. However, the hypervascularity and eversion of the endocervix will confuse the limits of the lesion. Mapping by preoperative colposcopy will clear the confusion. Bleeding from the hypervascular cervix can also obscure the operative site. A useful protocol is to place figure of eight sutures of polyglycolic acid at 3 and 9 o'clock. The sutures are left long for better visualization should late postoperative bleeding occur. They will reduce bleeding from the descending cervical branch of the uterine artery. The incision is started inferiorly so the blood will not obscure the field. Deep incision and invasion into the endocervix increase the risk of pregnancy wastage either by producing an incompetent cervix or by rupture of membranes. Once the specimen is removed, bleeding points must be individually ligated or cauterized. If traditional Sturmdorf sutures are used, they must be carefully placed to avoid rupture of membranes. Individual mattress sutures may be used, but the cervical os must be preserved. With either mattress or Sturmdorf closure, long-lasting polyglycolic sutures are recommended for hemostatis. The prophylactic use of Gelfoam at the operative site is not recommended because of the enhanced risk of infection in pregnancy.

Epinephrine and oxytocin should not be injected because of their effects on the pregnant uterus; epinephrine causes vasoconstriction and oxytocin causes uterine contractions. Strict limitation of activity for two to three weeks is recommended. Invasion of the vagina by coitus or tampons is interdicted. Excessive activity and lifting weights greater than 10 lbs are prohibited. The patient should report any temperature elevation, bleeding or flu-like symptoms and should be evaluated immediately. The follow-up visit is made in two to three weeks. Cytology and, if necessary, colposcopy should be repeated every two to three months postoperatively. Definitive therapy should be performed six weeks postpartum. Cone biopsy during pregnancy should be recognized as less effective treatment than in non-pregnant women. Hacker and co-workers (1982) reviewed 376 cone biopsies of pregnant women and found that 43% of patients had residual carcinoma in situ on histologic examination postpartum.

Postoperative Complications. Table 10–3 reviews selected series of cone biopsies during pregnancy. Although the first trimester spontaneous abortion rate is no greater than that in the general population, cone biopsy should be delayed until the second trimester. A sponta-

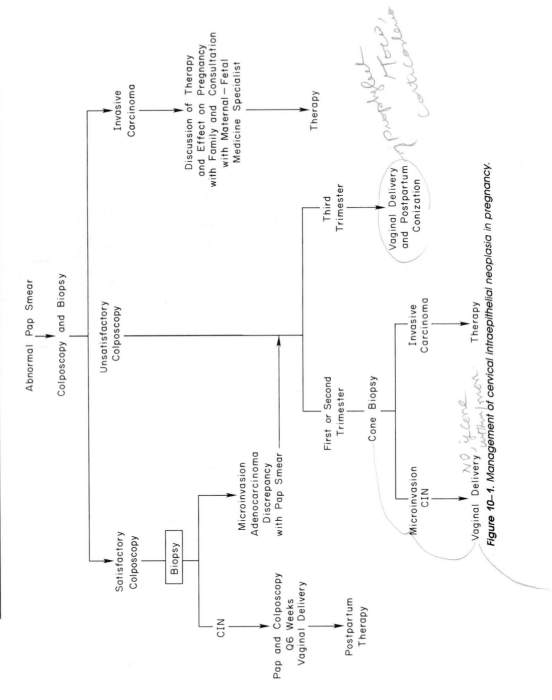

Figure 10–1. Management of cervical intraepithelial neoplasia in pregnancy.

COMPLICATIONS OF NON-OBSTETRIC OPERATIONS AND INTERVENTIONS

Table 10–3. Complications of Cone Biopsy in Pregnancy

Author	Abortion Rate	Perinatal Mortality Rate	Immediate Bleeding	Delayed Bleeding*	Transfusion	Premature Delivery	Cervical Laceration
Rogers & Williams (1967)	—	0/53	10/72	0/72	10/72	6/53	4/53
Daskal & Pitkin (1968)	2/12	4/68	4/77	4/77	4/77	13/68	2/68
Horowitz et al (1969)	0/7	1/36	4/37	0/37	0/37	3/36	—
Averette et al (1970)	8/30	8/162	5/180	8/180	17/180	28/162	13/162
Hannigan et al (1982)	0/7	3/68	10/82	3/82	2/82	10/68	8/68
Totals (%)	10/56 (18)	16/387 (4.1)	33/448 (7.4)	15/448 (3.3)	33/448 (7.4)	41/387 (10.6)	27/351 (7.7)

*After 5 days.

neous abortion through a recently sutured (and infected) cervix will confuse diagnosis and alter treatment and prognosis. Although prematurity and perinatal mortality rates seem to be slightly increased, these increases may be caused by demographic characteristics rather than the procedure itself. No studies have controlled for demographic differences, i.e., the frequency of low socioeconomic class and for pregnancy history.

The frequency of hemorrhage and preterm labor seems to be higher after third trimester cone biopsy. After 24 weeks the patient needs to be assessed for the risk of preterm delivery and subsequent death of a healthy child. Should cone biopsy be needed between 24 and 34 weeks, consideration should be given to 24 hours of preoperative corticosteroids to prevent respiratory distress syndrome in the event of preterm delivery. Most patients in this gestational age group will need prophylactic tocolysis. This may be accomplished by 48 hours of subcutaneous terbutaline or intravenous ritodrine. Oral ritodrine may be used when the patient can take medication by mouth. The mode of delivery after a cone biopsy during the antepartum period is uncertain. Labor in close proximity to the conization may lead to cervical laceration and hemorrhage. It is best to avoid vaginal delivery if the cone biopsy has occurred within a month of labor.

Perinatologists are frequently asked whether a prior cone biopsy will adversely affect the pregnancy. Several studies suggest an increasing risk of premature delivery by a factor of three to four (Jones et al, 1979; Leiman et al, 1980; Larsson et al, 1982; Moinian and Andersch, 1982). These studies have often had methodologic weaknesses (Weber and Obel,

1979), including lack of control for age, parity, smoking habits and previous pregnancy experience. Despite these weaknesses, the patient with prior cone biopsy should be managed as one at high risk for cervical incompetence. Some authors advocate prophylactic cerclage. In their study Moinian and Andersch (1982) described 82% term pregnancies after remote cone biopsy, and 18.9% required cerclage.

CESAREAN HYSTERECTOMY

Cesarean hysterectomy has a definite but limited role in the management of carcinoma in situ in pregnancy. The risks of cesarean section are increased and include more blood loss, urinary tract injury and decreased mother-infant bonding. However, the risk may be no greater than the combined morbidity of a vaginal delivery, postpartum cone biopsy and possible hysterectomy for definitive therapy. In addition, the patient managed conservatively must accept the responsibility for adequate postpartum follow-up. In the light of these arguments a cesarean hysterectomy should be considered in patients who desire sterilization, who have an obstetric reason for cesarean section and who have been adequately informed of the options and risks. The ideal patient would be one who has had several repeat classical cesarean sections.

Invasive Carcinoma

Fortunately, frank invasive carcinoma of the cervix is rare, 1 per 2,200 pregnancies. About 3% of all cases of carcinoma of the cervix are associated with pregnancy. There is a significantly increased risk of finding a higher stage in late pregnancy, although there is an equal incidence of carcinoma in all trimesters. About one half of pregnancy-associated carcinomas of the cervix are diagnosed in the postpartum period (Hacker et al, 1982).

The presence of the pregnancy complicates diagnosis. As with the non-pregnant patient, the most common symptom is painless bleeding. However, bleeding is also a prominent feature in many pregnancy complications such as threatened abortion or placenta previa. Thus, physician delay in diagnosis can occur in as many as 62% of cases of cancer of the cervix in pregnancy (Stander and Lein, 1960). Invasive carcinoma may be present even with a recent negative Pap smear. As many as 20% of screened patients who subsequently developed invasive carcinoma of the cervix had at least two negative Pap smears within three years of the diagnosis of cancer (Morell et al, 1982).

The management of carcinoma of the cervix in pregnancy is complicated by the presence of the fetus. In general, prior to 20 weeks, treatment should be begun promptly without regard to the fetus, since delay until viability might permit the cancer to grow beyond easy control. At 20 to 34 weeks some delay in therapy is appropriate to permit the fetus to mature, but each case requires individual consideration (see Table 10–2). After 34 weeks the fetus should be delivered by cesarean section and definitive treatment given as soon as possible.

The principles of treatment are similar to those for the non-pregnant woman. Although extrafascial hysterectomy is appropriate treatment for microinvasive (Stage IA) lesions, total excision or conization may be acceptable during pregnancy in some instances if the lesion is completely excised. Radical hysterectomy, recommended by some authors for Stage I disease, is complicated by the enlarged uterus and the increased blood supply to the pelvis. It is best to empty the uterus through a classical incision prior to the hysterectomy. Special care should be taken with hemostasis. If radiation therapy is to be used (suitable for all stages), abortion will usually occur spontaneously during external radiation therapy in the first or early second trimester. Hysterotomy prior to radiation therapy may avoid problems of managing complications such as abortion or intrauterine fetal death.

When inadvertent delivery occurs through invasive carcinoma there is no conclusive evidence that this worsens the prognosis (Hacker

et al, 1982). However, there is considerable risk of hemorrhage at the tumor site.

The clinical stage of invasive carcinoma of the cervix is the most important determinant of prognosis. Pregnancy does not seem to affect prognosis in Stages I and II. For more advanced disease the prognosis appears to be unfavorably affected by pregnancy. The complexity of dosimetry in a pregnant uterus and the increased interruption for genital infections may be related to this worse prognosis (Hacker et al, 1982). The prognosis for five year survival is 74.5% in Stage IB, 47.8% in Stage II, and 16.2% in Stages III and IV (Hacker et al, 1982) (see Chapters 7 and 14).

OPERATIONS ON THE OVARY

Ovarian tumors occur in between 1:500 and 1:1000 pregnancies (Buttery et al, 1973; Ballard, 1984). The most common size is 7.0 to 10.9 cm (59%), and 27% are greater than 10.9 cm in diameter. Pain is the most common symptom (48%), and torsion seems to occur more often in pregnancy—28.6% versus 7.3% (Buttery et al, 1973). The histology of ovarian tumors in pregnancy is listed in Table 10–4. As expected, neoplastic tumors are more common (86%) than functional tumors (14%). Two to 5% will be malignant.

The management of an ovarian mass in pregnancy is predicated on symptomatology, the

Table 10–4. Histology of Ovarian Tumors in Pregnancy*

Histology	Total	First Trimester	Mass >7 cm
Dermoid	55	33	12
Luteal cyst	50	5	17
Paraovarian cyst	11	6	4
Simple cyst	27	6	5
Endometrioid cyst	9	5	1
Mucinous cystadenoma	39	5	6
Serous cystadenoma	22	13	7
Fibroma	5	1	4
Brenner tumor	0	1	0
Dysgerminoma	1	1	0
Epithelial carcinoma	10	0	1
Choriocarcinoma	1	0	0
Granulosa cell	0	1	0
Total	221	79	57

*Data from Hill LM, Johnson CE, Lee RA: Am. J. Obstet. Gynecol. 122:565, 1975a; Ballard CA: Am. J. Obstet. Gynecol. 149:384, 1984; Beischer NA, Buttery BW et al: Aust. N.Z. J. Obstet. Gynaecol. 11:208, 1971; Buttery BW, Beischer NA et al: Med. J. Aust. 1:345, 1973.

chance of malignancy and the duration of the pregnancy. Ovarian enlargement is common in the first trimester, and a corpus luteum cyst is a likely diagnosis when the mass is less than 10 cm in diameter. The corpus luteum is essential for pregnancy survival in the first eight weeks (Csapo and Pulkkinen, 1978). The teratogenic risk of surgery and the necessary function of the corpus luteum dictate conservative management of a small (less than 10 cm) asymptomatic mass at less than 14 weeks' gestation. More aggressive attempts at diagnosis (i.e., laparoscopy or ovarian surgery) are warranted in a persistent cyst after 16 to 18 weeks' gestation, rapid growth or heterogeneous character of the mass on ultrasound.

Complications

IATROGENIC INFERTILITY

First trimester complications in an undiagnosed pregnancy will bring many young women under the care of general surgeons unfamiliar with obstetric problems. Conservative management should always be practiced. Oophorectomy is rarely indicated in pregnancy unless the tumor is large (> 10 cm in size), solid or there is evidence of malignancy. The incidental resection of a corpus luteal cyst at the time of laparotomy for other diseases should be discouraged as removal may cause abortion. Ovarian biopsy or cystectomy has a 35% incidence of iatrogenic postoperative adhesions (Goldstein et al, 1980). The incidence of subsequent infertility is hard to determine, but may be as high as 5 to 10%. When ovarian surgery is indicated, careful surgical technique is critical in reducing the risk of adhesions (Stangel, 1984). The essential points are:

1. Eliminate foreign particulate matter, such as starch, talc and lint, from the field.

2. Use magnification when necessary to allow controlled dissection.

3. Use fine 4-0 to 6-0 non-reactive absorbable sutures (polyglycolic acid).

4. Pay careful attention to the blood supply and hemostasis. Isolate the field using atraumatic material (rubber mat) rather than rough sponges.

5. Avoid traumatic tissue handling. Manual retraction is preferable to the use of metal instruments and retractors.

6. Avoid tissue dehydration. Frequent irrigation with normal saline will help.

The use of adjunctive procedures to decrease adhesions has been suggested. The most popular are the instillation of 50 to 100 ml of 32% dextran and administration of systemic steroids and antihistamines postoperatively. Theoretically, these procedures work by reducing contact adhesions and the inflammatory response. Unfortunately, well designed prospective studies are needed to define their efficacy in pregnancy. In addition, the risks to the fetus of dextran, steroids and antihistamines are not well defined.

LUTECTOMY

A bleeding corpus luteum cyst is a major differential diagnosis in the evaluation of a patient in early pregnancy with abdominal pain. Hibbard (1979) and Hallatt (1984) have described the clinical course of this frequent gynecologic-surgical problem. They advocate early pregnancy testing and culdocentesis. Culdocentesis with the finding of a hematocrit less than 12% is usually associated with a minimal amount of ovarian bleeding. The majority of fluids from ruptured ectopic pregnancies will have hematocrits greater than 12%. When the peritoneal hematocrit is > 12%, a diagnostic laparoscopy is usually indicated.

The corpus luteum is essential for hormonal (progesterone) support of the pregnancy until the placenta can support itself. Csapo and Pulkkinen (1978) have reviewed the endocrine details of this function. The corpus luteum is indispensable until about seven to nine weeks' gestation. Lutectomy prior to seven to nine weeks will result in spontaneous abortion. Csapo and Pulkkinen (1978) reported a group of seven patients who had lutectomy after 22 ± 2 days menstrual delay and who received 100 mg of progesterone I.M. b.i.d. for several days. After seven days they underwent a therapeutic abortion. In these cases the serum progesterone was maintained and abortion failed to occur. On the other hand, lutectomy patients with a menstrual delay of 19 to 22 days had spontaneous abortions. These data suggest that 100 mg of progesterone I.M. b.i.d. is valuable in the management of forced lutectomy in early gestation.

PRETERM LABOR

The stimulation of preterm labor by reproductive tract manipulations such as ovarian biopsy occurs in a small number of patients.

Prophylactic perioperative tocolysis is recommended in gestations over 24 weeks. Ritodrine is the only FDA approved tocolytic agent. However, subcutaneous terbutaline 0.25 mg Q 2 to 3 hours is easier and safe to manage. Magnesium sulfate may be used in patients in whom beta-adrenergic drugs are contraindicated, i.e., those with cardiac disease. After 24 weeks the fetal status must be followed in the perioperative period with periodic fetal monitoring.

OVARIAN MALIGNANCY

The diagnosis of ovarian malignancy is often a surprise and is always devastating. Unless directly involved with the tumor, the pregnant uterus is not an essential part of staging or surgical therapy. Hysterectomy or hysterotomy is not indicated. Otherwise, the patient should have a full staging procedure. This includes peritoneal washings, omentectomy, contralateral ovarian biopsy or oophorectomy, periaortic and pelvic lymph node biopsy and multiple peritoneal biopsies of the diaphragms, gutters and the pelvic peritoneum. As much neoplastic tissue should be removed as possible to reduce the residual tumor to nodules less than 1 cm in diameter. Adjuvant chemotherapy may be indicated in epithelial tumors. The risks to the fetus of chemotherapy are both teratogenic and carcinogenic (see Chapter 13). Successful pregnancy outcome has been reported in many cases in which chemotherapy has been used. However, the decision to use chemotherapy must involve consensus of the perinatologist, the gynecologic oncologist and the patient.

OPERATIONS ON THE UTERUS: LEIOMYOMA

Leiomyoma of the pregnant uterus is a common occurrence. However, complications are infrequently reported. The incidence of leiomyoma is between 5 to 25% in women of childbearing age; yet the incidence in pregnancy remains less than 1%. The difference is explained by the difficulty in diagnosis during pregnancy and the relative paucity of complications associated with leiomyoma. Ultrasonic examination has enabled prospective follow-up of symptomatic and asymptomatic leiomyomata (Muram et al, 1980). Only 42% of leiomyomata are diagnosed when the leiomyoma is less than 5 cm in diameter.

Maternal complications include aseptic necrosis, abdominal pain, and postpartum hemorrhage or infection. Perinatal complications include third trimester bleeding, preterm labor, obstruction of labor and placenta accreta (Fig. 10–2). Fetal complications include uteroplacental insufficiency, preterm delivery and deformities. The incidence of all these complications is hard to ascertain. Older literature tends to exaggerate it because asymptomatic leiomyomas are under-reported. Gainey and Keeler (1949), after an extensive review, made the following observations. First, the incidence of disturbance during pregnancy including aseptic necrosis, torsion of the pedicle and hemorrhage with abortion is 17.3%. Surgical intervention was required in 7.3%. Second, premature labor occurred in 12.3%. Third, non-cephalic presentation occurred more frequently but this was not controlled for preterm delivery. Fourth, postpartum hemorrhage occurred in 3 to 13% of cases. A more recent study by Muram and co-workers (1980) suggests that if the placenta lies over the fibroid, and especially if there is continuity between them, perinatal complications are drastically increased (10 of 13 patients) (Fig. 10–2).

During pregnancy pain due to aseptic necrosis or torsion of a leiomyoma is best managed

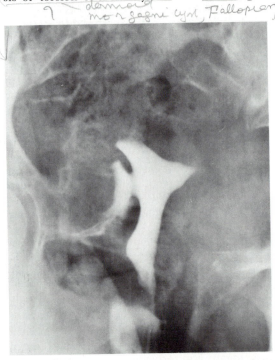

Figure 10–2. Postpartum hysterosalpingogram demonstrates an area of placenta increta with extravasation of dye around the leiomyoma.

conservatively with analgesics. Localized tenderness over a palpable fibroid or a rising serum creatine phosphokinase (CPK) level is suggestive of aseptic necrosis of a fibroid. Uncertainty of diagnosis and the presence of persistent peritoneal irritation or sepsis may indicate the need for surgical exploration.

Laparoscopy can be valuable in the first trimester, but is of limited value in later pregnancy. In other cases, an exploratory laparotomy should be performed through a midline incision. Only after other disorders are ruled out can the postoperative diagnosis be degenerating fibroid. Only rarely should myomectomy be performed during pregnancy. Incision and manipulation of the pregnant uterus will reduce uterine blood flow and may stimulate labor. Uterine incision is associated with increased blood loss, and the ability to control the bleeding is limited. Thus, myomectomy should be reserved for the rare leiomyoma with a small accessible pedicle. The pedunculated leiomyoma is isolated and the pedicle clamped. Hemostasis is secured with a fixed suture of 00 polyglycolic material. A broad-based pedicle may require more invasive surgical technique. An elliptical incision is made high on the pedicle. A cleavage plane is found, and the neoplasm is quickly removed. Hemostasis is obtained by ligating individual vessels and imbricating the surface myometrium with a "baseball stitch" of 00 polyglycolic suture. Bleeding from the incision site is a formidable problem during pregnancy. Epinephrine, oxytocin and uterine compression are hazardous because of their effects on uterine blood flow. Bleeding must be controlled by local pressure, suture ligature and the use of clotting adjuncts such as Surgicel or Avitene. Occasionally an omental graft will be needed to cover a broad surface of raw myometrium.

Preterm labor is the major postoperative complication of myomectomy during pregnancy. In the third trimester tocolytics should be given prophylactically at the time of myomectomy and continued for 72 hours postoperative. A useful protocol is to give antepartum steroids (Decadron 4 mg Q 8 hours) 24 to 48 hours preoperatively to prevent or limit hyaline membrane disease in the neonate should preterm labor result from the myomectomy. The mode of delivery after a myomectomy during pregnancy is determined by the findings at operation. Ligation of a small pedicle does not significantly compromise the integrity of the uterine wall. However, incision into the uterus

to shell out a neoplasm may place the uterus at risk for rupture during labor. In these cases cesarean delivery is indicated.

BREAST SURGERY DURING PREGNANCY AND POSTPARTUM

Breast Mass

About 15% of breast cancers occur in women younger than 41 years of age, and 1.5% in women less than 30 years of age. About 3% of breast cancers are diagnosed during pregnancy. The presence or absence of carcinoma of the breast is the most important issue in the management of a breast mass.

Figure 10–3 depicts the diagnostic algorithm for a breast mass in pregnancy. The physiologic response of the breast to pregnancy increases diffuse nodularity and makes mammograms and ultrasonographs more difficult to interpret. Diagnostic procedures are the same as in the non-pregnant patient, aspiration (and cytology) and biopsy (see Chapter 12). The former usually presents no additional complications in pregnancy. The latter is associated with three special complications. First, general anesthesia is not indicated (and not usually necessary) because of the possible danger to the fetus. Second, bleeding is common and heavier. Third postoperatively the presence of milk and milk stasis may predispose to infection, especially in the postpartum period.

The location of the incision and the technique of breast biopsy are somewhat different in pregnancy. In the non-pregnant patient, a cosmetic circumareolar incision is preferred by many surgeons. However, in the late pregnancy or in lactation a circumareolar incision may compromise lactation. Tissue swelling and oral contact with the incision will increase milk stasis and infection. A lateral incision parallel to the areolar edge is a better choice. Blunt dissection with a Kelly clamp is preferred to sharp dissection, which may injure vessels or milk ducts. Bleeding points should be individually isolated and ligated, because deep hemostatic sutures may compromise milk ducts. The skin may be closed using a subcuticular suture with fine absorbable synthetic material. Milk stasis can be a major problem in late pregnancy or in lactation. Engorgement in the postoperative period may be reduced by preoperative and postoperative breast drainage by feeding or breast pump.

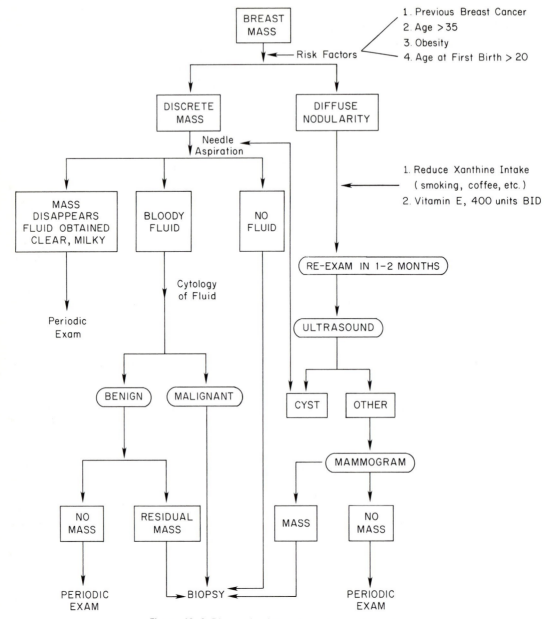

Figure 10–3. Diagnosis of breast masses in pregnancy.

Breast Infection

MASTITIS

Breast infection is a complication of lactation. Mastitis occurs most commonly two to three weeks postpartum and is characterized by localized redness, tenderness and swelling. Temperatures rising to 102 to 104 degrees F are common. Without treatment mastitis may progress to abscess formation, presenting a localized area of fluctuation. The incidence of breast infection is fairly constant at 1 to 3% of breast-feeding women. However, epidemics of mastitis can occur with incidences as high as 20%. These epidemics relate to virulent strains of penicillin-resistant *Staphylococcus aureus*. Epidemic mastitis is a nosocomial infection with employee to infant to mother transmission. Nipple fissuring is commonly felt to be a factor. However, nipple fissuring is present in fewer than 20% of women who develop mastitis. Nipple fissures may be reduced by proper positioning of the neonate. Nosocomial transmission can be reduced by hand washing between infant examinations and reduction of the number of hospital personnel caring for the infant. Rooming-in and early discharge accomplish the same goal.

Milk stasis or engorgement is common in hospitalized patients at three to four days postpartum in many institutions. Without adequate drainage infection has an excellent culture medium. The reduction of milk stasis is an important adjunct to the prevention of mastitis. The early initiation of milk production and the establishment of the let-down (ejection) reflex are required for adequate drainage of the milk ducts. Many factors inhibit the function of the let-down reflex. Among them are maternal anxiety, pain or drug exposure, neonatal drug exposure, delay in first feeding, arbitrary feeding schedules, negative attitudes toward breastfeeding by hospital personnel and family members, or nipple fissures from poor nursing positions. Hospital personnel and physicians must constantly examine all aspects of prenatal and postpartum care with the question: How is this practice helping or hurting the normal development of the let-down response?

Ninety-five percent of mastitis is due to *Staphylococcus aureus*. Therefore, the primary mode of treatment is by antibiotics that cover penicillinase-resistant organisms (e.g. dicloxacillin 250 mg q.i.d.) and continued breastfeeding from both breasts. The antibiotics should be continued for 7 to 10 days. Breastfeeding from a breast with mastitis is not associated with neonatal infection or adverse reaction to the antibiotics. The infant's feeding should start on the unaffected side so that his initial sucking will cause a let-down and easier removal of milk from the affected side.

BREAST ABSCESS

Occasionally mastitis progresses to parenchymal abscess. The presence of an abscess may be confirmed by needle aspiration or ultrasonography. Once an abscess is identified, incision and drainage are required. An abscess should be drained through an incision parallel to the areolar edge. The ductal compartment is then entered by a radial incision of the ductal system. Any loculation within the abscess should be broken up by blunt dissection. The cavity is packed with iodoform gauze for 24 to 48 hours. An intraoperative culture should be taken, and the patient should be started on appropriate antibiotics for 7 to 10 days. Again, milk retention needs to be prevented. The breast with

the abscess should be pumped pre- and postoperatively and then every two hours thereafter. Breastfeeding from the uninfected side is permitted. However, breastfeeding from the infected side is controversial. Some authors have suggested the development of lung abscesses in neonates feeding from an abscessed breast. Breastfeeding may be resumed on the affected side after purulent drainage has ceased and the infection has clearly responded to treatment.

Recurrent abscess formation can occur in as many as 20% of patients. Some authors (Benson and Goodman, 1970) contend that the incidence may be reduced by the initial technique. They recommend primary removal of the abscess wall and deep wide mattress sutures, and the cessation of breastfeeding. Recurrent and persistent abscess formation is again treated with incision and drainage. At this point it would be prudent to prohibit lactation on the affected side.

TRAUMA DURING PREGNANCY

Accidents are a common and important complication of pregnancy. Between 5 and 10% of pregnancies will be complicated by accidents (Table 10–5). Trauma is more likely to cause maternal death than the complications of pregnancy itself. The age adjusted death rate from accidents was 35.6 per 100,000 population in 1984, whereas maternal mortality was 6.7 per 100,000 births in 1984. (National Center for Health Statistics, 1985; Wegman, 1985).

The pregnant trauma victim presents unusual challenges to the emergency physician. The fetal risks demand consideration, but the emergency physician may be unfamiliar with the injury that causes fetal compromise (abruptio placentae) or with monitoring fetal distress. On the other hand, the obstetrician usually has little experience with the management of severe traumatic injury. As a result, diagnostic and therapeutic inaction may occur. This can lead to further maternal or fetal compromise and increased medicolegal risk.

Motor vehicle accidents are by far the most common source of injury during pregnancy. Crosby and Costiloe (1971) prospectively followed 441 pregnant victims of automobile collisions. When there was minor damage to the vehicle only 3 of 233 victims suffered injury and no placental separation occurred. However, when the damage to the vehicle was severe,

Table 10–5. Trauma During Pregnancy*

| Source | Trimester | | | Total | Rate per 1000 Pregnancies |
	1	2	3		
Vehicular accident	19	22	18	59	15.2
Accidental falls	12	26	22	60	15.4
Penetrating or cutting	13	9	5	27	7.0
Purposeful injury	5	1	3	9	2.3
Other	20	17	26	63	16.3

| Nature | Trimester | | | Total | Rate per 1000 Pregnancies |
	1	2	3		
Musculoskeletal	33	25	25	83	21.4
Lacerations	12	14	15	41	10.6
Superficial injury	13	9	8	30	7.7
Contusions	3	9	5	17	4.4
Burns	1	1	3	5	1.3
Internal injury	0	0	1	1	0.3
Other	7	10	7	24	6.2
No injury	9	12	19	40	10.3

*From Peckham CH, King RW: A study of intercurrent conditions observed during pregnancy. *Am. J. Obstet. Gynecol.* 87:609, 1963. Reprinted with permission.

more severe injury was to be expected. Fifteen of 208 pregnant victims (7.2%) died, and 26 of 193 (13.5%) survivors had major injury. Fetal death after 12 weeks' gestation occurred in 14 of 176 (8%) mothers surviving a severe collision. Except for cases of maternal death, first trimester loss could not be clearly explained by trauma. The most common causes of fetal death (at over 12 weeks) were maternal death, abruptio placentae and maternal shock. Abruptio placentae occurred in 3.4% of victims involved in severe accidents.

Falls, burns and penetrating injury to the abdomen occur less frequently. The incidence of fetal trauma is related to the extent of maternal injury and the location of the injury. A fractured pelvis from a fall or a knife or gunshot wound to the uterus has a greater fetal risk.

Management

GENERAL

All pregnant victims should be observed in a hospital equipped to monitor the mother and the fetus. When the patient is obviously pregnant, she should be transported on her side to avoid supine hypotension. A brief description of the severity of the accident and the status of the patient should be obtained from the ambulance attendant. A brief physical examination should focus on central nervous system function (neck injury), vital signs, chest wall motion and movement of extremities.

At this point diagnostic and monitoring stud-

ies should be performed. A large bore intravenous catheter (16 to 18 gauge) is placed peripherally; if intra-abdominal trauma is suspected or the patient is unconscious, a central venous pressure line should be placed. A complete blood count, urinalysis, electrolyte status and blood for typing and cross matching should be obtained. Tetanus toxoid (0.5 ml) should be given to all patients. Endotracheal intubation should be performed on all patients with respiratory failure or who are unconscious. A three-way Foley catheter should be placed in the bladder to follow hourly urinary output and identify hematuria. A nasogastric tube should be inserted to establish the integrity of the upper gastrointestinal tract and to empty the stomach of its contents. An external fetal monitor should be applied as soon as possible. The presence of fetal heart accelerations (greater than 15 BPM for greater than 15 seconds) is a good sign. During the placement of lines and monitors, a more complete history and physical examination should be performed.

The patient's vital signs should be monitored frequently, and a trained attendant should be with her at all times, including when she is taken for diagnostic x-ray studies. Young healthy patients will maintain their cardiovascular status up to a point at which shock develops very quickly.

X-ray studies and an obstetric ultrasound are important. No ordinarily indicated x-ray examination should be avoided during pregnancy. The irradiation of the fetus has little risk compared to the dangers of undiagnosed maternal trauma. Standard studies should focus on areas of injury. The obstetric ultrasound should confirm gestational age and fetal and placental position.

The fetal heart rate may act as a monitor not only for fetal well-being but for the adequacy of the mother's circulating blood volume. Fetal bradycardia (heart rate less than 120 BPM or late deceleration) may be due to maternal hypovolemia, abruptio placentae or uterine rupture. In pregnancies greater than 26 weeks, cesarean section should be considered for fetal distress. Fetal monitoring should continue for 24 to 48 hours, since signs of fetal compromise may occur up to 24 hours after injury.

In most trauma victims with multiple injuries or suspected intra-abdominal trauma, peritoneal lavage should be performed. The procedure can be used in all trimesters. In the first trimester the abdomen can be catheterized through the midline subumbilical percutaneous route. In obese patients a tap through the umbilicus may be easier. In the second or third trimester a semi-open technique is advised; the peritoneum is exposed under local anesthesia through a midline 3 to 4 cm incision. In either case the abdominal cavity is entered with a 16 to 18 gauge intravenous catheter. The catheter is advanced, and if there is no return of fluid, 200 ml of normal saline is infused over five minutes. The tubing and bottle are then placed on the floor and the fluid is allowed to siphon back to the bottle.

A positive lavage is suggested by an erythrocyte count greater than 100,000/cm², a leukocyte count greater than 500/cm², the presence of gastrointestinal contents or an elevated amylase level in the effluent. A rapid test is the ability to read newsprint through the effluent. Even with a negative test, significant injury can be present. However, a negative test means that laparotomy need not be performed as long as bowel sounds are present and the abdomen remains soft and non-tender.

The indications for exploratory laparotomy in trauma are a positive lavage, free air under the diaphragm (prior to lavage), progressive abdominal distension with a falling hematocrit, or cases in which the abdominal wall is disrupted or perforated. The intraoperative management of surgical trauma relates to the type of injury involved. The reader is referred to surgical textbooks for specific techniques.

Obstetric Complications of Traumatic Injury

Abruptio Placentae. Premature separation of the placenta, abruptio placentae, occurs in 2 to 5% of severe accident victims. The clinical characteristics are uterine tenderness, increased uterine tone, labor and vaginal bleeding. The separation of more than 30 to 50% of the placenta may result in fetal death, maternal hemorrhagic shock and disseminated intravascular coagulation (DIC). Significant abruption with hypotension and coagulopathy may occur without vaginal bleeding. This may cause confusion with other intra-abdominal disease.

Fetal monitoring and ultrasonographic findings will help define the obstetric management of vaginal bleeding or suspected abruptio placentae in association with trauma. Fetal and placental position are easily defined by ultrasound. Ultrasound is an insensitive examination for abruption, and can only identify one third to one fourth of cases. The major fetal risk of abruptio placentae is asphyxia. Except in unusual circumstances, labor should not be stopped in patients with trauma and vaginal bleeding, i.e., abruptio placentae. Labor is a stressful time for the fetus, and an otherwise compensated fetus may then deteriorate. The electronic fetal monitor is the best way to diagnose acute and chronic fetal hypoxia. An internal scalp electrode should be placed at the earliest possible time. The development of late decelerations with a scalp pH determination less than 7.20 indicates the need for delivery in the most expeditious manner. In most cases this is by cesarean section.

Coagulopathy and blood loss need to be followed carefully during labor with pad counts and clotting studies (CBC, fribrinogen and clot observation) every two to four hours. Significant blood loss or coagulopathy should be treated symptomatically with transfusions of blood and fresh frozen plasma. Since delivery is usually a cure for the hemorrhage and coagulopathy, labor should be augmented with oxytocin if it is not progressive. Placement of an intrauterine pressure catheter will allow accurate measurement of the strength and duration of contractions as well as baseline uterine tone. A coagulopathy should not be an indication for cesarean delivery unless there is a fetal reason. Luckily, abruption is usually associated with rapid labor, and symptomatic treatment is needed only for a few hours.

When the fetus has died, labor will normally ensue and is shorter than usual. However, coagulopathy is more common, and the surgeon-obstetrician is faced with the decision either to watch a worsening coagulopathy or to stop the coagulopathy with a cesarean delivery for a dead fetus. Vaginal delivery should be the goal. The use of prostaglandin vaginally (Prostin E₂ 20 mg) may hasten delivery. This should be used with caution, especially after 28 weeks' gestation. Maternal symptoms may be reduced by transfusion of blood and fresh frozen plasma. If the mother's cardiovascular system is unstable, cesarean section may be lifesaving.

At the time of cesarean section the appearance of the uterus may be quite striking. The traumatic injury may produce extensive ecchymosis over its surface and the broad ligaments. Abruptio placentae with the extravasation of blood into the myometrium (Couvelaire uterus) can appear quite similar to a hematoma of the uterus. In either case, if there is no uterine rupture or broad ligament hematoma, the uterus can be expected to contract and prevent bleeding. Hysterectomy is not indicated by the appearance of the uterus nor as a prophylaxis against bleeding.

Uterine Rupture. The pregnant uterus is rarely ruptured by severe blunt trauma. The force of the trauma is absorbed by the muscular and elastic wall of the uterus. Crosby and Costiloe (1971) reported only two uterine ruptures among 208 (1%) pregnant victims of severe automobile accidents. The use of automotive restraint systems does not seem to be associated with an increase in abruptio placentae or ruptured uterus. In fact, these restraints are clearly efficacious in reducing ejection from the vehicle, which is a very strong predictor of death in a motor vehicle accident.

When the uterus does rupture, shock, severe abdominal pain and an absent fetal heart beat are common. Other useful signs are easy palpation of fetal parts and demonstration of fetal parts below the maternal spine on a lateral abdominal x-ray. In cases of partial rupture, especially of an old uterine scar, point tenderness or hematuria may be critical signs. Peritoneal lavage will invariably be positive, and there may be copious amounts of fluid (amniotic fluid). The presence of vernix is diagnostic. Laparotomy should be performed immediately.

At operation the fetus and placenta are removed prior to management of the uterine rupture. Conservation of the uterus should be a high priority. Although a hysterectomy may be quicker and easier, especially with a supracervical technique, the postoperative period will be more difficult in the patient who has lost both her fetus and her uterus. Luckily, uterine rupture usually involves only one linear tear and requires only a two or three layer closure as in a cesarean section. Ligation of the uterine artery can be extremely useful in reducing hemorrhage from a fundal or upper segment laceration. Ligation is accomplished by placing an 0 chromic suture through a clear space in the broad ligament from anterior to posterior (see Chapter 11). The ureter, round ligament and fallopian tube are located outside the suture, and the suture is then brought posterior to anterior through the myometrium just above the insertion of the uterine artery into the uterus. This technique is used bilaterally and effects ligation of the ascending branches of the uterine artery. Bilateral ligation of the utero-ovarian anastomosis should also be performed (see Chapter 3, Fig. 3–2). In cases in which there is trauma to other pelvic organs, e.g., the bowel or bladder, hypogastric artery ligation may be needed. This technique is described in Chapter 3.

URINARY TRACT INJURY

During pregnancy the bladder rises out of the protective pelvis and is vulnerable to lower abdominal trauma. Bladder rupture is severe and life threatening. Early in the management of a trauma victim, a large three-way Foley catheter is inserted. If urethral injury is suspected (i.e., pelvic fracture or saddle injury), lubricating jelly should not be used. Extravasation of the jelly may lead to stricture formation. Easy passage of the catheter confirms urethral integrity, and the appearance of clear urine virtually rules out major trauma to the urinary tract. Bladder rupture may be confirmed by a cystogram using 150 to 500 ml of contrast dye. If bladder and urethral injury are ruled out, hematuria most likely results from kidney injury; ureteral injury is very rare. The Foley catheter serves two additional functions. It permits an accurate measure of urine output, and the extra port allows for irrigation to remove blood clots.

Bladder rupture is treated by operative repair in two layers by the technique described in Chapter 3. If there is urethral injury, repair should be delayed until the hematoma and edema surrounding the urethra has decreased. In both bladder and urethral injury, suprapubic catheterization may be useful. In bladder repair, the bladder should be drained for 7 to 10 days postoperatively with either a suprapubic or urethral (Foley) catheter.

Kidney injury is serious anytime but especially so during pregnancy. The increased blood flow (30 to 50%) can lead to massive hematuria or large retroperitoneal hemorrhage. Direct injury to the kidney may be suspected by several signs. Ecchymosis over the flank or periumbilically can be associated with a retroperitoneal hematoma. Hematuria requires that kidney injury be ruled out, even if bladder injury is present. A flat plate of the abdomen may reveal an obliteration of the psoas shadow by a hematoma. This sign is less valuable in late pregnancy because the fetus and uterus overshadow the muscle. If the patient's systolic blood pressure is greater than 70 mmHg, a two-shot intravenous pyelogram may be valuable. The absence of kidney function is probably due to trauma. However, an ultrasound examination of the renal bed must rule out unilateral renal agenesis. A retrograde cystogram and pyelogram will evaluate the integrity of the collecting system. Prior to surgery renal aortography is needed to delineate the extent of the vascular injury. The surgical management involves exploration, debridement of devitalized tissue and a watertight closure. Damage to the renal pedicle requires nephrectomy. Closed system drainage (Hemovac) of the renal bed is also necessary.

PENETRATING INJURIES

Stab and gunshot wounds are the most common major injuries to women other than those caused by automobile accidents. Violence against pregnant women often focuses on the pregnant uterus. Buchsbaum (1979) reviewed 199 gunshot wounds. Seventy percent of fetuses were injured, whereas only 28% of mothers had extrauterine injuries. The perinatal mortality was 64%, whereas only 3.2% of the mothers died.

The extent of internal injury must be evaluated in all penetrating wounds to the torso even if there is a clear entrance and exit wound. Most stab wounds that enter the thoracic or abdominal cavity need an exploratory operation. Penetration of the cavities may be documented radiographically. A catheter is placed deep in the wound and held in place with a purse string suture. Rapid injection of contrast material with subsequent x-rays will demonstrate entry. If entry has occurred, exploration is required. Gunshot wounds require more aggressive management because debris is often carried deep into the wound. Removal and debridement are essential to reduce infection. Anterior and posterior radiographs of the torso will demonstrate the position of radiopaque debris, i.e., bullet fragments.

If the mother's condition is stable, the fetus must be evaluated prior to exploration. An electronic fetal monitor is used to evaluate fetal health. Fetal heart rate reactivity (greater than 15 BPM for more than 15 seconds) shows the fetus to be healthy. Amniocentesis under ultrasound guidance should be performed. Bloody amniotic fluid suggests fetal injury and should indicate cesarean delivery if the pregnancy is greater than 26 weeks. If the fetus is at 30 weeks' gestation or greater, a rapid test of fetal lung maturity may be helpful in deciding on intraoperative cesarean delivery. The optical density at 650 nm of amniotic fluid is a valid and reliable test that can be performed in most hospitals. Specimens containing meconium or hemolyzed blood cannot be used. Otherwise the fluid is centrifuged at 2000 g for exactly ten minutes. Optical density measurements are made in a 1-cm light path curvette against distilled water at 650 nm in a spectrophotometer. Values greater than 0.15 are considered to indicate maturity (Cetrulo et al, 1980).

At the time of exploratory laparotomy the uterus is examined for penetrating injury. If the fetus is greater than 26 weeks and there is evidence of fetal injury (bloody amniotic fluid or abnormal fetal testing), cesarean delivery is indicated. Preterm deliveries should be attended by a pediatrician experienced in the management of premature infants. If the fetal lungs show maturity, cesarean delivery is indicated for any penetrating injury to the uterus. However, if the amniotic fluid is clear but shows immature lungs and the monitor indicates fetal wellbeing, the uterus may be repaired and the fetus left alone. Labor often ensues after recovery from anesthesia. In the absence of vaginal bleeding or fetal distress, labor may be suppressed with intravenous ritodrine. Penetrating injury to the uterus has a special risk of sensitization for the Rh negative women. Any patient with a penetrating injury to the uterus should have a serum alpha-fetoprotein determination and a Kleihauer-Betke test. The standard 300 mg dose of RhoGAM will cover a 30 ml fetal to maternal bleed. Only 0.1 ml of fetal blood is required for Rh sensitization.

Penetrating uterine injury at less than 26 weeks should be treated conservatively. Delivery would mean almost certain neonatal death from prematurity, and fetal fractures, stab wounds and bullet wounds may heal in utero. The only reason for hysterotomy would be maternal hemorrhage or fetal death in association with a uterine laceration that would preclude labor, i.e., a large fundal laceration. In general, vaginal delivery is preferable to hysterotomy in cases of fetal death even if delivery will occur soon after exploration.

BURNS

Pregnant women are rarely burned seriously but have special problems when this happens. The mother and fetus are at greater risk for fluid loss, hypoxemia and sepsis. The overall fetal and neonatal mortality rate is over 50% among pregnant patients with burns over greater than 60% of the maternal body (Taylor et al, 1976).

Fluid replacement, respiratory support and initial wound care are the emergency management goals in the pregnant burn victim. The loss of fluid through the denuded surface can be massive, and the amount is often underestimated in the pregnant patient. Upon arrival at the hospital and after the vital signs of the mother and fetus (monitor) are taken, a large bore (18 gauge) intravenous line is started. In cases in which the burn covers greater than 20% of the surface area, a central venous or Swan-Ganz catheter will provide a better guide to fluid replacement. Ringer's lactate is started at 200 ml per hour until the fluid replacement volume is calculated. A nasogastric tube should be inserted for burns involving greater than 20% of body surface area. Hospital admission is recommended for smoke inhalation, electrical burns, burns of both hands or both feet, partial thickness burns of greater than 10% of the surface area or full thickness burns of greater than 2% of the surface area.

The depth of the injury is estimated by appearance and sensation. Partial thickness (intradermal) injury appears red or pink with blister formation. Full thickness injury may be charred or marble gray in color, dry and anesthetic. Partial thickness burns may also be anesthetic because of neuropraxis of skin nerve endings in the burn area. Thus, pain response to stimulation is only valuable to indicate a partial thickness burn.

A rough estimate of the body surface area involved by a burn is determined by the rule of nines. The head and neck constitute 9% of the total body surface area, each upper extremity comprises 9%, the anterior torso 18%, the posterior trunk 18%, each lower extremity 18% and the genitalia 1%. Another method is to equate the number of palmar surfaces the burn entails, each palmar surface being equal to

1.25% of body surface. During late pregnancy 5% is added if the anterior abdomen is involved.

The fluid requirements for the first 24 hours after a burn injury are calculated by multiplying the percentage of surface area burned by 4 ml/kg body weight. Fluid requirements are met with Ringer's lactate solution. The metabolic requirements (500 ml) are supplied with 5% dextrose in water. Fifty percent of the replacement fluid is given in the first eight hours and the remainder over the next 16 hours. In the second 24 hours, colloids (albumin) are given to maintain the serum albumin above 3 gm/100 ml.

Fluid replacement is monitored by clinical and laboratory means. Systolic blood pressure should be above 110 mmHg, maternal heart rate less than 120 BPM, temperature below 38 degrees C and respiratory rate should be 12 to 24/minute. Central venous pressure should be about 10 cm saline and urine output should be above 0.5 ml/kg/hr. The initial laboratory work should include a CBC and determinations of electrolyte, glucose, albumin, blood urea nitrogen and serum creatinine levels. These parameters should be followed on a serial basis (Q 4 to 8 hours).

Smoke inhalation is a major cause of morbidity and mortality in burn victims. In pregnancy the fetus is at special risk because of its relatively hypoxic state (normal umbilical vein PaO_2 is 27 mmHg). The pathophysiology of inhalation injury relates to impaired maternal ventilation (upper airway obstruction from edema) increased diffusion distance (interstitial alveolar edema) and acute functional anemia from carbon monoxide poisoning. Carbon monoxide binds more efficiently to hemoglobin than oxygen. In addition to displacing oxygen, carbon monoxide impairs the release of oxygen from oxyhemoglobin. Very little carbon monoxide is needed to cause serious hypoxia. One part carbon monoxide per 1500 parts air can result in blood concentrations of carboxyhemoglobin of 5 to 10%. Car exhaust is 5 to 7% carbon monoxide. Carboxyhemoglobin values less than 15% are usually well tolerated, whereas values greater than 30% cause severe maternal and fetal effects, including maternal convulsions and syncope and fetal death.

Inhalation injury should be suspected in patients who have a history of closed-space fire, facial injury, carbonaceous material in the oropharynx or respiratory symptoms. Interstitial edema on chest x-ray, a carboxyhemoglobin level of greater than 10% or abnormal arterial blood gases would also aid the diagnosis of inhalation injury. Initial management of any burn patient should include an arterial blood sample for gases and carboxyhemoglobin and a chest film. The patient should be placed on 100% O_2 by mask for at least three hours or until the carboxyhemoglobin level is known. The patient should receive vigorous chest physiotherapy. Intubation and mechanical ventilation should be used early in the face of upper airway obstruction or oxygenation failure.

Sepsis is another major risk for the fetus and mother. Initial wound care can be instrumental in the prevention of these complications. Upon admission the wound is cleaned with bland soap and water, and all dirt and loose devitalized tissue are removed. Blisters may be left intact if they are smaller than 5 cm in diameter. When burns involve the scalp, axilla or pubic area, the hair should be clipped short until an adequate margin of unburned skin is obtained. After cleaning and debridement, a topical agent is applied with a bulky dressing. Silver sulfadiazine cream is most commonly used. However, the drug can be absorbed. The sulfa-derivative will cross the placenta and displace bilirubin. Should delivery ensue, hyperbilirubinemia will be a risk for the neonate. Silver nitrate (0.5%) is also used. This agent requires continuous soaking (Q 2 hours) and a bulky dressing. Tetanus toxoid (0.5 ml) should be given to all burn patients.

After the initial management of a severe burn patient, her care requires a team approach with the obstetrician acting as a consultant. Pregnant women with severe burns are best cared for in centers geared both to managing severe burns and to the possibilities of early delivery. The major long-term problems are healing, sepsis prevention, scar complications, nutritional support and rehabilitation. The various methods and problems of long-term care are beyond the scope of this book, and the reader is referred to a textbook on the management of burn victims.

OPERATIONS ON THE GASTROINTESTINAL TRACT

Appendectomy

DIAGNOSTIC COMPLICATIONS

Seventy percent of cases of appendicitis occur in women younger than 35 years of age. Thus, the ages of childbearing and appendicitis coincide. Despite progesterone-induced hypomobility of the intestinal tract, pregnancy does not seem to increase the incidence. Pathologically confirmed appendicitis occurs in approximately 1:1500 deliveries and is not clearly related to the stage of pregnancy. Appendicitis accounts for two thirds of the operations on the gastrointestinal tract in pregnancy. Biliary surgery and trauma account for an additional 24%.

The diagnosis of appendicitis in pregnant women is much more difficult than in the nonpregnant patient. In the first trimester, spontaneous abortion, ectopic pregnancy, pelvic infection and ovarian disease are a part of the differential diagnosis. In late pregnancy, chorioamnionitis, abruptio placentae, infarction of a leiomyoma and conditions such as cholecystitis, gastroenteritis or peptic ulcer can mimic appendicits. Changes in maternal physiology and anatomy alter the symptoms and signs of appendicitis. These contribute to delay in diagnosis and an increase in the incidence of perforation. Baer and co-workers (1932) marked by barium enema the location of the normal appendix at different stages of pregnancy. They noted a cephalic and posterior movement of the appendix. At three months the appendix is 4 to 5 cm cephalic to McBurney's point. By the fifth month it is at the level of the umbilicus and just over the iliac crest and has moved laterally approximately 3 cm. By the eighth month over 90% of appendices are two or more centimeters above the iliac crest. Often the appendix points in a subcostal direction. An important posterior displacement occurs. Initially the visceral pain produced by inflammation and distension of the appendix is referred to the umbilicus. Once suppuration occurs there is localized peritoneal tenderness. With posterior displacement less anterior localized peritonitis occurs. This probably accounts for the higher incidence of gangrenous or perforated appendices in late pregnancy.

The incidence of signs and symptoms of appendicitis in pregnancy are listed in Table 10–6. The most helpful are localized right lower quadrant pain, anorexia, tenderness and rebound tenderness. Equally important as distractors are pyuria, normal white blood count, no rectal tenderness or pulse less than 100. As the enlarging uterus displaces the appendix cephalad and posterolaterally, the physical signs become more obscure. For example, rebound tenderness is apparent in most cases of first trimester appendicitis, but in the third trimester it occurs in less than one half of cases.

Table 10–6. *Diagnosis of Appendicitis in Pregnancy**

Signs and Symptoms	Incidence (%)
Right lower quadrant pain	79
Vomiting	58
Anorexia	71
Rebound tenderness	
1st trimester	100
3rd trimester	43
Right lower quadrant tenderness	
1st trimester	100
3rd trimester	14
Right upper quadrant tenderness	
1st trimester	0
3rd trimester	57
Rectal tenderness	
1st trimester	60
3rd trimester	0
Temperature <37.5°C	42
Pulse <100 BPM	25
WBC >15,000	67
Pyuria (negative culture)	21
Hematuria (negative culture)	12

*From Weingold AB: Appendicitis in pregnancy. *Clin. Obstet. Gynecol.* 21:801, 1983. Reprinted with permission.

Perforation of the appendix and subsequent generalized peritonitis increases both maternal and fetal risks. Delay in diagnosis and gestational age are the major contributors to the incidence of perforation. In the first 24 hours of symptoms perforation occurs in 20%; after 48 hours the incidence is 70%. The incidence of perforation in the first and second trimester is 30.8% but in the third trimester it rises to 69.2%. The reasons for this may be delay in diagnosis caused by the obscure signs and symptoms, inhibition of omental migration, curtailment of the walling off process and the alteration of host response associated with the high steroid levels of pregnancy.

Babaknia and co-workers (1977) reviewed errors of diagnosis in appendicitis during pregnancy. Of 462 patients in whom laparotomies were done, 333 patients (72%) had appendicitis. Seventeen (4%) had other surgical disease, 22 (5%) had infection such as pyelonephritis or pelvic inflammatory disease and 46 (18%) had a normal appendix. The true incidence of missed diagnosis is probably underestimated. Many laparotomies are performed in cases in which no inflammation of the appendix is found and the appendix is not removed.

The question of removing a normal appendix in a case of missed diagnosis is controversial. On one hand, infectious complications and preterm labor can occur in about 1% of cases; on the other, the procedure is relatively easy, the operation coincides with the abdominal scar and the clinical diagnosis of a normal appendix may not agree with the histologic diagnosis. The incidence of abnormal appendices from incidental appendectomy at cesarean section is 0.5 to 25% (Sweeney, 1959; Onuigbo, 1981). Because of these issues, appendectomy is advisable when a lateral skin incision is made and an unexpectedly normal appendix is found.

OPERATIVE COMPLICATIONS

Choice of Incision: Obstetrical Concerns. The choice of abdominal incision depends on three factors: gestational age, the certainty of the diagnosis and the suspicion of perforation or abscess formation. If the diagnosis is in question during the first trimester a vertical lower abdominal midline incision is indicated. This incision will allow the best exposure to both adnexal regions. Appendectomy can usually be performed, although exposure is not ideal. In cases in which perforation or abscess formation has occurred, a midline incision has the disadvantage of allowing more peritoneal contamination. A pararectus incision (Battle's) should not be used. This incision does not provide the best exposure of the appendix when the diagnosis is clear, neither does it provide adequate exposure of the left adnexal region if the diagnosis is not clear. In addition, the pararectus incision is particularly prone to disruption or development of a ventral hernia if wound infection should occur.

In the second or third trimesters or when the diagnosis is clear, a muscle splitting incision over the point of maximal tenderness is the best choice. When the uterus is confined to the pelvis, this may be a classic McArthur-McBurney incision or a Rocky-Davis incision. The separation of the muscles in the direction of their fibers produces a wound that does not depend entirely upon sutures for restoration of tissue continuity. This is more important in pregnancy when the uterus increases intra-abdominal pressure. Exposure is increased and the risk of supine hypotension lessened by positioning all pregnant patients with a 30 degree tilt to the left side.

In the third trimester, advanced stages of appendicitis with perforation and generalized peritonitis demand critical decision making and more surgical expertise. One such decision is whether or not to do a concomitant cesarean delivery. Generalized septicemia and peritonitis can cause fetal damage or toxic intrauterine death through endotoxin transfusion. The actual incidence of this risk is not clear. Furthermore, weighed against it are the risks of premature delivery, e.g., respiratory distress, intraventricular hemorrhage, or necrotizing enterocolitis. Between 33 and 36 weeks about one in 200 live newborns will die from these complications. Prior to 33 weeks the risks of premature delivery by cesarean are prohibitive. After 34 weeks obstetric conditions may dominate the issue. Cesarean delivery may be indicated for abnormal fetal testing, abnormal fetal lie in labor, multiple gestation and third trimester bleeding. Concomitant cesarean section should only be considered at term. When a cesarean delivery is to be performed as part of the operation, a vertical midline incision is used. The cesarean is performed prior to the management of the appendix. Infectious contamination of the myometrium is a considerable risk if the peritoneum is entered. In these cases, an extraperitoneal cesarean section may be performed (Chapter 11).

Technique. Details of technique are given because the obstetrician may encounter appendicitis unexpectedly and the presence of a pregnant uterus complicates the usual procedure. In the first trimester a transverse incision is made 1 to 3 cm below the umbilicus and is centered on the midclavicular line. Later in pregnancy the incision will advance more cephalad and laterally as the uterus enlarges. The incision lies in the direction of the skin's wrinkle lines and yields a cosmetically superior scar. The length of the incision is about the width of the surgeon's hand. The aponeurosis and muscles are incised or split in the direction of their muscle fibers. The anterior rectus sheath, but not the enclosed muscle, is incised. This allows for improved retraction. The inferior epigastric artery, which lies on the posterior rectus sheath, must be carefully avoided or ligated.

Upon entry into the peritoneal cavity, cultures and a Gram stain of the peritoneal fluid should be obtained. In most cases in the first trimester, the appendix will be readily seen at the incision site. The anterior cecal taenia and the ileocecal junction are helpful anatomic landmarks. Entensive exploration should be avoided as necrotic, friable tissue may be involved. The mesoappendix is progressively clamped, cut and ligated with hemostats, Metzenbaum scissors and 00 polyglycolic sutures. In most cases this proceeds distally to proximally. In some cases of retrocecal appendices the direction is reversed. The free appendix is then crush clamped at its base and clamped distally, and a single 00 plain catgut ligature is placed in the groove. A second ligature is used if needed for control. The appendix is excised close to the clamp, and the knife and clamp are removed from the field. The use of phenol and alcohol or electrocautery on the stump probably does not affect outcome. In addition, phenol, if not neutralized with alcohol, may burn normal bowel if contact is made.

The management of the stump is controversial. The possible methods are inversion, ligation or ligation and inversion. Pushing the whole appendix inside out into the lumen of the cecum has regained some popularity. The advantage is that the bowel is not entered. The disadvantages are technical difficulty, limitations in cases of gangrenous appendicitis and confusion on later barium enemas. The traditional method is ligation with absorbable suture and inversion using 000 silk purse string or Z-type sutures. The advantages of this technique are security of the intramural branch of the appendiceal artery (ligation) and reperitonealization (inversion). However, the disadvantage is that the inversion of an infected stump into a closed cavity increases the risk of intramural abscess. If the ligation is done with fine plain catgut, this risk is minimal. Inversion without ligation endangers secure hemostasis. Ligation without inversion allows an infected surface to be free in the peritoneal cavity.

The appendiceal bed is then irrigated with saline, and purulent debris is removed. The use of antibiotics, i.e., cefoxitin, in the irrigant may be beneficial in preventing abscess formation. Although not always indicated in uncomplicated appendicitis in the non-pregnant patient, intravenous prophylactic antibiotics are recommended in pregnant patients. A second or third generation cephalosporin with anaerobic and Gram negative coverage is an appropriate choice. Antibiotics should be continued for five days.

The abdominal wall is closed in two layers. The peritoneum, muscle layers and fascia are closed with a single layer of monofilament nonabsorbable sutures (prolene) by a Smead-Jones technique. The skin is closed with interrupted mattress sutures or clips. In cases in which gross contamination exists, the skin is left open for delayed closure.

Appendiceal Abscess. In 30 to 70% of cases of appendicitis complicating pregnancy perforation has occurred. Perforation with abscess formation or diffuse peritonitis demands different intraoperative management. Occasionally in the non-pregnant patient with a fixed periappendiceal mass, expectant management with observation and intravenous antibiotics is advocated. Appendectomy is performed at a later date. However, the pregnant woman seems to be less able to contain the infection, and the risk to the fetus from endotoxins is high. Surgical management is always indicated in pregnancy.

The location of the abscess usually corresponds to that of the tip of the appendix. A transverse muscle splitting incision is made just medial to the crest of the ilium. The lateral edge of the peritoneum is exposed and the abscess is entered from its lateral and retroperitoneal aspect. Aerobic and anaerobic cultures are taken and loculations are broken down by gentle finger dissection. The adhesions walling off the abscess should not be disrupted for fear of further peritoneal spread. If the appendix is readily accessible, an appendectomy is performed.

A closed suction drainage system is then brought out through a separate flank incision (inside to outside). The wound and abscess cavity are irrigated with copious amounts of diluted antibiotic solution (2 gm of cefoxitin in 1000 ml NS). The fascia is closed with permanent sutures (nylon) using a Smead-Jones technique. The skin is packed open for delayed closure. The closed drain should be allowed to drain undisturbed for 24 to 48 hours after which, if it is draining less than 100 ml/24 hours, it may be rotated and removed two to four days later.

Systemic intravenous antibiotics should be continued for at least five days or until the patient has been afebrile for 24 hours (after five days). Continued fever suggests further abscess formation. Rectal examination may detect a developing pelvic abscess. Vaginal examination should be used only for detection of an obstetric complication, i.e., preterm labor. The head of the bed should be elevated 15 to 30 degrees. Although this will not prevent subphrenic abscess, it will promote drainage toward the pelvis.

When diffuse peritonitis or possible abscess formation due to appendicitis is suspected, management is by exploration and appendectomy. A midline abdominal incision is indicated. This allows for greater exposure for diagnosis and management of intra-abdominal abscesses. It is especially important in the third

trimester when the pregnant uterus seriously impedes the exploration of the left side of the abdomen. Localized collections of pus are drained by soft rubber drains, but the use of prophylactic drains is not indicated. These drains are rapidly walled off and thus defeat their purpose. The abdominal cavity is then irrigated with copious amounts of diluted antibiotic solution (see earlier discussion) and the abdominal wall is closed, in anticipation of wound infection, by permanent sutures using the Smead-Jones technique and delayed skin closure. Again close observation for developing abscess and positioning with the head of the bed elevated is important.

POSTOPERATIVE COMPLICATIONS

Postoperative complications occur in 5 to 10% of patients with early unperforated appendicitis, but in 30 to 50% of patients with perforated appendices. The major complications relate to the severity of infection and the effects of this infection and therapy on the gestation. Table 10–7 lists the major surgical and obstetric complications.

Wound infection, abscess formation and diffuse peritonitis are the chief maternal postoperative sequelae. Intraoperative techniques such as limited exploration, irrigation with antibiotics and delayed wound closure will limit these complications. Further management of infectious complications is discussed in Chapter 4.

Table 10–7. Complications of Appendicitis in Pregnancy*

General Surgical Complications	Incidence (%)
Minor wound	1–2
Wound sepsis	10–15
Pelvic abscess	1–2
Subphrenic and other abscess	<1
Fever of unknown origin	2–5
Ileus (>4 days)	0.5–1
Intestinal obstruction	1–2
Cardiac complications	0.5–1
Thromboembolism	0.5–1
Respiratory tract	0.5–1
Incisional hernia	0.5–1
Obstetric Complications	
Misdiagnosis	15–20
Perinatal mortality	5–8
Premature labor	15–20
Preterm delivery	10–15
Maternal death	0.1–0.5

*Data from Pieper R, Kager L, Nasman P.: *Acta Chir. Scand.* 148:51, 1982; Weingold AB.: *Clin. Obstet. Gynecol.* 21:801, 1983.

Preterm delivery and perinatal mortality are increased in appendicitis. The severity of the disease seems to be the critical factor rather than surgical intervention. Weingold (1983) reviewed 245 cases of appendicitis after 20 weeks of gestation. The perinatal mortality was 4.8% in cases with unperforated appendices and 27% in cases with perforation. With more extensive disease there is a greater release of prostaglandins and endotoxin and a wider area of localized uterine irritation. The transplacental transfusion of endotoxin may increase the risk of fetal death, and premature labor is stimulated by prostaglandins and uterine irritation. Premature delivery makes the largest contribution to perinatal mortality and is more likely to occur after 24 weeks' gestation. Early surgical intervention reduces the volume and source of prostaglandins and endotoxin and, thus, reduces the risk of prematurity.

The treatment of preterm labor in a patient with abdominal pain presumed to be appendicitis is a very difficult problem. On one hand, there are clear risks for preterm delivery; on the other, the intrauterine environment may not be ideal, and the treatment of preterm labor may exacerbate the effects of infection. Prior to the definitive diagnosis of appendicitis there are many conditions to be considered that have greater fetal risk (chorioamnionitis, abruptio placentae). These often mimic appendicitis. Tocolysis in the face of these diseases is not indicated. The cardiovascular effects of beta-adrenergic drugs (terbutaline, ritodrine) can exacerbate those of sepsis, i.e., vasodilatation and shock. Intravenous ritodrine has a 5 to 10% risk of serious cardiopulmonary complications such as pulmonary edema and significant subendocardial ischemia. Other tocolytic agents that involve calcium ion physiology ($MgSO_4$ and calcium channel blockers) have less significant but still disturbing cardiovascular effects in the face of sepsis. Prostaglandin inhibitors (indomethacin) are contraindicated for tocolysis as they mask the clinical signs of infection.

Keeping these problems in mind, the following management of preterm labor in appendicitis is suggested. First, uterine irritability is not labor until there is evidence of cervical effacement or dilatation. Any decision for tocolysis should await demonstration of cervical change. Prophylactic tocolysis is not indicated. Second, the presence of intrauterine disease should be determined by a sophisticated ultrasound and an amniocentesis. An amniocentesis under ultrasound guidance has many advantages. Chorioamnionitis is readily suggested by bacteria or sheets of WBC's on a highpower microscopic examination. Fetal lung studies and the OD 650 nm test may be rapidly performed in most institutions. However, the risk of third trimester amniocentesis must be kept in mind (Chapter 9). The special risk in this situation is amniotic fluid contamination if peritonitis is present. If peritonitis is present, an exploratory laparotomy should not be delayed by amniocentesis. Localized peritoneal contamination over the amniocentesis site cannot always be predicted. Amniocentesis should be performed away from the right lower quadrant or points of tenderness. An uncomfortable but good alternative is to perform a suprapubic tap through a full bladder under ultrasound guidance. This approach will avoid the peritoneum.

Once the diagnostic test or surgery has been performed and the mother's cardiovascular status is stable, the decision whether or not to inhibit labor can be made. Magnesium sulfate is the therapy of choice. The dose is 4 gm in 250 ml NS given intravenously over 15 minutes followed by 2 gm per hour by electronically monitored intravenous drip. The precautions and risks in use of this drug are discussed in Chapter 13. The fetus should have continuous fetal monitoring through the entire episode. Fetal distress should be aggressively diagnosed and treated. Magnesium sulfate should be continued for 12 to 24 hours after the operation. At that point the patient is weaned off the medication.

Cholecystectomy

Inflammation of the gallbladder, cholecystitis, is a relatively common diagnosis during pregnancy. In fact, cholecystectomy is second only to appendectomy in frequency of non-obstetric surgery during pregnancy; Hill and co-workers (1975b) found one to five cholecystectomies per 10,000 pregnancies. The reasons for this are the overall prevalence of cholelithiasis (10 to 15%) and the physiologic changes associated with pregnancy that increase the risk. Braverman and co-workers (1980) describe these changes as (1) increased cholesterol synthesis, (2) increased gallbladder volume after emptying, (3) increased concentration of cholesterol in the bile and (4) a decrease in circulating bile salt pool.

The clinical features of acute cholecystitis are similar in both pregnant and non-pregnant women. Mid-epigastric to right upper quadrant stabbing pain, eructation, heartburn, nausea, vomiting and fatty food intolerance are suggestive but not diagnostic. Tenderness over the right ninth costal cartilage upon inspiration (Murphy's sign) occurs in only 5% of pregnant women with cholecystitis. Jaundice suggests blockage of the common hepatic duct. However, cholecystitis and cholelithiasis account for only 5% of jaundice during pregnancy.

The differential diagnosis of right upper quadrant pain with gastrointestinal symptoms in the pregnant woman includes cholestasis of pregnancy among the other usual diagnostic possibilities. Over 50% of women undergoing cholecystectomy during pregnancy have known cholelithiasis prior to pregnancy. The presence of peritonitis, jaundice and sepsis suggests perforation, pancreatitis and ascending cholecystitis. These factors dramatically increase maternal mortality (15 to 20%) and perinatal mortality (60 to 70%).

Cholecystography is relatively contraindicated in pregnancy, but if perforation or intestinal obstruction is suspected, upright and left lateral decubitus films of the abdomen are indicated. Ultrasonography is the cornerstone of diagnosis of cholelithiasis, and its accuracy exceeds 90% (Fig. 10–4).

The management of biliary colic is conservative. The fetal risk of cholecystectomy outweighs the maternal risks of cholelithiasis unless infectious complications supervene.

Conservative treatment includes limitation of oral intake, nasogastric suction and intravenous fluids. Morphine should not be used as it may cause exacerbation of biliary colic. Antibiotics should be reserved for patients with signs of sepsis and for patients who are undergoing cholecystectomy. The use of bile acids in the medical management of gallstones during pregnancy has not been studied. Bile acids cross the placenta and may play a role in the high incidence of preterm delivery and intrauterine death in cholestasis of pregnancy. Thus, bile acid therapy is probably contraindicated.

The indications for surgery are repeated handicapping exacerbations, failure to respond to four to six days of conservative management and signs of serious complications such as sepsis, peritonitis or unremitting jaundice. When other disorders, such as perforated viscus or appendicitis, cannot be ruled out exploration is also indicated.

The surgical problems of cholecystectomy during pregnancy are exposure, positioning, uterine irritability and the possibility of pelvic contamination. Access to the right upper quadrant can be severely limited by an enlarged uterus. Excess traction on the liver may cause rupture, since the liver may be more sensitive to laceration during pregnancy. Excess traction on the uterus may stimulate uterine contractions. A vertical upper midline incision will allow greater exposure if the diagnosis is not clear but will further compromise hepatic exposure. A right subcostal incision allows the best exposure for a cholecystectomy. Left lateral positioning will facilitate this approach and will also prevent a supine hypotensive episode by decreasing the uterine compression of the maternal aorta and inferior vena cava. Concurrent elective appendectomy should not be performed in pregnancy; the contamination may stimulate labor. Uterine irritability and labor may be significant complications of cholecystectomy. Operations performed in the first and second trimesters are less likely to have this complication. In the third trimester the fetus needs to be monitored before and after the operation, and the need for tocolysis should be determined primarily by cervical change with contractions. Intravenous ritodrine is the treatment of choice in preterm labor, unless infection is present, when magnesium sulfate should be used.

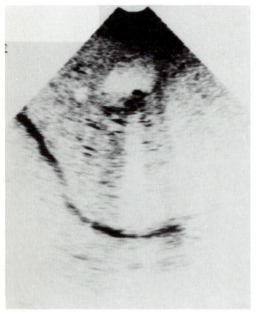

Figure 10–4. Ultrasonographic demonstration of cholelithiasis in pregnancy.

Intestinal Obstruction

In the presurgical era, pregnancy was complicated by intestinal obstruction very infrequently (Smith, 1944). Since 1940, there has been a dramatic rise in the occurrence of intestinal obstruction during pregnancy. Bowel obstruction now complicates one in every 2500 to 3500 deliveries (Davis and Bohon, 1983). This increase has been largely due to the greater frequency of laparotomy and postoperative pelvic adhesions. The rapid rise in the incidence of pelvic inflammatory disease with adhesions as a sequel is also partly to blame. Table 10–8 depicts the causes of intestinal obstruction. Adhesions are associated with 60% of intestinal obstructions and previous pelvic surgery with two thirds of those. Volvulus plays a larger role in bowel obstruction during pregnancy than it does in the non-pregnant population. The reasons for this are unknown, but may relate to the displacement of the bowel by the enlarging uterus. Intestinal obstruction seems to occur most frequently when the uterus becomes an abdominal organ at 12 to 14 weeks. At this time rapid uterine growth may cause the bowel to impinge on fixed pelvic adhesions. Obstruction also seems to occur frequently when the fetal head engages in the pelvis and in the early postpartum period when rapid decompression of the uterus changes the relationship of the bowel to fixed adhesions. A mild postpartum ileus may contribute to the development of the obstruction.

DIAGNOSTIC COMPLICATIONS

Unfortunately, gastrointestinal symptoms are common during pregnancy, and the differentiation between bowel obstruction and these symptoms is often difficult. Colicky abdominal pains every four to five minutes are characteristic of small bowel obstruction. Abdominal pain recurrent every 10 to 15 minutes suggests large bowel obstruction. Diffuse constant pain suggests bowel obstruction with bowel compromise or perforation. Uterine contractions can mimic colicky pain. Palpation of the uterus and cervical examination may diagnose labor. Labor may be the cause of the pain, but may also be coincident with bowel obstruction. The lack of uterine contractions in the presence of pain suggests gastrointestinal disease.

Nausea and vomiting are very common symptoms during pregnancy, but their sudden occurrence in the second or third trimester is unusual. High small bowel obstruction will lead to early violent vomiting of intestinal contents. Low colonic obstruction may produce little or no vomiting unless strangulation occurs. Vomiting of fecal material is diagnostic of colonic obstruction.

The passage of stool or flatus per rectum is an important sign. Chronic constipation is a common symptom of pregnancy, but absolute constipation without flatus is pathologic. The passage of flatus or stool does not rule out obstruction. In early cases of proximal obstruction the gas and stool distal to the blockage are cleared. Late in the course of obstruction little is passed. Auscultation of the abdomen may be helpful. Mechanical obstruction produces high pitched sounds, tinkles and rushes. However, bowel sounds may remain normal until strangulation occurs and, therefore, bowel sounds may be of little value in making the diagnosis of early obstruction.

Radiologic examination is an important adjunct to the diagnosis of bowel obstruction. In fact, serial studies at four- to six-hour intervals usually reveal progessive changes that confirm the diagnosis. Although there is a natural reluctance to order x-rays in the gravid patient, the benefits of diagnosis far outweigh the risks in terms of maternal and perinatal mortality. After the first trimester the risk of teratogenesis is remote, and radiation with less than 1 or 2 rads is not associated with significant carcinogenic risks. The radiologic examination of simple small bowel obstruction (Fig. 10–5) usually shows progressive dilatation with stepladder formation of the loops and air fluid levels in upright films. Large bowel obstruction can produce dilatation, loss of haustrations and accumulation of intraluminal fluid. The radiographic picture of a sigmoid obstruction is dilated segments of the sigmoid lying upright and parallel

Table 10–8. Causes of Intestinal Obstruction During Pregnancy

Cause	Incidence (%)
Adhesions	60
Appendectomy	38
Uterine or adnexal	28
Inflammation	18
Congenital	10
Other	6
Volvulus	25
Intussusception	4
Hernia	3
Other	8

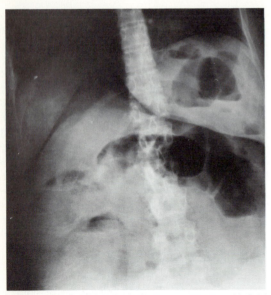

Figure 10–5. *Mid-gut volvulus in pregnancy. Air fluid levels in the upper abdomen are shown.*

on the left side of the abdomen. A visible column of air communicates between the segments at their apex. Two long air fluid levels are often seen on a decubitus film, with an air-fluid ratio in excess of 2:1.

Contrast studies are being used more frequently. The "bird of prey" sign evident with barium enema in large bowel obstruction shows the contrast material in the shape of a bird's bill. Use of a half barium and half Gastrografin solution may be valuable in differentiating mechanical obstruction from ileus and partial obstruction. This mixture minimizes the risk of full strength barium precipitating frank obstruction.

The treatment of intestinal obstruction in pregnancy is surgical exploration. The placement of a long tube may be valuable in partial small bowel obstruction in the non-pregnant patient, but in pregnancy long tubes may dangerously delay surgery and risk maternal and fetal health. A preoperatively placed short nasogastric tube is, however, essential in reducing air and fluid pressure above the obstructed bowel.

PERIOPERATIVE COMPLICATIONS

The perioperative concerns for the pregnant patient with intestinal obstruction are the rapid correction of fluid deficit, hypoxia and metabolic

acidosis, prevention of infection and maintenance of nutrition (see Chapter 4). The fluid deficit at the time of radiologic diagnosis is at least 1500 ml and may be as much as 4 to 6 liters. At this point uterine blood flow may be seriously reduced. Rapid resuscitation with Ringer's lactate solution is essential. Volume expansion and the addition of specific electrolytes (e.g., potassium) will help correct the metabolic deficits. The persistence of hypoxia and metabolic acidosis suggests sepsis. High flow oxygen by mask will raise the umbilical vein PaO_2 by 10 to 20 mmHg. Early surgery and antibiotics are needed to correct the infection and prevent choriaoamnionitis. Medical stabilization must be rapid, and if perforation or strangulation is suspected, immediate surgery is mandatory.

The abdominal incision should be vertical and large enough to allow for good exposure to the bowel and minimal manipulation of the uterus. The entire length of the bowel must be examined, since multiple sites of obstruction may be present. Many obstructions during pregnancy relate to fixed pelvic adhesions or sigmoid volvulus. Exposure of the posterior pelvis may be very difficult with a third trimester uterus. A cesarean section may be needed to gain adequate exposure. Harer and Harer (1958) in review of 33 cases of sigmoid volvulus in pregnancy noted 10 cases in which abdominal delivery was necessary to allow surgical therapy of the volvulus. Better maternal and fetal results are associated with repair of the obstruction without uterine manipulation. There is no justification for cesarean section solely out of concern for subsequent vaginal delivery in the early recovery period. A properly closed abdominal incision can withstand the stress of labor.

The actual surgical management is decided after complete exploration of the abdomen for the sites and types of obstruction. In most cases, simple division of adhesive bands or reduction of a volvulus may be all that is needed. Fixation and plication of redundant colon has been advocated by some authors to prevent recurrence of volvulus. Assessment of the viability of the bowel may be difficult (see Chapter 4). Nonviable bowel should be resected.

POSTOPERATIVE COMPLICATIONS

Prolonged starvation due to gastrointestinal disease can lead to intrauterine growth retardation. Parenteral nutrition must be considered. All patients should receive dextrose and intravenous multivitamins early in the recovery period. If the patient has had insufficient intake (less than 1000 cal/24 hours) for 72 hours, parenteral nutrition should be started. If support will be needed for less than 10 days, peripheral parenteral nutrition is indicated. An appropriate nutrient solution is the simultaneous use of 4.25% amino acid and 5% dextrose (1500 ml) with a fat emulsion (1500 ml of Intralipid) through a "Y" connector. This provides the patient with 3000 ml of H_2O, 64 gm of protein and 1950 calories in 24 hours. Electrolytes, trace elements and vitamins can be added to the protein solution. If support will be needed for longer than 10 days or if the patient's condition is particularly severe (recurrent Crohn's disease), total parenteral nutrition through a central venous catheter is needed. The reader is referred to Chapter 2 and to the works of Ghafouri and Miller-Doszpoly (1984) and Martin and Blackburn (1983) for further details.

The specific problems of parenteral nutrition during pregnancy are the increased metabolic needs (increase to 40 cal/kg/day and increase in protein by 30 to 50 gms/day). Hyperglycemia can be a greater risk, since pregnancy is normally a diabetogenic state. Consistent blood sugars above 120 mg/dl should be treated with insulin. Pregnancy is also a hyperlipidemic state, and there has been some theoretical caution about the use of lipid solutions. However, hyperalimentation is a replacement rather than a supplementation, and this caution may not be applicable. Like the gravida, the fetus must also be evaluated for growth and well being; non-stress tests are performed twice weekly and serial ultrasonograms for fetal growth should be obtained.

Despite improved operative techniques, antibiotics and anesthesia, maternal mortality remains at 5 to 15% from intestinal obstruction during pregnancy. The immediate causes of death include infection, shock and cardiac arrest. The fetus fares worse; premature labor or fetal death occurs in 50% of cases in the third trimester. Maternal hypotension and hypoxia are associated with the majority of fetal morbidity and mortality. Delay in diagnosis is a major contribution to severe maternal and fetal morbidity and mortality. Goldthorp (1966) found the average time was 3 to 5 days from the onset of symptoms to admission to the hospital and 2.8 days from hospitalization to operative intervention.

EXERCISE IN PREGNANCY

Despite the recent popularization of physical fitness, the physiology and outcomes of exercise in pregnancy have been incompletely studied. The need for study would seem apparent; the uteroplacental unit competes with the maternal body for oxygen and nutrients. The adverse effects of this competition could be measured in perinatal outcome, fetal growth, prematurity and mortality. Current evaluations of exercise in pregnancy have both theoretical and practical problems. Physiologic measurements require invasive and cumbersome equipment, i.e., surgical insertion of probes. Direct measurements have relied on chronically instrumented quadrupeds. The artificial nature of animal studies, including the untoward effects of anxiety and fear, limit their application to human subjects. Human studies are confined to indirect measurements made before and after weight-bearing exercise.

Patient selection is a second major problem of investigations concerned with exercise and pregnancy. Most studies are limited to small self-selected groups of patients of above average fitness and health. No current study has sufficient numbers of controls to assess the interactions among exercise and mother and fetus. Similarly, some groups would be impossible to study; individuals with poor obstetric histories are not likely to participate in a strenuous exercise study.

Lotgering and co-workers (1984) have reviewed the interaction of exercise and pregnancy and have focused on the third area of weakness: methodologic control. Pregnancy progressively changes many physical dimensions (weight, surface area, blood volume and composition) and variations in baseline values must be controlled for length of gestation. These physiologic changes may affect the physiologic burden of a given exercise. For example, in late pregnancy, resting and exercise hemodynamics in the sitting position are dominant factors that influence venous return, independent of physical fitness (Morton et al, 1985). Different individuals may have widely different responses to a fixed exercise regimen. This variation can be minimized by standardizing the exercise level to a percentage of the individual's maximum O_2 consumption. This type of standardization has not been widely used in pregnant women. Most studies rely on responses to a fixed exercise, i.e., a 1.5 mile run. Another methodologic hurdle is the establishment of interindividual control. In order to assess progressive changes during pregnancy, one must ascertain the level of pregravid fitness. Most studies rely on patient recall data rather than actual measurements.

Given the weaknesses in study design and the theoretical pitfalls, what are the effects of exercise in pregnancy? Lotgering and co-workers (1984) have made following observations:

1. Resting O_2 consumption rises by 16 to 32% at term. The increase is largely due to the increase in uterine tissue mass or, in other words, other maternal tissues are unaffected by pregnancy.

2. Oxygen consumption increases with both exercise and gestational age. Exercise in pregnancy will increase absolute values for oxygen consumption by 10% above non-pregnant values.

3. Exercise efficiency is not affected by pregnancy.

4. Training increases maximum oxygen consumption by 20 to 30%, similar to that in the non-pregnant individual. However, when weight gain is taken into account, the effect seems to be lessened (8 to 18%) (Collings et al, 1983).

5. Accurate uterine blood flow studies require instrumentation not available for human subjects. Most data come from weight-bearing forced exercise in large quadrupeds (sheep) (Lotgering et al, 1983; Clapp, 1980). During exercise stress, uterine blood flow decreases by 20 to 30%. The reduction of uterine blood flow suggests adverse fetal effects from exercise. However, compensating mechanisms allow maintenance of a consistent oxygen supply to the placenta. These mechanisms are hemoconcentration to increase the oxygen carrying capacity of maternal blood, a redistribution of uterine blood in favor of the placenta over the myometrium, and an increased fetal/placental extraction of oxygen.

6. Exercise increases total heat production as much as twenty times the resting values. Only 20% is used for external work. Exercise increases body temperature proportionately to the intensity and duration of the exercise. Maternal body temperature is the major determinant of fetal temperature (usually 0.5 degrees [C] higher than that of the mother). Maternal temperature rises by 2 to 3 degrees C with 40 minutes of training at 70% maximum oxygen consumption. Fetal temperature rises in similar fashion and takes at least one hour to return to normal.

Studies on fetal respiratory blood gas determinations must take into account the changes caused by temperature differences. If temperature is controlled, there is only minimal decrease in fetal oxygen tension and pH after 40 minutes at 70% maximum oxygen consumption.

The maternal benefits and risks of exercise during pregnancy are direct and indirect. Direct benefits stem from the training effect: an improved work capacity during labor or improved muscular efficiency in the second stage. The indirect benefits of exercise are lessened anxiety, an improved sense of control and the acquisition of better habits and diet necessary for a successful fitness program. The direct maternal risk of exercise in pregnancy is the possible trauma caused by the changes in balance, body weight and coordination that occur during pregnancy. The indirect maternal risk relates to failure to adjust the exercise program and diet to pregnancy and the danger of fetal compromise.

The adverse effects of maternal physical activity on perinatal outcome have been reported in both human and animal studies. The most commonly mentioned are the teratogenic effect of hyperthermia and low birth weight. Pleet and co-workers (1981) suggested hyperthermia in the first trimester as a cause of 28 cases of dysmorphism of unknown etiology. However, physical agents, such as subclinical viral infection, could not be ruled out. Central nervous system dysgenesis was produced in guinea pigs by increasing their core body temperature to 38.9 degrees C (102 degrees F). We do know that prolonged exercise, especially in hot humid weather, can cause temperature this high, but we do not know if intermittent exercise has the same dangerous potential.

Low birthweight in infants, caused by uteroplacental insufficiency (small for gestational age), and prematurity (premature, birthweight appropriate for gestational age) have both been associated with exercise during pregnancy. Animal studies (Lotgering et al, 1984) have shown an 8 to 20% decrease in birthweight when animals are forcibly exercised. However, one cannot exclude the possibility that the chronic "stress" of handling and forced exercise contributed to prematurity or growth retardation. Observations on human subjects have been conflicting. On the negative side, Clapp and Dickstein (1984) and Dale and co-workers (1982) noted a signifcant fall in average birthweight if endurance exercise was continued into the last trimester. Older data from the Collaborative

Perinatal Project (Naeye and Peters, 1982) suggest a similar finding when standing work is continued into the third trimester. Studies by Pomerance and co-workers (1974), Erkkola (1976) and Collings and co-workers (1983) suggest no adverse fetal effects.

Despite the lack of knowledge on exercise physiology in pregnancy and the weaknesses of outcome studies in humans, moderate exercise is well tolerated by the mother and her fetus. Extreme and prolonged exercise, i.e., greater than 40 minutes of continuous exercise at 70% maximum O_2 consumption, has its greatest risks of hyperthermia at 17 to 40 days postconception, and of low birthweight in the third trimester when venous return is limited by weight bearing exercise. Patients at high risk of fetal or maternal compromise should limit exercise (Table 10–9).

From these general observations the following clinical guidelines are useful for the average gravida:

1. Consider switching to non–weight bearing exercise such as swimming, cycling or rowing, especially in the third trimester.

2. Exercise regularly, at least three times a week.

3. Limit activity to shorter intervals: exercise 10 to 15 minutes, rest to a pulse rate less than 90, then exercise for another 10 to 15 minutes.

4. Decrease exercise level in the third trimester.

5. Monitor the intensity of the exercise. Ideally exercise should be maintained at 50 to 70% maximum O_2 consumption. The target zone concept is useful and can be approximated by measuring heart rate or ventilatory response. Heart rate should be 60 to 80% of maximum rate (120 to 140 BPM). The ventilatory target

Table 10–9. Absolute Limitations to Exercise in Pregnancy

History of two previous births of infants weighing less than 2500 grams.
History of incompetent cervix.
History of uterine anomalies with a history of poor obstetric outcome.
Multiple gestation, preeclampsia, or polyhydramnios in the current pregnancy.
Maternal disease.
  Retinopathy (> Stage I).
  Cardiac disease, especially pulmonary hypertension and mitral stenosis.
  Marfan's syndrome.
  Nephropathy.
  Hemoglobinopathies.
  Anemia (Hb <9 gm/dl)

zone is approximated by the ability to talk but not to sing comfortably while exercising.

ANTENATAL CLASSES

It is appropriate to review the possible complications of antenatal classes since they have become popular and widely available. The antenatal class is designed to educate the prospective parents about the physical and psychologic variables associated with pregnancy, labor, delivery and the early postpartum period. Such a program is usually shared by a number of couples, allowing for peer support, a self-help group. Another goal is to reduce the anxiety of hospitalization by demonstrating the various units of the hospital and the "normal" routine. "Normal" routine is often defined by the character of the individual providers practicing in that facility. This "normal" routine may vary from natural childbirth to epidural anesthesia, episiotomy and outlet forceps.

A consistent focus of childbirth classes has been the teaching of relaxation and psychoprophylactic techniques to reduce childbirth pain. The basic principle of these techniques is to create competitive and dominant physical or mental sensations in opposition to labor pain. The analgesic effectiveness of psychoprophylactic training methods has been well demonstrated in the laboratory (Stevens and Heide, 1977). However, their effectiveness in a clinical setting is much harder to assess. Early reports of antenatal preparation classes were descriptive, anecdotal and uncontrolled, but in the face of almost universal massive narcosis and general anesthesia for delivery the results were impressive. Thoms and Karlovsky (1954) reported on 2000 consecutive deliveries in which 34% and 29% were conducted without analgesia or anesthesia respectively.

One of the major weaknesses of research on the effectiveness of childbirth education is selection bias; the prepared and unprepared groups are not comparable. Beck and Hall (1978) and Beck and Siegel (1980) described the minimum essentials for an adequate trial of antenatal preparation: random assignments of subjects, the rater's unawareness of the subject's group membership and a three group design to include no-treatment controls and attention-placebo controls as well as the experimental subjects. The number of studies meeting these criteria are few in number and small in size. Timm (1979) studied a group of very low-income women in a prospective randomized fashion using the three groups. The group that attended the prenatal classes used significantly less pain medication than the two control groups. Despite the dearth of adequate scientific design, there is a consistent finding in most studies showing a decreased use of pain medication in the prepared patient.

The decreased use of medication may or may not reflect a true reduction in the intensity of pain. The patient may be more accepting of pain or have a greater fear of medication or anesthesia. The subjective measurement of pain intensity addresses the latter concern. Melzack and Taenzer (1981) addressed the problem of pain directly, using the McGill pain questionnaire. This discriminates between sensory, affective and evaluative aspects of pain as well as providing a total pain index. Although prepared childbirth was associated with lower pain scores, especially in primiparas, training and practice accounted for only 10% of the variance. This study points out that psychologic variables are subject to numerous confounding biases, such as personality, concurrent life stress or anxiety. These biases plus physical variables help explain the remaining variance in Melzack and Taenzer's study.

Antenatal classes have been given credit for a number of obstetrical advantages: decreased blood loss, decreased operative intervention, shortening of labor and improved outcome for the neonate. These observations come largely from studies with poor comparability between the prepared and unprepared populations. Any significant obstetric advantages shown are probably the result of a healthier prepared population and a reduction of analgesia or anesthesia in the prepared group. In the well-controlled study by Timm (1979) no obstetric advantage except for reduced medication was seen in the prepared group. A recent larger study by Bennett and co-workers (1985) also failed to show differences in the physical variables except for medication usage.

Antenatal classes have also been given credit for an enhanced feeling of self-esteem, a sense of achievement or a positive feeling about the birth experience (Huttel et al, 1972; Charles et al, 1978; Bennett et al, 1985). However, these studies and others rely on the patient's retrospective evaluation of the experience, for example, during the postpartum period, when confounding variables are the strongest. Ideally, psychologic evaluation should occur prospectively from preconceptual to prepartum to postpartum periods in a randomized group of prepared and unprepared women controlled for socioeconomic, educational and health variables.

The complications of antenatal classes are even harder to document than the purported benefits. The adverse effects of patient education are described by a collection of anecdotes and biased observations unencumbered by scientific study. The anecdotal cases often describe the woman or infant who suffered damage because the woman had been brainwashed by her childbirth educator into believing medication or all obstetric intervention was dangerous. Although patients may rarely become unreasonable about intervention or medication, the cause is more likely to be associated with the patient's personality than with the character of educational material given by the childbirth educator.

A real but inadequately studied complication of antenatal education is the psychologic effects of failure to meet expectations that may have been raised by it. Most antenatal courses state explicitly that the purpose of the class is to educate the patient about the process of pregnancy, birth and hospitalization but not to teach her how to avoid analgesia or anesthesia or intervention. However, unrealistic expectations and perceptions can occur in a success-motivated couple. When these perceptions and expectations are shattered by reality, feelings of anger, guilt or inadequacy may develop. Although some feelings of failure will develop in any couple when expectations are not met, the structure of antenatal classes can reduce the impact. The use of sensitive audiovisual material and the availability of childbirth educators who themselves have experienced birth can help address and avoid unrealistic expectations.

REFERENCES

Averette HE, Nasser N et al: Cervical conization in pregnancy. *Am. J. Obstet. Gynecol.* 106:543, 1970.

Babaknia A, Parson H, Woodruff JD: Appendicitis during pregnancy. *Obstet. Gynecol.* 50:43, 1977.

Baer JL, Reis RA, Arens RA: Appendicitis in pregnancy. *J. Am. Med. Assoc.* 98:1359, 1932.

Ballard CA: Ovarian tumors associated with pregnancy termination patients. *Am. J. Obstet. Gynecol.* 149:384, 1984.

Bavermann DJ, Johnson MI, Kern F Jr: Effects of pregnancy and contraceptive steroids on gallbladder function. *N. Engl. J. Med.* 302:363, 1980.

Beck NC, Hall D: Natural childbirth: a review and analysis. *Obstet. Gynecol.* 52:371, 1978.

Beck NC, Siegel LJ: Preparation for childbirth and contemporary research on pain, anxiety, and stress reduction: a review and critique. *Psychosom. Med.* 42:429, 1980.

Beischer NA, Buttery BW et al: Growth and malignancy of ovarian tumors in pregnancy. *Aust. N.Z.J. Obstet. Gynaecol.* 11:208, 1971.

Bennett A, Hewson D et al: Antenatal preparation and labor support in relation to birth outcome. *Birth* 12:9, 1985.

Benson EA, Goodman MA: Incision with primary suture in the treatment of acute puerperal breast abscess. *Br. J. Surg.* 57:55, 1970.

Buchsbaum HJ: Penetrating injury of the abdomen. In Buchsbaum HJ (Ed.): *Trauma in Pregnancy.* Philadelphia, W. B. Saunders Co., 1979.

Buttery BW, Beischer NA et al: Ovarian tumours in pregnancy. *Med. J. Aust.* 1:345, 1973.

Cetrulo CL, Sbarra A et al: Clinical application of amniotic fluid 650 nm optical density reading and neonatal respiratory outcomes. *Obstet. Gynecol.* 55:262, 1980.

Charles AG, Norr KL et al: Obstetric and psychological effects of psychoprophylactic preparation for childbirth. *Am. J. Obstet. Gynecol.* 131:44, 1978.

Clapp JF III: Acute exercise stress in the pregnant ewe. *Am. J. Obstet. Gynecol.* 136:489, 1980.

Clapp JF III, Dickstein S: Endurance exercise and pregnancy outcome. *Med. Sci. Sport. Exerc.* 16:556, 1984.

Collings CH, Curet LB, Mullin JP: Maternal and fetal responses to maternal aerobic exercise program. *Am. J. Obstet. Gynecol.* 145:702, 1983.

Crosby WM, Castiloe JP: Safety of lap seat restraint for pregnancy victims of automobile collisions. *N. Engl. J. Med.* 284:632, 1971.

Csapo AZ, Pulkkinen M: Indispensability of the human corpus luteum in the maintenance of early pregnancy. Lutectomy evidence. *Obstet. Gynecol. Surv.* 33:69, 1978.

Dale E, Mullinax KM, Bryan DH: Exercise during pregnancy: effects on the fetus. *Can. J. Appl. Sport Sci.* 7:98, 1982.

Daskal JL, Pitkin RM: Cone biopsy of the cervix during pregnancy. *Obstet. Gynecol.* 32:1, 1968.

Davis MR, Bohon CJ: Intestinal obstruction in pregnancy. *Clin. Obstet. Gynecol.* 26:832, 1983.

Edwards MJ: Congenital defects in guinea pigs following induced hyperthermia during gestation. *Arch. Pathol.* 84:42, 1967.

Erkkola R: The physical work capacity of the expectant mother and its effect on pregnancy, labor and the newborn. *Int. J. Gynecol. Obstet.* 14:153, 1976.

Gainey HL, Keeler JE: Submucous myoma in term pregnancy. *Am. J. Obstet. Gynecol.* 58:727, 1949.

Ghafouri I, Miller-Doszpoly JA: Artificial feeding and hyperalimentation. In Iffy L, Charles D (Eds.): *Operative Perinatology.* New York, MacMillan Publishing Co., 1984.

Goldenberg RL, Nelson KG et al: Delay in delivery: influence of gestational age and the duration of delay on perinatal outcome. *Obstet. Gynecol.* 64:480, 1984.

Goldstein D, Dechoenoky CJ et al: Laparoscopy in the diagnosis and management of pelvic pain in adolescents. *J. Reprod. Med.* 24:251, 1980.

Goldthorp WO: Intestinal obstruction during pregnancy and the puerperium. *Br. J. Clin. Pract.* 20:367, 1966.

Hacker NF, Berek JS et al: Carcinoma of the cervix associated with pregnancy. *Obstet. Gynecol.* 59:735, 1982.

Hallatt JG: Ruptured corpus luteum with hemoperitoneum: a study of 173 surgical cases. *Am. J. Obstet. Gynecol.* 149:5, 1984.

Hannigan EV, Whitehouse HH III et al: Cone biopsy during pregnancy. *Obstet. Gynecol.* 60:450, 1982.

Harer WB Jr, Harer WB Sr: Volvulus complicating pregnancy and puerperium. *Obstet. Gynecol.* 12:399, 1958.

Hibbard LT: Corpus luteum surgery. *Am. J. Obstet. Gynecol.* 135:666, 1979.

Hill LM, Johnson CE, Lee RA: Ovarian surgery in pregnancy. *Am. J. Obstet. Gynecol.* 122:565, 1975a.

Hill LM, Johnson CE, Lee RA: Cholecystectomy in pregnancy. *Obstet. Gynecol.* 46:291, 1975b.

Horowitz A, Sabatelle R et al: The risk of cone biopsy during pregnancy. *J. Reprod. Med.* 3:9, 1969.

Huttel FA, Mitchell I et al: A quantitative evaluation of psychoprophylaxis in childbirth. *J. Psychosom. Res.* 16:81, 1972.

Jones JM, Sweetnam P, Hibbard BM: The outcome of pregnancy after cone biopsy of the cervix: a case control study. *Br. J. Obstet. Gynaecol.* 86:913, 1979.

Larsson G, Grundsell H et al: Outcome of pregnancy after conization. *Acta Obstet. Gynecol. Scand.* 61:461, 1982.

Leiman G, Harrison NA, Rubin A: Pregnancy following conization of the cervix: complications related to cone size. *Am. J. Obstet. Gynecol.* 136:14, 1980.

Lotgering FK, Gilbert GD, Longo LD: Exercise responses in pregnant sheep: oxygen consumption, uterine flow, and blood volume. *J. Appl. Physiol.* 55:834, 1983.

Lotgering FK, Gilbert GD, Longo LD: Interaction of exercise and pregnancy. *Am. J. Obstet. Gynecol.* 149:560, 1984.

Martin R, Blackburn GL: Hyperalimentation during pregnancy. In Berkowitz RL (Ed.): *Critical Care of the Obstetric Patient.* Baltimore, Churchill Livingstone, 1983.

Melzack R, Taenzer P: Labor is still painful after prepared childbirth training. *Can. Med. J.* 125:357, 1981.

Moinian M, Andersch B: Does cervix conization increase the risk of complications in subsequent pregnancies? *Acta Obstet. Gynecol. Scand.* 61:101, 1982.

Morell ND, Taylor JR et al: False-negative cytology roles in patients in whom invasive cervical cancer subsequently developed. *Obstet. Gynecol.* 60:41, 1982.

Morton MJ, Paul MS et al: Exercise dynamics in late gestation: effects on physical training. *Am. J. Obstet. Gynecol.* 152:91, 1985.

Muram D, Gillieson M, Walters JH: Myomas of the uterus in pregnancy: ultrasonographic follow-up. *Am. J. Obstet. Gynecol.* 138:16, 1980.

Naeye RL, Peters EC: Working during pregnancy: effects on the fetus. *Pediatrics* 69:724, 1982.

National Center for Health Statistics. Births, marriages, divorces, deaths. Monthly Vital Statistics Report 33(12):1, 1985.

Onuigbo WZB, Chukudebelu WO: Appendices removed at cesarean section. Histopathology. *Dis. Col. Rect.* 24:507, 1981.

Peckham CH, King RW: A study of intercurrent conditions observed during pregnancy. *Am. J. Obstet. Gynecol.* 87:609, 1963.

Pieper R, Kager L, Nasman P: Acute appendicitis: a clinical study of 1018 cases of emergency appendectomy. *Acta Chir. Scand.* 148:51, 1982.

Pleet H, Graham JM, Smith DW: Central nervous system and facial defects associated with maternal hyperthermia at four to fourteen weeks gestation. *Pediatrics* 67:785, 1981.

Pomerance JJ, Gluck L, Lynch VA: Physical fitness in

pregnancy: its effects on pregnancy outcome. *Am. J. Obstet. Gynecol.* 119:867, 1974.

Rogers RS III, Williams JH: The impact of the suspicious Papanicolaou smear on pregnancy. A study of nationwide attitudes and maternal and perinatal complications. *Am. J. Obstet. Gynecol.* 98:488, 1967.

Stander RW, Lein JN: Carcinoma of the cervix and pregnancy. *Am. J. Obstet. Gynecol.* 79:164, 1960.

Stangel JJ, Nisbet JD, Settles H: Formation and prevention of postoperative abdominal adhesions. *J. Reprod. Med.* 29:143, 1984.

Stevens RJ, Heide F: Analgesic characteristics of prepared childbirth techniques: attention focusing and systematic relaxation. *J. Psychosom. Res.* 21:429, 1977.

Sweeney WJ III: Incidental appendectomy at cesarean section. *Obstet. Gynecol.* 14:588, 1959.

Taylor JW, Plumgott CD, McManus WF: Thermal injury during pregnancy. *Obstet. Gynecol.* 47:434, 1976.

Thoms H, Karlovsky ED: Two thousand deliveries under a training for childbirth program. *Am. J. Obstet. Gynecol.* 68:279, 1954.

Timm MM: Prenatal education evaluation. *Nurs. Res.* 28:338, 1979.

Weber T, Obel E: Pregnancy complications following conization of the uterine cervix. *Acta Obstet. Gynecol. Scand.* 58:259, 1979.

Wegman ME: Annual summary of vital statistics. *Pediatrics* 76:861, 1985.

Weingold AB: Appendicitis in pregnancy. *Clin. Obstet. Gynecol.* 21:801, 1983.

COMPLICATIONS OF OPERATIONS AND PROCEDURES FOR LABOR AND DELIVERY

11

EDWARD R. NEWTON

LABOR

Estimation of Gestational Age

Accurate dating is the cornerstone of many obstetric decisions, especially the timing of delivery. Inaccurate dating has significant risk to the neonate. In the mid to late 1970's, 10 to 15% of respiratory distress noted at teaching institutions was iatrogenic (Maisels et al, 1977). Cowett and Oh (1976) and Flakman and co-workers (1978) reported about a 3% risk of respiratory distress with elective cesarean section. Hack and co-workers (1976) noted that the obstetric estimate of gestational age was three or more weeks greater than the pediatric assessment in over 50% of these infants. Although these data have not adequately separated out maternal indications for delivery, it is safe to say that a significant problem exists.

Ideally the gestational interval should be defined by prospective study of a large number of regularly ovulating women in whom biochemical confirmation of pregnancy occurs prior to the second missed period (4 to 8 weeks' gestation). Much of the information about gestational interval is based on recall data at least four months old. Treloar and co-workers (1967) examined the gestational interval using prospectively recorded menstrual data obtained in a study on menstrual cycle variation. They found a mean of 277.9 ± 15.3 days as the gestational interval. Approximately 7.6% and 7.9% of patients will deliver prior to 38 weeks and after 42 weeks, respectively. This distribution describes the biologic variation to which any estimate of date of confinement must necessarily conform. Any method that purports to predict a due date with a standard deviation less than 10 days must be suspect. Numerous authors have described a regular last menstrual period recorded in the first trimester as the most accurate dating criterion (Jimenez et al, 1983).

A positive pregnancy test prior to the second missed period is an extremely valuable adjunct to dating. In fact, by ACOG standards,

315

any gestation at 33 weeks after a positive urine pregnancy test (slide test) or 35 weeks after a serum measurement of human chorionic gonadotropin should be considered mature. Timing of fetal heart tones heard by stethoscope can be good supporting data (Andersen et al, 1981). After 20 weeks of positive unamplified fetal heart tones the infant can be considered mature. Ultrasound can be used to date pregnancies in which the dates are in question. Crown-rump length at 8 to 10 weeks and biparietal diameter or femur length at 16 to 24 weeks are reliable parameters.

Pediatric estimates of gestational age are sometimes used by neonatologists as the gold standard to which the obstetricians' estimates are held. These estimates describe physiologic maturity not gestational interval. Dubowitz scoring and other methods can be quite inaccurate if used as exact gestational age estimates. Variation by greater than two weeks from known gestational age occurred in 33% of low birth weight infants (Spinnato et al, 1984). Another study (Van Vugt et al, 1981) evaluated two scoring methods and found 95% confidence levels to be ± 5 weeks. In extremely premature or small for gestational age neonates gestational ages were over-estimated, whereas in neonates who were appropriate for gestational age and who had respiratory difficulties gestational ages were underestimated.

If dating criteria supporting maturity are not certain, amniocentesis for fetal lung maturity studies is recommended prior to elective delivery. In cases in which amniocentesis is complicated and glucose tolerance is normal, a biparietal diameter greater than 9.3 cm can be considered an indication of maturity (Newton et al, 1983). Correct application of a dating protocol can reduce the complication of iatrogenic prematurity to less than 0.5% (Frigoletto et al, 1980).

Induction

Prior to 1965, elective induction occurred in 10 to 15% of pregnancies. However, a number of influential studies (Keettel et al, 1958; Niswander and Patterson, 1963) began to document the possible risks of elective induction. In these large series, the risk of iatrogenic prematurity was 3%, the risk of fetal death was 0.6% and neonatal death was about 0.4%. However, these studies have weaknesses: (1) there were no controls with which to compare outcome parameters within the same institution; (2) criteria for patient selection for induction were not well controlled and (3) most studies were performed prior to the advent of many important innovations in perinatal care such as continuous fetal monitoring, constant infusion pumps and neonatal resuscitation in the delivery room. More recent, better controlled studies have shown other important risks of elective induction—increased cesarean and forceps delivery rates and the increased use of epidural anesthesia (Smith et al, 1984). These studies show that strict adherence to dating criteria and the oxytocin protocol will reduce the risks of prematurity and hyperstimulation noted in the older studies.

In 1978, the United States Food and Drug Administration issued the following statement about oxytocin: "The Agency alerts doctors that they should not use this drug (oxytocin) for elective induction of labor. The reasons for this restriction are the risks of uterine hypertonicity, uterine rupture, fetal hypoxia and inadvertent prematurity." This admonition refers to elective induction but often there are situations in which the prolongation of pregnancy is dangerous for either the mother or the fetus and in which there is no contraindication to amniotomy or augmentation of contractions. Maternal indications include pregnancy-induced hypertension, fetal death and chorioamnionitis. Fetal indications might include progressive uteroplacental insufficiency (intrauterine growth retardation), post-date pregnancy, isoimmunization, hypertensive disease, chorioamnionitis, diabetes mellitus and premature rupture of membranes. Any fetal indication must be tempered by a recognition of the risks of prematurity (Barson et al, 1984).

Contraindications to the induction of labor include any condition in which spontaneous labor and delivery would be more dangerous for the mother or the fetus than abdominal delivery, such as fetal distress, abnormal fetal presentation, uncontrolled hemorrhage, placenta previa, unengaged fetal vertex and a previous vertical uterine incision. Caution should be employed in the following situations: grand multiparity (five or more previous pregnancies beyond 20 weeks' gestation), multiple gestation, suspected cephalopelvic disproportion, breech presentation, inability to adequately monitor the fetal heart rate during labor and a previous low transverse cesarean section.

Prior to the induction of labor all patients

must give informed consent so that they recognize: (1) the alternatives to induction and their risks and (2) the risks of induction, including the increase in operative delivery, the need for invasive monitoring and the possible risks of fetal distress, hyperbilirubinemia, increase in labor pain, prematurity and fetal trauma. The risk of prematurity can be estimated from a due date defined by good dating criteria or an amniocentesis for fetal lung maturity studies. Elective or indicated induction should be performed after 39.5 weeks. Prior to 39 weeks amniocentesis for fetal lung maturity studies is recommended.

Cervical Ripening. Successful labor requires mature biochemical and regulatory systems in the myometrium and cervix. Biochemical markers include adequate actinomyosin, appropriate changes in the progesterone/estrogen ratio, appropriate changes in prostaglandin synthesis and changes in the collagenous matrix of the cervix and uterus toward a more elastic character. Regulatory markers include adequate numbers of oxytocin/prostaglandin receptors and of gap junctions between myometrial cells. The exact state of readiness required for successful induction has not been defined as yet, but it is felt that evaluation of cervical readiness is a reflection of maturity of the whole system. Anderson and Turnbull (1969) have described the changes in the cervix as they relate to the onset of labor. For example, in a primigravida, if the internal os admits one finger at 32 weeks, 67% will deliver prior to the 40th week of gestation and only 8% will go longer than 42 weeks. On the other hand, if the internal os is closed at 32 weeks only 17% will deliver prior to 40 weeks and 32% will go past 42 weeks.

Bishop (1964) proposed a quantitative description of the cervix using a composite score of five different parameters: station, dilatation, effacement, consistency and position (Table 11–1). Friedman and co-workers (1966) applied the

Bishop score to the success of induction. They found that with scores of 0 to 4, 5 to 8 and 9 to 12 the failure rates were 19.5%, 4.8% and 0% respectively. Since that study, a variety of modifications have been proposed (Lange et al, 1982) without much change in predictive value. Cervical dilatation seems to be the most useful of the parameters.

The relationship between cervical score and the success of induction has led to a variety of interventions to improve the cervical score. The methods can be described as pharmacologic (prostaglandin, estrogen, relaxin), mechanical (laminaria, Foley catheter), or physiologic (breast stimulation). Intravaginal or intracervical prostaglandin has been the most widely studied pharmacologic agent. One to three milligrams of prostin E_2 in methylhydroxylethyl cellulose (Tylose) gel is inserted into the posterior fornix. This technique has been shown to improve the cervical score (Prins et al, 1983) and to induce labor with greater effectiveness than oxytocin (Ekman-Ordeberg et al, 1985).

Most patients note an increase in contractions soon after intravaginal insertion. Occasionally hypertonicity can be induced (0.1 to 1%). This may be related to the lack of control over the actual dose of prostaglandin. Most preparations are made by mixing a commercially prepared 20 mg preparation in gel and applying a portion of this mixture to the cervix. Incomplete mixing may allow for a larger dose than intended. Because of the possible stress to the fetus of hypertonicity, a non-stress test should be performed prior to the insertion, and the fetus should be monitored for a period of time (1 hour) after the insertion.

Oxytocin and prostaglandin affect the cervix by uterine contractions and by the secondary mechanical force of the presenting part upon the cervix. Relaxin appears to exert a direct effect upon cervical tissue and thus may have the advantage of achieving cervical change with-

Table 11–1. Bishop Score*

Parameter	Points Assigned			
	0	1	2	3
Dilatation (cm)	0	1–2	3–4	5–6
Effacement (%)	0–30	40–50	60–70	80
Station	−3	−2	−1/0	+1/+2
Consistency	Firm	Medium	Soft	
Position	Posterior	Mid	Anterior	

Total pelvic score is the sum of the points for individual parameters

*From Bishop EH: Pelvic scoring for elective induction. *Obstet. Gynecol.* 24:266, 1964. Reprinted with permission.

out stress on the fetus. Relaxin has been shown to effect significant change in cervical scores (MacLennan et al, 1980; Evans et al, 1983) and may become the best agent for cervical change if further studies support these findings.

The commonest mechanical agents are laminaria. Laminaria have been used successfully in therapeutic abortion to reduce cervical trauma. It would seem logical to use laminaria at term. Although laminaria are successful in improving cervical scores (Kazzi et al, 1982; Jagani et al, 1982; Rosenberg et al, 1980; Cross and Pitkin, 1978), the success in facilitating delivery has been mixed. The complications of laminaria are cervical trauma (Rosenberg et al, 1980) and infection (Kazzi et al, 1982). Cervical trauma occurs rarely (less than 1%) and can be reduced by direct cervical visualization and stabilization of the anterior lip of the cervix with a sponge forceps.

The report by Kazzi and co-workers (1982) deserves closer examination. In a retrospective review, the authors found a dramatically increased risk of endometritis (15 of 25) and neonatal sepsis (5 of 28) in laminaria-treated gravidas. Three of five septic neonates died. This study was poorly controlled and its definitions of sepsis are suspect, but the complications are dramatic enough to warrant caution. In patients with virulent organisms (group B streptococcus) present on their cervix or in those with compromised host response (chemotherapy, systemic steroids), laminaria should not be used.

Recently two reports have described breast stimulation to mature the cervix and prevent post-date pregnancy (Elliot and Flaherty, 1983, 1984). After the patients were screened for good dates and uteroplacental insufficiency (nonstress test) each breast was alternately stimulated for three hours a day. Significant improvement of Bishop scores was seen in three days, and a significant number of patients went into spontaneous labor. There was no increase in the incidence of meconium staining, fetal distress or low Apgar scores in the treated group. The recent use of the nipple stimulation contraction stress test indicates a significant risk of prolonged contractions (10%). It is not clear whether these contractions are detrimental to the neonate, but their occurrence warrants caution with breast stimulation. All patients should be screened for uteroplacental insufficiency prior to breast stimulation. The activity of the uterus with breast stimulation should be monitored initially by the obstetrician and subsequently by the patient. Contractions lasting longer than two minutes are of concern. Patients using breast stimulation should be followed by cervical examination and antepartum fetal testing every three days.

Induction Techniques. The maturity of the cervix predicts the success of induction. When the Bishop score is greater than 9, labor will be successful whether induced by amniotomy, prostaglandins or low dose oxytocin. Amniotomy has the disadvantages of prolonging rupture of membranes, the possibility of a prolapsed cord and rarely injury to fetal vessels. Caldeyro-Barcia and co-workers (1974) suggest an increase in fetal head molding and caput succedaneum with rupture of membranes prior to cervical dilatation of 5 cm.

The major disadvantage of the uterotonic drugs, prostaglandin and oxytocin, is hyperstimulation and subsequent fetal stress. When given as a bolus dose by way of vaginal absorption (prostaglandin E_2) or buccal mucosa (buccal oxytocin), hyperstimulation cannot be controlled. The advent of intravenous oxytocin given by infusion pump has helped minimize this risk.

The following guidelines will help reduce the risks of elective induction with intravenous oxytocin:

1. Follow guidelines as to the contraindications and precautions of induction.
2. The physician or other care providers starting the oxytocin administration should be familiar with its effects and complications and should be qualified to identify and treat both the maternal and fetal complications.
3. Monitoring parameters should be recorded and include:
   a. Continuous electronic fetal heart rate monitoring.
   b. The frequency and character of contractions by palpation and external tokodynamometer. At doses greater than 8 milliunits/minute, use of an intrauterine pressure catheter is recommended.
   c. The dose of oxytocin.
   d. Vital signs every half hour, or more frequently if needed.
   e. Intake and output of fluids.
4. The oxytocin solution is given in a concentration of one milliunit per milliliter of 5% dextrose and water or 0.5% normal saline.
5. The oxytocin is always given via a controlled infusion pump.

6. The rate of infusion is started at 0.56 milliunits/minute and the dose is doubled every 30 minutes.

7. The dose should be reduced for periods between contractions lasting less than 120 seconds, contractions exceeding 60 seconds in duration or uterine tonus exceeding 15 to 20 mmHg.

The goal is to establish a contraction pattern that will effect progressive effacement and dilatation of the cervix. The goal for uterine work activity has been defined by Seitchik (1981) as two ten-minute periods containing three contractions that averaged greater than 25 mm Hg amplitude, less than 240 second intervals and Montevideo units greater than 100. Once labor has been established (over 90 minutes), the dosage of oxytocin may be reduced. Most successful inductions will require dosages between 4 and 8 milliunits/minute.

Procedures During Labor

MONITORING OF LABOR

The ideal management of labor has the goal of aiding the delivery of a healthy baby from a healthy mother. It should interfere as little as possible with the normal physiologic process of labor. The goal of a healthy baby requires fetal monitoring. One key preventive measure is the identification of the 30% of pregnancies that are high risk. These contribute to the majority (75%) of perinatal mortality and morbidity. The high risk fetus will benefit most from continuous electronic fetal monitoring. Luckily the majority of pregnancies are low risk. Fetal monitoring during the stress of normal labor is no less important, but there can be more flexibility as to the technique. When the patient arrives on the labor and delivery floor, the health of the fetus is documented by external electronic fetal monitoring. For a short period of time, one-half hour, the tracing is observed for fetal reactivity, normal heart rate, good long-term variability and the absence of decelerations. These parameters confirm the health of the fetus at that point in labor. With this assurance fetal monitoring can be modified to auscultation every 15 minutes in the first stage or external electronic fetal monitoring for 15 minutes of every hour during labor. Intermittent monitoring necessitates one to one nursing care. Fetal tolerance of labor should be documented by another one-half hour period of monitoring at the onset of the second stage. Any intervention

such as amniotomy or anesthesia should initiate continuous electronic fetal monitoring. Any abnormality in the fetal heart rate pattern, such as loss of variability, tachycardia or decelerations, requires diagnosis and continuous electronic fetal monitoring.

The health of the mother is aided by monitoring for the signs of hypertension, infection, hemorrhage and normal progress in labor. Hypertension, infection and hemorrhage are associated with the majority of direct maternal deaths, and all are increased during labor. Maternal vital signs should be recorded every one-half hour during labor. Blood type, antibody screen and a complete blood count should be ascertained. Blood pressures above 140/90 should be considered abnormal. The intrapartum management of pre-eclampsia is described in obstetric textbooks. Chorioamnionitis occurs both prior to and during labor. The manifestations are maternal fever greater than 100.5 degrees F, maternal or fetal tachycardia and uterine tenderness. The maternal white blood count and differential are less helpful in labor because of the normal leukocytic response to labor. White blood cell counts of 20,000 to 30,000 are common in labor. The management of chorioamnionitis consists of parenteral antibiotics and augmentation of uterine activity if indicated. The antibiotic should cross the placenta to provide protective tissue levels in the fetus. Ampicillin (2 gm every 4 hours) is a reasonable choice. Any sudden vaginal bleeding must be investigated. The three most dangerous causes of bleeding are undiagnosed placenta previa, abruptio placentae and fetal hemorrhage. The most common source of mild to moderate bleeding is heavy bloody show. A loss of greater than 20 to 30 ml should initiate the following plan of action: (1) establish a large bore (16 to 18 gauge) intravenous line(s); (2) type and cross-match two or more units of blood; (3) obtain a complete blood count; (4) screen the mother for coagulopathy with laboratory tests (fibrinogen, platelet count, fibrin split products); (5) send a vaginal blood clot for an Apt test; (6) initiate continuous electronic fetal monitoring; (7) confirm a normal prenatal Pap smear; (8) document a normal placental position by ultrasound; (9) in the absence of a placenta previa (by ultrasound), a gentle sterile speculum examination should be performed to rule out a cervical lesion. The management of placenta previa and abruptio placentae is described in obstetric textbooks.

The development of hypertension, chorioamnionitis or hemorrhage does not indicate emer-

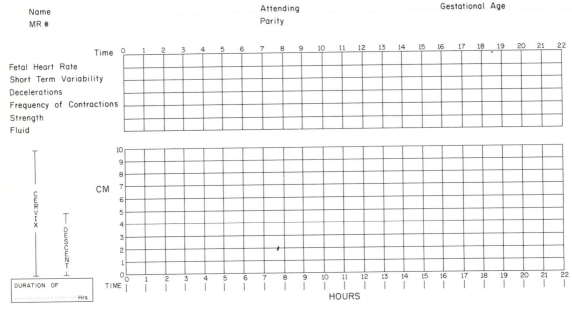

Name

MR #

Attending

Parity

Gestational Age

Time

Fetal Heart Rate
Short Term Variability
Decelerations
Frequency of Contractions
Strength
Fluid

CM

CERVIX

DESCENT

DURATION OF .... Hrs.

TIME

HOURS

Legend

Short Term Variability: (1) <5 BPM   (2) >5 BPM
Decelerations: (1) Early Decelerations
                     (2) Late Decelerations
                     (3) Variable Decelerations
                     (4) Suspicious Decelerations
Strength: (1) Mild or <50 mm H₂O
                     (2) Adequate or >50 mm H₂O
Fluid: (0) Not Ruptured
                     (1) Clear
                     (2) Meconium

Figure 11–1. Partogram.

gency delivery for fetal indications unless there is evidence of fetal decompensation by electronic fetal monitoring. In most cases the internal scalp electrode provides the best documentation of fetal health in the presence of preeclampsia or abruptio placentae. The presence of chorioamnionitis requires a more critical evaluation of the need for a scalp electrode because of the risk of scalp abscess. However, the scalp electrode should not be withheld for this reason alone.

Cervical dilatation and descent of the fetal presenting part are critical factors in labor. A clinically useful method is to plot dilatation and descent according to the hours of labor. Figure 11–1 depicts a partogram. The mean time intervals, speed of labor and the limits of normal are depicted in Table 11–2. Deviations from these guidelines are associated with increased operative delivery and perinatal mortality. The prognosis and management of specific arrest and protraction patterns are discussed by Fried-

Table 11–2. Duration of Normal Labor

Group	Latent Phase (hr)	Active Phase (hr)	Maximum Dilatation (cm/hr)	Maximum Descent (cm/hr)	Second Stage (hr)
Nulliparas (mean)	6.4	4.6	3.0	3.3	1.1
Upper limit*	20.1	11.7	1.2	1.0	2.9
Multiparas (mean)	4.8	2.4	5.7	6.6	0.4
Upper limit	13.6	5.2	1.5	2.1	1.1

*Limit = 95th percentile of distribution data.

man (1978); the reader is referred to this text-book for greater detail. The recognition of the type of pattern and the location of the fetal head are critical to intervention in the course of abnormal labor whether it be medical (oxytocin), instrumental (forceps or vacuum) or surgical (cesarean section).

POSITION IN LABOR

Continuous external electronic fetal monitoring is most reliable when the gravida remains quiet and in the supine position. This position allows the transducer to accurately fix points in the cardiac cycle in order to calculate rate. However, this labor position is the least desirable for both the mother and the fetus. The maternal variables affected by position are cardiovascular status, uterine efficiency, incidence of operative delivery and maternal discomfort. Fetal variables include abnormal fetal heart rate patterns, abnormal Apgar score or acid base status and long-term neurologic development.

Position can have profound effects on maternal cardiac function. In the supine position, the non-contracted uterus envelops the maternal spine and compresses the inferior vena cava and aorta. Venous return from the lower torso can be reduced by 60 to 80%, and the cross sectional area of the aorta is decreased as much as 40%. About 10% of gravidas have transient hypotension and subsequent stress to the fetus. As the uterus contracts it rises in front of the spine and blood flow returns. The contraction also expels 300 to 500 ml of blood from the uterine structures to increase venous return; thus cardiac output increases by 15%. When the parturient is lying on her side, the uterine contraction produces an average increase of only 8%.

Several randomized studies have demonstrated improved efficiency of contractions when the parturient is either lying on her side or is ambulatory. In the largest study, Diaz and co-workers (1980) examined 224 patients in each group. Labor was significantly shorter in both multiparous and primiparous women who were lying on their sides. Roberts and co-workers (1983), using each patient as her own control for supine, sidelying and vertical positions, demonstrated by internal pressure catheter measurements significant increases in uterine efficiency with sidelying and vertical positions. The improvement of uterine efficiency with a vertical position has been applied in a small randomized study comparing ambulation to oxytocin augumentation in the management of

hypotonic uterine contractions (Read et al, 1981). Ambulation improved uterine activity more quickly than oxytocin.

A reduction in operative deliveries would be expected as a result of improved uterine activity by vertical positioning. The number of cesarean births has not been reduced, but most studies show a consistent reduction in instrumental (forceps) deliveries. Maternal comfort seems to be improved with ambulation or the sidelying position by comparison of self-reported data and the use of analgesia or anesthesia. However, there is a significant bias against the supine parturient. The health care provider is much more likely to give potent narcotics to a recumbent woman than one who is ambulating.

The fetus seems to tolerate either position well. Although Flynn and co-workers (1978) showed significantly higher mean Apgar scores in infants of women in the ambulating group, this observation has not been consistent in all studies. Neurologic examinations of the neonates showed no differences in the ambulating versus the supine group (Diaz et al, 1980). These studies reassure the obstetrician that no harm will be done to the fetus by ambulating the mother.

AMNIOTOMY

Artificial rupture of membranes (amniotomy) is a very common procedure. It is usually performed for the diagnosis of meconium staining, placement of an internal monitoring system and to improve uterine efficiency. The most valid indication is the insertion of an internal scalp electrode or intrauterine pressure catheter; their accurate placement requires rupture of membranes. The diagnosis of meconium staining alerts the obstetrician to the possibility of uteroplacental insufficiency. An internal scalp electrode or fetal scalp blood sampling may be indicated in the presence of meconium. Meconium staining also indicates a need for DeLee suctioning of the oropharynx and trachea of the neonate at delivery. However, meconium staining has a benign outcome in 80 to 90% of cases.

Many obstetricians feel that amniotomy can stimulate labor or augment uterine activity during labor. Amniotomy can initiate labor when cervical dilatation is greater than 3 cm. However, amniotomy during the latent phase is not effective and, in fact, lengthens labor (Friedman, 1978). Amniotomy during labor has not been shown to incrase uterine efficiency (Friedman, 1978; Seitchik et al, 1985). These findings are in contrast to those of the prospective controlled trials by Laros and co-workers (1972) and Caldeyro-Barcia and co-workers (1974); in these studies the duration of labor was significantly shortened after rupture of membranes, especially in primiparas (Laros et al, 1972).

The performance of amniotomy requires a clear indication, which must be stated in the medical record. In addition, certain conditions must be fulfilled before amniotomy is undertaken: (1) vertex presentation, (2) the vertex at −1 station or lower, (3) no known source of virulent infection present, i.e., herpes or group B streptococcus, (4) the ability to provide immediate internal fetal monitoring, (5) absence of a low lying placenta or funic presentation.

Although prolonged rupture of membranes (greater than 24 hours) may be associated with maternal infection, the majority of the risks of amniotomy are fetal. Artificial rupture of membranes can lead to prolapse of the umbilical cord (0.5 to 1.0%). Fetal vessels (vasa previa) can be traumatized. Vaginal bleeding after amniotomy is cause for concern, and an Apt or Kleihauer-Betke test should be performed on a clot immediately. Injury to fetal vessels indicates prompt delivery. Intact membranes provide a uniform dilating wedge and protect against undue pressure on the fetal cranium. When amniotomy is performed at 4 to 5 cm versus greater than 9 cm cervical dilatation, there are significant increases in caput succedaneum (34% vs. 15%), disalignment of the cranial bones at birth (44% vs. 16%) and lower cord pH values (Caldeyro-Barcia et al, 1974).

PERINEAL SHAVING AND ENEMAS

Enemas and perineal shaving were common until the 1970's and are still used frequently today. These interventions are the extensions of the vigorous infection prevention policies of the early 1900's. Perineal hair was considered to be unsterile and to prevent adequate cleansing of the perineum and vagina. Stool was felt to contaminate the vagina and lead to childbirth fever and neonatal sepsis. Stool was considered to have the additional disadvantages of obstructing labor and "the shame and disgust from the involuntary expulsion of the feces during the last moments of labor."

Scientific evidence has failed to support either intervention. Shaving increases the incidence of infection and is associated with considerable discomfort, disappointment and itching (Romney, 1980). There is good evidence from surgical studies that the incidence of wound infection is actually increased with preoperative

shaving (Seropian and Reynolds, 1971). The routine use of enemas has come under less scrutiny than the perineal shave. Nonetheless, enemas have proved to be ineffective, uncomfortable and occasionally life-threatening. Romney and Gordon (1981) performed a controlled study of 274 women divided into enema and no enema groups. There were no significant differences in the incidence of contamination (38% vs. 34%), duration of labor or neonatal infection. Colitis, colonic perforation and anaphylactic shock have been reported as rare complications of enemas.

NUTRITION DURING LABOR

Aspiration of gastric material is the leading cause of anesthesia-related maternal death. Even after an 8 to 12 hour fast, 25% of women have sufficient volume and acidity of gastric contents to be at high risk for aspiration. The introduction of any food or fluid increases the risks. On the other hand, less than one half of laboring women will receive anesthesia that puts them at risk for aspiration. Of these patients, a minority will be at greatest risk for aspiration, i.e., those receiving general anesthesia. Labor is work that requires 200 to 300 calories per hour. Without a fluid or glucose source the patient can become dehydrated and ketotic. In the most common situation, fluid and sugar are supplied intravenously in a 5% dextrose and salt solution. This helps prevent dehydration but supplies only 50 grams (225 calories) of glucose per liter. This is inadequate as an energy source for labor.

A practical solution to this dilemma is a selective approach to oral supplementation during labor, limiting the character of oral intake, routine use of non-particulate antacid compounds and the use of anesthetic techniques to avoid aspiration on all gravidas requiring general anesthesia. Food intake should be interdicted in all high risk gravidas and in those in whom the use of conduction anesthesia is anticipated. Otherwise, in the latent phase, food should be confined to easily digested carbohydrates such as bread, fruit, rice or pasta and light proteins such as cheese or yogurt. As labor progresses the emphasis should change to high caloric non-particulate liquids. Water, "athletic" drinks and non-citrus fruit juices are good choices. Straight honey or sugar can provide calories. Eight ounces of fluid and 200 calories per hour is the optimum. The use of analgesia or conduction anesthesia precludes anymore oral intake. At that time and 10 to 45 minutes prior to anesthesia 30 ml of sodium citrate is given orally. If general anesthesia is required, a crash technique of induction and intubation is used. This technique is described in textbooks on obstetric anesthesia. The principal points include use of a antifasciculant (d-tubocurarine) prior to succinylcholine administration, digital pressure on the cricoid cartilage, rapid intubation with a cuffed tube and aspiration of gastric contents prior to extubation.

VAGINAL DELIVERY

Procedures

EPISIOTOMY

Episiotomy is the most common operation in women. Between 1.5 and 2.5 million episiotomies are performed each year in the United States. About 70% of primiparas and 30% of multiparas undergo episiotomies (Thacker and Banta, 1983). Obstetricians in the United States prefer midline incisions because of easier repair, better healing, less postpartum pain, less dyspareunia and reduced blood loss. The mediolateral incision is favored in Europe, because of the lower rate of extension into the rectum. Episiotomy is said to prevent perineal laceration, pelvic relaxation and damage to the fetal head. Episiotomy may be easier to repair than a perineal laceration. Thacker and Banta (1983) have reviewed the support for these contentions.

The efficacy of episiotomy in reducing perineal lacerations is hampered by inconsistent definitions of lacerations. Extension through the anal sphincter (third degree) or extension into the rectum (fourth degree) are more objective evidence of serious complications. Thacker and Banta (1983) reviewed the incidence of third and fourth degree lacerations by type of incision using 33 studies that were conducted between 1860 and 1980. The incidence of third degree extension in midline episiotomy was 3.6%, mediolateral episiotomy 0.6% and no episiotomy 2.0%. Coats and co-workers (1980) performed a prospective randomized trial of midline versus mediolateral episiotomies. Fourth degree extensions occurred in 5.5% of midline episiotomies and 0.4% of mediolateral episiotomies. However, midline episiotomy was associated with less discomfort and better anatomic recovery than mediolateral episiotomy. Beischer (1967) reported that 50% of his patients had

abnormal anatomic recovery from mediolateral episiotomy. Sleep and co-workers (1984) performed a randomized trial of 1000 patients divided into a restrictive versus a liberal policy toward episiotomy. The incidence of episiotomy was 10.2% and 51.4% respectively. The restrictive policy was associated with more perineal trauma but fewer episiotomy extensions. In summary, when compared with no episiotomy, midline episiotomy may increase and mediolateral episiotomy may reduce the risk of fourth degree extension. However, postoperative recovery is significantly more complicated in mediolateral episiotomy. Episiotomy produces a symmetrical laceration and reduces the incidence of other first and second degree lacerations of the perineum.

The prevention of pelvic relaxation is the second reason given for routine episiotomy. This reasoning has been based on older, poorly controlled retrospective reviews of pelvic relaxation (Nugent, 1935; Aldridge and Wootson, 1935). Adequate study of this subject would need to control for parity, age, medical conditions, fetal position, presentation, birth weight, method of delivery (forceps) and anesthesia. Fischer (1979) examined the factors associated with perineal lacerations; third and fourth degree lacerations were strongly related to low parity, young age, use of forceps and episiotomy and weakly related to weight gain over 30 pounds, anemia, long second stage and epidural and pudendal anesthesia. Buekens and co-workers (1985) noted that after control for birth weight and parity there was no association between mediolateral episiotomy and fourth degree laceration in spontaneous occiput anterior vaginal deliveries. Brendel and co-workers (1980) prospectively matched 50 women with and 50 women without episiotomies for many factors and examined them at least one year after their last delivery. There were no differences in pelvic symptomatology between the two groups. Regression analysis suggested that only 9 to 23% of the variance in the development of a cystocele or rectocele could be explained by the presence of an episiotomy or the severity of a laceration. Performance of Kegel's exercises prior to but not after delivery was associated with a reduction of symptoms. In the randomized study by Sleep and co-workers (1984), 19% of patients in the restrictive policy group and 19% of patients in the liberal policy group had involutary loss of urine after three months; 6% had to wear vulvar pads. Another randomized study of primiparas by Harrison and co-workers (1984) also failed to demonstrate differences at four weeks postpartum between the two groups. The reports by Fisher (1979), Brendel and co-workers (1980) and Beukens and co-workers (1985) also suggest that the study of the causes of pelvic relaxation is incomplete and indicate that episiotomy may have little effect on the prevention of pelvic relaxation.

The third reason for routine episiotomy has been to reduce the length of the second stage. Episiotomy may reduce the length of the second stage by 10 to 15 minutes. These minutes may be important if there is fetal distress (Wood et al, 1973). However, if fetal monitoring is normal, the length of the second stage is unrelated to fetal mortality or long-term morbidity (Cohen, 1977). A slower delivery of the head may also allow distension of the perineum without perineal laceration.

In summary, scientific reasoning does not support the routine use of episiotomy. The selective indications for the use of this operation include fetal distress, instrumental deliveries, macrosomic infants and abnormal presentation or position (breech or occiput posterior). Midline episiotomies are associated with less discomfort and improved healing but with a higher incidence of fourth degree extension than are mediolateral episiotomies.

Procedure. An episiotomy is best performed when the vertex distends the introitus 3 to 4 cm. An early incision will significantly increase blood loss (normal 100 to 200 ml). Major bleeding vessels should be clamped and ligated. Local pressure will reduce blood loss from the raw surface. If a midline incision is made, the superficial and deep transverse perineal muscles retract the cut structures laterally with little distortion of the anatomic architecture. Repair of midline episiotomy starts with closure of the vaginal incision with a continuous locked 3-0 polyglycolic suture on an atraumatic needle. The suture is continued to the introitus, brought out under the hymeneal ring and tied in the midline wound. Locking the hymeneal ring in a suture may cause dyspareunia. The base of the wound is closed with a row of interrupted 3-0 polyglycolic sutures. The most anterior suture reattaches the bulbocavernous muscles in the midline. All knots are buried to prevent perineal discomfort. At this point the rectum is examined. Sutures inadvertently passed into the rectum should be removed as they may create a rectovaginal fistula. The skin is closed with a subcuticular layer of 3-0 polyglycolic sutures. After the closure, two fingers are introduced into the introitus. The inability to introduce two fingers increases the risk of dyspareunia. The perineum is then cleansed and ice packs are used for one to two hours after delivery. Anesthetic ointment may be helpful. Sitz baths two to four times a day reduce discomfort.

When there is significant risk of a fourth degree extension (i.e., a short perineal body, large fetus, abnormal position or instrumental delivery), the midline incision should be extended in a mediolateral direction, a hockey stick incision. This type of incision protects the muscle body of the bulbocavernosus yet allows lateral extensions away from the anal sphincter and rectum. If the muscle of the bulbocavernosus or anal sphincter are cut, they retract and change their normal relationships. Repair is accomplished by grasping the ends of the muscles with an Allis clamp and stretching them back to their normal anatomic positions. The muscles are fixed in place by figure of eight sutures of 0 polyglycolic acid through their fascia.

Complications

EXTENSIONS INTO THE RECTUM. Fourth degree extension occurs in two situations. The first is when an episiotomy is performed prior to full distension of the perineum. In this case the rectal mucosa is entered behind the anal sphincter. A rectal examination prior to episiotomy repair will demonstrate the defect. If the defect is small, it may be repaired with two layers of inverting interrupted 4-0 polyglycolic acid sutures. If the defect is large, the laceration is converted to a complete fourth degree extension and repaired (Figure 11–2).

Preparation for the repair of a complete fourth degree laceration requires a clean field and adequate exposure. A surgical assistant is usually helpful. The apex of the rectal mucosa is identified, and its cut edge is inverted into the bowel by interrupted 4-0 polyglycolic acid sutures. This is reinforced by a second row of sutures taken in the surrounding perirectal fascia. The levator ani muscles are sutured with three or four stitches of interrupted 3-0 polyglycolic sutures and are held for tying after the sphincter repair. The ends of the severed sphincter are grasped with Allis clamps and brought to the midline. The fascia and muscle are reapproximated using figure of eight sutures of 2-0 polyglycolic acid. The levator ani sutures are tied, and the perineorrhaphy is completed in the usual fashion. Postpartum care requires no special diet or antibiotics. No mineral oil, rectal suppositories or enemas should be given. Frequent sitz baths are helpful. Stool softeners

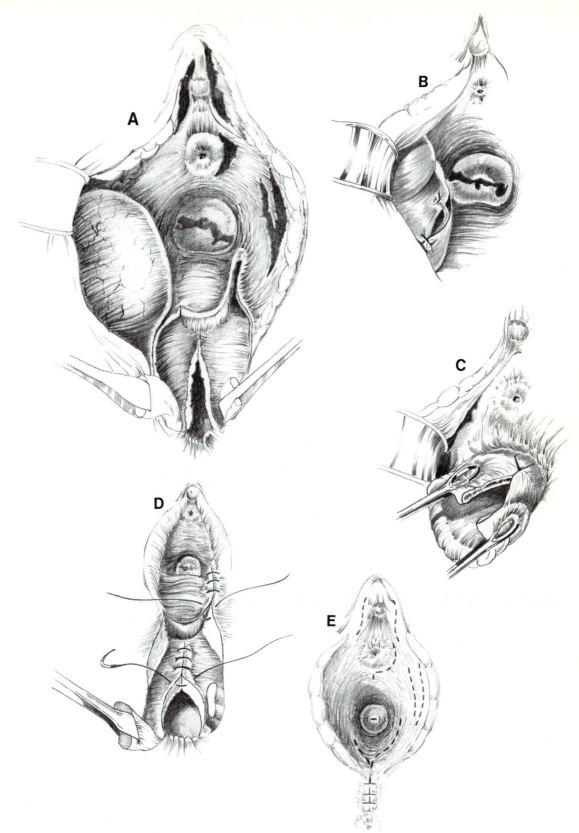

Figure 11–2. Genital tract trauma. A, Possible injuries: Labial lacerations, vaginal hematoma, vaginal lacerations, a fourth degree laceration, and cervical lacerations. B, Repair of a vaginal hematoma. C, Repair of a cervical laceration. D, Repair of a vaginal laceration and reapproximation of the rectal mucosa. E, Finished restoration of the perineal anatomy.

are started on the day of delivery, and milk of magnesia can be given on the second or third postpartum day. The wound should be inspected daily for three days.

The long-term prognosis for fourth degree lacerations is usually good. Between 1 and 5% of patients will have decreased sphincter tone, and one in 300 patients will develop a rectovaginal fistula (O'Leary and O'Leary, 1965; Harris, 1970). The rectovaginal fistula may develop as late as eight months postpartum (Cogan and Harris, 1966). The repair of a rectovaginal fistula is best performed after the defect has epithelialized and is relatively free of infection. The patient should have a workup for intrinsic bowel disease and bowel preparation prior to repair. Repair usually consists of excision of the fistulous tract and subsequent repair as in a fourth degree laceration (see Chapter 4).

INFECTION. Stitch abscesses and minor wound infections occur in between 0.5 and 3% of procedures (Thacker and Banta, 1983). The risk factors for perineal infection after episiotomy are unknown; the incidence of infection has not been compared to that after delivery without prophylactic episiotomy. The incidence is probably related to host factors (medical disease, smoking, steroid usage), delivery factors (blood loss, contamination) and postpartum care. Preventive measures include isolation and irrigation of the operative field, closure of dead space and frequent inspection and cleansing of the perineum during the early postpartum period. Therapy includes debridement, removal of sutures and sitz baths four times a day.

Rarely, maternal death occurs from systemic infection originating in an episiotomy (Shy and Eschenbach, 1979; Golde and Ledger, 1977; Ewing et al, 1979). These cases present on the third or fourth postpartum day with a history of a fourth degree laceration and increasing perineal pain. On physical examination there is perineal induration with asymmetric vulvar edema. Erythema of the lower abdomen, buttocks or thigh implies a fascial extension. Signs of systemic disease may be late; the patient's temperature may be greater than 38 degrees C and her WBC count may be greater than 25,000. The wound must be explored as soon as possible. Necrotic tissue must be excised until bleeding tissue is recognized. This may involve extensive surgery. High doses of antibiotics are given intravenously early in the treatment, for example, penicillin 10 million units Q 6 hours, gentamicin 1.5 mg/Kg and clindamycin 900 mg Q 8 hours. Septic shock can appear very rapidly, and the patient should

have constant surveillance and adequate intravenous access.

PERINEAL PAIN AND DYSPAREUNIA. Pain following episiotomy is universal. In fact, postepisiotomy pain has been used as a model for the evaluation of many pain relief compounds. Between 15 and 30% of patients have continued pain after three days (Thacker and Banta, 1983). One small study (Reading et al, 1982) reported a 15% incidence of perineal pain three months after an episiotomy. The study of perineal pain has been complicated by a lack of control for delivery factors such as anesthesia and mode of delivery. A controlled comparison of episiotomy pain versus laceration pain has not been performed. However, a study of women attending prenatal classes (Kitzinger and Walters, 1981) compared the two populations. Those with episiotomies experienced more perineal pain than those with lacerations (39% vs. 15%). Dyspareunia for longer than three months was also more common in episiotomy patients (19% vs. 11%).

The management of perineal pain and dyspareunia after three weeks requires close examination of the perineum. Pain may be related to persistent local skin infection or retained suture material. These can be treated with local therapy. Vaginal stenosis or constriction can be treated with dilatation. Lidocaine jelly may decrease the discomfort of dilatation. Perineotomy may be necessary if dilatation is unsuccessful. A vertical incision and transverse closure under local anesthesia may be all that is needed.

CORD CLAMPING

After delivery of the fetus there is a transfusion of placental blood to the neonate. The amount of blood transfused is related to the timing of cord clamping, the height of the neonate as compared with that of the placenta, the onset of respiration and intervening uterine contractions. Placental blood is a source of iron and can be useful in preventing anemia between three and six months of age. On the other hand, placental transfusion has theoretical risks such as fluid overload, increase in lung fluid and hyperbilirubinemia.

Philip (1973) randomly assigned neonates to early clamping (less than 15 seconds) and late clamping (after the onset of regular respirations). The mean time for cord clamping in the delayed group was 94 seconds. He found significantly lower residual placental blood volume per 100 grams placental tissue in the delayed clamping group. The volume of transfusion was about 10.4 ml per 100 grams of placental tissue. Newton and Moody (1961) have shown that the volume of maternal blood in the placenta (9 to 11 ml/100 gram placental tissue) does not change with delayed clamping. Philip (1973) also measured a number of biochemical and physiologic parameters in the first five days of life. There were no significant differences in bilirubin levels, hemoglobin, urine output or oral intake, but there was a 9% increase in hematocrit and a decreased reticulocyte count as a result of delayed clamping. The effect of delayed clamping on the incidence of anemia in the first year of life has not been studied.

MANUAL REMOVAL OF THE PLACENTA

After delivery of the baby, the uterus often undergoes a brief refractory period prior to the resumption of contractions. Upon contraction and separation of the placenta, there will be a lengthening of the cord, a rounding-up of the uterus, a sudden gush of blood and a protrusion of the placenta through the cervix. The third stage is usually completed within one-half hour. A third stage longer than 30 to 40 minutes increases the risks for hemorrhage, placenta accreta and inversion. These complications are discussed in subsequent sections.

After separation of the placenta, the delivery of the placenta is effected by placing the extended fingers of one hand just above the symphysis and then moving the hand toward the fundus while the umbilical cord is supported with gentle traction (Brandt-Andrews maneuver). Direct squeezing of the fundus with strong counter-traction on the umbilical cord (Crede maneuver) is not recommended because of the risk of uterine inversion and umbilical cord laceration. Delivery of the membranes should be performed with gentle twisting traction using ringed forceps. After delivery of the placenta and membranes, the uterus is encouraged to contract by breast feeding, gentle massage or the use of oxytocin. The placenta should be examined for size, completeness, number of fetal vessels, meconium staining and the presence of parenchymal abnormalities, i.e., infarction, thrombosis or abruption. With any deviation from a normal pregnancy or delivery the placenta should be examined by a pathologist.

If the placenta has not separated after 30 minutes, manual removal should be considered. The procedure should be a separate operation from the vaginal delivery. The prerequisites are a large bore intravenous catheter with an infus-

ing balanced salt solution, a recent complete blood count, two units of blood typed and cross-matched and adequate anesthesia (halothane). An individual qualified to resuscitate the mother should be involved in addition to the obstetrician. The procedure is performed in a clean field after perineal cleansing, redraping, regloving and regowning. The bladder should be emptied.

The procedure is performed in the following fashion. The operator holds the umbilical cord with the non-dominant hand and places the dominant hand into the uterine cavity. The plane between the placenta and the uterine wall is found and the separation is completed by a cupping maneuver underneath the placenta (Fig. 11–3). The placenta is then grasped and gently removed. After removal the uterus is examined for anatomic abnormalities and retained fragments of placenta or membranes. Adherent fragments may be removed by a large blunt curette. However, extensive sharp curettage in this situation may remove excess amounts of decidua and lead to intrauterine synechiae and Asherman's syndrome.

When the placental tissue remains tightly adherent to the uterine wall, a placenta accreta must be suspected. Excessive attempts at removal may further damage the uterus. In the face of continued hemorrhage, the obstetrician has no option but operation, usually involving hysterectomy. If oxytocic medications (oxytocin, Methergine or prostaglandin) are successful in preventing hemorrhage, a small amount of adherent placental tissue may be treated conservatively in order to preserve fertility. Conservative management includes prophylactic antibiotics, Methergine 0.2 mg PO Q 6 hours for eight doses, close postpartum follow-up and maintenance of the hematocrit at over 30%. The risks of conservative management are delayed postpartum hemorrhage and endometritis.

Some authors (Jones et al, 1966) previously advocated routine exploration of the uterus. In 5 to 10% of procedures, uterine abnormalities or retained products of conception were found. Routine uterine exploration was also credited with a reduction in postpartum bleeding without an increase in infectious morbidity. The resurgence of "natural" childbirth limits the ability to perform routine uterine exploration. Careful inspection of the placenta, vagina and cervix can provide adequate reassurance when no regional or general anesthetic has been used. Manual exploration when epidural anesthesia has been used probably has little risk. Antibiot-

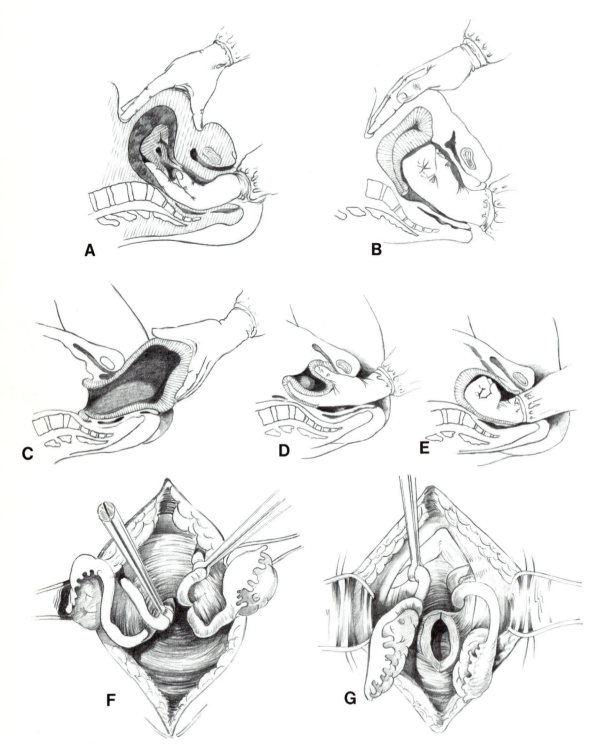

Figure 11–3. Complications of the third stage of labor. A, *Manual extraction of the placenta.* B, *Manual compression of the uterus.* C, *Inverted uterus: Fundus is cupped in hand.* D, *Inverted uterus: Pressure by hand effects traction by the round ligaments on inverted uterus.* E, *Inverted uterus: A clenched hand maintains normal anatomy until the uterus contracts.* F, *Huntington's operation.* G, *Haultain's operation.*

ics are used in patients in whom chorioannionitis, prolonged rupture of membranes, abnormal labor, instrumental delivery or retained products of conception have complicated the delivery.

PREVENTION OF POSTPARTUM HEMORRHAGE

The first 12 to 24 hours after delivery are considered by some obstetricians to be the fourth stage of labor, because of the serious complications that may occur during this period. The two most common are pre-eclampsia and early postpartum hemorrhage. Twenty to 40% of cases of eclampsia occur postpartum. Women at greatest risk are primigravidas, women with multiple births or gestational trophoblastic disease or women with medical diseases such as chronic hypertension, renal disease, diabetes or collagen disease. In these patients early postpartum discharge (less than 24 hours) should not be advised, and frequent blood pressure checks should be performed.

Although postpartum hemorrhage is defined as bleeding greater than 500 ml in the first 12 hours after delivery, 500 ml is actually the mean blood loss following an uncomplicated vaginal delivery (Newton et al, 1961; Pritchard et al, 1962). The measured blood loss is usually twice the estimated amount (Pritchard et al, 1962). Pregnancy increases blood volume by 1500 to 2000 ml, and thus the loss of 1000 to 1500 ml is well tolerated by the healthy gravida. The sources of postpartum hemorrhage are the episiotomy, lacerations, uterine atony, retained products of conception, uterine inversion and coagulopathy.

The vagina and cervix are systematically examined for lacerations or extensions after the delivery of the placenta. First, the episiotomy is examined for fourth degree extension, and the superior apex of any laceration is evaluated. Two or three extended fingers are used to depress the perineum and the lateral sulci are wiped dry with a sponge forceps. Sulcus tears or vaginal hematomas are most common over the ischial spines. The cervix is examined circumferentially by the use of sponge forceps. Lacerations are most often observed at 3 and 9 o'clock. The repair of lacerations is described in the discussion of complications of vaginal delivery.

Contraction of the uterus is the most important mechanism for the control of postpartum bleeding, and uterine atony is the most common cause of postpartum hemorrhage. Uterine atony is most likely to occur after prolonged labor,

distended uterus (multiple gestation, infant greater than 9 lbs), prolonged use of oxytocin, tocolytic medication (general anesthesia, $MgSO_4$) and abruptio placentae (Couvelaire uterus). Speedy contraction of the uterus is essential to prevent hemorrhage. Non-pharmacologic methods are gentle massage of the uterus and breastfeeding. The most common drugs are oxytocin (20 to 30 units I.V. in 1000 ml) and ergot derivatives such as Methergine (methylergonovine maleate) 0.2 mg I.V. or I.M. Sorbe (1978) compared the use of oxytocin and Methergine at the delivery of the anterior shoulder with controls in whom the drugs were given after the placenta was delivered. He found no differences in the length of the third stage but a decrease in blood loss in the experimental groups. Methergine was associated with a higher rate of trapped placenta. Ergot derivatives also have the additional risk of causing acute hypertensive crisis and the inhibition of lactation by disruption of prolactin secretion and milk ejection. If hemorrhage is severe, bimanual compression of the uterus may be necessary until the uterus contracts. A clenched fist is placed in the anterior fornix, and the body of the uterus is compressed against it by a hand placed behind the uterus through the abdominal wall (see Fig. 11–3).

Hemorrhage resulting from uterine rupture, retained products of conception, uterine inversion or coagulopathy is usually severe (greater than 1200 ml) with signs of hemodynamic compromise. The management of severe postpartum hemorrhage is described in the discussion of the complications of cesarean section.

BREECH DELIVERY

Few issues have generated as much controversy as the method of delivery in breech presentation. Crude perinatal statistics separated by presentation show a greater incidence of neonatal mortality, morbidity and long-term defects with breech delivery (Alexopoulos, 1973). However, breech presentation is more often associated with concurrent perinatal risks, i.e., prematurity, congenital abnormality, placental abnormality, multiple gestation, intrauterine growth retardation or uterine anomalies. More recent studies with better control for these factors suggest that delivery method has less effect on long-term development than previously thought (Faber-Nijholt et al, 1983; Rosen et al, 1985). Trauma and asphyxia have been related to the increase in the morbidity of vaginal breech delivery. Abnormalities of birth

Table 11–3. Selective Term Breech Management—Vaginal Versus Cesarean Delivery*

	Vaginal	Cesarean
Number of Patients	95	218
Maternal Outcome		
Infection	5	65
Transfusion	1	20
Hospital days	2.3	5.8
Infant Outcome		
Birth trauma (%)	4 (4.4)	1 (0.5)
Neonatal asphyxia (%)	9 (8.4)	6 (2.7)
Neonatal death	1	0

*Data from Collea JV, Chein C, Quilligan EJ. *Am. J. Obstet. Gynecol.* 137:235, 1980; Gimovsky ML, Wallace RC et al. *Am. J. Obstet. Gynecol.* 146:34, 1983.

weight (Rovinsky et al, 1973; Kauppila, 1975), presentation other than frank breech (Hall et al, 1965), pelvic inadequacy (Beischer, 1967; Todd and Steer, 1963; Kauppila, 1975) and hyperextension of the fetal head (Caterini et al, 1975) are associated with increased morbidity. Table 11–3 presents the cumulative statistics for two randomized, controlled studies evaluating method of delivery in breech presentation. The risk of short-term maternal morbidity is much higher in cesarean birth, yet the incidence of neonatal morbidity is higher in vaginal delivery. Table 11–4 presents the incidence of trauma and asphyxia in two older studies of unselected term vaginal breech deliveries consisting of 3,450 births (Rovinsky et al, 1973; Kauppilla, 1975). These statistics are compared to selected patients in Table 11–4 and reveal little difference.

Procedure. Currently, 60 to 80% of patients with breech presentation will have a cesarean birth. Many institutions perform cesarean sections for all breech presentations. In institutions in which a trial of labor is permitted, informed consent and a workup should be documented. A workup includes an ultrasonographic examination for congenital abnormalities and estimated fetal weight. Pelvimetry should be performed to define pelvic dimensions and the attitude of the fetal head. The criteria for trial of labor in breech presentation are listed in Table 11–5.

Table 11–4. Excess Perinatal Morbidity and Mortality in Term Vaginal Breech Deliveries

Parameter	Selected	Unselected
Number	95	3450
Trauma (deaths)	4.4% (1)	4% (15)
Asphyxia (deaths)	8.4% (0)	11% (28)

Table 11–5. Criteria for Trial of Labor in Breech Presentation

1. Adequate pelvic diameters	
Inlet diameters	
Transverse	>12 cm
Anterior/Posterior	>11 cm
Bispinous diameter	>10 cm
2. Estimated fetal weight 2000 to 3500 grams	
3. Biparietal diameter	<9.5 cm
4. Chest minus head circumference	<1.0 cm
5. Frank breech presentation	
6. Normal flexion of fetal head	
7. Normal fetal monitoring	
8. Normal progress in labor	

The four terms used for vaginal breech delivery are spontaneous breech delivery, assisted breech delivery, partial breech extraction and total breech extraction. The definition of each term involves an increasing amount of medical intervention. Assisted breech delivery involves only the assisted delivery of the fetal head. A partial breech extraction involves a spontaneous delivery to the umbilicus with subsequent assisted delivery of the shoulders and head. The complete removal of the fetus is total breech extraction.

Vaginal breech delivery requires a complete evaluation for pelvic adequacy and deflexion of the fetal head. Progress in labor should be normal, and electronic fetal monitoring should indicate fetal well being. The delivery is performed in a fully equipped delivery room. The bladder is emptied and the perineum cleansed. Breech delivery requires additional personnel, i.e. an additional obstetric attendant, a pediatrician and anesthesia standby.

Total breech extraction is associated with an increase in perinatal morbidity and mortality and has limited use in modern obstetrics. Total breech extraction may be considered in patients in whom delay for cesarean birth would significantly compromise the fetus, i.e., in cases of fetal distress or prolapsed cord. When total breech extraction is needed usually a leg is presenting, but, if not, one leg should be extracted by inward flexion at the knee through intrauterine manipulation. Once a leg is delivered, traction is applied with thumbs on the back of the leg. Traction should be directed downward toward the floor at a 45 degree angle until the anterior hip has passed the symphysis. At that point the traction is applied horizontally and eventually upward to facilitate delivery of the posterior hip. Traction should be coordinated with uterine contractions and maternal effort. Gentle pressure on the fetal head should be applied abdominally to maintain flexion of

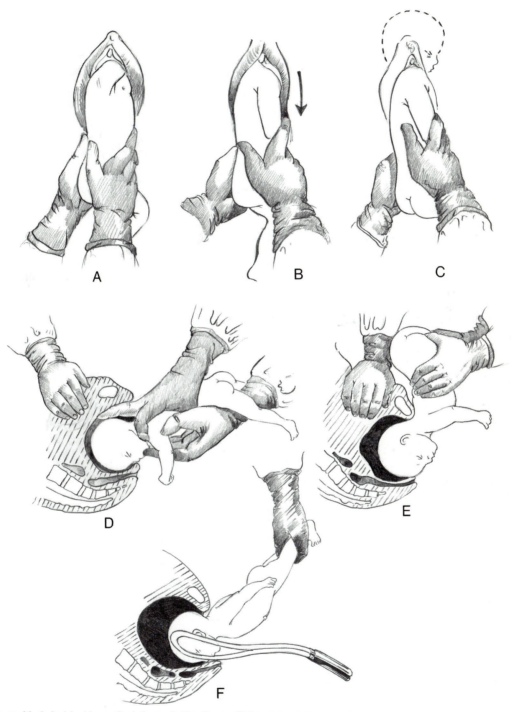

Figure 11–4. Assisted breech delivery. A, Traction until the scapulae and axilla are seen. B, Anterior arm is flexed at the elbow and is swept down across the fetal chest. C, The arm is then delivered. The same process is performed on the posterior arm. D, Mauriceau technique: Traction is supplied by the anterior hand. The fetal head is flexed by abdominal pressure and the index or middle finger of the supporting hand. The extended middle finger of the anterior hand also maintains flexion. E, Bracht's maneuver: Anterior abdominal pressure flexes the fetal head. Extension of the fetus over the maternal abdomen facilitates expulsion of the fetal head. F, Piper forceps are applied to an after-coming fetal head.

the fetal head. Once the pelvis has been delivered, two hands grasp the fetal pelvis with the two thumbs meeting over the sacrum. At this point, traction is changed to a downward direction. Normal rotation of the body is allowed. If the second leg fails to follow delivery of the first leg, no attempt is made to extract it; it will naturally follow the delivery of the trunk. Attempts at extraction may result in fracture.

In a more normal situation, the goal of vaginal breech delivery is to allow spontaneous delivery while assuring a short interval between the delivery of the umbilicus and delivery of the head. When this interval is four minutes or less the Apgar score is usually greater than 7 (Collea et al, 1980). In the course of a normally progressing breech delivery, patience is essential. Ill-advised manipulation or traction will cause deflexion of the head or nuchal arms. When the fetus has delivered spontaneously to the umbilicus, the delivery will be completed to the shoulders within two or three contractions. Gravity is used to facilitate the delivery. The fetus is not supported, although a tight umbilical cord may be loosened. Provided the cord is not occluded, spontaneous descent may be awaited for two or three contractions. If there is no progress or the cord is occluded, traction should be applied to effect a partial breech extraction. Traction is applied with two thumbs over the sacrum. Initially, the traction is downward, then upward to facilitate the delivery of the posterior shoulder. The delivery of the arms is performed in the sacral hollow. The right arm should be extracted by the operator's right hand, the left arm by the operator's left hand. The arms are flexed at the elbow and brought out in front of the fetus and never behind as this may cause fracture or brachial plexus injury.

Assisted delivery of the head is required in most cases of breech delivery and is performed without delay. Thus, most breech deliveries are by definition assisted breech deliveries. Three methods are equally effective and successful in experienced hands: Mauriceau's technique, Bracht's maneuver, and the Piper forceps technique (Fig. 11–4). In Mauriceau's technique, the body of the fetus is rested upon one arm of the operator. The index finger of the supporting hand is placed in the fetal mouth. This provides flexion, not traction, of the fetal head. Traction is supplied only by the upper hand with the first and third fingers placed over the shoulders of the fetus and the middle finger flexing the head. Traction is initially downward. Once the occiput clears the symphysis, the direction of traction gradually shifts upward.

Bracht's maneuver requires an empty bladder and two attendants, one to hold the fetus and one to exercise pressure over the lower abdomen upon the fetal head. The assistant simply supports the body of the fetus in an upward direction. The obstetrician places two fists above the symphysis to apply firm and continuous pressure on the fetal head.

Milner (1975) described the benefits of use of forceps to facilitate the delivery of the aftercoming head. This study noted a significant reduction in neonatal mortality with the use of forceps. Piper forceps are recommended because of their wide shank, fenestration, cephalic curve and reverse handle angle. In this case, the fetal body and arms are supported in the horizontal plane by the assistant. The operator kneels on the floor to place the left hand blade upward and diagonally across the introitus along the occipitomental line. The right hand blade is inserted in a similar fashion. A large episiotomy, an empty bladder and perineal relaxation are essential to prevent deflexion of the fetal head during introduction of the blades. Before locking the blades, the operator must be certain that the blades have been inserted to a depth sufficient for good traction on the fetal head. Traction is made in a downward continuous curve. The shanks of the forceps should not rise above the horizontal.

Complications.

NUCHAL ARMS. Occasionally one or both arms are caught behind the fetal head, thus blocking progress. Often nuchal arms result from intervention in a spontaneous delivery. Management of a nuchal arm is performed as follows (Fig. 11–5). The fetus usually presents with its shoulders in a transverse or oblique plane. The fetal body is then rotated so that the friction of the vaginal wall will disengage the nuchal arm. For example, when the right arm is behind the fetal neck counterclockwise rotation is necessary. Once the nuchal arm is freed, it is delivered prior to disengagement of the other nuchal arm. The other nuchal arm is disengaged by rotation of the body in the opposite direction.

PERSISTENT SACRUM POSTERIOR POSITION. The Prague maneuver is useful when the fetal head follows the delivery of the body in a persistent occiput posterior position. As the chin impacts on the symphysis, the fetal head extends and delivery is difficult. Prevention of this complication should be initiated prior to full delivery of the trunk. A fist may be used to displace the fetal chin to one side. A hand in the vagina may also help rotate the fetal head toward the desired position. If this technique fails, a reverse Prague maneuver may be tried

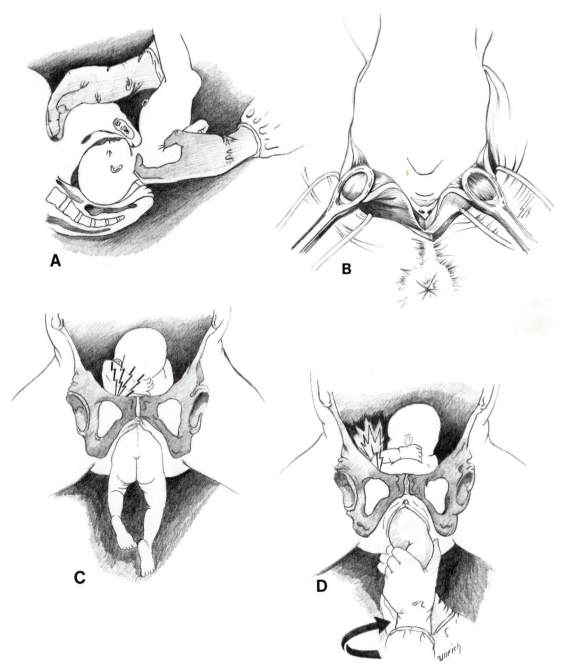

Figure 11–5. Management of complications of breech delivery. A, Reverse Prague maneuver in a persistent occiput posterior. B, Dührssen's incision at 6 o'clock in the management of cervical entrapment of fetal head. C, Nuchal arm. D, Rotation of the fetus relieves obstruction.

(Fig. 11–5). The fetus is lifted over the maternal lower abdomen, with traction applied by way of a vaginal hand over the fetal shoulders and back. Traction is directed downward, outward and then upward as the occiput presents. A large episiotomy facilitates this technique.

CERVICAL ENTRAPMENT OF THE FETAL HEAD. This catastrophic event happens most often when the breech delivers through an incompletely dilated cervix and when the diameter of the vertex exceeds that of the breech. Often these are premature infants whose risks are already great because of their prematurity. The premature fetus does not tolerate the trauma and asphyxia of this complication as well as a more mature fetus. Vaginal examination will readily identify this problem, and traction should not be applied to force the vertex through. Incisions on the cervix (Dührssen's incisions) are needed (Fig. 11–5). The operation is performed under adequate anesthesia when the cervix is greater than 6 to 7 cm dilated and nearly 100% effaced. Ring forceps are used to grasp the cervix. The first incision is made at 6 o'clock and is carried to the cervical-vaginal junction. Extension of the incision will enter the posterior wall of the uterus away from the uterine arteries, which are located at 3 and 9 o'clock. An anterior incision should not be used because of the risk of bladder injury. If delivery does not occur, further incisions are made at 2 and 10 o'clock. The incisions are repaired in one layer of 00 polyglycolic acid sutures. Extension beyond the cervical-vaginal junction suggests uterine rupture and potential hemorrhage. This may require laparotomy for full evaluation.

BIRTH TRAUMA. Birth trauma can occur in a completely spontaneous and normal birth. However, increasing manipulation is associated with increased risk of trauma. This is especially true of breech delivery. Total breech extraction has a prohibitively high rate of injury. Kauppila (1975) recorded the types of severe injury in 1,730 term vaginal breech births. He found intracerebral injury in 13, brachial plexus damage in 19, clavicular fracture in 13, and other injuries in 6. Death from trauma results from vertebral artery occlusion (Yates, 1959), posterior fossa hemorrhage (Wigglesworth and Husemeyer, 1977) or crush injury or muscle trauma (Ralis, 1975). Traumatic injury to the extremities is associated with an unusual amount of pressure on the long bone rather than the joint. Trauma to the neck occurs with excessive lateral traction or excessive traction on the body with a deflexed fetal head. The

Bracht maneuver and Piper forceps delivery are directed to avoid excessive body traction.

ACUTE ASPHYXIA. Kubli (1977) noted a 10% incidence of cord pH below 7.10 in breech labors, and low Apgar scores occur in about 8% of selected term infants of breech deliveries (Collea et al, 1980; Gimovsky et al, 1983). Umbilicus to head delivery times greater than 4 minutes are associated with a decrease in Apgar score (Collea et al, 1980). This may correspond to partial occlusion of the umbilical cord. However, healthy infants may tolerate a period of total occlusion up to 10 to 13 minutes (Myers, 1972). Long-term damage from hypoxia probably results from chronic uteroplacental insufficiency with a superimposed insult during delivery. For this reason, it is essential that electronic fetal monitoring be used to identify the fetus who might not be able to tolerate the additional hypoxic stress of a vaginal breech delivery. A physician able to resuscitate a depressed newborn should attend the neonate.

CIRCUMCISION

Circumcision is one of the most common operations performed on the reproductive organs in humans in the United States. In most cases, circumcision is performed by the obstetrician in the early neonatal period. Although it is a relatively easy procedure, the consequences of complications of circumcision may be medically and medicolegally severe. All too often circumcision is performed in a hurried fashion by the least experienced physician without the informed consent of the parents.

The natural history of the prepuce involves a rapid increase in retractability followed by a more gradual increase in complete separation of the preputial epithelium from the glans. Only 4% of prepuces are retractable at birth. The prepuce is retractable in 90 and 99% of boys by 3 and 17 years of age respectively. Complete separation of epithelium has occurred in 37 and 99% of boys by 5 and 17 years respectively. Smegma, on the other hand, is present in only 1% of uncircumcised 6-year-olds and in about 8% of uncircumcised 16-year-olds.

There are definite indications for circumcision, but none of these occur in the neonate. They include phimosis resulting in urinary retention, paraphimosis and recurrent inflammation of the glands (balanitis). Posthitis (inflammation of the prepuce) is a relative indication.

Newborn circumcisions are performed for religious purposes or for prophylaxis. Prophylactic reasons include prevention of penile cancer, prevention of cervical cancer and aid in preventing poor hygiene or social rejection. The prepuce is the common site for the development of carcinoma. Removal of the prepuce (foreskin) reduces the risk. However, carcinoma of the penis is very rare, and improved hygiene of the penis may accomplish the same result. Although early reports suggested an increase in cervical cancer among women with uncircumcised partners, subsequent study has not verified these findings. Genetic predisposition and sexual and hygienic behavior have a much greater effect. Approximately 1 to 2% of uncircumcised postnatal males will undergo circumcision during their life. However, this incidence is strongly related to lower socioeconomic class, poor hygiene, desert climate and medical disease such as diabetes. Herzog and Alvarez (1986) performed a retrospective controlled review of minor complications in circumcised and uncircumcised inner city children. Total complications were 14.3% in the uncircumcised group and 5.9% in the circumcised group (p less than .05). The difference in incidence of balanitis and phimosis did not reach statistical significance. Improved hygienic behavior in these individuals might reduce the incidence of subsequent infection and circumcision. Circumcision as a prophylaxis against peer ridicule is a vain hope. Vulnerable children are at risk for any difference. If the foreskin is not a focus of ridicule, some other difference will be used.

There are also strict contraindications to neonatal circumcision. First is the presence of any urogenital abnormality, i.e., hypospadias. In these cases the foreskin may be needed in the plastic repair of the defect. Second is a medical disease that increases the risk of surgery. Examples are prematurity and bleeding diathesis. A third contraindication is the possibility of neurologic disease in which urinary incontinence is a risk, i.e., myelomeningocele. An external catheter fits better with the prepuce present.

The American Academy of Pediatricians has reviewed the issue of circumcision and noted the lack of medical support for prophylactic neonatal circumcision (Thompson et al, 1975).

Procedure. Circumcision must be performed with the same care as any other operation. Knowledge and experience with the procedure are important. Aseptic techniques must be observed, and the operation should be done after a full pediatric evaluation. Neonatal circumcision is usually performed without anesthesia under the mistaken belief that the neonate has different sensations than the adult. However, Marshall and co-workers (1979) demonstrated

changes in sleep behavior patterns for at least 24 hours after circumcision. A dorsal nerve block of the penis is safe and effective local anesthesia (Kirya and Worthmann, 1978). The circumcision may be done free hand, but the procedure is facilitated by use of the Gomco clamp or the Plastibell.

Several general principles are valid in the prevention of surgical complications of circumcision.

1. The preputial epithelium must be completely separated from the glans prior to clamping or excision.

2. Clamping must be done under direct vision especially prior to incising a dorsal slit.

3. The amount of prepuce to be removed must be exact. Some surgeons advise marking the line of excision on the foreskin around the coronal sulcus.

4. The area of the prepuce near the frenulum must be avoided. This area is especially vulnerable to bleeding and subsequent scarring, which leads to painful erection and dyspareunia.

5. Clamps should be left in place a full five minutes prior to removal. Early removal often leads to bleeding.

6. Adequate removal of the preputial epithelium is essential. Failure to do so can result in a concealed penis.

7. Petrolatum gauze is applied lightly to the cut edge to protect from diaper friction.

Complications

BLEEDING. Excess bleeding occurs in 1 to 5% of circumcisions and is usually mild and not life-threatening (Table 11–6). The cut edge near the frenulum is the most common site. Unfortunately, over-zealous clamping and suture may jeopardize the penile urethra in this area, and subsequent scarring may tether the glans during erection. Initial therapy is firm digital pressure for five minutes. Occasionally Avitene or topical epinephrine in low concentration (1:100,000) may be helpful. Higher doses of epinephrine should not be used; vasoconstriction and slough of the penis have been reported. If these conservative methods are not successful, the bleeding points are individually clamped and tied with 4-0 chromic catgut. Suture ligature is used with caution. Continued bleeding should alert the operator to a bleeding diathesis.

INFECTION. Wound infection occurs in 5 to 10% of neonates (Table 11–6). Treatment is regular cleansing with an antiseptic solution. More serious infections (osteomyelitis of the pubis, septicemia, fasciitis, toxic shock syndrome) have been reported but fortunately are rare.

Meatitis and subsequent meatal stenosis are

Table 11–6. Complications of Circumcision*

	Incidence
Death	2 per million
Bleeding	0.1–10%
Infection	5–15%
Repeat circumcision	5–10%
Meatitis	8–31%
Other trauma	1%

*From Kaplan GW: Circumcision—an overview. *Curr. Probl. Pediatr.* 7:1, 1977. Reprinted with permission.

much more common in circumcised males. The incidence is 8 to 31% (Kaplan, 1977). Meatitis usually occurs in the first year of life, while the child is in diapers. The constant friction and inoculation from the diaper leads to infection of the sensitive meatal mucosa. Meatal stenosis is a long-term complication of meatitis. Berry and Cross (1956) defined adult meatal stenosis as a urethral meatus less than 20 French in circumference. Sixty percent of circumcised males and 25% of uncircumcised males had meatal stenosis.

OTHER TRAUMA. Many other case reports catalog the wide variety of trauma that complicates circumcisions. Often too little foreskin is removed and a repeat circumcision is necessary. When too much skin is removed plastic repair is much more difficult. A scrotal flap is often needed. Concealed penis, phimosis, urethral injury and removal of the glans have been reported. Fortunately these complications are rare and can be avoided by careful surgical technique. If they occur, a pediatric urologist should be consulted.

MOTHER-INFANT INTERACTION

Adverse environmental experiences during the birthing process can lengthen labor, increase perinatal mortality and disrupt mother-infant bonding. Scientific study of these complications has been performed by veterinarians and social scientists for at least 25 years (Newton et al, 1966; Newton and Newton, 1962). In the early 1970's Kennel and Klaus contributed greatly to the understanding of mother-infant bonding (Klaus and Kennell, 1976). Their studies and a review of the literature support the concept of a sensitive period immediately after birth. Many variables impact on this critical period (Siegel, 1982) but hospital and obstetric intervention may be the strongest. For example, the hospital intervention of separating the mother from the neonate in the first 12 hours has a significant negative impact on affectionate

behavior and breastfeeding success (Siegel, 1982). Obstetric variables such as fear, anger, exhaustion, incisional pain and medications may adversely impact on the mother during the sensitive period. The neonate may also be adversely affected by the stress of labor or by medications given to the mother during labor.

The study of the psychologic complications of obstetric intervention is in its infancy, and there are many obstacles to the scientific evaluation of this subject. First, psychologic measurement is very observer-dependent. Adequate controls with blinding of the observer and reliability testing are essential. Second, the identification of variables and the determination of their relative importance are yet to be done. For example, is early separation more important than the neonatal effects of maternal analgesia during labor? The use of multiple regression analysis will help define the variables and their relative strengths (Siegel, 1982). Third, how does early bonding relate to future social development? On one hand, poor bonding reduces breastfeeding success (Sosa et al, 1976; De Chateau and Wiberg, 1977). On the other hand, despite major disruption in maternal-infant bonding (intensive care admission) most human neonates develop normal social behavior. What factors counteract the negative influences of the early neonatal period?

Very few intervention studies have been performed. One such study was reported by Sosa and co-workers (1980). In healthy Guatemalan primigravidas, the presence or absence of a lay support person was randomized into two groups. The group with a supportive labor companion had fewer perinatal problems, shorter labors and better mother-infant bonding. Another example was reported by Nelson and co-workers (1980). Women were randomly assigned to either a Leboyer or a conventional delivery. No differences in maternal or neonatal morbidity or in neonatal behavior were noted in short- or long-term follow-ups.

Complications

SHOULDER DYSTOCIA

Shoulder dystocia is one of the obstetrician's greatest fears. It is often a surprise that the shoulders do not deliver soon after the head. The fetal chin retracts against the perineum (turtle sign) and traction on the head fails to deliver either shoulder. Often the delay is related to delay in the external rotation of the shoulders to an oblique plane. A hand inserted into the vagina may facilitate this rotation and effect delivery of the shoulders. However, in a true dystocia, the anterior shoulder is tightly impacted against the symphysis, and, more importantly, the posterior shoulder is impacted on the sacral promontory. In such a situation, the fetus becomes hypoxic with a fall in umbilical artery pH of 0.04 units per minute (Harris, 1984b). Anxiety increases the risk of trauma due to excess traction and manipulation. Bowes (1984) reviewed the perinatal morbidity of shoulder dystocia in 244 cases. He noted 20 (8.2%) fetal deaths, 31 (12.7%) brachial plexus injuries, and 16 (6.6%) fractured clavicles or humeri.

Fortunately shoulder dystocia is an uncommon event. The incidence is about one in 200 deliveries (Harris, 1984b). The frequency is increased with nulliparity, delayed second stage (more than 60 minutes), midpelvic deliveries and fetal macrosomia. When the fetus weighs more than 4000 grams, the incidence is 1.7%. If the fetal weight is more than 4500 grams, the incidence is 10% (Harris, 1984b). The incidence of shoulder dystocia after a midforceps delivery of the head is about 4% (Hughey et al, 1978). The combination of fetal macrosomia (greater than 4500 grams) and a second stage longer than one hour is especially hazardous; the incidence of shoulder dystocia was found by Sack (1969) to be 35%, with a 30% risk of fetal mortality.

The antenatal detection of a fetus at risk for shoulder dystocia allows the option of primary elective cesarean section. The evaluation is twofold: to select gestations at risk for a fetus weighing greater than 4000 grams and then to screen those patients with ultrasound. Patients at greatest risk for macrosomic neonates are those with previous neonate greater than 4000 grams, previous shoulder dystocia and a fundal height greater than 40 cm at term with normal

Table 11–7. Incidence of Birthweight > 4000 grams*

Maternal Variable	Incidence of Macrosomia (%)
Multipara 35 years or more	14.5
Pregnancy weight >70 Kg	19.8–22.6
Maternal height 170 cm or over	14.9
Ponderal index 0.016 or over	14.5–18.7
Weight gain >20 Kg	19.3
Post-dates 41 + weeks	16.0
Diabetes	22.0

*From Boyd ME, Asher RH et al: Fetal macrosomia: prediction risks and proposed management. *Obstet. Gynecol.* 61:715, 1983. Reprinted with permission.

amniotic fluid and an engaged head. Boyd and co-workers (1983) reviewed other maternal variables associated with fetal macrosomia (Table 11–7). In a high risk maternal population, ultrasound measurement of anthropometric variables identifies the actual at risk fetus. Modanlou and co-workers (1982) demonstrated that neonates experiencing shoulder dystocia had significantly greater shoulder-to-head and chest-to-head proportions than other macrosomic neonates delivered without this complication. Measurements that indicate high risk are an estimated fetal weight greater than 4000 grams, a chest-to-head circumference difference over 1.4 cm or a shoulder-to-head circumference difference over 4.8 cm. Primary cesarean section may be a reasonable option in patients whose fetuses have these characteristics.

The management of shoulder dystocia requires speedy but controlled maneuvers (Fig. 11–6). The steps are as follows:

1. A wide episiotomy is performed.

2. The McRoberts maneuver, consisting of sharp flexion of the maternal thighs onto her chest, is attempted. The superior rotation of the symphysis may free the impacted shoulder.

3. With the mother's legs hyperflexed, an assistant should apply firm suprapubic pressure on the anterior shoulder so as to disengage it.

4. If the previous methods have failed, Woods' maneuver should be attempted. The operator's hand is introduced into the vagina and pressure is applied to the antecubital fossa of the posterior arm. As the elbow flexes, the forearm and hand are drawn out of the vagina in the midline across the fetal chest. If delivery does not occur, the hand is introduced over the posterior chest and the posterior arm is rotated over the chest. This direction allows the shoulders to collapse forward onto the fetal chest and reduce the shoulder diameter. The posterior axilla may be rotated to rest under the symphysis.

5. Clavicular fracture is a last resort in shoulder dystocia. The fracture is produced by applying outward pressure on the midportion of the clavicle with a finger. The fracture allows collapse of the shoulder and a decrease in the shoulder diameter. Pneumothorax and subclavian vessel injury are common complications.

6. A pediatrician should be available for immediate resuscitation of the neonate.

MECONIUM

Meconium is first evident in the distal ileum by 16 weeks' gestation. Meconium is composed

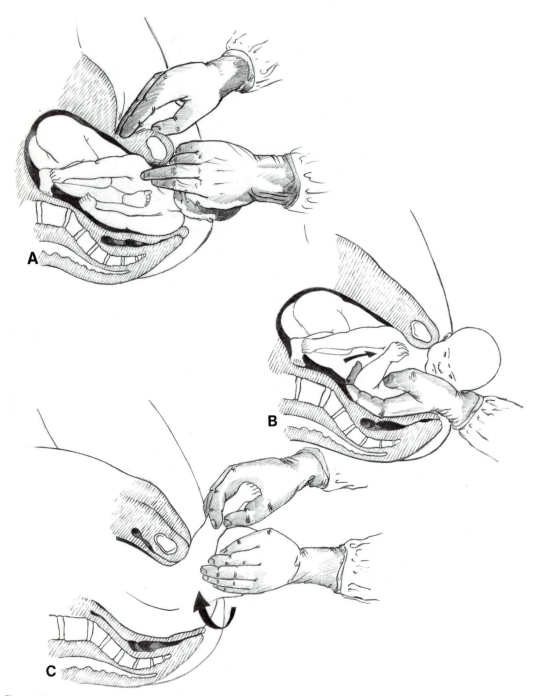

Figure 11–6. Management of shoulder dystocia. A, McRoberts' maneuver, pressure on the anterior shoulder and rotation to an oblique plane. B, Extraction of the posterior arm. C, Rotation of the posterior arm.

of gastrointestinal secretions and swallowed amniotic fluid. The control of its passage into the amniotic fluid is not well understood. Maturation and stimulation of the parasympathetic nervous system clearly play roles. The relationship between meconium passage and fetal distress is inexact (Woods, 1984). About one fifth of neonates with thickly meconium-stained amniotic fluid will have acid-base abnormalities. The frequency of meconium-stained amniotic fluid varies with gestational age—2 to 3% in the second trimester, 6 to 11% in the late third trimester and as many as 40% after 42 weeks. Intrapartum passage of meconium occurs in 1.5 to 18% of patients. The presence of meconium dictates the continuous use of electronic fetal monitoring. In animal models acidosis is associated with meconium passage more often than hypoxia. Thus fetal scalp sampling in the presence of an abnormal tracing may be especially appropriate for meconium staining. In the presence of an abnormal fetal heart tracing and thick meconium, the perinatal mortality rate is 3 to 22.2% and the neonatal morbidity rate is 7 to 50% (Woods, 1984).

Inhalation of meconium (meconium aspiration) severely compromises the resuscitation of the neonate. Ventilation abnormalities and coexistent hypoxemia combine to produce persistent fetal circulation and subsequent pulmonary hypertension. Meconium aspiration may occur within the first few breaths. However, in utero aspiration can happen and can result in death despite adequate airway management at birth (Davis et al, 1985).

The primary responsibility for the management of meconium rests with the obstetrician. Upon the delivery of the head, a DeLee trap is used to suction the upper airway, especially the nasal passages. The procedure is repeated after complete delivery. This simple procedure will clear the upper airway in 90% of cases. About 10% of neonates will have meconium in the trachea below the cords. Laryngoscopy with suction is necessary to clear this meconium. A large suction tube is used (No. 14 French

Table 11–8. Delivery Room Equipment for Neonatal Resuscitation

1. Laryngoscope (small handle preferred)
   Size 0/1 blade
2. Endotracheal tubes appropriate for infant size
2.5 mm	<1000 gram
3.0 mm	1000–1500 gram
3.5 mm	1500–2200 gram
4.0 mm	>2200 gram
3. Suction apparatus: DeLee trap, No. 14 French catheter, bulb syringe
4. Bag and mask set
   non-rebreathing, pressure relieving elbow
   1 liter breathing bag
   conductive rubber masks
5. Orogastric tubes (sizes 5 and 8)
6. Oxygen source and flow meter
7. Intravenous tubing for transfusion
8. Intravenous catheters 20–25 gauge
9. Drugs
   D10
   D5W
   NaHCO$_3$
   Epinephrine (1:10,1000)
   Atropine (0.4 mg/ml)
   Naloxone (0.2 mg/ml)

catheter) to remove large particles. It is preferable that no positive pressure be applied until the first suction is complete. However, ventilation support should be given shortly thereafter.

DEPRESSED NEWBORN

The incidence of a severely depressed neonate (Apgar score 0 to 3) is 0.5 to 1%, and rapid and effective resuscitation is instrumental in long-term recovery. Any delivery room attendant may be called upon to provide resuscitation and, thus, must be skilled in the technique. Adequate equipment is essential for timely resuscitation. Table 11–8 depicts the necessary delivery room supplies.

The Apgar score (Table 11–9) was developed to direct and follow the resuscitation of the depressed neonate. Apgar scores are the cumulative scores reached at 1 and 5 minutes. If

Table 11–9. Components of the Apgar Score

Sign	Score		
	0	1	2
Heart rate	Absent	<100 beats/min	>100 beats/min
Respiratory effort	Absent	Slow, irregular	Good cry
Color	Cyanotic, pallid	Acrocyanotic	Pink
Muscle tone	Limp	Minimal	Active
Reflex response	Absent	Minimal	Active

the score is below 6 at 5 minutes, a 10 minute score is calculated. Apgar scores of 7 to 10 indicate a normal infant. Scores of 4 to 6 are associated with moderate depression. Severe depression (scores 0 to 3) requires a major resuscitative effort.

Regardless of the Apgar score, hypothermia is a problem for all neonates and results from several factors. Rapid heat generation is needed in the first minutes after birth. Heat loss is affected by a large surface to mass ratio, limited oxygen and glucose supplies, compromised catacholamine stimulation of brown fat and depression by drugs or asphyxia of neurologic responses necessary for heat production and conservation. Hypothermia may initiate anaerobic metabolism and, thus, metabolic acidosis. Physiologic responses are further inhibited by this acidosis. In particular, surfactant production is depressed when the core temperature falls below 36.5 degrees C.

A neonate may lose body heat by evaporation, convection, conduction or radiation. In the immediate newborn period evaporation is the major route. A neonate's skin temperature can decrease at a rate of 0.3 degrees C/minute unless preventive measures are initiated. The neonate should be dried, its head covered and it should be placed in a warm environment. If the infant is cold-stressed, vasoconstriction of the peripheral vessels ensues; acrocyanosis and mottled skin appear.

Moderately depressed neonates (Apgar scores 4 to 6) are not as responsive as normal neonates. These neonates have adequate cardiorespiratory response but require support since they have less reserve. The airway is cleared and supplemental oxygen is given by mask. With these supports and close observation, the neonate usually recovers quickly.

Narcotics are a common cause for a moderately depressed neonate. Narcotics given intramuscularly within one and a half to two hours or intravenously within one-half to three-quarters of an hour prior to delivery can significantly depress the neonate. Narcotic depression is treated with naloxone 0.01 mg/Kg. The neonate's tone and respiratory effort will rapidly improve. If they fail to do so, other diagnoses must be suspected (asphyxia, shock, sepsis, CNS bleeding). Acute drug withdrawal is a potential risk in infants whose mothers have used narcotics or other substances extensively during pregnancy.

Hopefully, the delivery of a severely depressed neonate (Apgar score 0 to 3) has been anticipated and a resuscitation team of two or three persons and equipment have been gathered. The resuscitation of a floppy and cyanotic neonate should be initiated prior to one minute after birth. The cord is clamped and cut and the neonate is transferred to a warmed neonatal table. An umbilical artery blood gas determination can be helpful. A large base deficit indicates a long-standing asphyxia. The principles of neonatal resuscitation are depicted in Table 11–10.

The neonate without meconium staining is ventilated initially with a bag and mask with a 40 to 50% oxygen source. A tight seal from the mask will deliver continuous positive airway pressure (CPAP) and oxygen. If spontaneous breathing is not initiated by CPAP within a few seconds, ventilation is started at 40 to 60 breaths per minute with a peak pressure of 20 to 25 mmHg. A high ventilation rate in the beginning helps correct the acidosis and reduce the need for alkali therapy.

Proper use of the bag and mask will effectively ventilate the neonate. Intubation is performed when it can be done quickly and easily. Intubation is performed with the neonate in a straight position without hyperextension of the neck. The laryngoscope with a 0 or 1 straight blade is held in the left hand and advanced into the neonate's mouth to the right of the midline. The blade is placed between the base of the tongue and the base of the epiglottis. As the tip is slightly advanced, the epiglottis is raised and the vocal cords are visualized. The endotracheal tube is held in the right hand and advanced through the vocal cords from the right side. The tube is advanced only one or two centimeters prior to checking for bilateral breath sounds. Ventilation is established at 40 breaths per minute with a maximum pressure of 20 to 25 mmHg.

Acute fetal bleeding or a tight nuchal cord with early clamping can result in hemorrhagic shock in the neonate. Intravascular volume can be rapidly restored with a 5% albumin solution

Table 11–10. The ABC's of Neonatal Resuscitation

Airway:	suction nose and mouth
	endotracheal suction for meconium or blood
Breathing:	bag and mask with pressure valve
	40 breaths/minute, maximum pressure 25 mmHg
	intubation
Circulation:	external compression 100–120/minute
	place thumbs over sternum, use chest encircling technique

or Plasmanate given through an umbilical line in a dose of 4 ml/Kg. Placental blood may also be used. The blood is obtained in a heparinized syringe. The blood is then anticoagulated and passed through a blood filter prior to transfusion.

BIRTH TRAUMA

Over the last 25 years research and development in obstetrics have been directed to reducing the morbidity and mortality from intrapartum asphyxia and birth trauma. Advances in fetal monitoring have reduced the incidence of intrapartum fetal death from asphyxia. Cesarean section has replaced traumatic obstetric operations, i.e., high forceps delivery and internal podalic version. Cyr and co-workers (1984) examined the trends in severe birth asphyxia and birth trauma over a 20-year period. A significant fall in severe birth asphyxia was noted, but there was a rise in birth trauma. The authors felt that the increase was the result of an increase in midforceps operations as a result of an increase in epidural anesthesia.

Clavicular fracture, facial nerve palsy, brachial plexus injury and cephalohematoma are the most common birth injuries (Table 11–11). The risk factors for birth injury are primigravidity, fetal macrosomia (over 4000 grams), prematurity, second stage over 60 minutes, vaginal breech delivery, forceps operation and shoulder dystocia. Levine and co-workers (1984) used logistic regression analysis to develop a risk assessment score using these variables. Their model predicted 50 to 75% of the injured neonates. Neither spontaneous vaginal delivery nor cesarean birth completely protects the fetus from injury. Hepner (1969) argued that facial nerve palsy resulted as much from compression of the facial nerve against the maternal spine as from forceps operations. Brachial plexus injury and humeral fractures have been reported in cesarean birth (Cyr et al, 1984; Collea et al, 1980). Coexisting asphyxia may predispose to brachial plexus injury, since it causes hypotonia and allows excess lateral flexion and traction by the anxious obstetrician.

The presence of one injury signals the possibility of others. The incidence of skull fracture in the presence of a cephalohematoma is 10 to 25% (Painter and Bergman, 1982). Brachial plexus injury is associated with fracture of the clavicle or humerus (9%), diaphragmatic paralysis (5 to 9%) or facial paralysis (5 to 10%) (Painter and Bergman, 1982). The incidence of

Table 11–11. Birth Injury*

Injury	Rate/1000 Births
Clavicular fracture	3.96
Facial palsy	3.61
Brachial plexus injury	2.60
Cephalohematoma	2.50
Intracranial injury	0.85
Skull fracture	0.84
Soft tissue laceration	0.58
Humeral fracture	0.45

*Data from Painter MJ, Bergmann I. *Semin. Perinatol.* 6:89, 1982; Rubin A. *Obstet. Gynecol.* 23:218, 1964; Gresham EL. *Pediatr. Clin. North Am.* 22:317, 1975; Levine MG, Holroyde J et al. *Obstet. Gynecol.* 63:792, 1984; Yonekura ML, Teberg A et al. Society of Perinatal Obstetricians, Abstract No. 119, 1984.

coexisting soft tissue injury is underestimated yet contributes significantly to morbidity and mortality. Hemorrhage into the subperiosteal space (cephalohematoma) or into subcutaneous tissue can lead to anemia and hyperbilirubinema. Ralis (1975) describes the crush injury syndrome as the major cause of traumatic death in vaginal breech delivery. In these cases, parenchymal hemorrhage, disseminated intravascular coagulation and renal failure are responsible.

In general, the prognosis is quite good in most cases of injury. Fractures and soft tissue injury heal normally. In most cases, nervous system injury recovers as well. Complete recovery is expected in 70 to 92% of brachial plexus injuries, 50 to 60% of cases of diaphragmatic paralysis and 90 to 95% of cases of facial paralysis (Painter and Bergman, 1982). Improvement within two weeks is a good prognostic sign, and complete function returns by five months. Partial recovery will continue for at least 18 months. Early diagnosis and physiotherapy are felt to improve the prognosis.

The key to management of birth trauma is the recognition of the patient at risk, i.e., primiparas, gestational diabetes, fetal macrosomia, prolonged second stage and abnormal fetal lie. Midpelvic forceps deliveries should be used with caution when a timely cesarean section may provide a large degree of protection. Unfortunately, 20 to 40% of difficult vaginal deliveries cannot be predicted. When a difficult vaginal birth is occurring, the obstetrician must recognize the limits of traction. Figure 11–7 illustrates the errors leading to birth injury. They include traction on the long bones in a limb extraction, hyperextension of the fetal head and lateral traction on the fetal head.

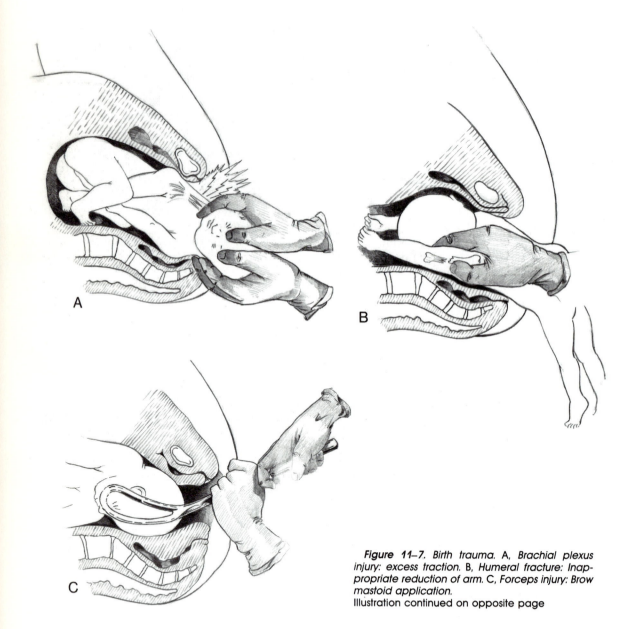

Figure 11–7. *Birth trauma.* A, *Brachial plexus injury: excess traction.* B, *Humeral fracture: Inappropriate reduction of arm.* C, *Forceps injury: Brow mastoid application.*
Illustration continued on opposite page

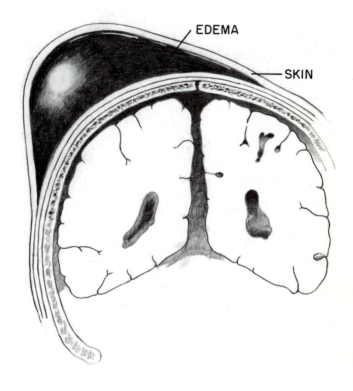

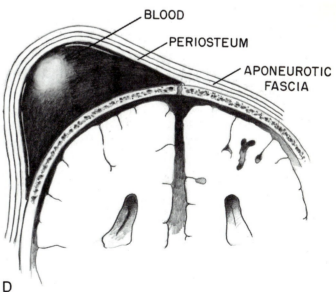

Figure 11–7 Continued D, *Scalp injury: Caput succeedaneum (top) subdermal edema which extends beyond suture lines. Cephalohematoma (bottom) subperiosteal hematoma limited by suture lines.* Illustration continued on following page

D

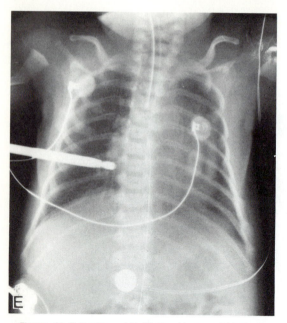

Figure 11–7 Continued E, Bilateral humeral fractures.

ACUTE PUERPERAL INVERSION OF THE UTERUS

Uterine inversion has been classified in two ways, by extent and by time. Classification by extent is incomplete when the dome of the uterus is at or above the internal os, complete when the dome of the uterus extends into the vagina and prolapsed when the inverted uterus extends through the introitus. The classification by time is acute if inversion occurs between delivery and contraction of the cervical ring, subacute if it occurs from the formation of a cervical constriction ring until four weeks postpartum or chronic if it occurs after four weeks. The incidence of inverted uterus varies considerably but is around 1:2000 to 5000 (Harris, 1984b; Watson et al, 1980; Van Vugt et al, 1981; Platt and Druzin, 1981). The most consistent predisposing factors are a previous history of an inversion, traction on the cord with fundal pressure (Crede maneuver), uterine atony (MgSO$_4$) and primigravidity (Platt and Druzin, 1981).

The classic symptom is shock out of proportion to blood loss. This may relate to strong vagal stimulation as the cervix dilates. Shock is present in 25 to 40% of patients (Watson et al, 1980; Platt and Druzin, 1981). Although blood loss may be considerable (1200 to 1800 ml), shock may not be relieved by fluid replacement until the uterus is replaced. Pain is not a leading symptom and is usually seen in chronic inver-

sion. Subacute and chronic inversion usually present with infection, thrombosis, urinary complaints or disseminated intravascular coagulation. The most common sign of acute inversion is palpation immediately after delivery. Maternal mortality is less than 10% (Van Vugt et al, 1981).

The prognosis is improved by speedy diagnosis and rapid replacement. The following procedures are recommended (see Fig. 11–3).

1. When an inversion is detected just after delivery, the placenta is rapidly removed. Replacement is first attempted by indenting the fundus in its center with three to four fingers. The fundus may readily reinvert if no constriction ring is developing. The procedure should not be delayed for general anesthesia if it can be accomplished easily. At the time of diagnosis, the labor and delivery suite should be mobilized for a potential resuscitation. Rapid infusion of Ringer's lactate solution through at least two large bore intravenous lines should be started. Two or more units of blood should be typed and cross matched, and anesthesia personnel should be summoned.

2. If the first procedure does not work, the following maneuver may be attempted. The patient is given general anesthesia with a uterine relaxant (halothane). The fundus is grasped with the palm, and the fingers are extended into the sulcus between the cervix and fundus (see Fig. 11–3). Pressure is exerted through the vagina and pelvis toward the umbilicus. This effects traction on the round ligaments, which can help in the reinversion.

3. If replacement is successful, a hand should be kept in the uterine cavity until the uterus contracts strongly under the influence of oxytocin (20 to 30 units) and Methergine (0.2 mg I.M. or I.V.) (Fig. 11–3).

4. If all efforts at replacement from below are fruitless, surgical repositioning must be undertaken. The Huntington procedure (see Fig. 11–3) is most commonly used. The abdomen is opened through a vertical midline incision. The operator and assistant grasp the uterine wall within the inversion funnel and pull upward on either side. Traction on the round ligaments and vaginal elevation may facilitate the reinversion. Occasionally the constriction ring prevents this. At this point a Haultain's procedure (see Fig. 11–3) is used. A midline posterior incision is made through the ring in order to widen its diameter. After the reinversion, the uterine incision is repaired in the same way as a classic uterine incision.

5. Perioperatively the patient is given antibiotics and is maintained on ergot derivatives for two to three days.

GENITAL TRACT TRAUMA

Perigenital hematomas and lacerations are classified into four types: vulvar, paravaginal, vulvovaginal and supravaginal. Extension of the episiotomy and cervical trauma are common lacerations. A variety of conditions predispose to the development of genital tract injury: young primipara, fetal macrosomia, abnormal presentation (occiput posterior, breech), precipitous labor, abnormal pelvic structure (narrow subpubic angle, straight sacrum), abnormal soft tissue (scar), obstetric manipulation and uncontrolled delivery. The incidence is difficult to ascertain because of population differences and the differences in accuracy of definitions, evaluation and recording. One recent study (Sleep et al, 1984) randomized 1000 patients between two perineal management protocols involving the liberal and conservative use of episiotomy. Posterior trauma (sulcus tears) was recorded in 43.7% and anterior trauma (labial tears) was recorded in 21.8%. Fourth degree extension or upper vaginal trauma occurred in only 0.5%.

Maternal death from genital tract trauma is uncommon unless uterine rupture is involved. However, a variety of morbidity risks can occur. Blood loss is the most acute and can be associated with hemorrhagic shock. In most cases this complication is heralded by external blood loss in the face of a contracted uterus. Occasionally intrafascial blood loss is occult, from a paravaginal, ischiorectal or parauterine hematoma (see Fig. 11–2). Perineal pain and rectal pressure may be the only symptoms prior to shock.

Other risks associated with genital tract trauma are perineal infection, dyspareunia, urinary stress incontinence and fistula formation. Sleep and co-workers (1984) reported that 90% of their patients returned to sexual relationships within three months postpartum. However, 20% complained of dyspareunia at that time. Nineteen percent of women had involuntary loss of urine at three months postpartum. However, a long-term prospective study of stress incontinence and genital tract trauma has not been performed. This type of study would need to control for age, parity, maternal and fetal size, length of labor, position of the presenting fetal part and the presence of manipulation. In addition, medical diseases that affect tissue integrity need to be studied.

Fistulas of the urinary tract or bowel are a rare complication of delivery. They are related to pressure necrosis or trauma. Prolonged obstructed labor causes pressure necrosis 7 to 10 days after delivery. Anteriorly, the fetal head compresses the trigone, bladder neck and upper urethra against the symphysis, and a fistula forms as the necrotic tissue sloughs. Less frequently, a similar complication occurs posteriorly; the rectum is compressed against the sacral promontory and a high rectovaginal fistula occurs.

The incidence of obstetrically related fistulas has dropped with the advent of safer cesarean section. Destructive manipulation of a dead fetus and complicated forceps operations have been largely eliminated, and rarely is obstructed labor neglected for days in Western countries. In Third World countries fistula formation from pressure necrosis remains a problem in rural obstetrics.

After a difficult forceps procedure, bloody urine should be investigated, as hematuria is a sign of traumatic injury. If a laceration or hematoma extends anteriorly, a cystoscopy should be performed to rule out bladder trauma. Acute injury to the rectal mucosa is identified during the routine rectovaginal examination performed with episiotomy repair. Rectal mucosal injury can occur above the rectal sphincter without sphincter involvement. Acute injuries of the bladder or rectum are repaired as described earlier in this chapter and in Chapter 4. If the injury is over eight hours old when it is first identified, it is best to delay repair until infection and swelling have subsided (one to two months). Prolonged bladder catheterization may allow a small bladder laceration to heal spontaneously.

Anterior lacerations of the perineum usually involve stretch tears of the labia (see Figure 11–2). The urethral meatus and clitoris may be involved. Individual vessels are clamped and ligated. A general ooze may be treated with ice and pressure after the skin repair. When bleeding occurs close to the clitoris it is important not to place a suture into the body of the clitoris, as a hematoma and subsequent dyspareunia may result. The skin and mucosa are reapproximated to restore normal anatomic relationships.

Posterior lacerations of the fourchette and vagina are classified by the degree of injury. First degree lacerations involve only the mucosa. Second degree lacerations involve the bulbocavernous and superficial and deep transverse perineal muscles. Third degree lacerations involve the rectal sphincter and fourth degree lacerations involve the rectal mucosa. European literature includes rectal mucosal injury in third degree lacerations.

The repair of posterior lacerations is directed at restoration of normal function and anatomy (see Fig. 11–2). The important points are the identification and repair of rectal mucosa injury, restoration of the sphincter and prevention of hematoma formation. Prior to the repair of a posterior laceration a rectovaginal examination is performed with a double gloved hand. The integrity of the mucosa, rectovaginal septum and ischiorectal fossa is established. The repair of a fourth degree laceration has been described in the discussion of episiotomy. The vessels of the perineum are engorged during delivery and are only loosely attached to the underlying structures. When these vessels are lacerated they can retract well away from the wound edge. If this is not recognized, a hematoma can form. The loose areolar/fat tissue offers little resistance to hematoma formation. Repair of perineal lacerations and hematomas must be directed to securing these vessels. Individual bleeding points are clamped and ligated whenever possible (see Fig. 11–2). In repair of a laceration or episiotomy one should pay careful attention to the apex. The first stitch of a mucosal repair is placed well above the apex of the laceration (see Fig. 11–2); a simultaneous rectal examination will help prevent rectal mucosal injury with the apical suture. Dead space is closed with interrupted 3-0 polyglycolic acid sutures. The vaginal mucosal edges are reapproximated by a running locking 3-0 polyglycolic stitch.

The incidence of perigenital hematomas is difficult to determine. It varies a great deal with the care with which this complication is examined and reported. Older studies with a higher incidence of instrumental deliveries showed a large incidence. Sotto and Collins (1958) examined 47 consecutive perigenital hematomas in great detail. Their study revealed an incidence of 1:309 deliveries. Twenty-one of 47 (45%) were perineal or vulvovaginal and 25 of 47 (53%) were paravaginal. Perineal hematomas often resulted from a bleeding vessel within the episiotomy site. Paravaginal hematomas tended to occur over the ischial spines and were related to instrumental delivery. Thirty-two of 47 (68%) occurred on the right side, and 31 of 47 (66%) were between 2 and 4 inches in diameter. The most common symptoms were rectal pain and

pressure with radiation to the coccyx. Thirty-six (77%) were diagnosed within eight hours of delivery, although four of 47 (8.5%) were found 5 to 10 days postpartum. One supravaginal hematoma was diagnosed 10 days postpartum and was complicated by anemia and abscess formation. Nine of 47 (19%) patients developed shock and 20 of 47 (43%) received blood transfusions.

The management of a perigenital hematoma depends on the timing, location and severity of symptoms. A hematoma of the episiotomy site developing within four to six hours should be opened, the vessel ligated and the episiotomy resutured. A small (less than 5 cm) paravaginal hematoma should be watched carefully for enlargement. The patient should have serial hematocrit determinations, rectovaginal examinations and determination of vital signs. Enlargement or hemodynamic instability indicates a need for surgical exploration. With the patient under adequate anesthesia, a longitudinal mucosal incision is performed over the hematoma (see Fig. 11–2). Transverse incisions may lead to vaginal constriction from scar formation. The hematoma is evacuated and the individual vessels are ligated. The dead space and mucosa are closed with simple sutures of 3-0 polyglycolic acid. The vagina is tightly packed for 12 hours, and a Foley catheter is placed to relieve urinary tract obstruction.

A supravaginal hematoma is an extension of a hematoma from the paravaginal area or more commonly from broad ligament trauma with uterine rupture or cesarean section. The management often requires exploratory laparotomy. The presence of a cervical or vaginal laceration extending beyond the fornix is an indication for immediate laparotomy. Occasionally, a non-expanding broad ligament hematoma can be observed. Continued bleeding is treated with supportive transfusion and exploration.

Cervical lacerations are related to three factors—prior surgery, cervical manipulation during transition (late first stage of labor) and instrumental delivery. Cerclage and cone biopsy are the most common antecedent operations. Precipitous delivery in the present of a cerclage can lead to the annular amputation of the cervix. Often bleeding will be minimal, otherwise a running locking stitch of 3-0 polyglycolic acid will accomplish hemostasis. Cervical lacerations that occur during cervical manipulation or intrumental deliveries are linear and extend toward the vaginal reflection at 3 and 9 o'clock (see Fig. 11–2). After a vaginal delivery the cervix should be assessed for laceration. When there is adequate anesthesia, the cervix is progressively visualized with ring forceps. In an unmedicated vaginal delivery, perineal discomfort may prohibit this. Palpation of the cervical ring can then be used to screen for lacerations. In cases of postpartum hemorrhage, the vagina and cervix should always be examined.

Linear cervical lacerations are repaired only if they are bleeding or extend into the upper one third of the vaginal cervix. The cervix is stabilized with ring forceps and repaired with interrupted through and through sutures of 2-0 vicryl (see Fig. 11–2). If the laceration extends beyond the vaginal reflection, a full exploration is recommended.

POSTPARTUM DEPRESSION

Psychotic postpartum depression is a real and dangerous complication of delivery. Infanticide has been reported as the fourth and most common traumatic cause of death for children under one year of age in the United Kingdom (D'Orban, 1979). The incidence of psychotic depression varies between 0.1%, based on hospital inpatient records, and 12% when non-hospitalized patients are included. Table 11–12 lists the symptoms of depression. The women at greatest risk are those with a history of an affective disorder, family history of postpartum depression (23%) or a previous episode of postpartum depression. Recurrence may be as high as 30 to 50% (Braverman and Roux, 1978).

The most important differential diagnoses of postpartum psychotic disease are drug effects

Table 11–12. Symptoms of Postpartum Depression

Emergency Symptoms
  Suicidal thoughts
  Paranoid delusions
  Threats of violence toward the infant
Classic Symptoms
  Insomnia
  Anorexia
  Weight loss
Moderate Depression
  Listlessness
  Apathy
  Increased irritability
  Emotional lability
  Self-derogatory feelings
  Despair and hopelessness
  Indecisiveness
  Inability to concentrate

or medical diseases. Antihypertensive agents such as reserpine, Aldomet, hydralazine, and beta blockers reduce the ratio of noreprinephrine to dopamine and, thus, cause depression. Narcotic potentiators and antinauseant drugs (Phenergan and Compazine) can produce a catatonic-like state that can be confused with schizophrenia. Drug abuse, overdose or withdrawal can produce psychiatric symptoms. Sleep deprivation, hypoxia, thyroid disease, collagen disease or primary neurologic disease may be confused with postpartum psychosis.

Violent or suicidal ideation demands emergency psychiatric intervention. The mother and infant are temporarily separated and constant companionship is provided. Organic disease must be ruled out. A review of the medication record and a physical examination including neurologic evaluation is performed. A drug screen, thyroid function tests and arterial blood gases are helpful.

HEMORRHAGE AND INFECTION

Hemorrhage and infection are among the most common causes of postpartum morbidity. Both complications are more common after operative vaginal delivery or cesarean section. These complications are discussed in the context of cesarean section.

INSTRUMENTAL VAGINAL DELIVERY

Instrumental deliveries, forceps and vacuum extraction, have had a much smaller role in the delivery of obstetric care in the last 10 to 15 years. Two sources have contributed to this decline. First, an increasing awareness and monitoring of both neonatal and maternal outcome have better defined the safety of instrumental delivery. A second equally important reason is the radical shift in the public's attitude toward obstetric health care. In the 1950's and 1960's the public requested and the practitioners desired a well medicated labor and delivery. The heavy use of analgesia and anesthesia, including general anesthesia, both facilitated and created the need for instrumental delivery. Recently, the consumer has become more aware of the deleterious effects of medication and has become more receptive to labor and delivery without medication.

Friedman (1978) has delineated and amplified the risks of instrumental delivery, especially in

Table 11–13. Perinatal Mortality and Labor Pattern*

Labor Pattern	Delivery Method			
	Spontaneous	Low Forceps	Mid-Forceps	Total
Normal	2	3	11	5
Protraction disorder	0	12	29	15
Arrest disorder	16	24	38	31
Total	2	6	19	10

*Perinatal deaths per 1000 term births.

the case of labor abnormalities. Table 11–13 depicts the relationship between abnormal labor, method of delivery and perinatal mortality. However, the connection between instrumental delivery and fetal safety is not as clear as depicted in Table 11–13. The reader is referred to an excellent review of the methodologic weaknesses of studies (Richardson et al, 1983) on the safety of instrumental delivery. First, fetal status has not been delineated prior to operative delivery. Many studies occurred before the advent of continuous electronic fetal monitoring. Second, labor status has not been well standardized. For example, the fetal prognosis for a primipara after a primary arrest pattern followed by midforceps delivery is clearly different from the prognosis of midforceps delivery subsequent to a normal first stage and a long second stage secondary to excessive conduction anesthesia. Third, the definition of forceps operations has been confused. A midforceps operation has a rotational component (occiput transverse) and a station component. Rotation or high midforceps operations may have a different prognosis than low midforceps operations. Fourth, the indications for instrumental delivery have not been standardized. It is hard to compare studies in which one institution has a 40% instrumental delivery rate and another has a rate of 3%. Fifth, prospective controlled studies comparing maternal and neonatal morbidity in instrumental versus spontaneous vaginal deliveries have not been performed.

Instrumental delivery will always have an appeal to the obstetrician. In given situations the operation provides a rapid and safe option without having to rely on other personnel. For example, second stage bradycardia can occur suddenly and unexpectedly. Mobilization for a cesarean section may require a potentially dangerous delay in delivery. Another attractive aspect of instrumental delivery is the reduction of the maternal morbidity found in cesarean

section. Two examples are uterine inertia in the late second stage and maternal disease in which Valsalva's maneuvers would be risky (cardiac disease or vascular abnormalities of the central nervous system).

Procedures

GENERAL GUIDELINES

The safe conduct of an instrumental delivery and the prevention of complications involve careful selection, preparation, application, extraction and inspection. Forceps and vacuum extractors are the instruments used for instrumental deliveries. The principles of selection, preparation and inspection are essentially the same for the two operations.

The proper selection of a patient for an instrumental delivery is perhaps the most important variable in determining the morbidity and mortality of instrumental delivery. First, the course of labor must be reviewed. An arrest of descent despite adequate contractions defined by an intrauterine pressure catheter is a caution. Davidson and co-workers (1976) evaluated the degree of difficulty of forceps delivery in relation to the duration of 7 to 10 cm cervical dilatation. If the duration was less than two hours, an easy delivery could be expected. The greater the time lapse over two hours, the greater the difficulty of the forceps maneuver. Documentation of adequate uterine contractions is important, since oxytocin augmentation rather than instrumental delivery may be prudent.

Second, the status of the fetus should be evaluated. Fetal macrosomia will increase the risks of instrumental delivery. Shoulder dystocia seems to be more common after midforceps operations (Hughey et al, 1978a). The fetal heart rate pattern should be reassuring, i.e., normal short-term and long-term variability without tachycardia. Late decelerations with good variability may be an indication for instrumental delivery. Any question as to the heart rate pattern should initiate a scalp stimulation test or fetal scalp sample for acid-base status. In the presence of fetal acidosis, instrumental delivery, with the possible exception of a rapid outlet forceps delivery, may involve greater fetal risk than prompt cesarean section.

Third, the position and station of the fetal head must be known. The misapplication of forceps or vacuum can lead to severe birth trauma or increased difficulty in extraction. The station of the biparietal diameter is more important than the station of the presenting caput or molding cranium. The palpation of the fetal head above the pubis precludes an attempt at instrumental delivery (Crichton, 1974). In these cases the biparietal diameter is above the ischial spine (high forceps operation).

The preparation for instrumental delivery involves anesthesia selection and sterile preparation of the patient. The depth of anesthesia must be balanced between causing a painless relaxation of the vagina and perineum and allowing continuing uterine contractions and expulsive efforts by the patient. Complete subarachnoid block will maximize relaxation but allows little voluntary expulsive effort. On the other hand, pudendal anesthesia allows maximum expulsive effort, but only variable pain relief and relaxation. Vacuum-assisted deliveries can be performed fairly easily under pudendal block. Epidural anesthesia or a subarachnoid block with a lower dose of lidocaine will give adequate anesthesia yet allow some expulsive effort. Prior to the use of conduction anesthesia the patient is hydrated with 1000 ml of a balanced salt solution to blunt the hypotensive episode that may be associated with sympathetic blockage in 20 to 40% of cases.

Instrumental deliveries are normally performed with the patient in the dorsolithotomy position. Elevation of the mother to a semisitting position will add to the expulsive force. The clinician must adjust to a more downward direction of the pelvic canal. A perineal shave or enema will not facilitate a successful instrumental delivery, but clipping of excessive pubic hair may be appropriate. The perineum is gently scrubbed and rinsed. The bladder is catheterized to reduce the risk of trauma. Rupture of membranes is confirmed. The presence of another physician and DeLee suction equipment is recommended for instrumental deliveries other than outlet forceps.

FORCEPS

Choice of Instrument. There are many different forceps available. An obstetrician's choice is guided by his experience and a knowledge of the clinical situation. An accurate broad-based bimalar-biparietal application is essential. The position over the malar eminences avoids trauma to the eyes and ears of the fetus. A broad-based application prevents uneven pressure points during traction. In order to prevent uneven pressure application the instrument should have a cephalic curve to simulate the shape of the head. Elliot-type forceps have a tighter cephalic curve, and the long overlapping shanks are useful on small round fetal heads. On molded heads Elliot-type forceps cause pressure points on the zygoma and the parietal bone which may result in injury to these areas. In addition, some Elliot-type forceps do not have fenestrations (Tucker-McLane) and may slip because of lack of anchorage below the malar eminences. Luikart's modification, in which the fenestration is preserved on the inner surface of the solid blade, minimizes the disadvantages of the solid blade.

Simpson-type forceps have a long tapering cephalic curve to adjust for molding, and fenestrations in the blade allow for better traction. The separated shanks reduce the possibility of fetal head compression, but the separation distends the perineum and can create perineal lacerations. Fenestrated blades provide a good grip on the fetal head but often leave significant marks on the fetal face and increase vaginal lacerations (see Fig. 11–7).

Correct Application of Forceps. The posterior fontanelle, the sagittal suture and the fenestration of the blade are the three landmarks used in checking the correct placement of forceps. In anterior positions, the posterior fontanelle should be one finger's breadth anterior to the plane of the shanks and an equal distance from the blades (Fig. 11–8). When the distance from the blades to the posterior fontanelle is greater than one finger's breadth, the blades are too far back on the fetal face. Traction is likely to cause deflexion of the fetal head. If the posterior fontanelle is less than a finger's breadth away, the blades ride forward on the face. This causes overflexion and may injure the eye socket.

The plane of the sagittal suture should be perpendicular to the midplane of the shanks. Misapplication results in undesirable brow/mastoid traction. This increases the difficulty of the extraction and the risk of slippage and subse-

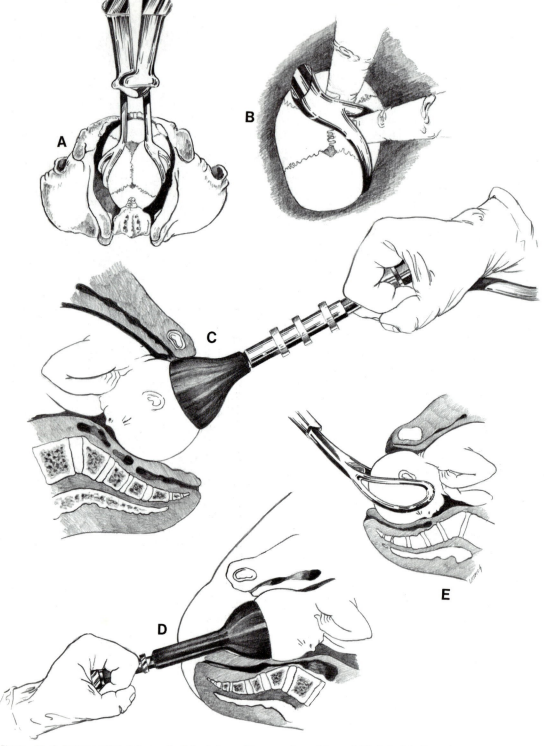

Figure 11–8. Instrumental delivery. A, Orientation of forceps to pelvis and fetal skull. B, Examination for forceps placement: One finger breath below posterior fontanelle and a finger tip's exposure of fenestration. C, Correct application of Silastic vacuum: Placement over the posterior cranium allows flexion of the fetal head. D, Downward traction is needed for mid-pelvic deliveries. E, Upward and outward traction extends and delivers the head in an outlet delivery.

quent fetal trauma. The location and amount of fenestration can also warn of slippage. It should be possible to insert no more than the tip of one finger into the lower end of the fenestration in advance of the head (Fig. 11–8). If excess fenestration is palpated, the blades have not been inserted deeply enough to anchor the malar eminences. If traction is applied, dangerous slippage may occur. The amount of palpable fenestration should be monitored during traction. Traction should cease immediately if slippage occurs.

Readjustment of the blades may be done without their being removed. It is more easily accomplished by rotation of the head to an occiput anterior position. The blades are unlocked and their position changed individually with a hand in the vagina. Readjustment from the handle may exert too much force and displace the fetal head to a higher station. The application of the forceps should be evaluated periodically throughout the traction.

Technique of Application. The technique of forceps application varies with the position and station of the fetal head and the type of forceps used. The discussion of individual techniques is found in articles and textbooks on forceps delivery (Dennen, 1964, 1965). The basic principles are:

1. Displacement of the fetal head should be avoided. The use of a lubricant and gentle fundal pressure prevents displacement.

2. The blades are applied after the obstetrician has visualized the position in which they will be when applied to the fetal head.

3. The handle of the left blade, held in the operator's left hand, is inserted to the left side of the mother's pelvis in front of the baby's left ear. The right hand and the right side of the pelvis are used when dealing with the right blade. In left-sided positions of the occiput, the left ear is posterior, and in right-sided positions the right ear is posterior.

4. When the sagittal suture is in an oblique diameter of the pelvis, the posterior blade is applied first. The posterior blade provides a splint for the head and prevents backward rotation. With the right occiput position, proper placement requires overlapping the blades to lock them. When the sagittal suture is directly occiput anterior, the left blade is applied first in order to facilitate locking the blades.

5. The direction of the blade is marked by placement of the appropriate index finger and forefinger over the parietal bone of the corresponding side. The handles follow the cephalic curve as they are applied. For example, the left handle starts in the left side of the groin area and rotates across the midline and down to about a 4 o'clock position.

6. The blades are inserted with only the force generated by the thumb on the heel of the vaginal blade. Force on the handle is too strong and uncontrolled and may lead to injury.

Traction and Delivery. The operator sits directly in front of the patient in such a way as to brace against any sudden movement and somewhat below the perineum to facilitate downward traction; the higher the station, the lower the stool. For low or low midforceps operations, the operator sits chin-high to the patient's symphysis. The plane of traction is similar for all forms of instrumental delivery and is illustrated in Figure 11–8. The initial traction is downward and follows the path of least resistance. If the direction of the traction is changed too soon, the symphysis and subpubic angle obstruct progress; if changed too late, the coccyx impedes it. Axis traction is accomplished using a two-handed grip. The handles rest on the palm of the right hand and are grasped at their junction with the shanks. Thus, the force of traction is applied to the lock instead of the handles where head compression is maximized. The left hand grasps the shanks from below at the vulva. The left hand exerts a downward force, which allows the head to avoid the symphysis and reduces anterior vaginal wall injury. The right hand provides traction in an outward fashion. Manual axis traction is sometimes replaced by handles that drop below the plane of the shank. These handles mechanically provide the proper angle of traction to follow the pelvic curve.

Traction is applied with a steady crescendo-descrescendo intensity corresponding to uterine contractions. The amount of force varies from case to case but in general is 34 to 45 pounds for a primigravida and 24 to 29 pounds for a multigravida. The traction is from a flexed forearm only, and the elbows are held close to the body. This technique protects against sudden slippage and limits the amount of traction. Between periods of traction, the handles are unlocked and separated, and the fetal heart tones are evaluated. The correct application is checked prior to the next period of traction.

As the occiput rides under the symphysis, the traction takes a more outward and upward direction. The fetal head is then extended by raising the handles to about 45 degrees above the horizontal. An episiotomy is performed as the head distends the perineum. After extension the fetal chin is grasped with the left hand

and the blades are removed with the right hand. They are removed by a reversal of the motion used in applying them. The blades should be removed with little resistance. If resistance is encountered, it is advisable to deliver the head with one or both blades still applied.

VACUUM EXTRACTION

The contraindications to vacuum extraction are absolute cephalopelvic disproportion, face presentation and after-coming fetal head. Relative contraindications include birthweight less than 2000 grams, previous scalp sample, high fetal head or an incompletely dilated cervix.

There are two basic types of vacuum instruments, the classic metal Malmstrom's vacuum extractor and the newer Silastic cup vacuum (see Fig. 11–8). Both work by the same principle. The instrument is attached by suction to the occiput. Traction will use the fetal spine as a fulcrum to allow optimal flexion.

Application. The equipment and technique needed for use of the Malmstrom vacuum extractor are well described by Malstrom and Jansson (1964). The cup sizes are 30, 40, 50 and 60 mm in diameter, and the largest cup size is best, since traction force is proportional to the cup size. The cup is lubricated with a sterilized soap solution and is inserted into the vagina. Pudendal anesthesia often provides enough pain relief for vacuum extraction. The cup is placed over the occiput and a finger is swept around the circumference to determine whether maternal tissue has been incorporated under the cup. Once the cup is free, the pressure is reduced in decrements of 0.2 Kg/cm² at intervals of two to three minutes until a vacuum of 0.6 to 0.8 Kg/cm² is reached (Table 11–14). The gradual increase (more than 10 minutes) in suction allows edematous tissue, a chignon, to envelop the rim of the cup to produce an adequate area for traction and prevent slippage.

The Silastic vacuum has significant advantages and differences. The cup size is a standard

Table 11–14. Vacuum Strength

mmHg	Inches Hg	lb/in²	Kg/cm²
760	29.9	14.7	1.03
700	27.0	13.5	0.95
600	23.6	11.6	0.82
500	19.7	9.7	0.62
400	15.7	7.7	0.54
300	11.8	5.8	0.41
200	7.9	3.9	0.27
100	3.9	1.9	0.13

65 mm in diameter and is collapsible to allow easy placement in the vagina. The blue line on the shaft is oriented to the plane of the sagittal suture. This provides a guide for rotation. The rim of the cup is checked prior to traction. Rather than a delay in suction, full suction of 600 mmHg (0.82 Kg/cm²) can be applied immediately and traction initiated. Unlike the Malmstrom vacuum, the suction in the Silastic vacuum can be reduced through a trumpet valve in the handle. The suction is released between contractions. This adaptation reduces the incidence of scalp trauma and increases the usefulness in emergency situations, e.g., late second stage bradycardia.

Vacuum Traction and Delivery. The principle of vacuum extraction is to augment the primary forces generated by the uterus. The operator's dominant hand holds the handle or chain and applies traction in the direction of the pelvic curve (see Fig. 11–8) during contractions. The operator's other hand presses the traction cup and fetal head posteriorly against the sacral concavity. This hand can follow the rotation of the fetal head and correct any tendency of the cup to become detached. Usually 5 to 10 applications of traction synchronized with uterine contractions are sufficient for delivery. An increase in scalp damage has been suggested when suction time exceeds 30 minutes with the Malmstrom extractor. Time limitation may not be a issue with the Silastic cup, since suction is applied only during contractions.

Vacuum extractors cannot develop the amount of tractional force that can be developed with forceps. Approximately 10 to 15 Kg of force can be applied to a cup without detachment, whereas forces in excess of 25 Kg can be generated with forceps. This can be seen as an advantage; difficult and traumatic instrumental deliveries are avoided in vacuum extraction. A similar traction of 10 Kg by vacuum extractor or by forceps produces considerably different pressures on the fetal head (Mishell and Kelly, 1962). Intracranial pressure was 1500 Kg/cm² for forceps and 75 Kg/cm² for vacuum, with a traction force of 98 Kg/cm² for forceps and 58 Kg/cm² for vacuum.

Complications

The major complications of instrumental delivery are traumatic injury to the fetus and mother. Luckily those injuries are rarely lifelong and usually heal completely within weeks.

Table 11-15. Maternal Trauma and Method of Delivery*

	Method of Delivery			
Injury	Spontaneous	Low Forceps	Mid-Forceps	Vacuum
Number	303	470	234	785
Perineal trauma (%)	70(23)	207(44)	145(62)	99/785(12.6)
Anemia (%)	64(21)	85(18)	122(52)	32/193(16.5)
Transfusion (%)	6(2)	61(13)	9(4)	2/540(0.4)

*Data from Gilstrap LC, Hauth JC et al. *Obstet. Gynecol.* 63:681, 1984; Berkus MD, Ramamurthy RS et al. *Obstet. Gynecol.* 66:503, 1985; Baerthlein WC, Moodley S et al. *Obstet. Gynecol.* 67:594, 1986; Maryniak GM, Frank JB. *Obstet. Gynecol.* 64:431, 1984; Nyirjesy I, Hawks BL et al. *Am. J. Obstet. Gynecol.* 85:1071, 1963.

In the long run, the complications of instrumental vaginal delivery must be compared with those of cesarean delivery. However, this is not easy. First, cesarean delivery is reserved for complicated pregnancies, and the potential for long-term problems is greater. Second, the complications of instrumental delivery are related to many different factors including the fetal status, station, labor progress, fetal size, gravidity, instrument and operator experience. Third, there is potential for reporting bias. The infants delivered vaginally by instruments are more carefully evaluated for damage. Ultimately, a prospective randomized trial is needed to help answer this question.

GENERAL STATISTICS

Tables 11–15, 11–16 and 11–17 depict representative statistics for maternal and fetal trauma occurring with instrumental deliveries. In general, there is an increase in complications associated with increasing manipulation—midforceps deliveries have more complications than low forceps. Forceps are more often associated with maternal reproductive tract trauma, especially that unrelated to episiotomy. Vacuum

extraction is more related to scalp injury, with the Malmstrom extractor having a greater risk than soft cup extractors. Only recently have investigators begun to separate out the indication for operative vaginal delivery as an important factor (Gilstrap et al, 1984, Dierker et al, 1985, 1986). In general, the indication for operative delivery is as important as the type of delivery. Ultimately, prospective randomized trials with adequate control for medication and adequate fetal/neonatal evaluation will give important answers. One unanswered question is the extent of operator experience as an outcome variable in instrumental deliveries.

MATERNAL COMPLICATIONS

Genital Tract Trauma. The incidence of genital tract trauma varies with the type of instrument, degree of manipulation, incidence of routine episiotomy and consistency with which genital tract trauma is recorded. Overall, extension of the episiotomy through the sphincter or into the rectum occurs about 40% of the time. Other genital tract trauma such as cervical lacerations, high vaginal tears or hematomas occurs about 15% of the time. Genital tract trauma, especially other than episiotomy exten-

Table 11-16. Recent Retrospective Reviews of Instrumental Delivery*

	Method of Delivery		
Outcome	Midcavity Malmstrom Vacuum	Midcavity Forceps	Silastic Vacuum
Number of patients	161	195	431
Maternal injury (%)			
Sphincter tear	41(25)†	88(45)	—
Other lacerations	10(6)†	42(22)	20(5)
Fetal injury (%)			
Cephalohematoma	35(22)†	20(10)	26(6)
Nerve palsy	1	3	0
Other	5	4	6
1 min Apgar 5 or less	—	—	20(5)
Jaundice (phototherapy)	—	—	8(2)

*Data from Baerthlein WC, Moodley S et al. *Obstet. Gynecol.* 67:594, 1986; Maryniak GM, Frank JB. *Obstet. Gynecol.* 64:431, 1984.
†p <.05

Table 11–17. *Recent Randomized Trials of Vacuum Versus Forceps Delivery*

	Method of Delivery			
Outcome	Malmstrom Vacuum†	Forceps†	Soft Cup Low Vacuum††	Low Forceps††
Number of patients	152	152	73	45
Number of spontaneous deliveries	10	8	4	1
Failures of method (%)	19/142 (13)	15/144 (10)	10/69 (14)*	2/44 (5)
Maternal trauma (%)				
Sphincter tear	9 (6)	24 (16)*	10 (14)	18 (40)*
Other laceration	9 (6)	15 (10)*	7 (10)	25 (34)*
Fetal trauma (%)				
Cephalohematoma	14 (9)*	8 (5)	11 (15)*	1 (2)
Facial palsy	0	1	0	0
Seizures	1	0	0	0
1 min Apgar 7 or less	42 (28)	46 (30)	6	2
Jaundice	36 (24)*	21 (14)	2	0
Subgaleal hemorrhage	1	0	0	0
Other soft tissue injury	6 (4)	13 (9)*	33 (45)	23 (51.1)*

*p <0.05

†Data from Vacca A, Grant A et al. *Br. J. Obstet. Gynaecol.* 90:1107, 1983.

††Data from Dell DL, Sightler SE et al. *Obstet. Gynecol.* 66:624, 1985.

sion, is consistently more common in forceps than in vacuum operations (Tables 11–15, 11–16, and 11–17). Low pelvic (outlet) deliveries are complicated by genital tract trauma at a rate one-half that of midpelvic rotational instrumental deliveries. The studies comparing vacuum to forceps deliveries vary considerably in the incidence of genital tract trauma (Tables 11–16 and 11–17). The variance reflects the institutional policy toward routine episiotomy, the care in observing and recording trauma and operator experience. Routine episiotomy and decreased operator experience significantly increase the incidence of genital tract trauma complicating instrumental delivery.

Forceps operations are more often complicated by trauma than vacuum operations for a variety of reasons. Forceps increase the delivery diameters and further distend the perineum. Forceps allow greater traction and more stable manipulation, often at the cost of trauma. Operator inexperience may be compounded in a forceps operation; the limits of force and manipulation are not recognized. The most common injuries are cervical lacerations, bilateral vaginal sulcus tears, hematomas over the ischial spines, and extension of the episiotomy. Irregular excessive traction in an inappropriate direction often leads to these injuries.

Anemia. Given the increase in genital tract trauma it is not surprising that anemia is more common after forceps delivery. Greis and co-workers (1981) described a fall in hemoglobin concentration of over 2 gm/dl in 30% of patients who had forceps deliveries and in only 4% of those who had Malmstrom vacuum extractions. A comparison group of cesarean deliveries had a 72% incidence of anemia. Berkus and co-workers (1985) reported a prospective study of silastic vacuum deliveries compared to consecutive forceps and spontaneous vaginal deliveries. Birth canal trauma occurred in 27% of spontaneous, 25% of vacuum and 59% of forceps deliveries (p less than 0.001). A greater than 2 gm/dl fall in hemoglobin level occurred in 17.3%, 27.3% and 43% of spontaneous, vacuum and forceps deliveries, respectively (p less than 0.05).

Failed Instrumental Deliveries. Failed forceps delivery occurs in 0.08% to 7% of cases (Dell et al, 1985; Hughey et al, 1978b). In the past, this complication was associated with excessive maternal and fetal mortality and morbidity. For example, Law (1953) reported fetal mortality of 24.3% and maternal morbidity of 27%. The morbidity and mortality of failed forceps operations will always be high because of the high risk indications for the operation—failure to progress or fetal distress. However, older statistics contained significant bias. The incidence was underreported and the worst cases were more likely to be recorded. The statistics failed to control for fetal status prior to the operation; electronic fetal monitoring was not used. Recent randomized studies of forceps versus vacuum extraction (Vacca et al, 1983; Dell et al, 1985) indicate that the increase in incidence of failed forceps or vacuum has been accompanied by a minimal increase in morbidity.

Failed vacuum extraction occurs more frequently—12.8% with Malmstrom's extractor (Nyirjesy et al, 1963) and 15% with the soft cup vacuum (Dell et al, 1985). A failed vacuum extraction means failure to deliver with 30 minutes of traction because of pelvic resistance (cephalopelvic disproportion), uneven application (caput succedaneum) or failure to apply perpendicular traction. Slippage and failure of the Malmstrom extractor have been associated with scalp trauma. This risk may not occur with the Silastic cup vacuum. When vacuum extraction fails, subsequent use of forceps is risky. Ahuja and co-workers (1969) reported a 3.3% incidence of dangerous subaponeurotic hemorrhage in infants delivered by the Malmstrom vacuum extractor, but seven of the 13 had a failed vacuum extraction followed by midcavity forceps traction. This report was also unusual in that the majority of the neonates had abnormal coagulation studies. Nyirysey and co-workers (1963) reported one ruptured uterus following a failed Malmstrom vacuum extraction and a subsequent forceps delivery.

Failure of instrumental delivery is an indication for immediate cesarean section. The key to reducing maternal and fetal morbidity is the appropriate selection of patients and recognizing the limits of traction. Vacuum extraction is automatically limited; the cup detaches with traction in excess of 10 to 15 Kg. This protection is not present in forceps deliveries, and tremendous traction can be exerted. Experience with forceps helps the clinician recognize a failed forceps extraction prior to maternal or fetal damage.

Future Deliveries. One of the many potential adverse consequences of a difficult delivery is the mother's fear of future childbirth. Will she conceive again and is she likely to repeat a risky delivery? Steer (1950) found that 62% of women continued childbearing after a spontaneous first birth, whereas only 32% of women continued after a first birth complicated by a midcavity delivery. Kadar and Romero (1983) noted that after a midcavity delivery the second delivery was spontaneous in 75% and required cesarean section for dystocia in 11.2% despite an increase in birthweight in 50% of the subsequent neonates. The mean increase in birthweight was 560 grams.

FETAL COMPLICATIONS

Scalp Injuries. The vacuum extractor can exert four vectors of force: suction, traction, circular force and shearing force. Suction and traction are always present. Circular force occurs with rotation and shearing force occurs with traction applied at other than a right angle to the scalp. Suction force produces an effusion into the subcutaneous tissue, the chignon. The Malmstrom extractor uses the chignon to facilitate traction. Prolonged suction can cause ecchymosis. The other vectors of force have the potential to injure scalp vessels and tissue. Traction and circular forces abrade and lacerate the skin. Scalp abrasion or laceration occurs in 12.6% of Malmstrom vacuum extractions (Plauche, 1979). These lesions appear to be less common (0.2%) when the silastic vacuum extractor is used (Maryniak and Frank, 1984). Significant hemorrhage has been reported when the Malmstrom extractor was placed after a scalp sample had been obtained (Roberts and Stone, 1978). This represents a relative contraindication to vacuum extraction.

Shearing forces can disrupt scalp vessels and produce subperiosteal or subaponeurotic bleeding. Subperiosteal bleeding occurs with disruption of a diploic or emissary vein and is commonly limited to one bone (usually the right parietal bone). Subperiosteal bleeding (cephalohematoma) presents as a indentable soft mass with a clean edge limited by a suture line. These resolve gradually over several weeks, and jaundice or anemia are minor complications (see Fig. 11–7).

Cephalohematomas are reported in 6.0% (range 2.3 to 25%) of vacuum extractions (Plauche, 1979; Maryniak and Frank, 1984) and in 2 to 3% of forceps deliveries (Baerthlein et al, 1986; Berkus et al, 1985). One of the major factors affecting the incidence is the accuracy of clinical diagnosis. Plauche (1979) noted that many cephalohematomas attributed to vacuum extraction are atypical; they are diffuse, not limited by suture lines, and are reabsorbed more readily than classic cephalohematomas. Berkus and co-workers (1985) noted that only three of 12 clinically diagnosed cephalohematomas were confirmed by ultrasonographic examination.

Subaponeurotic hemorrhage is a much more serious complication. Subaponeurotic or subgaleal hemorrhage collects in the loose aerolar tissue in the space between the periosteum of the skull and the galea aponeurotica. The subgaleal space extends without interruption from the orbital ridges to the nape of the neck. If this space is filled to 1 cm thickness, a total of 260 ml of blood can accumulate. Plauche (1980) reviewed the literature on this complication. In 123 cases, prematurity, macrosomia, prolonged labor, cephalopelvic disproportion, primiparity, male sex and African lineage were risk factors. A coagulopathy was present in 29%, and the mortality was 22.8%. Although Ahuja and co-workers (1969) relate this complication to vacuum delivery, the degree of risk from vacuum extraction is not clear. Subgaleal hemorrhage was found to occur with spontaneous delivery in 35 of 123 cases (28.4%), with forceps in 17 of 123 (13.8%), with cesarean section in 11 of 123 (8.9%) and with vacuum extraction in 60 of 123 (48.8%) (Plauche, 1980).

The management rests on early diagnosis of this insidious complication. A coagulation profile of the neonate is recommended after midcavity instrumental deliveries. Treatment consists of a pressure bandage, vitamin K and transfusion of 30 to 40 ml of fresh whole blood.

Intracranial Bleeding. The incidence of intracranial bleeding has been confused by faulty definitions. Traumatic intracranial bleeding is largely epidural or subdural, whereas intraventricular bleeding is probably more related to prematurity, bleeding diathesis or prenatal asphyxia. Plauche (1979) reported an incidence of intracranial bleeding of 0.35% for vacuum extraction. Recent comparisons of vacuum versus forceps deliveries reported an 0.44% incidence of intracranial bleeding with forceps deliveries (Vacca et al, 1983; Dell et al, 1985).

Two recent reports from the same author and institution (O'Driscoll et al, 1981, 1983) provide a caution for modern obstetrics. In one study the authors reported an extremely low cesarean section rate (O'Driscoll and Foley, 1983). Yet, in the other study of the same population, they describe 27 deaths from traumatic intracranial hemorrhage from forceps and vaginal breech delivery occurring during the same time period (O'Driscoll et al, 1981). When cesarean section rates fall this low, should we accept an excess of deaths (and more morbidity) from traumatic intracranial hemorrhage which occurs with the subsequent increases in difficult vaginal deliveries?

Skull Fracture. Skull fracture is another rare event whose incidence is obscure. Most skull fractures are asymptomatic, and many go undiagnosed. Approximately 10 to 25% of classic cephalohematomas are associated with parietal skull fractures (Gresham, 1975). The fractures are usually linear and occasionally of the "ping-pong" type. In this case the flexible bone is just depressed, not broken. Forceps delivery, maternal trauma and pressure from maternal pelvic bones have been implicated as risk factors. Management includes neurosurgical consulta-

tion, ultrasonography or CT scan of the head and follow-up with skull x-rays in two or three months. Separation of the fracture line on follow-up skull films is consistent with the diagnosis of a leptomeningeal cyst.

Retinal Hemorrhage. Prospective and controlled studies have documented an increase in retinal hemorrhage in infants delivered by vacuum extraction (Egge et al, 1981; Ehlers et al, 1974). However, Berkus and co-workers (1985), in a prospective study of forceps, Silastic vacuum and spontaneous deliveries, noted no significant differences in the incidence of severe retinal hemorrhage. The incidence of this complication was 13%, 18% and 18% in forceps, vacuum and spontaneous deliveries, respectively. These incidences compare to 6%, 3% and 7% in the respective delivery methods reported by Egge and co-workers (1981).

The implications of retinal hemorrhage are unclear. Peripheral retinal hemorrhage has no influence on subsequent function of the eye (von Barsewisek, 1979). However, macular injury has the potential for prolonged recovery. The incidence of macular injury was 2 to 3% in spontaneous or vacuum deliveries (Berkus et al, 1985). The concern is the possible relationship between retinal hemorrhage and other intracranial injury. Short-term prospective studies have not demonstrated an association (Berkus et al, 1985), but long-term follow-up is needed.

Neonatal Acidosis. Older reports cited midforceps operations as a cause of low Apgar scores (Friedman, 1978; Chiswick and James, 1979). However, more recent studies have controlled for fetal heart rate abnormalities and indications for delivery (Gilstrap et al, 1984; Dierker et al, 1985). These studies have not shown differences in short-term morbidity by method of delivery when indications for operative delivery were examined. In fact, when cesarean deliveries were studied, low Apgar scores were more common than for indicated forceps deliveries. Gilstrap and co-workers (1984) also noted no differences in neonatal depression or acidosis following elective forceps compared with spontaneous delivery. Maryniak and Frank (1984) reviewed 431 Silastic vacuum deliveries and found an incidence of one minute and five minute Apgar scores less than 5 to be 5% and 0.002%, respectively. Baerthlein and co-workers (1986) demonstrated no significant differences in Apgar scores between midcavity vacuum deliveries and midforceps deliveries.

Long-Term Prognosis. Long-term outcome is more often determined by genetic, antepartum and postnatal factors than by intrapartum factors. Yet controversy remains as to the effect of midforceps deliveries on later development. Friedman and co-workers (1984) used matched pair analysis to evaluate data from the National Collaborative Perinatal Project conducted in the late 1950's and 1960's. They emphatically stated, "on balance, therefore, unless one can provide justification in the form of documentable benefit on a case by case basis to counterbalance the potential risk, midforceps procedures should no longer be done." The methologic weakness of older studies have been reviewed by Richardson and co-workers (1983). More recent data, which controlled for fetal heart rate patterns and the indication for operative delivery, failed to demonstrate a deleterious effect based on the method alone (Dierker et al, 1986). Also, long-term follow-up of neonates delivered by vacuum extraction does not show increased risk (Plauche, 1979; Bjerre and Dahlin, 1974).

CESAREAN OPERATIONS

Cesarean section rates have risen more than three fold since 1970 after remaining constant at 4 to 6% since 1965 (Fig. 11–9). The indications of previous cesarean delivery and dystocia dominated the rise (25 to 30%). The indications

of breech presentation and fetal distress have contributed to 10 to 15% of the rise (Table 11–18). The rapid increase in cesarean section rates has generated much controversy. Newspaper, television and radio advertisements by malpractice lawyers add anxiety to the physician's decision-making process. If a cesarean section is performed, it is believed that medicine has done everything possible to prevent intrapartum damage to the fetus. Biostatisticians have examined the feasibility and benefits of prophylactic cesarean section at term (Feldman and Freiman, 1985). On the other hand, epidemiologists discuss controlling the cesarean section rate by the dissemination of information from vital records (Williams and Chen, 1983). Lay authors seem to argue strongly for an adversarial relationship between doctor and patient, thus controlling the cesarean section rates (Cohen and Esther, 1983).

The NIH publication *Cesarean Childbirth* (1981) and more recent studies by Davis and co-workers (1984) and Higgins (1985) have reviewed the epidemiologic factors related to cesarean birth rates. They include the following observations:

1. In 1981 cesarean birth rates were highest in the northeast (17.6%) and lowest in the north central region (13.9%) of the United States.

2. Prepaid insurance has an independent attentuating impact on the cesarean birth rate.

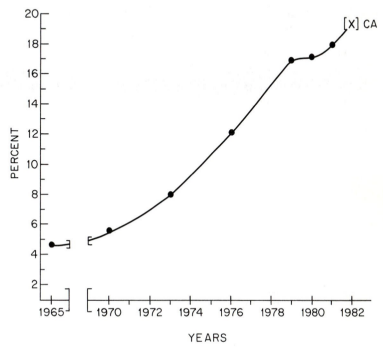

Figure 11–9. Cesarean section rates U.S.A. (1965–1982). [×] CA = California data.

Placek (1980, 1981), Petitte (1985)

Table 11–18. Contribution of Diagnosis to Cesarean Section Rate*

Indication	Percent Of All Cesareans Done For This Indication (1978)	Percent Contribution To Rise In Rate
Dystocia	31	30
Repeat cesarean	31	20–25
Breech presentation	12	10–15
Fetal distress	5	10–15

*Data from *Cesarean Childbirth*. NIH Publication No. 82-2067, U.S. Department of Health and Human Services. October 1981.

3. When high risk factors are controlled, the hospital's teaching status and the availability of a neonatal intensive care unit attenuate the cesarean birth rate.

4. There is little, if any, relationship between the type of hospital ownership and the cesarean rate.

5. Physician specialization does not seem to affect the cesarean birth rate.

6. Personal monetary gain by the physician seems to have little or no impact (Phillips et al, 1982; Higgins, 1985).

7. Certain maternal and fetal characteristics will increase the likelihood of cesarean birth. These include previous cesarean birth, maternal age over 35, low socioeconomic class, abnormal presentation, low birthweight and high birthweight.

Despite these variables, many factors are unknown. In a study of first births in Massachusetts in 1981 only 30% of the variation between regional cesarean section rates could be explained by high risk or epidemiologic factors (Davis et al, 1984). The unknown factors may include variation in individual provider practice, fear of malpractice, patient attitudes or differences in anesthetic technique.

Procedure

INDICATIONS AND CONTRAINDICATIONS

The indications for cesarean section vary according to the relationship between maternal and fetal risks. Cesarean birth is a major operation with maternal mortality and morbidity risks four to ten times greater than for a vaginal birth. Cesarean birth has some independent risks to the fetus when other risk factors are controlled. However, the stress and trauma of a vaginal delivery may contribute to long-term disability of the fetus. The balance between maternal and fetal risk provides the indication for cesarean section. For example, fetal distress in early labor provides a strong fetal indication

despite the maternal risks of cesarean delivery. The increased maternal risks of cesarean section in the face of severe chorioamnionitis may counterbalance lesser fetal risks. Absolute cephalopelvic disproportion and placenta previa have combined maternal and fetal indications. Unfortunately when the maternal diagnosis (failure to progress) and the fetal diagnosis (fetal distress) are inexact, the indications for cesarean section can be abused.

Progress in labor always plays an important role in the indication for cesarean birth. A rapid vaginal delivery may be more advantageous than a delay for a cesarean section. For example, in many community hospitals personnel and equipment cannot be mobilized for cesarean birth within 30 minutes to one hour. A properly performed midcavity instrumental delivery may be the indicated method of delivery. One concept that is slowly changing is the need to perform a crash cesarean section for fetal distress. A rapid emergency cesarean section is always indicated for a viable fetus in the presence of an incompletely dilated cervix when there is a prolapsed cord or a prolonged bradycardia. However, the long-term morbidity associated with classic fetal distress probably does not change with variation of delivery time by 30 minutes to one hour. Fetal distress that is identified upon admission probably has been present for hours, and damage may have already occurred; a crash cesarean section will not change the outcome. Fetal distress developing during labor usually has a large time margin (at least two to four hours) before damage occurs (Adamson and Meyers, 1977; Fleischer et al, 1982). In a fetus with pre-existing risk factors such as growth retardation or prematurity, the time margin may be narrowed.

Failure to progress, cephalopelvic disproportion and dystocia are terms used to describe a pathologic condition of delayed dilatation or descent during labor. In its extreme, failure to deliver increases maternal risk of sepsis and pelvic trauma. Ultimately the fetus decompensates under the stress. Friedman (1978) has described the increase in perinatal mortality associated with labor disorders. Perinatal mortality rises from 5 per 1,000 births with a normal spontaneous birth to 16 per 1,000 births for spontaneous delivery after an arrest disorder. In the presence of an arrest disorder and a midforceps delivery the perinatal mortality rate rises to 38 per 1,000 births (see Table 11–13).

Unfortunately, the dystocia category includes many unknown factors involving passage, passenger and powers. Pure absolute contraction of the pelvis (passage) is rare and is usually related to bone disease. The most common cause of dystocia is multifactorial, for example, a large infant with a minor malpresentation (occiput posterior) and ineffective uterine contractions secondary to maternal anxiety or exhaustion. Seitchik and Rao (1982) reviewed in detail the first labor and delivery and subsequent trial of labor after a primary cesarean section for failed oxytocin augmentaton. With the trial of labor, 40 of 58 women delivered vaginally. All first labor parameters, such as birthweight difference, dose of oxytocin, cervical dilatation on admission prior to oxytocin administration and before cesarean section, the clinical or radiologic estimation of pelvic dimensions failed to predict success or failure in a subsequent trial of labor.

The method of delivery in breech presentation is a very controversial subject. Approximately 60% of patients with breech presentations will be selected for cesarean delivery by strict criteria (Table 11–19). Vaginal breech delivery has a small but definable risk of trauma and asphyxia to the newborn. Ten to 15% of breech deliveries will be difficult, and successful fetal outcome will depend on the control and skill of the obstetrician. Appropriate training in vaginal breech delivery has been lacking in some training programs. All of these factors lead to an increased medicolegal risk of vaginal breech delivery. These factors as well as patient request will foster the decision to perform a cesarean section. The use of external version may significantly reduce the incidence of breech presentation in labor.

Previous cesarean section is a frequent indication for cesarean birth. In the United States approximately 95% of patients with a previous cesarean section will have a repeat cesarean birth. Computer-assisted decision analysis has strongly favored a trial of labor when the chances of success are greater than 45% and risks of rupture remain constant (Shy et al, 1981). Reviews of the literature by Lavin and co-workers (1982) and Flamm (1985) have also supported the safety of a trial of labor. The success rate varies according to the indication for cesarean birth (Table 11–20) but averages 79% (Flamm, 1985). The incidence of uterine rupture among 3,214 trials of labor was 0.7%, and the incidence of perinatal mortality due to the ruptured uterus was 0.93% (Lavin et al, 1982). The reader is referred to these reviews and a recent symposium (Paul, 1984) for a detailed discussion of management issues. The American College of Obstetricians and Gynecologists published in February 1985 the following guidelines for vaginal delivery after a previous low transverse uterine incision.

1. Informed consent should be given early in pregnancy.

2. Absolute cephalopelvic disproportion and previous classic uterine incisions are contraindications to a trial of labor.

Table 11–19. Maternal Mortality U.S.A. 1978*

Selected Complications	CDR‡	Percent of All Births	Cesarean‖	Vaginal‖
No mention	0.2	54.4	‡	4.9
Abnormal labor†	33.5	18.5	43.1	11.5
Previous cesarean	98.9	4.6	18.4	§
Breech	60.1	2.8	9.8	73.0
Multiple pregnancy	24.3	1.6	241.5	38.0
Fetal distress	59.0	1.4	51.8	§
Antepartum hemorrhage	48.1	1.1	122.4	127.0
Total	14.7		41.0	9.8

*Data from U.S. Department of Health and Human Services: *Cesarean Childbirth.* NIH Publication No. 82-2067, October 1981. Total births = 1,199,215.

†Abnormal labor: cephalopelvic disproportion, failure to progress, abnormal pelvis, malposition (OP), prolonged pregnancy, premature rupture of membranes, preterm labor.

‡Cesarean delivery rate (%).

§Too few births to provide stable estimate of rate.

‖Rate is number of maternal deaths per 100,000 deliveries.

Table 11–20. *Prior Indication and Success of Trial of Labor After Cesarean Section*

Prior Indication	Vaginal Delivery (%)
Breech	80–90
Third trimester bleeding	80–90
Fetal distress	70–80
Failure to progress	60–80
Cephalopelvic disproportion	25–50
Overall	70–90

3. There should be only one fetus, and the estimated fetal weight should be less than 4000 grams.

4. Continuous electronic fetal monitoring and 24 hour blood banking capabilities should be available. The patient's blood should be typed and screened for irregular antibodies upon admission to the labor and delivery area.

5. A physician who is capable of evaluating labor and performing a cesarean delivery should be immediately available.

6. The facilities and personnel should be available to perform an emergency cesarean birth within 30 minutes.

7. The risk of labor has not been assessed for patients with more than one prior cesarean birth, with a low vertical uterine scar or with breech presentation. The guidelines do not apply to these situations.

CHOICE OF ABDOMINAL WALL INCISION

Midline vertical incisions offer rapid entry and good exposure. However, vertical incisions are structurally and cosmetically inferior to transverse incisions. Limited exposure during a transverse incision can be predicted in well-muscled, large-boned women who have a narrow deep forepelvis (android pelvis). A wider and more cephalad skin incision can help overcome the difficulties in exposure; additional exposure may be obtained by incising the recti muscles transversely, using electrocautery. The ascending branch of the inferior epigastric vessels should be carefully avoided on the lateral aspect of the recti muscles. Another method is to separate the recti muscles off the pubis (Cherney's modification). Restoration of the recti muscles is accomplished by pulley suture of permanent material from the remaining severed aponeurosis on the pubis or to the fascia just above the pubic bone.

CHOICE OF UTERINE INCISION

The lower transverse uterine incision is the most popular and the best to perform in most situations. The visceral peritoneum is incised and bluntly separated from the lower uterine segment over the area of the proposed uterine incision. Excess separation should be avoided as it creates a potential space for hematoma formation or infection. The transverse uterine incision is centered to correct for uterine rotation and is started just below the point of reflection of the vesical peritoneum onto the uterus. A common mistake occurs after prolonged labor, i.e., deep transverse arrest. In these cases the lower uterine segment, cervix and upper vagina are greatly dilated and a contraction ring (Bandl's ring) may exist at the junction of the lower uterine segment and the fundus. The mistake is made when the incision is too low on the uterus. The surgeon may find that his incision is in the cervix or upper anterior vaginal fornix. Delivery of the fetus can be difficult and may necessitate a "T" extension.

Two techniques are commonly employed to open the uterus, a curvilinear incision and lateral fracture with the fingers after a scoring incision. The finger fracture technique has the advantage of less instrumentation and speed. The technique is adequate when there is a widely dilated lower uterine segment. However, the major disadvantage is the possibility of extension into the lateral vessels. This concern can seriously limit the length of the incision and create a difficult delivery of the fetus. The problem is of particular concern with a very premature fetus when little labor has occurred. Extension of the uterine incision using bandage scissors helps avoid these problems. Two fingers inside the uterine cavity guide the incision and protect against fetal injury. A curvilinear incision is performed to increase the opening and reduce the risk of lateral vessel injury in the event of extension.

The lower uterine segment should be utilized because incision in this area reduces blood loss, allows better healing, lessens the risk of uterine rupture in future pregnancies and can be covered by bladder peritoneum. In cases in which the transverse incision is not feasible because of limited space, a low vertical incision may have to be performed. When cesarean section occurs at 32 weeks or less, the incidence of vertical uterine incisions is 30% (Newton et al, 1986). The technique of making a vertical uterine incision is similar to that of making a low transverse incision, except that the bladder is reflected off to a greater degree inferiorly than laterally. Most low vertical incisions involve a portion of the upper segment. Thus, a trial of labor is not recommended in subsequent pregnancy.

A vertical upper segment uterine incision (classic) is rarely performed. The disadvantages are greater intraoperative blood loss, greater risk of pelvic/fundal adhesions and increased chance of uterine rupture with subsequent pregnancy. However, there are occasions when a classic incision is preferred, for example, in a scheduled cesarean hysterectomy, in cases of cervical cancer, when myomas are obstructing the lower uterine segment, in anterior placenta previa and in a transverse fetal lie with the back down. The technique involves a midline incision with extension superiorly and inferiorly with bandage scissors.

DELIVERY OF THE INFANT

The fetal head is delivered by cupping the operator's most caudad (dominant) hand over the occiput. The fetal head is gently flexed into the uterine wound. Traction should be in a midline plane. Oblique traction leads to extension of the uterine wound laterally. Oblique traction is encouraged by extraction with the cephalad hand or the use of the nondominant hand. Once the fetal head is in the uterine wound, fundal pressure accomplishes delivery.

A cesarean breech delivery is very similar to a vaginal breech extraction. The breech is delivered into the wound as in a vertex presentation. Traction is applied to the hips with two hands over the pelvis and the thumbs meeting over the sacrum. Once the fetal scapulae are fully exposed, the fetal arms are reduced and delivered by flexing at the elbow and sweeping them out along the ventral midline. A nuchal arm can be reduced by rotation of the fetus in the direction in which the nuchal hand points. The head is delivered by extension of the fetal body caudad and fundal pressure to maintain flexion of the fetal head.

REPAIR

After delivery the uterus may or may not be exteriorized. The angles are inspected and clamped with atraumatic clamps. Angle sutures of 0 polyglycolic acid are placed prior to delivery of the placenta in order to reduce blood loss.

After delivery of the placenta, the uterine wall is closed in two layers (Figs. 11–10C, D). A Lembert suture is valuable when the bladder is adherent near the uterine incision line. The horizontal nature of this stitch allows a better purchase on the myometrium with less risk to the bladder. A broad-based suture and gentle perpendicular traction, with a snug but not strangulating knot, help prevent tissue tearing and bleeding.

Post-cesarean hysterography has been used to measure the quality of healing and examine the effects of suture technique (Waniorek, 1967, Poidevin, 1961, Van Vugt, 1979). In general, 20% of uteri will have a regular outline, 55% will have small defects (4 mm or less) and 25% will have defects larger than 4 mm. Early investigators related these defects to the inclusion of the decidua in a single layered closure (Poidevin, 1961) or the use of multiple sutures to obtain hemostasis (Waniorek, 1967). However, a more recent study (Van Vugt, 1979) suggests that hysterographic defects more often reflect the thickness of the myometrium at the time of cesarean section rather than suture technique or the presence or absence of postoperative complications (endometritis). Moreover, it is not clear whether even a large defect has a significant risk for future pregnancy other than to make the obstetrician nervous about the risk of labor.

The bladder peritoneum is used to cover as much of the uterine incision as possible. Invariably, a portion of a vertical uterine incision is exposed. In vertical incisions, a third layer of stitches should endeavor to reduce the amount of suture and raw myometrial surface exposed to the bowel and omentum. This can be accomplished by the traditional Lembert suture or by a baseball type of suture. Fine (3-0 or 4-0) polyglycolic acid suture material is used for this layer.

The abdominal wall is closed in three or four layers. The first layer is a continuous running suture of 2-0 polyglycolic acid that is used to close the peritoneum. The sutures are placed so as to exclude the cut peritoneal edge from the abdominal cavity. The fascia is closed by interrupted figure of eight sutures of 0 polyglycolic acid for a vertical incision and by three lengths of running locking suture of 0 polyglycolic acid for a Pfannenstiel incision. In patients at risk for dehiscence, the abdominal incision should be closed by the Smead-Jones technique, using permanent synthetic suture (0 proline).

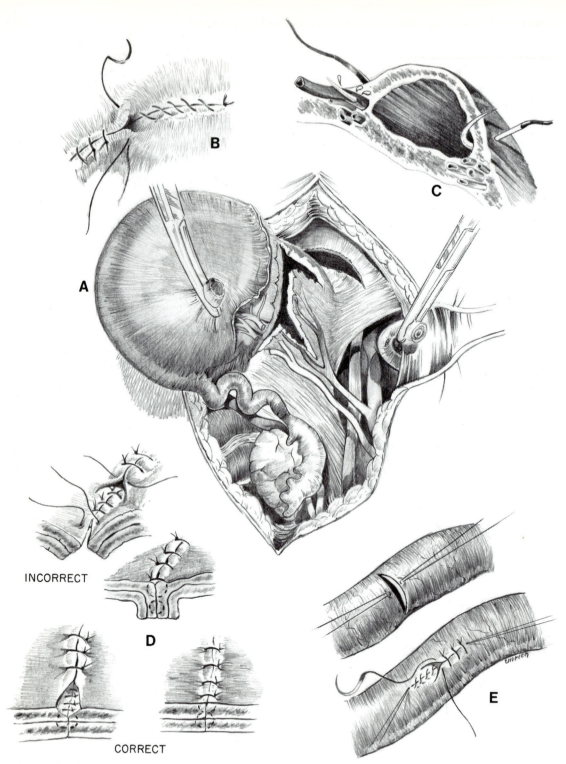

Figure 11-10. Intraoperative complications of cesarean section. A, Uterine lacerations: Extension of the uterine incision can occur laterally and inferiorly. Inferior extension is associated with bladder injury. Repair of lateral or broad ligament lacerations is facilitated by division of the round ligaments. B, Two-layered closure of bladder injury. C, Placement of angle suture. Incorrect placement of the angle suture endangers the uterine vessels (left). Correct placement maintains a plane perpendicular to the endometrial cavity and includes the endometrial cavity (right). D, Closure of the uterine wall. Incorrect: inclusion of the serosa on the first stitch initiates inversion of the raw myometrial surfaces into the endometrial cavity. Correct: the first row of partial thickness stitches restores anatomic layers and reduces blood loss. E, Repair of bowel injury. A complete laceration is closed in two layers in the longitudinal axis of the bowel to avoid constriction.

PREVENTION OF POSTOPERATIVE ENDOMETRITIS

The leading maternal risk of cesarean section is postoperative endometritis. Approximately 10 to 20% of post-cesarean section patients will show evidence of infection, and infection remains a leading cause of maternal death (see Tables 8–2, 11–21). The risk of endometritis can be dramatically reduced by hospital controls against nosocomial infection (Iffy et al, 1979), surgical technique and selected use of prophylactic antibiotics. Hospital control of nosocomial infection includes the organization of an infection control committee, active involvement of an infection control nurse or practitioner and an active medical epidemiologist (Allen, 1984; Haley et al, 1981). The establishment of policies, procedures, monitoring instruments and enforcement mechanisms is critical to the effectiveness of the infection control committee. One critical role is to provide the individual practitioner or caretaker with information about the infection rates in his or her patients. The reader is referred to the articles cited previously and the *Guidelines for Infection Control* published by the Centers for Disease Control for specific recommendations.

Operative techniques can be as important to the prevention of infection as the use of prophylactic antibiotics. These techniques include (1) surveillance and classification, (2) preparation of the patient, (3) preparation of the surgical team, (4) ventilation and air quality in the operating room, (5) cleaning and culturing, (6) intraoperative technique, (7) postoperative wound care and (8) prophylactic antibiotics. The details of these guidelines are found in Chapters 2 and 4 and in the Centers for Disease Control recommendations (Polk et al, 1983).

Intraoperative technique in the prevention of postoperative infection involves working as efficiently as possible, handling tissues gently, preventing bleeding, eradicating dead space and minimizing devitalized tissue and foreign material remaining in the wound. Techniques specific to cesarean section include the following:

1. Rarely is the need for cesarean section so acute as to limit the usual preparation of the operating room, instruments, patient and personnel.

2. Subcuticular bleeders should be clamped and tied prior to the fascial incision unless there is fetal distress or general anesthesia.

3. The surgeon should double glove and then remove one pair after the contamination that occurs with the delivery of the infant. The first pair of gloves should be removed prior to the delivery of the placenta.

4. The peritoneal gutters should be packed with moist laparotomy sponges to isolate the upper abdomen from contaminated blood and amniotic fluid. These sponges are removed after the visceral peritoneum is repaired.

5. Prior to the closure of the uterine incision the wound is irrigated, cleaned with a new suction tip and isolated with fresh drapes placed over the old drapes.

6. After each layer is closed, the operative field is irrigated liberally with warmed saline. This reduces the size of the innoculum and removes excess blood clots.

7. The wound is covered with sterile gauze prior to removal of the drapes and cleansing of the abdomen. A new clean bandage is placed after these procedures.

Prophylactic antibiotics have been shown to be highly effective in reducing the infectious morbidity of cesarean section (Swartz and Grolle, 1981). Cumulative statistics have shown a reduction in febrile morbidity from 52% in controls to 20% in antibiotic-treated groups. Prophylactic antibiotics seem to be most effective in reducing endomyometritis, with less but still significant reductions in wound and urinary tract infections. A number of observations can be made concerning prophylactic antibiotics.

1. The patients who benefit most from prophylactic antibiotics are those with rupture of membranes in labor. The use of internal fetal monitoring systems adds only a slight risk when compared to other factors. The value of prophylactic antibiotics is less clear when a high socioeconomic class patient without labor and without rupture of membranes undergoes cesarean section. A patient whose labor has been complicated by prolonged labor, prolonged use of internal monitoring systems and difficult cesarean birth may benefit from a prolonged (five days) course of antibiotics because of her excessive risk for endomyometritis despite prophylactic antibiotics.

2. Any antibiotic with a wide spectrum of coverage is equally effective in preventing endomyometritis. An antibiotic with anaerobic coverage has theoretic appeal. However, a recent, large, randomized study comparing cefoxitin and cefazolin failed to show a difference in the incidence of genital tract infection after prophylaxis (Stiver et al, 1983). Currently the surgeon should choose the cheapest single dose antibiotic with broad spectrum coverage.

3. The duration of therapy does not improve prophylaxis. One dose after cord clamping is as effective as other regimens.

4. Unless the operation is prolonged (greater than 2 hours) the timing of the dose does not change the effectiveness. The use of prophylactic antibiotics prior to cord clamping can lead to excessive neonatal intervention and increased cost (Cunningham et al, 1983).

5. Intraoperative irrigation with an antibiotic-containing solution (cefamandole nafate, 2 gm in 800 ml normal saline) can be effective in reducing endomyometritis (Rudd et al, 1981).

6. The use of antibiotic prophylaxis is safe for the mother. Occasionally an allergic reaction may appear. A theoretic risk is a shift in genital tract flora toward more resistant organisms (Stiver et al, 1984).

7. Pseudomembranous colitis has been reported following prophylactic antibiotics (Block et al, 1985; Arsura et al, 1985).

EXTRAPERITONEAL CESAREAN SECTION

Prior to the use of antibiotics, the extraperitoneal cesarean section was developed to reduce the risks of peritoneal contamination by inoculated amniotic fluid. Despite good theoretic appeal, there have been few controlled studies of its effectiveness (Perkins, 1980; Hanson, 1984). This has prevented the teaching and use of the technique. The success of various antibiotic regimens has also reduced the indications for this potentially valuable operation.

The technique may still have a place in the management of certain patients. The operation was developed to exclude the clean peritoneum from an infected uterus. The presence of chorioamnionitis after a long labor would be an excellent situation for extraperitoneal cesarean section. The operation may also be used to exclude a "clean" uterus from an infected peritoneum, i.e., cesarean section prior to laparotomy for appendicitis.

The following selection criteria should be evaluated prior to an extraperitoneal cesarean section:

1. The estimated fetal weight should be greater than 3000 grams and the cervix should be 5 cm or more dilated. This assures a well dilated lower uterine segment.

2. Previous cesarean section markedly increases the difficulty of the operation.

3. A placenta previa is a contraindication to extraperitoneal cesarean section because of the risk of bleeding.

4. The operator should have observed and

assisted in at least 10 procedures as training for the procedure.

5. The presence of fetal distress or general anesthesia is prohibitive.

The technique most commonly used is a modified Norton technique, well described by Durfee (1960). The bladder is partially filled with sterile milk (infant formula) to highlight bladder injury should it occur. A Pfannenstiel abdominal incision is used to expose the left side of the bladder. The fascial incision should extend at least 5 cm lateral to the recti muscles. More exposure can be obtained by removal of the recti muscles from the pubis (Cherney's modification). The perivesical space (space of Borgros) is explored, and the bladder is swept off the peritoneum and lower uterine segment by blunt disection. It can be helpful to ligate and incise the obliterated umbilical arteries and urachus. The endopelvic fascia on the lower uterine segment is then incised transversely and reflected inferiorly with a Doyen retractor. This maneuver protects the bladder inferiorly. A transverse uterine incision and delivery are performed in the usual fashion. Repair usually takes less time because no peritoneal repair is needed. Most authors recommend closed drainage of the perivesical space for 24 hours.

The dangers of the procedure are related to the proximity of the lateral vessels, bladder and ureter. Atherton and Williamson (1954) published pessimistic results. Among 68 patients there were 29 technical errors, including 14 peritoneal perforations and one major urinary tract injury. One technical error occurred in the comparison group of 75 transperitoneal cesarean sections. Durfee (1960) reported 125 attempts at extraperitoneal cesarean section. There were nine failures. The average skin to delivery time was 11 minutes. The peritoneum was accidentally entered five times and no bladder or major vessel damage occurred. Approximately 20% of patients were catheterized after 24 hours. A recent review by Hanson (1984) confirmed Durfee's older data. Peritoneal perforation can be repaired easily by a purse string suture of fine polyglycolic acid. Bladder injury is repaired in two layers as described in Chapter 3.

PERIPARTUM HYSTERECTOMY

Hysterectomy in the peripartum period has the potential for serious complications. Massive blood loss, distorted anatomy and associated pathology (hematoma or uterine laceration) create a catastrophic situation that the obstetrician long remembers. Often these are emergency operations associated with inadequate instruments and less experienced personnel. Blood loss and surgical field contamination contribute to major morbidity.

In spite of this, most cesarean hysterectomies are elective (75%) (Chestnut et al, 1985; Park and Duff, 1980). The common indications for elective cesarean hysterectomy are sterilization (28%), neoplasia of the cervix (33%) and leiomyoma (27%). The major indications for emergency peripartum hysterectomy are uterine rupture (45%), placenta previa/accreta (18%), uterine atony (18%) and laceration at the time of cesarean section (11%) (Chestnut et al, 1985).

Recent data from elective cesarean hysterectomies suggest a decreasing morbidity risk: transfusion (19%), febrile morbidity (6%), bladder injury (6%), broad ligament hematoma (5%) and postoperative ileus (2%) (McNulty, 1984). The guidelines for elective cesarean hysterectomy include:

1. Obstetric need for cesarean birth.
2. Desire for sterilization.
3. Informed consent, including the option of a tubal ligation.
4. The presence of accepted indications such as leiomyoma or cancer of the upper female reproductive tract. Carcinoma in situ of the cervix can be an indication in selected cases. The options of cryotherapy, laser therapy and cone biopsy should be discussed.
5. Technical ability to repair the bladder or manage severe obstetric hemorrhage.

Procedure. Blood loss, hematoma formation and bladder injury are the major intraoperative complications of peripartum hysterectomy. The essential factor in reducing blood loss is quick control of the major blood supply to the uterus. When anatomy has been grossly distorted by uterine rupture or hematoma formation, a drier, safer operative field may be attained by a hypogastric artery ligation. The four major pitfalls of this procedure include misidentification and ligation of the external iliac artery, laceration of the iliac vein or artery, injury to the ureter and retroperitoneal hematoma. The first complication is identified by palpation of the femoral pulse before and after the ligation. Ureteral injury can be avoided by entry into the retroperitoneum lateral to the external iliac artery and by clear identification and medial retraction of the ureter during ligation of the artery. Injury to the veins and retroperitoneal hematoma are avoided by close application of the tip of the right angle clamp to the artery and passage of the tip from lateral to medial. Elevation of the

artery with a large Babcock clamp facilitates this maneuver. Ligation of the artery decreases the pulse pressure and helps limit distortion of the operative field by hematoma formation (see Chapter 3).

The sources of excessive intraoperative blood loss include uterine atony, blood loss from the uterine wound, and operative management of the utero-ovarian anastomosis, cardinal ligaments and angles of the vagina. Massage and oxytocin will limit uterine atony. Ergotrate or Methergine 0.25 mg I.V. or I.M. may be given if no contraindications are present. One layer partial closure of the opened uterus will reduce wound bleeding. A small opening for finger assessment of the vaginal angles should be maintained in the midline. Double clamping and delayed ligation of the adnexal pedicles have the effect of allowing the operator to ligate an area much reduced in circumference and vascularity. Double ligation using an all-encompassing tie of 0 polyglycolic acid followed by a transfixing suture of the same material reduces the risk of late bleeding. The posterior leaf of the broad ligament often has persistent bleeding from small utero-ovarian anastomoses. Caution should be used in control of these bleeders because the ureter is dangerously close.

Once the round ligament and adnexal pedicles are cut and ligated, quick control of the uterine blood flow is essential. A clamp-cut-and-tie-later technique is used. Retrograde bleeding from the lateral uterine wall is controlled with medial clamps. Once the uterine arteries have been controlled, the bladder flap is developed. Midline dissection with pressure toward the uterus may decrease bladder injury and inadvertent trauma to the venous plexus of Santorini.

Dissection of the cardinal ligament is another area of technical difficulty and increased blood loss. Pregnancy softens ligamentous attachments and pedicles, which can be easily torn from the lateral uterine wall. Small bites with generous pedicles and gentle traction can avoid this difficulty. It is better to err by incorporating a small amount of cervical tissue in the bites than to venture laterally. The hypertrophied uterosacral ligaments are cut separately and ligated with 0 polyglycolic acid. Later these sutures will be incorporated into the angle for vaginal support.

The identification of the vaginal fornices can be difficult. The apex of the vagina can be found by introducing a double-gloved forefinger through the uterine wound and grasping the cervix between the thumb and forefinger. At this point the vagina can be entered. The last clamp on the cardinal ligament can readily be directed toward the vaginal finger. The vagina is often entered with this clamp. This ensures that the angle wil be transfixed by the 0 polyglycolic suture. If the vagina has not been entered at the angle, it is best to enter the fornix posteriorly. Prior to vaginal entry the field is isolated with wet laparotomy pads, and prompt suction is performed to reduce the size of the innoculum from the contaminated vaginal secretions and lochia. Irrigation is also a valuable adjunct.

Proper closure of the vaginal cuff is essential to reduce infection and postoperative bleeding. Backflow of vaginal fluid may be blocked by placing a sponge in the vagina for removal immediately after the procedure. The surgeon then changes gloves and continues with closure. Hemostasis of the cuff is obtained with a running, locking suture of 0 polyglycolic acid. Vaginal support is maintained by incorporation of the uterosacral ligaments or the round ligament with separate sutures through the angle. The contaminated field and blood loss create a maximum risk for cuff cellulitis and pelvic abscess. For these reasons, the vaginal cuff may be left open with closed "T" tube drainage.

Urinary tract injury is a consistent problem in both elective and emergency peripartum hysterectomies. Bladder injury occurs most often as the bladder flap is developed. The presence of adhesions from a prior cesarean section is a common predisposing factor. Careful sharp dissection is recommended. The bladder flap is developed only enough for each progressive bite down the cardinal ligament. Advancing further will initiate bleeding at a site where control is difficult.

Inadvertent suture of the bladder into the anterior vaginal cuff is a frequent cause of injury. These injuries are often undetected during the operation and present as a fistula in the postoperative period. Vaginal contamination and subsequent cuff cellulitis must also play a major role, since a small uninfected bladder injury usually heals spontaneously. Careful suture technique can avoid this complication. Prior to closure of the pelvic peritoneum, the bladder may be filled with sterile milk (infant formula) or a dilute solution of indigo carmine. Bladder and ureteral injuries are discussed in Chapter 3.

COMPLICATIONS OF PERIPARTUM HYSTERECTOMY

Maternal Mortality. About one in 200 women will die in association with peripartum hyster-

ectomy (Table 11–21). However, this statistic is significantly biased. Many operative deaths occurred prior to the development of modern blood banking, anesthesia techniques and antibiotic usage. Only large teaching hospitals with their indigent populations can develop meaningful numbers to report the incidence of complications. The lower general health and fragmented prenatal care in these patients add to the risks. Furthermore, mortality and morbidity may be more related to the obstetric catastrophe than to the operative technique. Clark and co-workers (1984) reviewed 70 peripartum hysterectomies. The mean blood loss prior to the decision to perform a hysterectomy was 2,125 ml, and about 30% of patients had undergone arterial ligation as well. The mean blood loss during surgery was 2,183 ml. The one maternal death in this series resulted from an amniotic fluid embolism.

Urinary Tract Injury. The incidence of urinary tract injury is 3.8% (Table 11–21). This complication occurs with equal frequency in elective and emergency cesarean hysterectomies (McNulty, 1984; Chestnut et al, 1985) (see previous discussion). Vesicovaginal fistula formation (0.6%) may occur because of inclusion of the bladder in the suture of the anterior vaginal cuff. Ureteral injury is related to abnormal anatomy caused by pregnancy, broad ligament hematoma or congenital malformation. The ureter may be traumatized during control of the uterine arteries or closure of the pelvic

Table 11–21. Complications of Cesarean Hysterectomy*

Major Complication	Percent	
	Mean	Range
Maternal mortality	0.7	0–10.1
Infectious morbidity		
Febrile morbidity	26.5	7.0–39.7
Wound	3.3	0.4–11.6
Cuff cellulitis	7.4	0.6–15.3
Pelvic abscess	1.8	0.3–3.8
Pulmonary	2.7	0.4–6.3
Urinary	9.8	1.2–28.1
Hemorrhagic morbidity		
Transfused	44.0	19.0–82.0
Reoperation	0.8	0–2.1
Traumatic morbidity		
Hemorrhage requiring unilateral oophorectomy	2.9	0–10.0
Bladder laceration	1.7	–
Ureteral injury	0.3	–
Urinary fistula	0.6	–
Thromboembolism	1.7	0.20–3.0

*Data from Plauche WC. *Clin. Obstet. Gynecol.* 29:318, 1986; Park RC, Duff WP. *Clin. Obstet. Gynecol.* 23:601, 1980.

peritoneum. Accurate knowledge of the location of the ureter and the careful placement of each clamp or suture are essential to avoid injury.

Infection. The potential for infection postoperatively is great. Emergency hysterectomy is often associated with labor, ruptured membranes, a compromised host, a bloody field and gross bacterial contamination. Postoperative infection occurs in 15 to 25% of patients. Reviews by Park and Duff (1980) and Plauche (1986) found wound infection in 3.3%, cuff cellulitis in 7.4%, pelvic abscess in 1.8% and septic pelvic phlebitis in 0.8%. Urinary tract infection and pulmonary infection occurred in 9.8% and 1.7% of patients, respectively. Prophylactic antibiotics, isolation of the pelvis, copious irrigation, double-glove technique and good perioperative surgical techniques are recommended as preventive measures. High dose broad spectrum antibiotics with anaerobic coverage are recommended to treat a pelvic cellulitis. Pelvic examination and perhaps a CT scan should be used to rule out abscess formation. Localized areas of infection should be treated surgically (see Chapter 4).

Hemorrhage. The definition of hemorrhage is seriously biased. First, blood loss is notoriously underestimated. Second, much of the blood loss occurs as a part of the primary obstetric disease, i.e., placenta previa or accreta. Third, statistics that combine the results of elective and emergency cesarean hysterectomies add important errors.

Despite these weaknesses, peripartum hysterectomy is a bloody procedure, both theoretically and practically. Approximately 5 to 20% of patients will have a significant loss (more than 1800 ml). The blood flow to the placental bed is 400 to 600 ml/min with large, distorted and tortuous veins returning the blood. Often the anatomy is distorted by uterine rupture, extension of the uterine incision and broad ligament hematoma. Elective cesarean hysterectomy is also associated with a risk of hemorrhage. Two recent series (McNulty, 1984; Chestnut et al, 1985) reported a 19% and 66% incidence of transfusion during elective cesarean hysterectomy, respectively. The incidence of intraoperative hypotension during elective cases was 2.7% (Chestnut et al, 1985).

Complications of Cesarean Section

Society and physicians have become somewhat cavalier about cesarean birth and its complications. Prior to the advent of modern anesthesia, surgical techniques, blood banking facilities and antibiotics, cesarean section had a very morbid and often fatal outcome. Modern medicine has reduced the risk of death to less than one in 2000 procedures, and most women do not suffer permanent morbidity from the operation.

Despite the usually good outcome in the individual patient, the burden of psychologic, physical and economic morbidity is ever-increasing, as one quarter of all births are performed by cesarean operations. Although the focus of this section is to catalog and review the management of cesarean complications, the best way to reduce maternal morbidity is to carefully

Table 11–22. Obstetrical Statistical Cooperative 1973–1977: Puerperal Complications*†

Complication	Cesarean Delivery (%)	Vaginal Delivery (%)
Endometritis	16.11	1.40
Wound infection	3.16	0.10
Pyelonephritis	4.56	0.41
Thrombophlebitis	0.60	0.13
Respiratory	1.89	0.21
Wound dehiscence	0.74	0.01
Post-spinal syndrome	0.79	0.12
Psychosis	0.21	0.07

*Data from U.S. Department of Health and Human Services: *Cesarean Child Birth.* NIH Publication No. 82-2067, October 1981.
†Total deliveries: cesarean, 23,169; vaginal, 142,030.

Table 11–23. Postoperative Cesarean Section Morbidity (1,391 Operations)*

	No. of Patients (%)
Minor Complications (11.5%)	
1. Paralytic ileus 3 to 5 days	3
2. Endometritis†	87 (6.6)
3. Urinary tract infection	41 (3.1)
4. Superficial wound infection	21 (1.6)
Major Complications (3.0%)	
1. Reoperation for bleeding or infection	12 (0.9)
2. Hysterectomy	1
3. Delayed hemorrhagic shock	1
4. Major infection (sepsis, peritonitis, parametritis, pneumonia)	25 (1.9)
5. Urethral catheter 5 days or more	2
6. Paralytic ileus over 5 days	2
7. Thrombosis	1
8. Pneumothorax	1

*From Nielson TF, Hokegard KH: Postoperative cesarean section morbidity: a prospective study. *Am. J. Obstet. Gynecol.* 146:911, 1983. Reprinted with permission.
†No prophylactic antibiotics were given

Table 11–24. Causes of Maternal Death Sweden 1956–1980*

Cause	1956–1960	1966–1970	1970–1980
Sepsis	3.2	1.8	0.3
Hemorrhage	6.2	1.7	0.2
Eclampsia/preeclampsia	6.0	2.2	1.3
Dystocia/trauma	5.4	1.7	0.4
Abortion	6.4	2.9	1.3
Embolism	3.8	3.9	3.5

*From Hogberg V, Joelsson I: The decline in maternal mortality in Sweden 1931–1980. *Acta Obstet. Gynecol. Scand.* 64:583, 1985. Reprinted with permission.
Per 100,000 live births.

and accurately select the patient for whom the risks of cesarean birth are exceeded by the risks of vaginal birth for the mother or the infant. The comparison of maternal mortality and morbidity risks of cesarean section versus vaginal delivery are displayed in Tables 11–19 and 11–22. Table 11–23 describes a prospective review of the major and minor postoperative morbidity of 1,391 cesarean sections (Nielson and Hokegard, 1983).

MATERNAL MORTALITY

One of the major achievements of modern civilization has been the dramatic reduction in maternal mortality. Hogberg and Joelsson (1985) detailed and reviewed maternal deaths in Sweden between 1931 and 1980. Their review encompassed 5,034 maternal deaths from direct obstetric causes. Individual charts were reviewed in 84% of cases between 1950 and 1980 with only three missing charts in the last 10 years. By 1970 maternal mortality had fallen to one fiftieth of the 1930 rate. Since the mid 1970's mortality has leveled off. This fall closely corresponds to the development of antibiotics, blood transfusion and hospital deliveries and antenatal care for 90% of women. Fifteen to 30% of the decline was related to a shift in age distribution; more births occur in the low risk age group (20 to 30 years old). Table 11–24

depicts the fall in the maternal death rate by cause of death. This fall may be caused by a decrease in the incidence or severity of the complications, e.g., eclampsia (Table 11–25), or by an improvement in the case fatality rate, e.g., abruptio placentae (Table 11–25). In theory, improved prenatal care will reduce the incidence and severity of a disease (pre-eclampsia) and improved operative management will improve the case fatality rate. A review of individual cases revealed a fall in the incidence of preventable factors from 40% in the 1950's to 20% in the 1970's. Eighty percent of the preventable factors in maternal death are professionally related.

The dramatic fall in maternal deaths from the diseases of pregnancy and birth has set the stage for a major reordering of the principal causes of death. Improved case identification (Rubin et al, 1981) and a rise in the cesarean section rate play a major role in the relationship of operative complications of cesarean birth to maternal death. Thromboembolism has now become the leading cause of maternal death in the United States (Kaunitz et al, 1985). The ratio of thrombophlebitis, hemorrhage and infection between cesarean and vaginal deliveries is 4 to 12:1. Thus the risk of death attributable to the the complications of cesarean section is increased.

Petitti and co-workers (1982), in the United

Table 11–25. Incidence and Case Fatality Rate Sweden 1956–1980*

Cause	1956–1960	1966–1970	1971–1980
Eclampsia			
Incidence	1.25	0.45	0.22
Case fatality rate	2.4	2.2	3.1
Abruptio placentae/placenta previa			
Incidence	7.9	5.3	8.1
Case fatality rate	0.4	0.2	0.02

*From Hogberg V, Joelsson I: The decline in maternal mortality in Sweden 1931–1980. *Acta Obstet. Gynecol. Scand.* 64:583, 1985. Reprinted with permission.
Incidence = cases per 1,000 live births.
Case fatality rate = deaths per 100 diagnosed cases.

States, examined in-hospital mortality as related to time and method of delivery. Maternal mortality associated with cesarean section fell from 113.8/100,00 deliveries in 1970 to 40.9/100,000 deliveries in 1978. Maternal mortality associated with vaginal delivery fell from 20.4/100,000 to 9.8/100,000 deliveries during the same period. The fall in maternal mortality related to cesarean section may reflect improved technique or the inclusion of healthier patients in the cesarean group by a tripling of the cesarean section rates.

The actual differences in the risks may be greater than these broad population statistics would suggest. First, the vaginal delivery death rate includes those deaths in which cesarean section would not have been a viable option (i.e., intrauterine fetal death and abruptio placentae) but would contribute to mortality. Second, hospital records underestimate the risk of death from cesarean section. Death from pulmonary embolism usually occurs 10 to 14 days after an operation. This happens well after the post-cesarean section patient has gone home.

Rubin and co-workers (1981) demonstrated this effect by linking death certificates with live birth certificates in Georgia between 1975 and 1977. They identified 36% more total maternal deaths and 45% more maternal deaths after cesarean sections than by analysis of death certificates alone. The authors found the cesarean-attributed maternal mortality rate to be 59.3/100,000 cesarean deliveries. Benedetti and co-workers (1985) also demonstrated significant under-reporting (112%) in Washington. In this review, death from hypertensive disease as well as pulmonary embolism was under-reported.

INTRAOPERATIVE COMPLICATIONS

Multiple Repeat Cesarean Section. A postpartum history of four or more previous cesarean sections is a clear risk factor for intraoperative complications. Thein and McSweeney (1964) and Fons and Brennan (1967) reviewed the clinical course of patients undergoing four or more cesarean sections. In a combined total of 396 patients, the complications were severe intraperitoneal adhesions in 22.3%, significant hemorrhage in 6.8%, placenta previa in 7.4%, placenta accreta in 1.8%, bladder injury in 1.5% and hysterectomy in 4.0%.

Preoperative preparation can reduce the risk of these complications. An ultrasonographic examination should identify placental position. The patient should give informed consent concerning hysterectomy and sterilization. Preoperative correction of anemia and an adequate blood supply for the operation are important. Intraoperatively, the bladder should be assessed for trauma.

Uterine Laceration. Difficulties in delivery of the fetal head often lead to extension of the uterine incision. This complication is associated with deep transverse arrest of labor, occiput posterior presentation, prolonged labor, failed forceps delivery and fetal macrosomia. The most usual location for extension is laterally into the broad ligament and down the lateral wall of the uterus (see Fig. 11–10). Occasionally, the laceration can extend inferiorly and damage the bladder (see Fig. 11–10). This is more common with repeat cesarean section or vertical uterine incisions. Intraoperative hemorrhage often exceeds 1500 ml and, in fact, 10% to 20% of cesarean hysterectomies are performed for uterine lacerations at cesarean section.

The keys to the management of this complication include:

1. Quick control of bleeding. Uterine and utero-ovarian artery ligation can be instrumental in reducing operative blood loss and facilitating repair. Uncontrolled suture or clamping can endanger the ureter.

2. Accurate estimation of the extent of the laceration. The laceration may extend down the cervix and the lateral wall of the vagina. Accurate reapproximation of the structures may require a vaginal examination and repair in the severe cases.

3. Adequate exposure. Repair and control of a broad ligament extension or hematoma can be aided by division of the round ligament and blunt dissection of the broad ligament (Fig. 11–10A). This procedure allows better visualization and localization of the ureter and uterine vessels.

4. Repair by placing an Allis clamp at the apex and using two layers of 00 polyglycolic acid suture.

5. Prophylactic antibiotics. If the procedure exceeds two hours, another dose should be given.

Hysterectomy is not the solution to a failure to understand the anatomy of uterine laceration or extension. Unless the damage is outlined and exposed, hysterectomy may not control the bleeding, and it unnecessarily endangers the other pelvic organs. In most cases, hysterectomy should be reserved for failure to control uterine atony despite conservative management and when repair may leave a uterus unsafe for future childbearing. In the latter case, a tubal ligation will accomplish the same purpose without the risks of hysterectomy.

Urinary Tract Injury. Eisenkop and co-workers (1982) reviewed the incidence and management of urinary tract injury at cesarean section. The incidence of bladder injury during primary and repeat cesarean section was 0.19% and 0.6%, respectively (total incidence 0.31%). Adhesions of the bladder flap from prior cesarean section were related to 8 of 13 bladder injuries during repeat cesarean section. The incidence of ureteral injury was 0.09%, and two thirds of the injuries were identified at the time of surgery. In difficult cases involving uterine laceration or hysterectomy, the integrity of the bladder should be checked with the instillation of indigo carmine or sterile milk through a three-way Foley catheter. Ureteral injury should be checked after extensive lateral or inferior uterine laceration, broad ligament dissection, hysterectomy or hypogastric ligation. Ureteral function can easily be determined by efflux of blue-tinted urine after intravenous injection of indigo carmine. A bladder repair involves a water-tight, two-layer closure as shown in Figure 11–10B. Further discussion on the diagnosis and management of urinary tract injury is given in Chapter 3.

Other Intraoperative Procedures and Complications. Tubal ligation is often performed in conjunction with cesarean delivery. Tubal ligation in the puerperium seems to have a higher failure rate, especially when the Pomeroy technique is used. Fimbriectomy or techniques that bury the proximal tube (Uchida, Irving) are recommended. Silastic ligature is often difficult secondary to the edematous tube, and tubal lacerations often result.

Occasionally, an obstetrician or surgeon will have to consider a post-mortem cesarean section because of brain death or severe trauma in the mother. This is often a "no win" situation: a maternal death and a great likelihood of a stillborn or damaged neonate. Although the exact incidence is not clear—failures are buried—no more than 15% to 20% of neonates survive intact when the operation is performed within 15 to 20 minutes of maternal death (Weber, 1971; Arthur, 1978). Sudden maternal death favors neonatal survival, whereas long-standing maternal disease reduces survival. In sudden maternal death, the medicolegal risk is great, and operative permission is often impossible to obtain.

The management of this crisis requires a generally accepted definition of death. The individual hospital should make this determination. The American Medical Association published the following definition of death (JAMA, 1968).

1. No response to painful stimuli.

2. No muscular movement or respiration for one hour (or three minutes off a respirator).

3. No reflexes, occular movements or blinking and the presence of fixed and dilated pupils.

4. A flat isoelective electroencephalogram repeated twice over a 24-hour period.

5. The preceding must be unrelated to deep barbiturate intoxication or hypothermia.

The following guidelines are suggested for post-mortem cesarean section:

1. If the pregnancy is over 26 weeks' duration, a cesarean section is justifiable.

2. The fetal heart motion must be documented, preferably by ultrasound.

3. The procedure should be carried out by classic incision as rapidly as possible.

4. Cardiopulmonary resuscitation should continue until the birth of the fetus.

5. Maximum resuscitation of the neonate should be performed.

6. Any critically ill patient in the third trimester of pregnancy should have a surgical kit immediately available.

7. Permission for the procedure should be obtained in advance, if possible, but failure to obtain approval should not prohibit the operation.

Bowel injury occurs very rarely and usually in patients with a history of previous operation(s). It most often happens upon entry into the peritoneum. If the injury is recognized prior to the uterine incision, the bowel should be rapidly isolated with laparotomy pads. If readily available, gently clamped rubber-shod clamps can be used to prevent further spillage. The uterine field is then isolated and irrigated to remove gross contamination. The surgeon should quickly regown and glove prior to the uterine incision. After the delivery and closure of the peritoneum, the bowel can be repaired as described in Chapter 3 and depicted in Figure 11–10E. After the procedure, the peritoneum should be irrigated with warmed saline. Antibiotics with anaerobic coverage should be used prophylactically.

IMMEDIATE POSTOPERATIVE COMPLICATIONS

Many of the immediate postoperative complications of cesarean delivery are similar to those that have been covered in Chapter 4.

These include atelectasis, pneumonia, paralytic ileus, urinary tract infection, urinary retention and superficial wound infection.

Puerperal Infection. Infection is the most common complication of cesarean section or vaginal delivery. The incidence is reviewed in Tables 11–23 and 11–24. Some type of infection occurs in 15 to 20% of post-cesarean patients; endometritis is the most common (15%). About 10 to 20% of these infections are serious, including septicemia, pelvic cellulitis, septic pelvic thrombosis, abscess formation and pneumonia. The most important single factor in predicting a puerperal infection is the presence of a uterine wound. The relative risk of endometritis after the following procedures is: internal monitoring, 1.0; multiple vaginal examinations 2.2; rupture of membranes, 2.6; and labor, 4.0 (Gibbs et al, 1978, Gibbs, 1985; Eschenbach and Wager, 1980). Many other factors also contribute to the development of puerperal infection. The roles of host response, facultative organisms, preexisting subclinical amnionitis and surgical techniques are actively under investigation at the present time.

Puerperal infection results from a multi-organism invasion of vaginal flora (Table 11–26). Endometrial cultures show 70% of the isolates to be aerobic. Gram negative rods (*E. coli*), group B streptococcus and group D enterococci predominate. Eighty percent of the isolates will have anaerobic organisms as well (*Bacteroides* and anaerobic *Streptococcus* species). *Chlamydia* and *Mycoplasma* will be present in 5 and 15% of cultures, respectively. However, the role of these organisms is not clear. They may be important as permissive organisms. *Chlamydia trachomatis* is associated with 25% of

late-occurring endometritis after a vaginal delivery (Wager et al, 1980). This observation has not been verified by the examination of post-cesarean section patients (Blanco et al, 1985). The acute morbidity of cesarean section may mask the low-grade symptoms of the infection; unfortunately, infertility may be the consequence.

The diagnosis of a postoperative puerperal infection can be difficult. Normal postoperative pain and postpartum contractions obscure the discomfort from mild infection. The clinical markers are fever, uterine tenderness, foul-smelling lochia, uterine subinvolution and a persistent paralytic ileus. Standard febrile morbidity is the occurrence of two elevations of temperature greater than 100.4 degrees F on at least two days taken by standard technique at least four times a day and occurring between the second and tenth postpartum days. Despite the definition, fever in the first 24 hours should not be ignored, and its source should be sought by complete physical examination and appropriate tests (see Chapter 4). Possible causes include pulmonary atelectasis, mild transient bacteremia and febrile response to the transfusion of foreign proteins by placental separation and delivery. It is important to remember that pregnancy and delivery may be coincident with various infectious diseases. Incentive spirometry and increased activity will facilitate pulmonary recovery. Antipyretics should not be used, as they may mask a more serious infection. A high fever in the first 24 hours (equal to 101.3 degrees F or more) is highly predictive (93%) of subsequent clinical infection (Filker and Monif, 1979). Patients with this sign should have a complete fever workup and appropriate therapy. Occasionally, early high fever can be associated with extremely virulent organisms such as aerobic *Streptococcus* species and *Clostridia*.

Unfortunately, fever is not always present in endometritis. Approximately one third to one half of patients with clinical infection will have temperatures of less than 100.4 degrees (Eschenbach and Wager, 1980). In these cases, the other clinical signs are useful. A physical examination is most important in localizing an infection, and a thorough pelvic examination is essential. Another important function is to provide a baseline to mark progress in the management of the infection. Antibiotic therapy should not be started without a complete examination.

The initial laboratory evaluation is critical in the diagnosis and management of postoperative

Table 11–26. *Microbiology of Post-Cesarean Infection*

Organism	Percentage of Cultures
Aerobic	70
Gram negative	
Escherichia coli	30
Klebsiella	5
Proteus mirabilis	5
Other	5
Gram positive	
Group B Streptococci	15
Group A Streptococci	1
Group D Enterococci	25
Anaerobic	80
Bacteroides, Peptococcus, Peptostreptococcus	
Genital Mycoplasmas	13

infection. Laboratory data should include a complete blood count and differential count and serum blood urea nitrogen and serum creatinine determinations. A urinalysis should be obtained. A gram stain of the lochia should be obtained in patients with a high fever within the first 24 hours. Sheets of gram positive cocci or gram positive rods with fragments of muscle are of great concern and point to streptococcal or clostridial infection. The patient should have a complete set of cultures: urine, two or three sets of blood cultures, a cervical and a transcervical culture of the endometrial cavity. The results of the cultures can significantly alter the cost and management of postoperative infection. The sensitivities of the organisms within the particular hospital population help to limit the use of potentially toxic antibiotics (aminoglycosides). Positive blood cultures occur in 10 to 20% of patients with endometritis. The identification of *Staphylococcus aureus* should lead to a prolonged course of antibiotics to prevent metastatic infection. The isolation of aerobic streptococci may indicate a need for high-dose penicillin therapy. The isolation of enterococci indicates a change in antibiotics, especially if the primary drug is a cephalosporin.

Antibiotic therapy is the cornerstone of treatment for puerperal endometritis. As the infection is polymicrobial, an antibiotic with a broad spectrum of action, including anaerobic coverage, is recommended. The combination of clindamycin (900 mg) and gentamicin (1.5 mg/Kg) intravenously every eight hours is considered the therapeutic standard for comparison. The weighted average cure rate in post-cesarean section endometritis in seven studies was 92% (Gibbs, 1985). Unfortunately, this antibiotic combination has some disadvantages. First, early infections (less than 48 hours) are often associated with gram positive organisms (streptococci). In these cases, penicillin (4 million units Q 4 hours) should be added to the regimen. Second, both drugs have potentially serious side effects. Diarrhea (6 to 8%) can occur with clindamycin. Aminoglycoside therapy has the potential for nephro- or ototoxicity. Therapeutic aminoglycoside levels may be difficult to obtain in obstetric patients using a standard dosing regimen. Testing aminoglycoside levels are recommended for patients with poor response, obesity or renal disease. Third, cost concerns are becoming more important. Many drugs, frequent doses and concurrent laboratory testing make this combination less appealing financially (Iams and Chawla, 1984).

Some of the newer synthetic penicillins and cephalosporins may have a place in the treatment of endometritis. Cefoxitin, cefotetan, piperacillin, cefotaxime, and cefoperazone have favorable activity against genital tract flora. Single-drug therapy, infrequent dosing (cefotetan) and a wide margin of safety are attractive features. The weighted average cure rates with these drugs approach 85 to 90% (Gibbs, 1985). However, the research on them is incomplete. The current studies involve a relatively low number of patients, and conclusions may be biased by patient selection (post-vaginal vs. post-cesarean endometritis), study methodology (definitions of failure) and dosage definition.

The management of endometritis also includes serial examinations to evaluate response. The temperature curve is a critical monitor. The patient should have a clear response within 48 hours after initiation of therapy and should be afebrile by the third or fourth day. The breasts, wound, intravenous sites and uterus should be examined daily. Uterine tenderness will also improve over a 48 to 72 hour period. Antipyretics should be used in a one-time dose only to treat symptoms. Fever, per se, has an important antimicrobial function. Intravenous antibiotics should be continued until the patient has been afebrile for 48 hours. A total of four to five days of intravenous therapy is recommended. Oral antibiotics are not needed if intravenous therapy has been adequate. In cases in which bacteremia has occurred, a short course (five days) of oral antibiotics may be used, although there is no scientific support for this management.

Antibiotic failure should be considered after 48 to 72 hours of persistent high fever. The causes of antibiotic failure include: (1) wound infection; (2) pelvic hematoma, "plegmon," or abscess; (3) resistant organisms; (4) septic thrombophlebitis; (5) inadequate drug dose or improper route of administration; (6) non-genital infection; (7) a non-infectious source of fever, such as a drug reaction. The patient should be thoroughly examined to rule in or out these diagnoses and the workup includes:

1. Thorough physical examination, including a pelvic examination.

2. Check of cultures and sensitivity.

3. Review of dose, route and levels of antibiotics.

4. A pelvic ultrasonograph or a computerized axial tomographic study can be helpful in the diagnosis of abscess, hematoma or retained products of conception.

The management of failed antibiotic therapy should consist of "triple" therapy: an aminoglycoside, clindamycin, and penicillin. This may include adding penicillin to the combination of clindamycin and aminoglycoside or discontinuing a cephalosporin and starting "triple" therapy. In patients with a fever, in whom other signs or symptoms are minimal, a drug fever can be suspected. The presence of eosinophilia can be helpful in making a diagnosis. In this case, the drugs may be stopped and the patient observed for 48 hours. If fever recurs, the patient should have a complete set of cultures, and triple therapy should be initiated. Surgical intervention is indicated in patients with abscess, myonecrosis or septic pelvic thrombophlebitis who are not responding to heparin and antibiotics.

If a triple therapy regimen has not improved the clinical picture within 24 to 48 hours, septic thrombophlebitis must be suspected. Intravenous heparin is started in conjunction with antibiotic therapy. The partial thromboplastin time (PTT) should be maintained at one and one-half to two times the control. Response should occur within 48 hours, and treatment should be continued for 10 to 14 days.

Postpartum Hemorrhage. Postpartum hemorrhage remains a significant risk despite the technologic advances of modern obstetrics. Hemorrhage accounts for 13.4% of maternal deaths and is the third leading cause of maternal death (Kaunitz et al, 1985). Hemorrhage is the chief reason for peripartum hysterectomy. Postpartum hemorrhage is a problem after normal vaginal delivery as well. Without the use of oxytocic drugs in the fourth stage, 12.2% of women require aggressive management of perceived excessive postpartum bleeding (Howard et al, 1964).

Estimates of postpartum blood loss are very inaccurate. Table 11–27 depicts the incidence of blood loss of over 500 ml after vaginal delivery with increasing sensitivity of the technique of blood loss measurement. Newton and co-workers (1961) noted that when the physician estimated the blood loss to be greater than 500 ml, his estimate was on average 34% less than the actual loss. A variety of factors affect the incidence of blood loss associated with delivery. These include primiparity ($+179$ ml), episiotomy (mediolateral, $+153$ ml) and parity of six or more ($+176$ ml) (Newton et al, 1961). Oxytocin and ergot derivatives significantly reduce blood loss (Sorbe, 1978; Howard et al, 1964). By using intravascular volume measurements, Pritchard (1965) reported significant changes related to the number of fetuses and the method of delivery. The mean blood loss for vaginal delivery of a single fetus was 505 ml; vaginal delivery of twins, 905 ml; repeat cesarean section, 905 ml; and repeat cesarean hysterectomy, 1435 ml.

The maternal physiologic response to acute blood loss results in an activation of the sympathetic nervous system and a release of stress hormones. Activation of the sympathetic nervous system increases peripheral vascular resistance and cardiac output. The release of antidiuretic hormone and mineralocorticoids increases water and salt conservation by the kidney. Intravascular hypovolemia stimulates the renin-angiotensin system, which, in turn, increases peripheral vascular resistance and fluid retention. As intravascular hypovolemia increases, vasoconstriction and hypoperfusion of non-essential tissue result in lactic acidosis, capillary injury and microaggregate coagulation. Endothelial damage allows the escape of protein-rich fluid into the extravascular spaces. This potentiates the hypovolemia and lactic acidosis. The release of tissue thromboplastin from damaged capillary beds activates the coagulation cascade, further increasing peripheral vascular resistance and tissue hypoperfusion. The release of catecholamines, glucagon, growth hormone and glucocorticoids stimulates gluconeogenesis and inhibits insulin secretion. Concurrent lipolysis increases the concentration of free fatty acids in serum, which, in turn, inhibits insulin-mediated glucose uptake by the cells. Intracellular hypoglycemia stimulates anaerobic metabolism. Hypoperfusion potentiates the buildup of lactic acid. Local tissue hypoxia

Table 11–27. *Measurement of Postpartum Hemorrhage after Vaginal Delivery*

Author	Technique	Percentage with Hemorrhage ≥ 500 ml
Howard et al (1964)	Physician estimate	3.2
Newton (1966)	Direct collection	22.0
Pritchard et al (1962)	Red cell volume loss	39.0

and acidosis ultimately result in failure of the cardiovascular system, and cardiac output falls.

Risk factors for postpartum hemorrhage include prolonged labor, induced labor, multiple gestation, fetal macrosomia, chorioamnionitis, leiomyoma, low placental implantation and retained products of conception. Unfortunately, postpartum hemorrhage often occurs silently, acutely and without warning. It has few symptoms and changes in sensorium may be masked by analgesia or the lingering effects of anesthesia. Sheets and blankets can cover considerable blood loss. Pritchard (1965) noted that 50% of blood loss was absorbed into sheets rather than the bucket. Fortunately, the recently postpartum patient is protected by the normal expansion of the blood volume in pregnancy by 1500 to 2000 ml. Usually, blood loss up to 1500 ml is well compensated.

The signs and symptoms of postpartum bleeding of more than 1000 ml relate to the sympathetically mediated cardiovascular response (pallor, diaphoresis), hypovolemia (syncope, orthostatic changes) and tissue hypoperfusion and hypoxia (anxiety, confusion, oliguria, dyspnea, tachypnea). Orthostatic changes, tested by rechecking blood pressure and pulse with the patient in the sitting position, are a reliable indicator of severe blood loss. A postural drop of more than 10 mmHg in systolic blood pressure or a postural increase in heart rate by 10 BPM suggests a 10 to 15% decrease in circulating blood volume. Postural changes are insufficient grounds for the diagnosis of shock unless they are accompanied by evidence of tissue hypoxia.

Postpartum bleeding should be managed as follows:

1. Massage the fundus.

2. Establish adequate large bore intravenous access.

3. Administer oxytocin at 20 units per 1000 ml of Ringer's lactate in a 500 ml fluid challenge. Methergine, 0.2 mg I.M., may be given if there is no hypertension.

4. Examine the rectum, vulva, vagina and cervix for lacerations and hematomas. Often blood clots in the lower uterine segment inhibit adequate uterine contraction. These may be manually expressed.

5. If atony persists, give prostaglandin. Prostaglandin E_2, 20 mg vaginal suppositories, placed in the vaginal fornix can be effective. However, washout can limit its use. Fifteen-methyl analogues of prostaglandin F_2, 0.25 mg, can be given intramuscularly or intramyometrially. Until the uterus contracts, manual

compression of the uterus (see Fig. 11–3B) will limit blood loss. Ultrasonography can be very useful in persistent postpartum hemorrhage. Lee and co-workers (1981) noted an empty uterus in 42 of 56 patients with postpartum bleeding. In these cases, curettage would not be helpful and might delay more definitive surgery.

The management of hemorrhagic shock is discussed in Chapter 4; it is summarized as follows:

1. Monitor CBC, blood chemistry and bleeding profile and arterial blood gases.

2. Replace adequate amounts of fluid. Crystalloids such as 5% dextrose in lactated Ringer's solution help maintain acid-base status and hemostatis. Colloid transfusion in the form of the freshest available blood replaces the oxygen-carrying capacity and intravascular oncotic pressure. Fresh frozen plasma helps correct the dilutional coagulopathy secondary to massive transfusion of banked blood.

3. Monitor hemodynamic changes adequately. A Swan-Ganz catheter provides the best measure of intravascular pressure and cardiovascular function.

4. Monitor arterial blood gas determinations to measure ventilation and tissue hypoxia/acidosis. Oxygen is given at 4 to 6 liters/minute by mask in all cases.

5. Attempt to rapidly diagnose lacerations, and treat uterine atony pharmacologically, with oxytocin, Methergine and prostaglandins.

Pharmacologic support of the cardiovascular system can be vital to provide time for conservative or surgical control of hemorrhage. However, these drugs do not replace adequate volume expansion, especially in the usual patient with postpartum hemorrhage. The best pharmacologic manipulation of the cardiovascular system is based on adequate measures of preload, afterload and ventricular contractility. Swan-Ganz catheterization is essential for these measurements. The preload is measured by the pulmonary artery wedge pressure (adequate = 6 to 12 mmHg). The afterload is estimated by the systemic vascular resistance (normal = 800 to 1200 dynes/sec/cm^{-5}). Left ventricular stroke work index (normal = 51 to 61 gm/beat/M^2) gives a rough estimate of left ventricular contractility. In patients with a systole blood pressure greater than 90 mmHg, peripheral hypoperfusion (increased systemic vascular resistance) and an elevated "wedge" pressure, a vasodilator such as nitroprusside, nitroglycerine or hydralazine may be helpful. If contractility or excess vasodilatation is an issue, dobutamine HC1, dopamine HC1 or epinephrine may be valuable. The coordination of pharmacologic therapy of shock and hemodynamic monitoring is discussed in a review by Prough and co-workers (1985).

Occasionally, inotropic agents (dopamine) have been used empirically prior to adequate hemodynamic monitoring. This decision implies the need to establish monitoring as soon as possible and indicates that further administration of a volume expander will not improve cardiac output or tissue perfusion. Dopamine HC1 is one of the most commonly employed drugs for shock states. In the dose range of 0.5 to 2 microgram/Kg/min, the drug facilitates kidney perfusion. In doses of 2 to 10 microgram/Kg/min, increasing beta adrenergic effects are observed. Above 20 microgram/Kg/min, dopamine causes alpha-receptor–mediated peripheral constriction.

If postpartum bleeding persists after the appearance of shock and conservative management fails, surgical control must be initiated without delay. Older techniques, such as uterine packing (Hester, 1975; Lester et al, 1965) and intrauterine lavage (Fribourg et al, 1973) are primarily temporizing methods. Although they may be effective, they may also delay more definitive surgical therapy. In institutions where skilled arteriography is available, selective pelvic artery embolization may be a preferred technique because (1) the bleeding site may be obscure at the time of surgery, (2) surgical injury to other pelvic organs is avoided, (3) a hysterectomy may be avoided, (4) hypogastric artery ligation may fail because of a rich collateral supply and (5) continued extravasation of blood can be visualized by fluoroscopy (Glickman, 1983; Pais et al, 1980). Selective embolization may be highly effective. The success rate was reported to be about 90% in a heterogeneous group of patients (Glickman, 1983; Pais et al, 1980). The complications include ischemia in the distribution of the blocked artery, embolization of non-target arteries (3 to 5%), toxic effects of the contrast material on a hypoperfused kidney, radiation dose and delay of definitive surgery in the case of uterine rupture.

Classic surgical control of hemorrhage may be the only way to save a rapidly deteriorating patient. The surgical approach involves (1) sequential bilateral uterine and utero-ovarian artery ligation, (2) bilateral hypogastric artery ligation and (3) hysterectomy. The primary function of artery ligation is to reduce the pulse pressure rather than actual flow, because of collateral circulation. Uterine artery ligation is helpful only with fundal bleeding; bleeding from cervical or vaginal lacerations will not be controlled.

Thrombophlebitis. Pregnancy increases the risk of thrombophlebitis. The normal physiologic response to pregnancy increases coagulation factors I, II, VII, IX and X. There is increased platelet adhesiveness, and the placenta and amniotic fluid are rich in tissue thromboplastin. Dextrorotation of the enlarged uterus compresses the right ovarian and uterine veins against the ureter and pelvic brim. The resultant stasis compounds the risk of thrombophlebitis. When the vascular injury and infection associated with cesarean section are added, the patient is at special risk of thrombophlebitis.

Thrombophlebitis can occur as a classic deep venous thrombosis in the legs or as pelvic or ovarian vein thrombosis. Deep venous thrombosis of the legs presents either with a painful leg or with the unpredicted complication of pulmonary embolism, up to six weeks postpartum. Physical signs of thrombosis of the legs include asymmetric leg enlargement (more than 2 cm difference in circumference), palpation of a tender cord or leg tenderness. Peripheral venous thrombosis is diagnosed by impedence plethysmography, Doppler ultrasound or venography. These issues are discussed in Chapters 2 and 4.

Septic pelvic thrombophlebitis complicates 1 to 2% of cases of post-cesarean endomyometritis (Duff and Gibbs, 1983). In these cases, bacterial endotoxin or direct infection initiates thrombosis in the uterine and ovarian veins. A right-sided predominance is predictable from angiographic documentation of greater venous return on the right side. Septic pelvic thrombophlebitis has two features—acute ovarian vein thrombosis and "enigmatic fever." Ovarian vein thrombosis presents suddenly two to four days postoperatively. The patient appears acutely ill with right-sided abdominal and pelvic pain. Physical examination reveals a mild to moderate temperature elevation and constant tachycardia. A right-sided pelvic mass can be palpated in 60 to 70% of cases. Signs of paralytic ileus and pulmonary disease may be present. On the other hand, "enigmatic fever" appears slowly four to eight days postoperatively in a less ill-appearing patient. The fever curve displays intermittent high spikes. The patient's examination is often unremarkable with minimal tenderness and no masses or ileus.

Diagnostic confirmation of pelvic thrombophlebitis is difficult. Right ovarian vein thrombosis can occasionally be diagnosed by ultrasound or CT scan. This shows a tubular mass extending from the ovary toward the retroperitoneum. Often the diagnosis of ovarian vein thrombosis is made at the time of laparotomy for suspected abscess, appendicitis or ovarian torsion. Otherwise, the diagnosis of septic pelvic thrombosis is a diagnosis by exclusion and a rapid response to anticoagulant therapy.

The danger of thrombophlebitis is pulmonary embolism. Untreated deep venous thrombosis of the legs with subsequent pulmonary embolism has a 10 to 20% mortality. Pulmonary embolism from septic pelvic thrombophlebitis has an even higher risk because of possible metastatic infection. Approximately one third of patients with septic pelvic thrombophlebitis will have abnormal ventilation-perfusion lung scans (Duff and Gibbs, 1983). The diagnosis of pulmonary embolism is suspected with the sudden appearance of dyspnea, tachycardia and tachypnea. Physical examination reveals cyanosis, abnormal breath sounds and, occasionally, signs of right ventricular strain. The key diagnostic test is an arterial blood gas determination. Ninety percent of patients with pulmonary emboli will have a PaO_2 less than 80 mmHg and almost all have a PaO_2 less than 90 mmHg.

Radiologic confirmation includes a chest x-ray, ventilation-perfusion lung scan and pulmonary arteriography. These techniques are discussed in Chapter 4. There are several important considerations in the post-cesarean section patient. In most cases the parturient woman has little pulmonary disease. Discrepancies between the ventilation-perfusion (V/Q) scan and the chest x-ray are less likely to be explained by prior lung disease: the V/Q scan may therefore be more sensitive. Pulmonary emboli from septic pelvic thrombophlebitis often involve smaller vessels than do the classic deep venous thrombosis of the leg. A shower of small emboli may be missed by pulmonary arteriography; the sensitivity of this test may be decreased.

The primary therapy for septic pelvic thrombophlebitis is therapeutic heparin for 10 days with concomitant broad spectrum antibiotics. Unless the bacteria, especially anaerobes, are treated, clot formation will persist and heparin therapy will fail. Anticoagulant therapy is discussed in Chapter 4. The length of anticoagulation is quite different in the post-cesarean patient than in the gynecologic patient. In the postpartum period, hypercoagulopathy and venous stasis disappear completely by six to ten

weeks. As soon as endothelial repair and clot organization have occurred, the post-cesarean patient is at minimal risk for recurrent thrombosis. On the other hand, anticoagulation has a clear risk for ovarian hemorrhage once ovulation returns. In most cases of septic pelvic thrombophlebitis anticoagulation beyond 10 to 14 days of heparin therapy is not needed. However, if the patient has a previous history of thrombosis or has had pulmonary emboli, anticoagulation should be extended for six weeks. In cases in which the patient has a history of thrombosis while not on birth control pills or pregnant, anticoagulation should be considered for three to six months.

Surgical therapy for septic pulmonary thrombophlebitis should be reserved for those in whom heparin and antibiotic therapy have failed, and for those who experience pulmonary emboli while on therapeutic doses of heparin. In these cases, the infected vein should be ligated. The vena cava should be ligated only if the clot extends to this vein or if the patient has experienced recurrent emboli. In the peripartum period, the ovarian veins should be ligated as well as the vena cava. Thrombectomy is not performed unless there is clear abscess formation or the renal veins are involved. If ovarian vein thrombosis is found after exploratory laparotomy, the veins should not be ligated and heparin should be initiated postoperatively.

Adverse Effects on the Neonate. The popular conception is that cesarean section is less traumatic for the neonate than vaginal delivery. Indeed, this may be true when the clinical situation has excessive fetal risks such as prolonged arrest pattern in labor or fetal distress. However, population studies have suggested that cesarean section has some neonatal risk. Benson and co-workers (1969) reported on the neonatal risks of 43,219 prospectively studied births in relation to mode of delivery. Neonates of 37 to 40 weeks' gestation from elective cesarean deliveries and multiparous vaginal deliveries were compared. The results showed that cesarean birth was associated with an increase in low birth weight (2500 grams or less), neonatal asphyxia (Apgar scores 0 to 3) and neonatal mortality. General anesthesia and inaccurate dating were used to explain these differences. Increased respiratory disease among premature and term neonates delivered by cesarean section has been confirmed by several authors (Hjalmarson et al, 1982; Cohen and Carson, 1985; Newton et al, 1986; Bowers et al, 1982; Heritage and Cunningham, 1985). Iatrogenic prematurity does not explain all the risks of respiratory disease in term elective cesarean section (Schreiner et al, 1982). A number of possible explanations include the lack of the following:

1. Labor-stimulated lung fluid absorption.

2. Labor-stimulated lung maturation and surfactant release.

3. Labor-induced diminution of pulmonary vascular resistance (Milner et al, 1978; Callen et al, 1979; Jacobstein et al, 1982).

The practical aspect of allowing labor to occur prior to elective cesarean section is that labor seems to reduce the respiratory risk significantly (Bowers et al, 1982; Cohen and Carson, 1985).

The increased incidence of low Apgar scores in cesarean-delivered babies is harder to confirm. Many factors can lead to low Apgar scores. Some of these include antepartum risk factors, gestational age, type of anesthesia or duration of uterine incision time. No study has adequately controlled these factors. Gilstrap and co-workers (1984) compared primary cesarean section to indicated forceps delivery with control for indication for the procedure and found a significantly increased risk of Apgar scores of 6 or less in the cesarean-delivered group. However, an umbilical cord pH of less than 7.20 did not differ with the method of delivery. This discrepancy may relate to decreased fetal activity from cesarean anesthesia or a bias toward low Apgar scores when neonates are evaluated after cesarean delivery.

The blood volume of the neonate can be significantly affected by management of the neonate prior to cord ligation. Sisson and co-workers (1973), in a prospective study, compared the time of cord clamping and altitude of the fetus. When the fetus was held for 180 seconds at 15 cm above the maternal abdomen there was a significant fall in the blood volume and hematocrit at four hours of age. The largest blood volumes and highest hematocrits were found in infants held 15 cm below the maternal abdomen.

Several other neonatal effects have been attributed to cesarean section. Neonatal trauma can occur at cesarean section. Fracture of long bones and peripheral nerve injuries have been reported with difficult breech extraction at cesarean section. The presenting part can be incised upon entry into the uterus if caution is not observed. In an occiput posterior position, the fetal face and eyes are at risk during the uterine incision. Caution is also warranted during the volume expansion prior to anesthesia. The preoperative infusion of dextrose or hyponatremic solutions correlates with neonatal hypoglycemia and hyponatremia (Grylack et al, 1984). Volume expansion with Ringer's lactate is recommended.

Disruption of Mother-Infant Bonding. Numerous authors have proposed and demonstrated a "maternal sensitive period" lasting for about 12 hours after birth (Klaus and Kennell, 1976). Separation of the mother-infant dyad has significant effects on neonatal neurobehavioral activity, maternal behavior and breastfeeding rates. Cesarean delivery has the potential of delaying and blunting bonding behavior. McClellan and Cabianea (1980) performed a randomized intervention study involving elective cesarean section deliveries and mother-infant contact within the first 12 hours. In the experimental group the mother-infant dyad was given 5 to 15 minutes of visual contact in the delivery room and extensive skin-to-skin contact in the recovery room. The control group had the routine management, which included less than 5 minutes visual contact in the delivery room and complete separation in the recovery room. The experimental dyads showed significantly more bonding behavior than did those in the control group. The implications of this study are obvious: mother-infant contact needs to be maximized even in the cesarean section patient.

Other Immediate Postoperative Complications of Cesarean Section. Wound infection, urinary tract infection, urinary retention and paralytic ileus are discussed in detail in Chapter 4. High progesterone levels during pregnancy are associated with smooth muscle relaxation. This contributes to a larger amount of bowel gas in the immediate postpartum period. Bowel gas patterns have been prospectively studied by Lawaetz and Jansen (1976). Among 100 patients who had radiography on the third and fifth postoperative days, the mean cecal diameter was 6.4 cm, and 90% of the free subdiaphragmatic air had disappeared by the fifth day after the cesarean section.

LONG-TERM COMPLICATIONS OF CESAREAN SECTION

The long-term adverse effects of cesarean section include repeat cesarean section, placenta previa, placenta accreta, dysfunctional uterine bleeding, possible infertility from postoperative infection and adverse psychologic effects. Most reviews concerning the risk of cesarean section and subsequent trial of labor fail to evaluate these long-term dangers.

The greatest risk of a primary cesarean section is the likelihood of a repeat cesarean section. Despite the recent interest in and support for a trial of labor, the frequency of elective repeat cesarean section has not changed except in teaching hospitals (Petitti, 1985). Currently over 95% of subsequent pregnancies after cesarean delivery are terminated by repeat cesarean section. The operative complications of repeat cesarean section vary with the presence of medical and obstetric disease, rupture of membranes, gestational age and the presence or absence of labor. In general, the mortality and morbidity risks of elective repeat cesarean section are about one-half those of non-elective primary cesarean section. One exception is that intraoperative trauma to the bladder seems to double with each successive cesarean section. Another is the possible neonatal risk of respiratory disorders secondary to prematurity or lack of labor.

Previous cesarean section is a risk factor for both symptomatic (Singh and Gupta, 1981; Clark et al, 1985) and asymptomatic midtrimester placenta previa (Newton et al, 1984). Clark and co-workers (1985) found the incidence of placenta previa to rise linearly with the number of previous cesarean sections: 0 cesareans, 0.26%; 1 cesarean, 0.65%; 2 cesareans, 1.8%; 3 cesareans, 3% and 4 or more cesareans, 10%. More importantly, the incidence of placenta previa or placenta accreta also rises with the number of previous cesarean sections. When placenta previa was associated with 2 or more cesarean sections, 11 of 21 patients had placenta accreta. Overall, 82% of patients with placenta previa and placenta accreta underwent cesarean hysterectomy.

Infertility subsequent to pelvic infection is always a concern. Despite the frequency of post-cesarean endometritis, little has been written about the subsequent fertility of these patients. Hurry and co-workers (1984), in a retrospective review of 1,131 potentially fertile post-cesarean women over a five year period, found that 89% became pregnant. Endometritis and pelvic cellulitis did not affect the conception rate. However, if endometritis was complicated by pelvic abscess (2.7%), the conception rate fell to 43% after five years. Zdeb and co-workers (1984) performed a prospective population study (in upstate New York) to examine the effect of primary cesarean section on frequency, spacing and outcome of pregnancies subsequent to primary cesarean section. A cohort of 5,513

women in whom pregnancy was terminated by a primary cesarean section were followed for five years. They were matched by race, maternal age, maternal education and complications of pregnancy to a similar group of women who had an uncomplicated vaginal delivery. The loss of follow-up caused by outmigration was not considered to affect the cesarean group differentially. The pregnancy rate in the cesarean group was 11% less than in the vaginal group, yet the spacing was not significantly different. The fall in the fertility rate can be explained by medical and psychologic factors. Tubal disease resulting from clinical or subclinical endometritis could account for it. An alternative explanation would be psychologic trauma secondary to a difficult birth or the feeling of failure (Cohen and Esther, 1983). However, one would expect a spacing effect as well if psychologic trauma was major.

The disruption of uterine architecture can contribute to dysfunctional uterine bleeding, for example, with leiomyoma. Previous cesarean section scar(s) may disrupt the normal hemostatic function of the myometrium. Weed (1959) suggested a high incidence of subsequent non-pregnancy hysterectomy after one or more previous cesarean sections. Among those patients followed for eight years or more after cesarean section, 27% had hysterectomy. The indications for the hysterectomy seemed to be more often related to menstrual abnormalities and seemed to be more common after previous classic uterine incisions. Although the data were provocative, the study suffered from methodologic weaknesses and loss of follow-up. More recently the relationship between cesarean section and adenomyosis has been examined (Harris et al, 1985). In hysterectomy specimens, 15% of old cesarean section scars had adenomyosis. Although hysterectomy for menstrual abnormalities seemed common, many cases had other abnormalities (leiomyoma) to explain the indications for hysterectomy.

REFERENCES

Adamson K, Meyers RE: Late deceleration and brain tolerance of the fetal monkey to intrapartum asphyxia. *Am. J. Obstet. Gynecol.* 128:893, 1977.

Ahuja GL, Willoughby MLN et al: Massive subaponeurotic hemorrhage in infants born by vacuum extraction. *Br. Med. J.* 3:743, 1969.

Aldridge AH, Wootson P: Analysis of end results of labor in primiparas after spontaneous versus prophylactic methods of delivery. *J. Obstet. Gynecol.* 30:554, 1935.

Alexopoulos KA: The importance of breech delivery in the pathogenesis of brain damage and results of a long-term follow-up. *Clin. Pediatr.* 12:248, 1973.

Allen JR: Nosocomial obstetric infections and hospital epidemiology. In Iffy L, Charles D (Eds.): *Operative Perinatology: Invasive Obstetric Technique.* New York, MacMillian Publishing Co., 1984.

Ali Z, Lowry M: Early maternal child contact: effects on later behavior. *Dev. Med. Child Neurol.* 23:337, 1981.

Andersen HF, Johnson TRB et al: Gestational age assessment. I. Analysis of individual clinical observation. *Am. J. Obstet. Gynecol.* 139:173, 1981.

Anderson ABM, Turnbull AC: Relationship between length of gestation and cervical dilatation, uterine contractility and other factors during pregnancy. *Am. J. Obstet. Gynecol.* 105:1207, 1969.

Arsura EL, Fazio RA, Wickremesinghe PC: Pseudomembranous colitis following prophylactic antibiotic use in primary cesarean section. *Am. J. Obstet. Gynecol.* 151:87, 1985.

Arthur RK: Postmortem cesarean section. *Am. J. Obstet. Gynecol.* 132:175, 1978.

Atherton HE, Williamson PJ: A clinical comparison of extraperitoneal cesarean section and low cervical cesarean section for potentially or frankly infected parturient. *Am. J. Obstet. Gynecol.* 68:1091, 1954.

Baerthlein WC, Moodley S et al: Comparison of maternal and neonatal morbidity in midforceps delivery and midpelvic vacuum extraction. *Obstet. Gynecol.* 67:594, 1986.

Barson AJ, Tasker M et al: Impact of improved perinatal care on the causes of death. *Arch. Dis. Child.* 59:199, 1984.

Beischer NA: Pelvic contraction in breech presentation. *J. Obstet. Gynaecol. Br. Commonwlth.* 66:421, 1966.

Beischer NA: The anatomical and functional results of mediolateral episiotomy. *Med. J. Aust.* 2:189, 1967.

Benedetti TJ, Starzyk P, Frost F: Maternal deaths in Washington State. *Obstet. Gynecol.* 66:99, 1985.

Benson RC, Berendes H, Weiss W: Fetal compromise during elective cesarean section II. A report from the Collaborative Project. *Am. J. Obstet. Gynecol.* 105:579, 1969.

Berkus MD, Ramamurthy RS et al: Cohort study of silastic obstetric vacuum cup deliveries. I. Safety of the instrument. *Obstet. Gynecol.* 66:503, 1985.

Berry CD Jr, Cross RR Jr: Urethral meatal caliber in circumcised and uncircumcised males. *Am. J. Dis. Child.* 92:152, 1956.

Bishop EH: Pelvic scoring for elective induction. *Obstet. Gynecol.* 24:266, 1964.

Bjerre I, Dahlin K: The long-term development of children delivered by vacuum extraction. *Dev. Med. Child Neurol.* 16:378, 1974.

Blanco JD, Diaz KC et al: *Chlamydia trachomatis* isolation in patients with endometritis after cesarean section. *Am. J. Obstet. Gynecol.* 152:278, 1985.

Blanco JD, Gibbs RS: Infections following classical cesarean section. *Obstet. Gynecol.* 55:167, 1980.

Block BS, Mercer LJ et al: Clostridum difficile associated diarrhea follows perioperation prophylaxis with cefoxitin. *Am. J. Obstet. Gynecol.* 153:835, 1985.

Bowers SK, MacDonald HM, Shapiro ED: Prevention of iatrogenic neonatal respiratory distress syndrome: Elective repeat cesarean section and spontaneous labor. *Am. J. Obstet. Gynecol.* 143:186, 1982.

Bowes WA: Clinical aspects of normal and abnormal labor. In Creasy RK, Resnick R (Eds.): *Maternal Fetal Medicine.* Philadelphia, W. B. Saunders Company, 1984.

Boyd ME, Asher RH et al: Fetal macrosomia: prediction

risks and proposed management. *Obstet. Gynecol.* 61:715, 1983.

Braverman J, Roux JF: Screening for the patient at risk for postpartum depression. *Obstet. Gynecol.* 56:731, 1978.

Brendel C, Peterson G, Mehl LE: Routine episiotomy and pelvic symptomatology. *Women Health* 5:49, 1980.

Buekens P, Lagasse R et al: Episiotomy and third degree tears. *Br. J. Obstet. Gynaecol.* 92:820, 1985.

Caldeyro-Barcia R, Schwarcz R et al: Adverse perinatal effects of early amniotomy during labor. In Gluck L (Ed.): *Modern Perinatal Medicine.* Chicago, Yearbook Medical Publishers, 1974.

Callen P, Goldsworth S et al: Mode of delivery and lecithin/sphingomyelin ratio. *Br. J. Obstet. Gynaecol.* 86:965, 1979.

Caterini H, Langer A et al: Fetal risks in hyperextension of the fetal head in breech presentation. *Am. J. Obstet. Gynecol.* 123:632, 1975.

Cesarean Childbirth. NIH Publication No. 82-2067, U.S. Department of Health and Human Services. October 1981.

Chestnut DH, Eden RD et al: Peripartum hysterectomy: a review of cesarean and postpartum hysterectomy. *Obstet. Gynecol.* 65:365, 1985.

Chiswick ML, James DK: Kielland's forceps: association with neonatal morbidity and mortality. *Br. Med. J.* 1:7, 1979.

Choate JW, Lund CJ: Emergency cesarean section: an analysis of maternal and fetal results in 1,770 operations. *Am. J. Obstet. Gynecol.* 100:703, 1968.

Clark SL, Koonings PP, Phelan JP: Placenta previa/accreta and prior cesarean section. *Obstet. Gynecol.* 66:89, 1985.

Clark SL, Yeh SY et al: Emergency hysterectomy for obstetric hemorrhage. *Obstet. Gynecol.* 64:376, 1984.

Coats PM, Chan KK et al: A comparison between midline and mediolateral episiotomies. *Br. J. Obstet. Gynaecol.* 87:408, 1980.

Cogan JE, Harris JW: Rectal complications after perineorrhaphy and episiotomy. *Arch. Surg.* 93:634, 1966.

Cohen M, Carson BS: Respiratory morbidity benefit of awaiting onset of labor after elective cesarean section. *Obstet. Gynecol.* 65:818, 1985.

Cohen NW, Esther LD: *Silent Knife: Cesarean Prevention and Vaginal Birth After Cesarean.* Boston, Bergmen and Gravey, 1983.

Cohen WR: Influence of duration of second stage labor on perinatal outcome and puerperal morbidity. *Obstet. Gynecol.* 49:266, 1977.

Collea JV, Chein C, Quilligan EJ: The randomized management of term frank breech presentation: a study of 208 cases. *Am. J. Obstet. Gynecol.* 137:235, 1980.

Cowett RM, Oh W: Foam stability prediction of respiratory distress in infants delivered by repeat cesarean section. *N. Engl. J. Med.* 295:1222, 1976.

Crichton D: A reliable method of establishing the level of the fetal head in obstetrics. *S. Afr. Med. J.* 48:784, 1974.

Cross WG, Pitkin RM: Laminaria as an adjunct in induction of labor. *Obstet. Gynecol.* 51:606, 1978.

Cunningham FG, Leveno KJ et al: Perioperative antimicrobials for cesarean delivery: before or after cord clamping. *Obstet. Gynecol.* 62:151, 1983.

Cyr RM, Usher RH, McLean FH: Changing patterns of birth asphyxia and trauma over 20 years. *Am. J. Obstet. Gynecol.* 148:490, 1984.

Davidson AC, Weaver JB et al: The relationship between the ease of forceps delivery and the speed of cervical dilatation. *Br. J. Obstet. Gynaecol.* 80:279, 1976.

Davis LK, Rosen SL et al: Cesarean births in Massachusetts. Boston, *Mass. Dept. Public Health*, October, 1984.

Davis RO, Phillips JB et al: Fatal meconium aspiration syndrome occurring despite the airway management considered appropriate. *Am. J. Obstet. Gynecol.* 151:731, 1985.

De Chateau P, Wiberg B: A study of factors promoting and inhibiting lactation. *Dev. Med. Child Neurol.* 19:575, 1977.

Dell DL, Sightler SE et al: Soft cup vacuum extraction: a comparison of outlet delivery. *Obstet. Gynecol.* 66:624, 1985.

Dennen, EH: *Forceps Deliveries*, Ed. 2. Philadelphia, F. A. Davis Company, 1964.

Dennen EH: Technique of application for low forceps. *Clin. Obstet. Gynecol.* 8:834, 1965.

Diaz AG, Schwarcz R et al: Vertical position during the first stage of the course of labor and neonatal outcome. *Eur. J. Obstet. Gynecol. Reprod. Biol.* 11:1, 1980.

Dierker LJ, Rosen MG et al: The midforceps: maternal and neonatal outcomes. *Am. J. Obstet. Gynecol.* 152:176, 1985.

Dierker LJ, Rosen MG et al: Midforceps deliveries: Long-term outcome of infants. *Am. J. Obstet. Gynecol.* 154:764, 1986.

D'Orban PT: Women who kill their children. *Br. J. Psychiatry* 134:560, 1979.

Duff P, Gibbs RS: Pelvic vein thrombophlebitis: diagnostic dilemma and therapeutic challenge. *Obstet. Gynecol. Surv.* 38:365, 1983.

Durfee RB: Elective extraperitoneal cesarean section. *Surg. Obstet. Gynecol.* 110:173, 1960.

Egge K, Lyng G, Maltau JM: Effect of instrumental delivery on the frequency and severity of retinal hemorrhage in the newborn. *Acta Obstet. Gynecol. Scand.* 60:153, 1981.

Ehlers N, Jensen JK, Hansen KB: Retinal hemorrhage in the newborn. Comparison of delivery by forceps and by vacuum extraction. *Acta Opthalmol.* 52:73, 1974.

Eisenkop SM, Richman R et al: Urinary tract injury during cesarean section. *Obstet. Gynecol.* 60:591, 1982.

Ekman-Ordeberg G, Uldbjerg N, Ulmsten U: Comparison of intravenous oxytocin and vaginal prostaglandin E_2 gel in women with unripe cervices and premature rupture of membranes. *Obstet. Gynecol.* 66:307, 1985.

Elliot JP, Flaherty JF: The use of breast stimulation to ripen the cervix in term pregnancies. *Am. J. Obstet. Gynecol.* 145:553, 1983.

Elliot JP, Flaherty JF: The use of breast stimulation to prevent post-date pregnancy. *Am. J. Obstet. Gynecol.* 149:628, 1984.

Eschenbach DA, Wager GP: Puerperal infection. *Clin. Obstet. Gynecol.* 23:1003, 1980.

Evans MI, Dougan MB et al: Ripening of the human cervix with porcine ovarian relaxin. *Am. J. Obstet. Gynecol.* 147:410, 1983.

Ewing TL, Smale LE, Elliott FA: Maternal deaths associated with postpartum vulvar edema. *Am. J. Obstet. Gynecol.* 134:173, 1979.

Faber-Nijholt R, Huisjes HJ et al: Neurological follow-up of 281 children born in breech presentation in a controlled study. *Br. Med. J.* 286:9, 1983.

Feldman GB, Freiman JA: Prophylactic cesarean section at term? *N. Engl. J. Med.* 312:1264, 1985.

Filker R, Monif GRG: The significance of temperature during the first 24 hours postpartum. *Obstet. Gynecol.* 53:358, 1979.

Fischer SR: Factors associated with the occurrence of perineal lacerations. *J. Nurse-Midwif.* 24:18, 1979.

Flakman RJ, Vollman JH, Benfield DG: Iatrogenic prematurity due to elective termination of the uncomplicated pregnancy: a major perinatal health care problem. *Am. J. Obstet. Gynecol.* 132:885, 1978.

Flamm BL: Vaginal birth after cesarean section. Controversies old and new. *Clin. Obstet. Gynecol.* 28:735, 1985.

Fleischer A, Schulmann H et al: The development of fetal acidosis in the presence of an abnormal heart rate tracing. I. The average for gestational age fetus. *Am. J. Obstet. Gynecol.* 144:55, 1982.

Flynn AM, Kelly J et al: Ambulation in labor. *Br. Med. J.* 2:591, 1978.

Fons JW, Brennan JJ: Multiple cesarean sections. *Obstet. Gynecol.* 29:287, 1967.

Fribourg SRC, Rothman LA, Rovinsky JT: Intrauterine lavage for control of uterine atony. *Obstet. Gynecol.* 41:896, 1973.

Friedman EA: Patterns of labor as indicators of risk. *Clin. Obstet. Gynecol.* 16:172, 1973.

Friedman EA: Prognostic outlook. In *Labor: Clinical Evaluation and Management*. New York, Appleton-Century-Crofts, 1978.

Friedman EA, Niswander KR et al: Relation of prelabor evaluation to inductability and the course of labor. *Obstet. Gynecol.* 28:495, 1966.

Friedman EA, Sachtleben-Murray MR et al: Long-term effects of labor and delivery on offspring: a matched pair analysis. *Am. J. Obstet. Gynecol.* 150:941, 1984.

Frigoletto FD, Phillippe M et al: Avoiding iatrogenic prematurity with elective repeat cesarean section without the routine use of amniocentesis. *Am. J. Obstet. Gynecol.* 137:521, 1980.

Gibbs RS: Infection after cesarean section. *Clin. Obstet. Gynecol.* 28:697, 1985.

Gibbs RS, Jones PM, Wilder LJY: Internal fetal monitoring and maternal infection following cesarean section. *Obstet. Gynecol.* 52:193, 1978.

Gilstrap LC, Hauth JC et al: Neonatal acidosis and method of delivery. *Obstet. Gynecol.* 63:681, 1984.

Gimovsky ML, Wallace RC et al: Randomized management of the non-frank breech presentation at term: a preliminary report. *Am. J. Obstet. Gynecol.* 146:34, 1983.

Glickman MG: Pelvic artery embolization. In Berkowitz RL (Ed.): *Critical Care of the Obstetric Patient*. New York, Churchill Livingstone, 1983.

Golde S, Ledger WJ: Necrotizing fasciitis in postpartum patients: a report of four cases. *Obstet. Gynecol.* 50:670, 1977.

Gower RH, Toraya J, Miller JM: Laminaria for preinduction cervical ripening. *Obstet. Gynecol.* 60:617, 1982.

Greis JB, Bieniarz J, Scommegna A: Comparison of maternal and fetal effects of vacuum extraction with forceps or cesarean deliveries. *Obstet. Gynecol.* 57:571, 1981.

Gresham EL: Birth trauma. *Pediatr. Clin. North Am.* 22:317, 1975.

Grylack LJ, Chu SS, Scanlon JW: Use of intravenous fluids before cesarean section: effects of perinatal glucose, insulin and sodium homeostasis. *Obstet. Gynecol.* 63:654, 1984.

Hack M, Farnaroff AA et al: Neonatal distress following elective delivery. A preventable disease? *Am. J. Obstet. Gynecol.* 126:43, 1976.

Haley RW, Culver DH et al: Progress report on the evaluation of the efficacy of infection surveillance and control programs. *Am. J. Med.* 70:971, 1981.

Hall JE, Kohl SG et al: Breech presentation and perinatal mortality. *Am. J. Obstet. Gynecol.* 91:665, 1965.

Hanson HB: Current use of the extraperitoneal cesarean

section: a decade of experience. *Am. J. Obstet. Gynecol.* 149:31, 1984.

Harris BA: Acute puerperal inversion of the uterus. *Clin. Obstet. Gynecol.* 27:134, 1984a.

Harris BA: Shoulder dystocia. *Clin. Obstet. Gynecol.* 27:106, 1984b.

Harris RE: An evaluation of the median episiotomy. *Am. J. Obstet. Gynecol.* 106:660, 1970.

Harris WJ, Daniell JM, Baxter WJ: Prior cesarean section: a risk factor for adenomyosis? *J. Reprod. Med.* 30:173, 1985.

Harrison RF, Brennan M et al: Is routine episiotomy necessary? *Br. Med. J.* 288:1971, 1984.

Hayashi RH, Castillo MS, Noah ML: Management of severe postpartum hemorrhage with a prostaglandin F_2 alpha analogue. *Obstet. Gynecol.* 63:806, 1984.

Hepner WR: Some observations on facial paresis in the newborn infant: etiology and incidence. *Pediatrics* 8:494, 1969.

Heritage CK, Cunningham MD: Association of elective repeat cesarean delivery and persistent pulmonary hypertension of the newborn. *Am. J. Obstet. Gynecol.* 152:627, 1985.

Herzog LN, Alvarez SR: The frequency of foreskin problems in uncircumised children. *Am. J. Dis. Child.* 140:254, 1986.

Hester JD: Postpartum hemorrhage and reevaluation of uterine packing. *Obstet. Gynecol.* 45:501, 1975.

Higgins CS: *Cesarean Section: Do economic incentives matter?* Doctor of Philosophy Thesis. Department of Economics, Baltimore, University of Maryland, 1985.

Hjalmarson O, Krantz ME et al: The importance of neonatal asphyxia and cesarean section as risk factors for neonatal respiratory disorders in an unselected population. *Acta Paediatr. Scand.* 71:403, 1982.

Hogberg V, Joelsson I: The decline in maternal mortality in Sweden 1931–1980. *Acta Obstet. Gynecol. Scand.* 64:583, 1985.

Howard WF, McFadden PR, Keettel WC: Oxytocic drugs in the fourth stage of labor. *J. Am. Med. Assoc.* 189:411, 1964.

Hughey MJ, McElin TN et al: Forceps in perspective I. Midforceps rotation operation. *J. Reprod. Med.* 20:253, 1978a.

Hughey MJ, McElin TN et al: Forceps operations in perspective II. Failed operations. *J. Reprod. Med.* 21:177, 1978b.

Hurry DJ, Larsen B, Charles D: Effects of postcesarean section febrile morbidity on subsequent fertility. *Obstet. Gynecol.* 64:256, 1984.

Iams JD, Chawla A: Patient cost in the prevention and treatment of postcesarean section infection. *Am. J. Obstet. Gynecol.* 149:363, 1984.

Iffy L, Kaminetzky HA et al: Control of perinatal infection by traditional preventive measures. *Obstet. Gynecol.* 54:403, 1979.

Jacobstein MD, Hirschfeld SS et al: Neonatal circulation changes following elective cesarean section: an echocardiographic study. *Pediatrics* 69:374, 1982.

Jagani N, Schulman H et al: Role of the cervix in the induction of labor. *Obstet. Gynecol.* 59:21, 1982.

Jagani N, Schulman H et al: Role of prostaglandin induced cervical changes in labor induction. *Obstet. Gynecol.* 63:225, 1984.

JAMA: Report of the ad hoc committee of the Harvard Medical School to examine the definition of brain death. *J. Am. Med. Assoc.*, 205:337, 1968.

Jander HP, Russinovich NAE: Transcatheter Gelfoam embolization in abdominal, retroperitoneal, and pelvic hemorrhage. *Radiology* 136:337, 1980.

Jimenez JM, Tyson JE, Reisch JS: Clinical measures of gestational age in normal pregnancies. *Obstet. Gynecol.* 61:438, 1983.

Jones RF, Warren BL et al: Planned postpartum exploration of the uterus, cervix and vagina. *Obstet. Gynecol.* 27:669, 1966.

Kadar N, Romero R: Prognosis for future childbearing after midcavity instrumental deliveries in the primigravida. *Obstet. Gynecol.* 62:166, 1983.

Kaplan GW: Circumcision—an overview. *Curr. Probl. Pediatr.* 7:1, 1977.

Kaunitz AM, Hughes JM et al: Causes of maternal mortality in the United States. *Obstet. Gynecol.* 65:605, 1985.

Kauppila O: The perinatal mortality in breech deliveries and observations on affecting factors. *Acta Obstet. Gynecol. Scand.* 54(S39):9, 1975.

Kazzi GM, Bottoms SF, Rosen MG: Efficacy and safety of laminaria digitata for preinduction ripening of the cervix. *Obstet. Gynecol.* 60:440, 1982.

Keettel WC, Randall JH, Donnelly MM: The hazards of elective induction of labor. *Am. J. Obstet. Gynecol.* 75:496, 1958.

Kirya C, Worthmann MW: Neonatal circumcision and penile dorsal nerve block, painless procedure. *J. Pediatr.* 92:998, 1978.

Kitzinger S, Walters R: *Some Women's Experiences of Episiotomy.* London, National Childbirth Trust, 1981.

Klaus MH, Kennell JH: *Maternal-Infant Bonding.* St. Louis, C. V. Mosby, 1976.

Kubli F: Risk of vaginal breech delivery. *Contrib. Gynecol. Obstet.* 3:80, 1977.

Landesmann R, Graber EA: Abdominovaginal delivery: modification of the cesarean section operation to facilitate delivery of the impacted head. *Am. J. Obstet. Gynecol.* 148:707, 1984.

Lange AP, Secher NJ et al: Prelabor evaluation of inducibility. *Obstet. Gynecol.* 60:137, 1982.

Laros RK, Work BA, Witting WC: Amniotomy during the active phase of labor. *Obstet. Gynecol.* 39:702, 1972.

Lavin JP, Stephens RJ et al: Vaginal delivery in patients with a prior cesarean section. *Obstet. Gynecol.* 59:135, 1982.

Law RG: Failed forceps: a review of 37 cases. *Br. Med. J.* 2:955, 1953.

Lawaetz O, Jansen HK: Survey radiography of the abdomen following cesarean section, with particular reference to caecal diameter and the presence of free subdiaphragmatic gas. *Acta Obstet. Gynecol. Scand.* 55:311, 1976.

Lee CY, Madrazo B, Drukker BH: Ultrasonic evaluation of the postpartum uterus in the management of postpartum bleeding. *Obstet. Gynecol.* 58:227, 1981.

Lester WM, Bartholomew RA et al: Reconsideration of the uterine pack in postpartum hemorrhage. *Am. J. Obstet. Gynecol.* 98:321, 1965.

Levine MG, Holroyde J et al: Birth trauma: incidence and predisposing factors. *Obstet. Gynecol.* 63:792, 1984.

MacLennan AH, Green RC et al: Ripening of the human cervix and induction of labor with purified relaxin. *Lancet* 1:220, 1980.

Maisels MJ, Rees R et al: Elective delivery of the term fetus. An obstetrical hazard. *J. Am. Med. Assoc.* 238:2036, 1977.

Malmstrom J, Jansson I: Use of the vacuum extractor. *Clin. Obstet. Gynecol.* 8:893, 1964.

Marshall RE, Stratton WC et al: Circumcision: effect upon newborn behavior. A control blind observation study. *Pediatr. Res.* 13:334, 1979.

Maryniak GM, Frank JB: Clinical assessment of the Kobayashi vacuum extractor. *Obstet. Gynecol.* 64:431, 1984.

McClellan MS, Cabianea WA: Effects of early mother-infant contact following cesarean birth. *Obstet. Gynecol.* 56:52, 1980.

McNulty JV: Elective cesarean hysterectomy—revisited. *Am. J. Obstet. Gynecol.* 149:29, 1984.

Milner AD, Saunders RA, et al: Effects of delivery by cesarean section on lung mechanics and lung volume in the human neonate. *Arch. Dis. Child.* 53:545, 1978.

Milner RDG: Neonatal mortality of breech deliveries with and without forceps to the after-coming head. *Br. J. Obstet. Gynaecol.* 82:783, 1975.

Mishell D, Kelly JV: The obstetrical forceps and vacuum extractor and assessment of their compressive forces. *Obstet. Gynecol.* 19:204, 1962.

Modanlou HD, Komatsu G et al: Large for gestational age neonates: anthropometric reasons for shoulder dystocia. *Obstet. Gynecol.* 60:417, 1982.

Munsat TL, Neerhout R, Nyirjesy I: A comparative clinical study of the vacuum extractor and forceps. II. Evaluation of the newborn. *Am. J. Obstet. Gynecol.* 85:1083, 1963.

Myers RE: Two patterns of perinatal brain damage and their conditions of occurrence. *Am. J. Obstet. Gynecol.* 112:246, 1972.

Nelson NM, Enkin MW et al: A randomized clinical trial of the Leboyer approach to childbirth. *N. Engl. J. Med.* 302:655, 1980.

Newton ER, Barss V, Cetrulo CL: The epidemiology and clinical history of asymptomatic midtrimester placenta previa. *Am. J. Obstet. Gynecol.* 148:743, 1984.

Newton ER, Cetrulo CL, Koza DL: Biparietal diameter as a predictor of fetal lung maturity. *J. Reprod. Med.* 28:480, 1983.

Newton ER, Haering WA et al: Effect of mode of delivery on morbidity and mortality of infants at early gestational age. *Obstet. Gynecol.* 67:507, 1986.

Newton M: Postpartum hemorrhage. *Am. J. Obstet. Gynecol.* 94:711, 1966.

Newton M, Moody AR: Fetal and maternal blood in the human placenta. *Obstet. Gynecol.* 18:305, 1961.

Newton M, Mosey LM et al: Blood loss during and immediately after delivery. *Obstet. Gynecol.* 17:9, 1961.

Newton N, Foshee D, Newton M: Experimental inhibition of labor through environmental disturbance. *Am. J. Obstet. Gynecol.* 27:3, 1966.

Newton N, Newton M: Mothers' reaction to their newborn babies. *J. Am. Med. Assoc.* 181:206, 1962.

Nielson TF, Hokegard KH: Postoperative cesarean section morbidity: a prospective study. *Am. J. Obstet. Gynecol.* 146:911, 1983.

Niswander KR, Patterson RJ: Hazards of elective induction. *Obstet. Gynecol.* 22:228, 1963.

Nugent FB: The primiparous perineum after forceps delivery. *Am. J. Obstet. Gynecol.* 30:249, 1935.

Nyirjesy I, Hawks BL et al: A comparative clinical study of the vacuum extractor and forceps. Part I. Preliminary observations. *Am. J. Obstet. Gynecol.* 85:1071, 1963.

O'Driscoll K, Foley M: Correlation of decrease in perinatal mortality and increase in cesarean rates. *Obstet. Gynecol.* 61:1, 1983.

O'Driscoll K, Meagher D et al: Traumatic intracranial haemorrhage in first born infants and delivery with obstetric forceps. *Br. J. Obstet. Gynaecol.* 88:577, 1981.

O'Leary JL, O'Leary JA: The complete episiotomy: analysis of 1,224 complete lacerations, sphincterectomies, and episiproctotomies. *Obstet. Gynecol.* 25:235, 1965.

Painter MJ, Bergman I: Obstetrical trauma to the neonatal central and peripheral nervous system. *Semin. Perinatol.* 6:89, 1982.

Pais SO, Glickman M et al: Embolization of pelvic arteries for control of postpartum hemorrhage. *Obstet. Gynecol.* 55:754, 1980.

Park RC, Duff WP: Role of cesarean hysterectomy in modern obstetric practice. *Clin. Obstet. Gynecol.* 23:601, 1980.

Paul RH (Ed.): Pregnancy management after prior cesarean section. *J. Reprod. Med.* 29:1, 1984.

Perkins RD: Role of extraperitoneal cesarean section. *Clin. Obstet. Gynecol.* 23:583, 1980.

Petitti DB: Present trends in cesarean delivery rates in California. *Birth* 12:25, 1985.

Petitti DB, Cefalo RC et al: In-hospital maternal mortality in the United States: time-trends and relation to the method of delivery. *Obstet. Gynecol.* 59:6, 1982.

Philip AGS: Further observations on placental transfusion. *Obstet. Gynecol.* 42:334, 1973.

Phillips RN, Thornton J, Gleicher N: Physician bias in cesarean section. *J. Am. Med. Assoc.* 248:1082, 1982.

Placek PJ, Taffel SM: Trends in cesarean section rates for the United States 1970–1978. *Public Health Rep.* 95:540, 1980.

Placek PJ, Taffel SM, Moien M: Cesarean delivery rates: United States, 1981. *Am. J. Public Health* 73:861, 1983.

Platt LD, Druzin ML: Acute puerperal inversion of uterus. *Am. J. Obstet. Gynecol.* 141:187, 1981.

Plauche WC: Fetal cranial injuries related to delivery with the Malmstrom's vacuum extractor. *Obstet. Gynecol.* 53:750, 1979.

Plauche WC: Subgaleal hematoma: a complication of instrumental delivery. *J. Am. Med. Assoc.* 244:1597, 1980.

Plauche WC: Cesarean hysterectomy—indications, techniques and complications. *Clin. Obstet. Gynecol.* 29:318, 1986.

Plauche WC, Wycheck JG et al: Cesarean hysterectomy at Louisiana State University 1979–1981. *South Med. J.* 76:1261, 1983.

Poidevin LOS: The value of hysterography in the predictions of cesarean section wound defects. *Am. J. Obstet. Gynecol.* 81:67, 1961.

Polk HC, Simpson CJ et al: Guidelines for prevention of surgical wound infection. *Arch. Surg.* 118:1213, 1983.

Prins RD, Bolton RN et al: Cervical ripening with intravaginal prostaglandin E_2 gel. *Obstet. Gynecol.* 61:459, 1983.

Pritchard JA: Changes in blood volume during pregnancy and delivery. *Anesthesiology* 26:293, 1965.

Pritchard JA, Baldwin RM et al: Blood volume changes in pregnancy and the puerperium. II. Red cell loss and changes in the apparent blood volume during and following vaginal delivery, cesarean section plus total hysterectomy. *Am. J. Obstet. Gynecol.* 84:1271, 1962.

Prough DS, Johnston WE et al: Recent advances in critical care pharmacology. Part III: Treatment of shock. *Hosp. Formul.* 20:40, 1985.

Ralis ZA: Birth trauma to muscles in babies born by breech delivery and its possible fatal consequences. *Arch. Dis. Child.* 50:4, 1975.

Read JA, Miller FC, Paul RH: Randomized trial of ambulation versus oxytocin for labor enhancement: a preliminary report. *Am. J. Obstet. Gynecol.* 139:669, 1981.

Reading AE, Sledmere CM et al: How women view postepisiotomy pain. *Br. Med. J.* 284:243, 1982.

Report of the ad hoc committee of the Harvard Medical School to examine the definition of brain death. *J. Am. Med. Assoc.* 205:337, 1968.

Richardson DA, Evans ME, Cibils LA: Midforceps delivery—a critical review. *Am. J. Obstet. Gynecol.* 145:621, 1983.

Roberts IF, Stone M: Fetal hemorrhage: complication of vacuum extraction after fetal blood sampling. *Am. J. Obstet. Gynecol.* 132:109, 1978.

Roberts JE, Mendez-Bauer C, Wodell DA: The effects of maternal position on uterine contractility and efficiency. *Birth* 10:243, 1983.

Romney ML: Predelivery shaving: an unjustified assault? *J. Obstet. Gynecol.* 1:33, 1980.

Romney ML, Gordon H: Is your enema really necessary? *Br. Med. J.* 282:1269, 1981.

Rosen MG, Debanne S et al: Long-term neurological morbidity in breech and vertex births. *Am. J. Obstet. Gynecol.* 151:718, 1985.

Rosenberg LA, Tejani NA et al: Preinduction ripening of the cervix with laminaria in the nulliparous patient. *J. Reprod. Med.* 25:61, 1980.

Rovinsky JJ, Miller JA, Kaplan S: Management of breech presentation at term. *Am. J. Obstet. Gynecol.* 115:497, 1973.

Rubin A: Birth injury: incidence, mechanism and end results. *Obstet. Gynecol.* 23:218, 1964.

Rubin GL, Peterson HB et al: Maternal death after cesarean section in Georgia. *Am. J. Obstet. Gynecol.* 139:681, 1981.

Rudd EG, Long WH, Dillon MB: Febrile morbidity following cefamandole nafate intrauterine irrigation during cesarean section. *Am. J. Obstet. Gynecol.* 141:12, 1981.

Sack RA: The large infant. *Am. J. Obstet. Gynecol.* 104:195, 1969.

Schreiner RL, Stevens DC et al: Respiratory distress following elective repeat cesarean section. *Am. J. Obstet. Gynecol.* 143:689, 1982.

Seitchik J: Quantitating uterine contractility in clinical context. *Obstet. Gynecol.* 57:453, 1981.

Seitchik J, Holden AEL, Castillo M: Amniotomy and the use of oxytocin in nulliparous women. *Am. J. Obstet. Gynecol.* 153:848, 1985.

Seitchik J, Rao VRR: Cesarean delivery in nulliparous women for failed oxytocin-augmented labor: route of delivery in subsequent pregnancy. *Am. J. Obstet. Gynecol.* 143:393, 1982.

Seropian R, Reynolds B: Wound infections after preoperative depilatory versus razor preparation. *Am. J. Surg.* 121:251, 1971.

Shy KK, Eschenbach DA: Fatal perineal cellulitis from an episiotomy site. *Obstet. Gynecol.* 54:292, 1979.

Shy KK, Logerfo JP, Karp LE: Evaluation of elective repeat cesarean section as a standard of care: an application of decision analysis. *Am. J. Obstet. Gynecol.* 139:123, 1981.

Siegel E: Early and extended maternal-infant contact: a critical review. *Am. J. Dis. Child.* 136:251, 1982.

Singh PM, Gupta AN: Placenta previa and previous cesarean section. *Acta Obstet. Gynecol. Scand.* 60:367, 1981.

Sisson TRG, Knutson S, Kendall L: Blood volume of infants. Part IV: Infants born by cesarean section. *Am. J. Obstet. Gynecol.* 117:351, 1973.

Sleep J, Grant A et al: West Berkshire perineal management trial. *Br. Med. J.* 289:587, 1984.

Smith LP, Nagourney BA et al: Hazards and benefits of elective induction of labor. *Am. J. Obstet. Gynecol.* 148:579, 1984.

Sorbe S: Active pharmacologic management of the third stage of labor. A comparison of oxytocin and ergotmetrine. *Obstet. Gynecol.* 52:694, 1978.

Sosa R, Kennell JH, Klaus M: The effect of early mother-infant contact on breastfeeding, infection and growth. In: *Ciba Foundation Symposium No. 45, Breastfeeding and the Mother,* Amsterdam, Elsevier, 1976.

Sosa R, Kennell J, Klaus M: The effect of a supportive companion on perinatal problems, length of labor and mother-infant interaction. *N. Engl. J. Med.* 303:597, 1980.

Sotto LSJ, Collins RJ: Perigenital hematomas. *Obstet. Gynecol.* 12:249, 1958.

Spinnato JA, Sibai BM et al: Inaccuracy of Dubowitz obstetrical age in low birth weight infants. *Obstet. Gynecol.* 63:491, 1984.

Steer CM: Effect of type of delivery on future childbearing. *Am. J. Obstet. Gynecol.* 60:395, 1950.

Stiver HG, Forward KR et al: Multicenter comparison of cefoxitin versus cefazolin for the prevention of infections, morbidity after nonelective cesarean section. *Am. J. Obstet. Gynecol.* 145:158, 1983.

Stiver HG, Forward KR et al: Comparative cervical microflora shifts after cefoxitin or cefazolin prophylaxis against infection following cesarean section. *Am. J. Obstet. Gynecol.* 149:718, 1984.

Swartz WH, Grolle K: The use of prophylactic antibiotics in cesarean section. *J. Reprod. Med.* 26:595, 1981.

Thacker SB, Banta HD: Benefits and risks of episiotomy: an interpretative review of the English language literature, 1860–1980. *Obstet. Gynecol. Surv.* 38:322, 1983.

Thein W, McSweeney DJ: Multiple repeat cesarean section. *Am. J. Obstet. Gynecol.* 90:913, 1964.

Thompson HC, King LR et al: Report of the ad hoc task force on circumcision. *Pediatrics* 56:610, 1975.

Todd WD, Steer CM: Term breech: review of 1006 term breech deliveries. *Obstet. Gynecol.* 22:583, 1963.

Treloar AE, Behn BG, Cowan DW: Analysis of gestational interval. *Am. J. Obstet. Gynecol.* 99:34, 1967.

Vacca A, Grant A et al: Portsmouth operative delivery trial: a comparison of vacuum extraction and forceps delivery. *Br. J. Obstet. Gynaecol.* 90:1107, 1983.

Van Vugt PJH: The protrusions from the cervical canal of the scar of a previous cesarean section. *Acta Obstet. Gynecol. Scand.* 58:327, 1979.

Van Vugt PJH, Baudoin P et al: Inversio uteri puerperalis. *Acta Obstet. Gynecol. Scand.* 60:353, 1981.

Vogt H, Haneberg B et al: Clinical assessment of gestational age in the newborn infant. *Acta Paediatr. Scand.* 70:669, 1981.

von Barsewisek B: *Perinatal Retinal Hemorrhages.* New York, Springer-Verlag, 1979.

Wager GP, Martin DH et al: Puerperal infectious morbidity: relationship to route of delivery and to antepartum *Chlamydia trachomatis* infection. *Am. J. Obstet. Gynecol.* 138:1028, 1980.

Waniorek A: Hysterography after cesarean section for evaluation of suture technique. *Obstet. Gynecol.* 29:192, 1967.

Watson P, Besch N, Bowes WA: Management of acute and subacute puerperal inversion of the uterus. *Obstet. Gynecol.* 55:12, 1980.

Weber CE: Postmortem cesarean section: review of the literature and case reports. *Am. J. Obstet. Gynecol.* 110:158, 1971.

Weed JC: The fate of the postpartum uterus. *Obstet. Gynecol.* 14:780, 1959.

Wigglesworth JS, Husemeyer RP: Intracranial birth trauma in vaginal breech delivery. *Br. J. Obstet. Gynaecol.* 84:684, 1977.

Williams RL, Chen PM: Controlling the rise in cesarean rates by the dissemination of information from vital records. *Am. J. Public Health* 73:863, 1983.

Wood C, Na KH et al: Time—an important variable. *J. Obstet. Gynaecol. Br. Commwlth.* 80:295, 1973.

Woods JR: Significance of amniotic fluid meconium. In Creasy RK, Resnick R (Eds.): *Maternal Fetal Medicine.* Philadelphia, W. B. Saunders Co., 1984.

Yates, PO: Birth trauma to the vertebral arteries. *Arch Dis. Child.* 34:436, 1959.

Yonekura ML, Teberg A et al: Birth associated mechanical injury. A contemporary review. Society of Perinatal Obstetricians, Abstract No. 119, 1984.

Zdeb MS, Therriault GD, Logrillo VM: Frequency, spacing and outcome of pregnancies subsequent to primary cesarean childbirth. *Am. J. Obstet. Gynecol.* 150:205, 1984.

COMPLICATIONS OF GENERAL AND GYNECOLOGIC PROCEDURES

12

MICHAEL NEWTON

GENERAL PROCEDURES

Venous

VENIPUNCTURE

Drawing blood from an arm vein for testing is now a routine medical procedure that is performed by many different individuals and generally accepted by patients as a necessary part of diagnosis. Complications are minor and uncommon. They include pain, bleeding, hematoma formation, thrombosis and infection.

Pain depends on the site of venipuncture and the size and sharpness of the needle. Flexor surfaces are generally more likely to give rise to pain than extensor surfaces, although individuals vary greatly in their anticipation of and susceptibility to pain. Repeated attempts to obtain blood obviously increase apprehension and pain. The use of local anesthesia for venipuncture does little good, since the injection of the local anesthetic causes almost as much discomfort as the venipuncture itself. Bleeding from the puncture site rarely occurs in women whose coagulation factors are normal, provided that adequate pressure is maintained over the vein. Deep bleeding with hematoma formation may occur if the needle penetrates the posterior wall of the vein. Pressure and, if necessary, the application of an icebag minimize the hematoma. Thrombosis is rare following simple venipuncture. Infection is very unusual unless the patient has a generalized infection.

The legal responsibility for pain and bleeding or hematoma formation may be important. In general, the hospital, in the case of a nurse or technician employed by it, or the physician, in the case of an office employee, may be considered liable. However, the individual drawing the blood has a responsibility according to the level of skill that he or she may be expected to possess. In all cases the patient's oral consent must be obtained, although it is not customary to describe all the possible eventualities. If blood is to be drawn as part of a research study, this procedure has to be approved by the appropriate Institutional Review Board (for the protection of human subjects) and must be included in the informed consent form signed by the patient prior to the investigation.

Complications from venipuncture may be prevented by observing a few, relatively simple guidelines:

1. Selection of a good vein. If necessary, the hand or arm should be immersed in hot water for five or more minutes prior to venipuncture.

2. Cleansing of the skin with an antiseptic. Seventy percent alcohol is generally used; the skin should be allowed to dry.

3. Use of a sharp needle of the smallest size (21 or 22G) compatible with obtaining enough blood quickly.

4. Insertion of the needle with the bevel up to prevent its passage through the posterior wall of the vein.

5. Removal of the tourniquet and needle before applying pressure to the puncture site; this procedure decreases pain.

6. Maintenance of pressure on the puncture site until bleeding has ceased even with movement of the arm and hand.

Occasionally it may not be possible to obtain blood from an arm or hand vein. In this case the internal jugular, subclavian or femoral vein may be used. Complications associated with the first two are discussed later. Those of obtaining blood from the femoral vein include inability to identify the vein and puncture of the femoral artery. Both can be avoided by knowledge of the anatomic relationships (Fig. 12–1).

PERIPHERAL INTRAVENOUS THERAPY

The intravenous route is used for the immediate injection of medications or for the prolonged administration of fluids, electrolytes and colloids. Hand or forearm veins are generally used. Veins in the legs and feet should not be used, because of the necessity of immobilizing the patient and the danger of thrombosis. Complications may be related to the drugs used or to the technique of insertion and maintenance of the needle or catheter. Intravenous injection of drugs may result in complications because the drugs may cause sclerosis or thrombosis of the veins themselves or because they irritate the surrounding tissue if extravasation occurs. Specific drug effects will be considered in Chapter 13.

The complications of insertion and maintenance of a peripheral intravenous line include (1) pain, (2) infiltration of the surrounding tissues, (3) reflux of blood and development of clots in the system, (4) inflammation of the vein (phlebitis), (5) contamination of the injected fluid and (6) fever and infection.

Holland and co-workers (1982) studied complications following insertion of 254 peripheral intravenous cannulas by anesthesiologists before elective operations (18% gynecologic). The overall incidence of complications is shown in Table 12–1. There were some differences between the four different catheters used. Three important observations were made: (1) removal

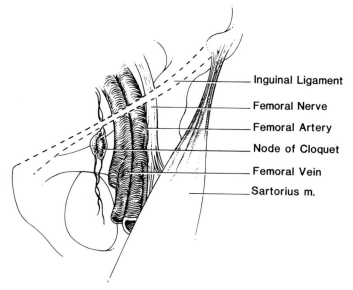

Figure 12–1. Anatomical relationships of the femoral vein.

Inguinal Ligament

Femoral Nerve

Femoral Artery

Node of Cloquet

Femoral Vein

Sartorius m.

Table 12–1. Complications of Venous Cannulas in 254 Patients*

Complication	No.	Percent
Phlebitis or thrombophlebitis	51	20
Extravasation	20	8
Blockage	6	2
Total	77	30

*Adapted from Holland RB, Levitt MW et al: Intravenous canulas. Survey of their use in patients undergoing elective surgery. Copyright 1982, *The Medical Journal of Australia*. Reprinted with permission.

of a catheter for complications increased sharply after 48 hours and again after 72 hours, (2) fewer complications were found with catheters in the dorsum of the hand than with those in the forearm and (3) the addition of blood, antibiotic agents and potassium chloride to the infusion increased the complication rate.

Pain occurs with the insertion of the needle or catheter; its degree depends upon the individual's tolerance to pain, the site of the injection, the number of attempts at puncture and the amount of probing used at each attempt. In the apprehensive patient, pain may be lessened by an unhurried, careful approach to the procedure. The use of local anesthesia (1% lidocaine) may be helpful, particularly if a large needle is used, although it tends to obscure the vein. The choice of the best vein and skill in venipuncture do most to decrease pain. The arm on the side of a previous mastectomy should be avoided. It is important to select at first the most peripheral vein available on the dorsum of the non-dominant hand (at a point where two veins join) and to warm the arm sufficiently to dilate the veins. In general, a catheter is preferable to a needle. The date and time of insertion should be written on the tape holding the catheter or tubing in place.

Infiltration of intravenous fluid into the extravascular space may occur because the vein wall is thin (as in older women), permitting fluid to pass through it, or the needle or catheter has come out of the vein. Swelling occurs around the site of injection, and the patient notices pain. The swelling can become large especially in the semiconscious, postoperative patient. If blood can be drawn back into the tubing, it may be possible to continue the infusion for a time if medication is not being given. If blood cannot be drawn back, the infusion should be restarted elsewhere. Swelling caused by infiltration of the commonly used fluids and electrolytes subsides in 24 to 48 hours. Application of ice may help.

Reflux of blood and clotting in the system usually occur as a result of a kink in the tubing or failure to replace an empty bottle of fluid. Attempts to aspirate and flush out the system may permit the infusion to be continued. Otherwise the infusion has to be restarted in another vein. This complication can be lessened by appropriate taping of the tubing and by consistent nursing care.

Phlebitis or thrombophlebitis may be caused by inflammation alone or by inflammation associated with infection. The former is more common. It appears as a painful red streak along the vein, occasionally with swelling in the surrounding tissue. Detachment of clots from an arm vein occurs very rarely, but the thrombosis will persist for many weeks and continue to be slightly painful. Initially, local heat will help. Antibiotics are not necessary unless there is evidence of spreading infection. If possible, the infusion site should be changed before phlebitis occurs. As a general rule, this means that one vein should be used for no more than 48 to 72 hours. Removal of microparticles by an in-line filter significantly reduces the phlebitis rate, according to data from six studies totaling 760 cases, and is clearly cost effective (Rapp and Bivins, 1985).

Fever associated with intravenous infusions may be due to pyrogens in the fluids, a rare event with modern aseptic preparation, or to a bloodstream infection. This may result from a contaminated solution or the introduction of infection from the puncture site, especially in debilitated patients, and septic shock may occur. The incidence of sepsis related to peripheral vein catheters was calculated by Collignon and co-workers (1984) to be about 0.1%. Clinical evidence of thrombophlebitis was noted in the majority of cases, and in a large proportion the catheter had been left in place for over 48 hours. If sepsis from the catheter is suspected, the infused solution should be discontinued and returned to the pharmacy for culture and study of other similarly prepared solutions. Blood cultures and appropriate multiple antibiotic therapy are indicated. When blood or blood products are infused, there is risk of transmitting infections, especially hepatitis or AIDS. This is also a special danger from the indiscriminate intravenous self-injection of substances by drug-dependent persons.

CENTRAL VENOUS INFUSIONS

During the past 20 years, the use of catheters in large central veins has become widespread.

Although they are not ordinarily necessary in gynecology and obstetrics, they are important for short-term use in the occasional patient in whom venous pressure must be measured (as in hemorrhage), when cardiorespiratory monitoring (Swan-Ganz catheter) is needed, or when other venous access is unavailable. Over the longer term central venous infusions are used for hyperalimentation and for intermittent administration of chemotherapy.

The subclavian and internal jugular veins are most commonly used, the femoral vein rarely. In some patients alternate sites may be necessary. These alternatives are discussed by Parsa and Tabora (1985). The central catheter may be inserted through a peripheral vein, such as those in the antecubital fossa, the cephalic, the external jugular or, rarely, the long saphenous vein. Insertion may be done percutaneously or through use of a cut-down technique. The chief problems of the peripheral route are the necessity of inserting a catheter long enough to reach the superior vena cava, and, in the case of the arm veins, the constant movement of the catheter, which causes inflammation and eventual thrombosis of the axillary vein. This usually limits the use of the peripheral approach to five to seven days. Direct insertion of the catheter into the internal jugular vein is often used during operations. Its disadvantage is that it is uncomfortable for the patient if the catheter is kept in place for more than two to three days. The subclavian vein is the most convenient for the patient and for long-term use, and it will be the one primarily considered here. Insertion may be by the supraclavicular route into the junction of the internal jugular and subclavian veins or by the infraclavicular route directly into the subclavian vein. Insertion on the left side is perhaps easier for the right-handed operator and vice versa, but the right side may be more commonly used because of the possible danger of injuring the thoracic duct on the left.

Many different needles and catheters have been described (see list in Peters, 1983), and modifications in design and techniques are constantly being made. Catheters may contain one, two or three lumens, depending on where they are to be placed and the need for sampling or infusion. For long-term use, catheters of the Hickman-Broviac type are commonly inserted. They have a Dacron cuff (for increased fixation) and may be tunnelled under the skin of the chest wall to come out 6 to 10 cm below the entry into the vein, usually the subclavian.

Central venous catheters may be introduced directly (1) through a needle, (2) over a guidewire or (3) through a cannula. The first and original method requires the needle to be withdrawn and carries the risk of shearing off the catheter. The second method permits a smaller needle to be used for venipuncture, but the catheter or its introducer must be stiff enough to enlarge the guidewire tract; the guidewire technique is useful for replacing a catheter. Insertion through a cannula permits the use of a soft catheter; there is no danger of shearing it off, since the catheter does not come in contact with the needle. Whatever method is used, attention to the technique of insertion materially reduces complications. Important principles are as follows:

1. The patient should be relaxed.
2. Her head is tilted down in a 20 to 30 degree Trendelenburg position.
3. Her shoulders are extended over a folded towel or sandbag placed between her scapulae.
4. Her head is turned to the opposite side.
5. Her arms lie alongside her chest.
6. Full aseptic precautions are followed, including gowning and masking of the operator and thorough wide skin preparation.
7. Local anesthesia is used at the puncture site and beneath the clavicle.
8. The needle with attached syringe is inserted beneath the clavicle at the junction of its medial and middle thirds and advanced cautiously with repeated aspirations in a horizontal plane toward the top of the sternoclavicular joint on the same side (Fig. 12–2).
9. The needle is rotated from bevel up to bevel down as it enters the vein to avoid perforating the posterior wall and to permit smooth insertion of the catheter or guidewire.
10. The patient must hold her breath whenever there is a chance that air may enter the vein.
11. Op-site or other occlusive dressing should be used.

Insertion of a central venous catheter is an invasive procedure and carries important risks and complications. These relate to (1) the general condition of the patient, since many patients are acutely ill (Cotton and Benedetti, 1980); (2) the skill and experience of the physician who inserts the catheter; (3) faults in catheter design; (4) the actual procedure of insertion; and (5) catheter maintenance and use. Reliable current data on complications are difficult to obtain because of the variety of equipment and techniques of insertion. An audit of 225 subclavian catheter placements by house

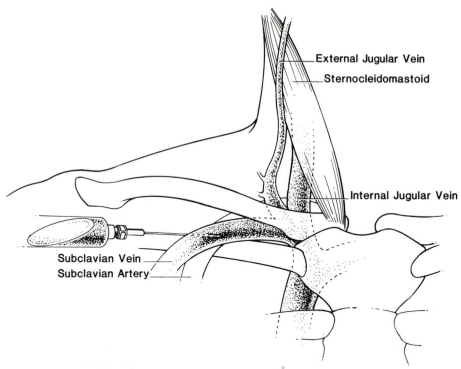

Figure 12–2. Right subclavian vein catheterization

staff in a teaching hospital during 1983 and 1984 showed an overall complication rate of 12% (Fares et al, 1986). Although some complications are related to insertion and can be attributed in part to the experience of the operator, the number of complications can be reduced but not completely eliminated. On the other hand, later complications increase according to the complexity of the techniques used and the length of time the catheter is in place. Pessa and Howard (1985) noted a 34% complication rate after the placement of 157 Hickman-Broviac catheters over a four year period. It is reasonable to expect a complication rate of less than 5% for the initial insertion and management, with a variable increase depending upon the length of time the venous access is maintained.

Complications of Insertion. The immediate complications of subclavian catheterization through the percutaneous route are listed in Table 12–2. If the subclavian artery (the usual vessel involved) has been punctured, bright red blood enters the syringe with force. The needle should be removed and firm pressure applied over the artery (against the first rib) for at least five minutes with the patient sitting up. Fortunately, this procedure is usually effective.

Serious difficulties requiring prompt surgical exploration arise if the cannula or needle penetrates another major vessel or, in addition, the pleura. The occurrence of arterial puncture can be reduced by careful attention to the technique of insertion.

Pneumothorax is the most common complication, accounting for up to 30% of those reported in the literature. It is usually small and occurs immediately, although delayed pneumothorax has been reported. Since pneumothorax cannot be detected easily, a post-insertion chest x-ray is required; in addition, the x-ray is needed to determine the position of the catheter. No treatment is needed if less than 15% of the lung volume is involved, since the air will be absorbed. However, x-rays should be repeated within several hours, since the pneumothorax may increase. If the pneumothorax is large or the patient is in respiratory

Table 12–2. Immediate Complications of Percutaneous Subclavian Catheter Insertion

Arterial entry
Pneumothorax
Thoracic duct injury
Misdirection of catheter

distress, the air can then be released by inserting, under local anesthesia, a large venous catheter in the sixth intercostal space (above the rib) in the mid-axillary line and connecting it to underwater drainage. This procedure needs to be followed by the insertion of a chest tube.

Air embolism is a rare complication (Lambert, 1982). The patient is acutely distressed. A sucking noise may be heard, and a cogwheel murmur may be present over the chest. The patient should be placed on her left side and given oxygen. Air should be aspirated if possible through the catheter or from the heart. The outcome is fatal in over 50% of patients. Air embolism can be prevented largely by placing the patient in a 20 to 30 degree head-down position during the insertion and by asking her to perform a Valsalva maneuver (forced expiration against resistance) at any time a cannula or catheter may even momentarily be left open to the air.

Injuries to the thoracic duct (mostly on the left side but also on the right) occur very rarely. If injury to the thoracic duct is not recognized, lymph may continue to flow out along the catheter tract. This may produce fluid under the dressing and potentiate infection. The catheter should be removed and local pressure applied for 30 minutes; a suture should be used at the skin puncture site if leakage continues (Parsa and Tabora, 1985).

Embolism of a portion of the catheter may occur if a piece breaks off during insertion. Accurate localization and removal by the venous route is necessary.

Misdirection of a catheter occurs in about 5% of insertions (Peters, 1983), and the rate is higher the further the insertion is from the central vein. Extravascular insertion may result in infusion of fluid into the mediastinum or pleural cavity. Intravascular misdirection may result in the catheter entering the internal jugular vein rather than the superior vena cava. This is a not a problem if the purpose of the catheter is to measure venous pressure or to give crystalloids. However, hyperosmolar solution infused into the internal jugular vein may cause thrombosis and intracranial problems. Misdirection of the catheter can be detected by the prompt use of a post-insertion x-ray, conducted at the bedside. Miller and Broom (1983) found that cephalad deviation of the guidewire after removing it and laying it flat indicated misplacement into the internal jugular vein. If the catheter is misdirected, it must be replaced; a guidewire is often helpful.

Delayed Complications. Late complications of central venous catheter use include (1) air embolism, (2) catheter "failure," (3) central vein thrombosis, (4) vascular perforation and (5) infection.

The danger of air embolism is present as long as the catheter is used, especially when its connections are changed. The diagnosis and management are the same as described earlier.

Catheter failure means either that fluid can no longer be infused or that blood can no longer be withdrawn from the catheter. This usually indicates that the catheter is kinked, compressed or, possibly, outside the vein, or that there is a clot in it. The diagnosis of kinking or compression can be supported by an improvement in the flow of fluid with changes in position of the arm. An x-ray examination may demonstrate a constriction in the catheter (Aitkin and Minton, 1984) or suggest the extravascular position of the tip. Although clots may develop in the catheter during continuous use, they are more likely to occur when hyperalimentation or chemotherapy is given. To clear the line streptokinase or urokinase (10,000 IU in 5 ml saline) is injected into the catheter and left in place for one to four hours before further infusion is attempted (Gilligan et al, 1979). No ill effects seem to occur from this therapy. If attempts to clear the catheter fail and if the catheter is still needed, it must be replaced, preferably over a guidewire. Flushing the catheter with heparin and a heparin lock is widely used to prevent clotting, but it is unclear how often the catheter should be flushed. Gillies and Rogers (1985) suggest that flushing of any sort may be unnecessary except after drawing blood, transfusion or chemotherapy. Catheter failure may not be completely preventable, but it can be reduced by meticulous nursing care. The team approach, especially in continuing hyperalimentation or chemotherapy, is of great value.

The incidence of thrombosis in the subclavian vein is reported to vary from less than 1% (Smith and Hallett, 1983) to as high as 42% (Lokich and Becker, 1983). Since thrombosis may be partial and undiagnosed, the actual incidence may well be higher than 1%. Polyvinyl catheters are more prone to generate thrombi than those made of silicone, fluoroethylene propylene or polyurethane. Kinks and loops in catheters predispose to thrombosis formation as does the length of time the catheter is in place. Thrombosis in the internal jugular vein is uncommon, possibly because of the straight course of the vein and the high rate of blood flow. Central venous thrombosis is frequently asymptomatic. When present, the clinical picture consists of arm and shoulder pain and later swelling of the arm, neck or face with prominence of the jugular vein system (superior vena cava syndrome). Confirmation can be obtained with Doppler flow studies or a venogram. Because of the danger of pulmonary embolism the catheter must be removed and the patient treated with heparin (see Chapter 4). Elevation of the arm and analgesics are helpful. Prophylactic daily intermittent injections of low-dose heparin (3000 to 5000 units) appear to reduce the incidence of thrombosis.

Infection is the most serious complication of indwelling central venous catheters. Predisposing factors include:

1. The patient's poor general condition and the severity of the disease.

2. The presence of pathogenic (often antibiotic-resistant) microorganisms in the hospital environment.

3. The possibility of contamination from stomas or other sources in seriously ill and immobilized patients.

4. The use of antibiotics that may predispose to colonization with unusual organisms, e.g., *candida*, in place of the patient's own usual bacteria.

5. The number of caregivers handling the patient, which increases the possibility of staff to patient or patient to patient cross infection.

6. The length of time the catheter is in place.

7. The scrupulousness of the precautions taken against infection in the care of the patient and the catheter.

The reported incidence of infection varies considerably. Press and co-workers (1984), summarizing 18 series of cases, noted infections in 14% of patients (13% of insertions) who had indwelling Hickman catheters for long periods. The range of infections reported was from 0 to 56%. Clearly, infection is less frequent when a catheter is used temporarily for an acute problem. The incidence of infection in gynecologic or obstetric patients is not established; most of the infections reported occurred in patients receiving hyperalimentation or chemotherapy for other medical or surgical conditions.

The primary symptoms of infection are redness at the exit site and fever. The former is a warning sign and may be handled initially by changing the dressing, by careful cleaning of the skin (peroxide and povidone-iodine) and replacing the dressing preferably with Op-site or a similar plastic film (Vasquez and Jarrard, 1984). If fever of over 101 degrees F (38.4 degrees C) persists for six hours, thorough investigation of all causes is indicated before it is concluded that catheter sepsis is responsible, since replacement of the catheter may not be easy and may involve temporary discontinuation of necessary therapy. Once the studies are underway multiple antibiotics should be started (for antibiotic choices, see Chapters 4 and 13). If there is no bacteremia, if the study results are negative and the fever and evidence of exit site inflammation disappear, antibiotics may be discontinued after the temperature has been normal for 48 hours; the catheter need not be removed. If an infection is found elsewhere, it should be treated appropriately and the catheter left in place. Removal of the catheter is indicated if bacteremia is present, there is no evidence of infection elsewhere and clinical evidence of catheter infection persists. Replacement of the catheter should await control of the infection. If a tunnel infection is found, catheter removal is generally needed (Press et al, 1984). Once a catheter infection has occurred, all members of the team as well as hospital infection control personnel should carefully review all the technical steps associated with catheter insertion and management.

TUNNELLED CATHETERS

Apart from the complications characteristic of all subclavian catheters, several problems arise with the use of tunnelled catheters. First, the insertion takes longer and may be painful. Second, the need for the regular injection of heparin as an anticoagulant by the nurse or the patient herself makes occlusion more likely and third, the chance for infection is greater since the catheter is left in place for many weeks. Removal of these catheters may require local anesthesia and an operative procedure to remove the Dacron cuff unless, as often happens, it is loose.

Arterial

Arterial puncture in gynecology and obstetrics is used primarily to obtain arterial blood for gas studies and to measure arterial pressure. In related radiologic procedures it is used to obtain contrast studies of the pelvic vessels for sites of hemorrhage or increased blood flow, as in trophoblastic disease. For the former the radial or, less commonly, the brachial artery is generally used, for the latter the femoral or axillary artery.

The complications of arterial puncture are related to the procedure itself and to the contrast materials injected; the latter are considered in Chapter 13. A single arterial puncture may cause pain or extravasation of blood. Pain can be decreased by using local anesthesia in the skin and on each side of the artery. Firm pressure over the artery for at least five minutes after removal of the needle will usually prevent significant extravasation of blood, although a small hematoma around the artery is not unusual. Arterial occlusion rarely occurs after a single puncture, but this remote possibility dictates using the radial rather than the brachial artery when possible because of the collateral circulation from the ulnar artery (this should be checked). When an arterial cannula has to be left in place to obtain repeated blood samples, the danger of occlusion is increased. Occlusion has no ill effects, except that the radial pulse cannot be obtained after it occurs.

Intramuscular and Subcutaneous Injection

Intramuscular and subcutaneous injections are given by various medical personnel. They are so common that the complications tend to be forgotten. However, they may be a source of continuing concern to patients. Complications may be related to the site and technique of injection as well as to the substance injected.

Intramuscular injections are usually given in the large muscles of the buttocks (glutei) or arm (deltoid). The upper outer quadrant of the buttocks (to avoid the sciatic nerve) and the thickest part of the deltoid are generally used. Apart from reactions caused by the injected substances (see Chapter 13), the two chief complications are pain and bleeding (hematoma). Pain varies with the medication used, the depth of the injection (usually the deeper the injection, the less the pain), the number of injections and the proximity of the injection site to nerves. Pain may be lessened by deep, slow injection. After the injection heat may be useful in relieving pain. Hematoma formation or bleeding may be a serious complication in the presence of a coagulation deficiency. Firm pressure should be maintained over the injection site for at least three to five minutes. When coagulation is normal, bleeding is not often appreciated at the time of injection. It later appears as a tender, usually self-limited, swelling at the injection site. The patient can be assured that it will usually disappear, and it can be improved by gentle massage or heat. Sometimes a hard, persistently painful nodule remains for several weeks.

Similar complications (i.e., pain and bleeding) occur with subcutaneous injections, which are usually given in the outer arm, outer thigh or abdominal wall. Bleeding appears on the surface of the skin and is obvious to the patient, but is usually self-limited.

Infection at intramuscular or subcutaneous injection sites should be very rare if aseptic precautions are used, except in debilitated patients who already have infections elsewhere. Local heat is usually helpful, and antibiotics are not needed unless a major local or a generalized infection develops.

GYNECOLOGIC PROCEDURES

Diagnostic

The diagnostic procedures performed from the vaginal approach on the vulva, vagina, cervix and uterus have been discussed in Chapter 5. Gynecologic patients may also require biopsies of extrapelvic lymph nodes, aspiration of the peritoneal cavity (culdocentesis), aspiration or biopsy of intraperitoneal or parametrial masses or diagnostic procedures on the breast.

In considering any diagnostic test in gynecology, the specificity and sensitivity of the test are important, since the complications of failing to make a diagnosis or of making the wrong diagnosis may be serious (see Chapter 9).

BIOPSIES

Biopsy of an inguinal or scalene lymph node may be a necessary part of the gynecologic diagnostic workup. Biopsy of other lymph nodes or skin nodules occasionally comes within the scope of gynecology or obstetrics. Biopsy of inguinal lymph nodes is usually performed under local anesthesia. Complications include injury to the structures in the femoral triangle (the femoral nerve, artery and vein), hematoma formation, breakdown of the incision and development of a collection of lymph (lymphocele). Injury can be avoided by excising only superficial nodes or, if necessary, the superficial part of a node mass. Frequently, needle aspiration will give enough cells or tissue for diagnosis. Breakdown of the incision can be obviated by placing it parallel to the inguinal ligament. Small collections of lymph usually disappear over several weeks. Large and persistent collections may require one or more aspirations.

Scalene node biopsy (Fig. 12–3) is occasionally part of the workup of a patient with gynecologic cancer. Complications include damage to the internal jugular or the subclavian vein or to the thoracic duct. These structures can be avoided by careful dissection. Small hematomas usually disappear spontaneously; collections of lymph may require aspiration.

Culdocentesis is usually performed in order to obtain a specimen of peritoneal fluid, especially if intraperitoneal bleeding is suspected, for example, in ruptured ectopic pregnancy. Culdocentesis is sometimes used to sample peritoneal fluid for bacteria or malignant cells. The procedure involves pulling the posterior lip of the cervix downward and forward by means of a tenaculum and puncturing the peritoneum of the posterior cul-de-sac with a needle attached to a 10 ml syringe. Complications include pain, inability to obtain fluid, penetration of intestine and intraperitoneal bleeding. Culdocentesis is usually painful. Unfortunately, injection of local anesthetic solution into the cervix at the sites of insertion of the tenaculum requires additional time in a patient who is often already in distress. Moreover, it may not be effective. Furthermore, it is difficult to anesthetize the peritoneum at the site of the puncture, and the injection of anesthetic may be as painful as the puncture itself. The best way to lessen pain is to do the procedure quickly, use a good light source and use the smallest long (spinal) needle compatible with obtaining bloody fluid easily (No. 18 or No. 20). Failure to obtain fluid may be due to a retroflexed uterus or to adhesions in the cul-de-sac. Careful examination in advance may obviate these types of failures. Penetration of the intestine is indicated by the aspiration of brown material, which smells of feces if it comes from the colon. Conservative treatment is indicated; untoward results are not likely to follow. Intraperitoneal bleeding from the uterus or from another pelvic organ such as a pelvic kidney may occur, and a hematoma of the rectal serosa has been reported by Anasti and co-workers (1985).

NEEDLE ASPIRATION

Needle aspiration has simplified the diagnosis of solid intraabdominal and other masses. Using

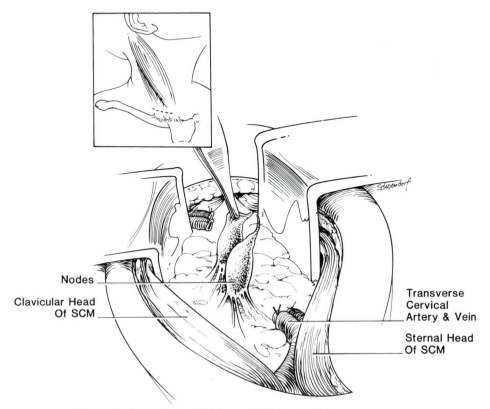

Nodes

Clavicular Head
Of SCM

Transverse
Cervical
Artery & Vein

Sternal Head
Of SCM

Figure 12–3. Scalene node biopsy. SCM, sternocleidomastoid muscle.

a long, fine (22 gauge) needle, with or without localization by ultrasound or CT scan, a tissue sample satisfactory for cytologic examination can be obtained. This is usually sufficient to distinguish malignant from benign cells and often to identify the cell type. A second aspiration is indicated if the first is unproductive and the establishment of a diagnosis is important. A second failure may lead one to use a larger needle and obtain a bigger tissue specimen (Trucut needle) or to perform an open biopsy.

Complications of needle aspiration are few even though the needle may traverse various intraabdominal organs. In a collected series of 11,700 patients, not solely gynecologic, Livraghi and co-workers (1983) reported one death and six major complications. These all occurred following upper abdominal aspirations. In the same series, 0.49% of patients had other less severe complications. In a series limited to aspiration for gynecologic indications, no complications were reported in 90 cases by Belinson and co-workers (1981). Fortier and co-workers (1985) reported that three of 32 patients had pneumothoraces following lung aspiration but none of 50 patients who had aspirations of other sites had any complications. When aspiration was performed on pelvic and para-aortic lymph nodes that showed abnormalities on lymphangiographic examination, nine of 50 patients (18%) were reported by McDonald and co-workers (1983) to have complications. One patient had an apparent retroperitoneal hematoma, one had a subcutaneous hematoma of the anterior abdominal wall, four had pain and three had probable hypersensitivity (rash and fever) to the ethiodized oil used for lymphangiography. Conservative treatment (observation) was used successfully in these patients, and this should be the primary principle of management.

Biopsy of the parametrium with a Vim-Silverman or Trucut needle is often performed in gynecology in preference or in addition to aspiration in order to obtain an adequate tissue sample for staging of carcinoma of the cervix or for the diagnosis of persistent or recurrent disease. Complications are similar to those of needle aspiration. Bleeding from the puncture site is common, especially in patients who have received radiation therapy. It can easily be controlled by simple pressure on the vaginal wall. Among 89 patients studied by Selim and Beck (1984), full thickness of the small intestine was obtained in one biopsy specimen, whereas retroperitoneal hematomas were observed in

two. All were managed conservatively. Close observation is essential, however, because of the possibility of intraperitoneal bleeding or infection, as occurred in one of the author's patients whose radiated small intestine was fixed to the parametrium.

Other types of aspiration that are occasionally used in gynecology and obstetrics include paracentesis (aspiration of the peritoneal cavity) and thoracentesis (aspiration of the pleural cavity). Paracentesis is indicated to determine the nature of intraperitoneal fluid, i.e., blood, pus or ascites (from benign or malignant lesions). It is usually performed in either lower quadrant at about the middle of a line joining the umbilicus to the anterior superior iliac spine or in the midline about half way between the umbilicus and the symphysis pubis. The bladder is emptied, the skin prepared with an antiseptic, and the skin, subcutaneous tissue, muscle and peritoneum infiltrated with local anesthetic. If only a small sample of fluid is needed for diagnosis, this may be obtained with a No. 18 or No. 20 needle. If a large amount of fluid is present owing to an ovarian tumor, removal may be necessary for the patient's comfort. This can usually be done without risk of fluid or electrolyte disturbances. However, if the ascites is due to cirrhosis, removal of more than a small amount of fluid at a time may result in serious changes in plasma volume. When ascites is to be drained as completely as possible, a large trocar and cannula should be used at the sites mentioned in order to speed the removal. A small skin incision is necessary; this can be closed with a stitch after the cannula is withdrawn.

The complications of paracentesis with a smaller needle are few. They include (1) bleeding from the puncture site, (2) perforation of the intestine, (3) subsequent leakage of fluid and (4) infection. Bleeding is a serious problem only in patients with coagulation defects. Perforation usually does not result in serious complications, and fluid leakage stops promptly. Infection is only likely to occur if a patient has generalized sepsis. With a large trocar and cannula, prior aspiration with a small needle, possibly the one used for local anesthesia, is a wise precaution to ensure that fluid is obtained. Perforation of the intestine is more serious with the use of the trocar and cannula. Perforation is more likely to occur in a patient who has widespread cancer or whose abdomen has been previously radiated, thus leading to adhesions and fixed loops of intestine. If perforation is suspected, the procedure should be terminated and the patient carefully observed for signs of intraperitoneal infection. More fluid may leak through the puncture site after the use of a cannula; it will usually stop eventually. If leakage is excessive and dressings do not contain it, a stoma bag with a Karaya seal is helpful.

Thoracentesis may be necessary to determine the nature of an effusion or to remove fluid that is embarrassing respiration. Prior to the procedure the presence and amount of fluid should be ascertained by physical examination and chest x-ray. Generally, thoracentesis should be performed in the mid or posterior axillary line in the seventh, eighth or ninth intercostal space. The patient sits and leans forward with her arms on a bed-side table or similar object. The skin is prepared, and a local anesthetic is injected above the appropriate rib and into the muscle and pleura. Aspiration is performed with a closed system, and the skin puncture is occluded with a firm dressing.

The complications of thoracentesis include mediastinal shift, pneumothorax and pain. Mediastinal shift may occur with the removal of large amounts of fluid. The consequent respiratory distress usually subsides with oxygen therapy; respiratory support is seldom necessary. This complication can usually be avoided by removing no more than 1000 ml at one time. Pneumothorax may result from air leaking into the aspiration system. A chest x-ray is essential after thoracentesis. Management follows the lines described previously for complications of subclavian venipuncture. Pain following thoracentesis subsides in 48 to 72 hours and can be controlled with oral analgesics.

BREASTS

Until recently biopsies and excision biopsies of breast lumps were usually performed as in-patient procedures by general surgeons, who often planned to proceed to mastectomy if cancer was found on frozen section examination. Four factors have changed this situation. First was the finding that a modest delay (less than 30 days) in definitive treatment following biopsy did not affect prognosis (Bertario et al, 1985); second, out-patient procedures were recognized as being more cost-effective; third, needle biopsy and aspiration cytology were found to be effective diagnostic techniques; and, fourth, gynecologists recognized their responsibility for the diagnosis of breast disease as part of the general and routine examination of women.

Aspiration of breast masses or cysts using a 22 gauge needle is a safe initial diagnostic test. It has an accuracy of 92%, a sensitivity of 78% and a specificity of 100% according to a review of 369 biopsy specimens by Somers and co-workers (1985). Complications have not been reported (Hindle and Navin, 1983). A positive report indicates the need for referral for removal of the mass and definitive treatment. If fluid is removed, the mass disappears and cytologic studies are negative, the lesion can generally be considered benign, and no further operative treatment is indicated. If the lesion is solid and cytologic data are equivocal or negative, more tissue must be obtained by core needle or open biopsy. There is no technical reason why either of these out-patient procedures cannot be performed by a well-trained gynecologist; from the patient's point of view it is probably better psychologically, but among physicians interdisciplinary hostility is provoked (Mitchell and Homer, 1982). The complications of core (Trucut) needle biopsy are few. In a report on 158 cases, Minkowitz and co-workers (1986) related one instance of ecchymosis larger than 1 to 2 cm and two instances of severe pleuritic pain lasting 10 minutes and several hours respectively. The complications of open biopsy are minimal and were reported by Badder and Nahrwold (1977) to include ecchymosis (8%), hematoma (5%) and others (3%). None of these complications required more than conservative treatment.

DIAGNOSTIC RADIOLOGY

Imaging techniques used in gynecology and obstetrics include (1) radiologic examinations of specific organs such as the breast (mammogram), abdomen and pelvis; (2) special radiologic studies with or without the use of contrast material, such as computed tomography (CT scans), angiograms, lymphangiograms, hysterosalpingograms or studies of neighboring organs such as the gastrointestinal or urinary tract; and (3) other techniques such as ultrasonography and magnetic resonance imaging (MRI).

Effects of Radiation. In the last 30 years there has been great professional and public concern about the possible effects of radiation on the female genital tract. This has been caused, in part, by greater knowledge of and interest in genetics and in part by confusion with the known side effects of therapeutic radiation. However, in diagnostic radiology, the dose of radiation is usually small, and it is becoming even smaller with the use of newer machines.

The effects of small amounts of radiation on the tubes, uterus, cervix, vagina and vulva appear to be minimal. In the case of mammograms the possible effect of radiation on the later development of breast cancer has been widely discussed, particularly in the late 1970's when the use of mammography became more widespread. Retrospective studies of young women whose breasts were exposed to 100 rads or more of radiation from repeated fluoroscopies for tuberculosis, exposure to atomic bomb radiation or radiation therapy for puerperal mastitis show that radiation may be a causative factor in the development of breast cancer, usually after a latent period of several years (Swartz and Reichling, 1977). It can be calculated that the risk of breast cancer among American women exposed to breast radiation after age 35 is 0.6 excess cancers/million women/rad/year. Early mammography involved a dose of 1 to 5 rads or more per exposure. Thus, repeated examinations were of concern. However, recent advances in techniques have resulted in a mean dose of 66 to 450 millirads per two-film examination (Dodd, 1984). At this dose, if a 35-year-old woman has a 9% life-time risk of developing breast cancer spontaneously, the risk would rise to 9.75% if she had annual mammograms up to age 70. It is reassuring to note that the chance of a woman developing a cancer of the breast from a 250 millirad dose of radiation during a mammogram is 1 to 666,664. This risk is more than outweighed by the benefit resulting from the early detection of a large number of breast cancers. An important proviso is that mammography should be performed with up-to-date machines that have been shown to give a low dose of radiation. Screen-film techniques result in less radiation exposure than does xeromammography, although which technique produces better images is debatable. Recently, magnification mammography has been helpful in clarifying equivocal findings obtained from conventional mammography.

Another concern is the possible effect of diagnostic radiation on the ovary and its genetic material. Estimated radiation to the maternal and fetal gonads during various radiologic examinations is shown in Table 12–3. It should be noted that doses may vary considerably, depending upon the length of exposure, the thickness of the patient's body wall and the quality of the radiographic equipment used. Also, prolonged fluoroscopy, for example in

Table 12–3. Typical Radiation Doses by Millirads*

Chest	5
Cholecystogram	300
Upper GI	330
Intravenous pyelogram	585
Abdomen	185
Pelvimetry	750
Lower GI	465
Pelvis, lower spine	390
Hip, upper femur	100

*From Swartz HM, Reichling BA: Hazards of radiation exposure in pregnant women. *J. Am. Med. Assoc.* 239:1907. Copyright 1978, American Medical Association. Reprinted with permission.

upper or lower gastrointestinal examinations, may add considerably to the dose given. It is theoretically possible that even a very small amount of radiation may affect the genetic material in the ovaries. A high incidence of damage occurs at doses of 50 to 100 rads, but the level at which the danger becomes significant is not known. Dangers to the fetus are covered in Chapter 9. In the non-pregnant woman of reproductive age diagnostic radiologic examinations involving the pelvis should be performed only when the necessary information cannot be obtained in any other way. In the woman who has not been sterilized and who is not taking birth control pills regularly, studies should preferably be performed in the first part of the menstrual cycle, i.e., within 10 days after the onset of menstruation. If possible, the pelvis and abdomen should be shielded when diagnostic examinations are performed on neighboring organs. If the patient is pregnant, the indications should be much more stringent, but with proper radiologic techniques examinations, when they are essential to diagnosis and management, should be obtained.

Special Radiologic Procedures. Special procedures, including CT scans, tend to take longer and require more films than those in which no contrast material is used. Thus, a higher dose of radiation is given to the maternal gonads and to the fetus. In addition, the techniques of inserting or injecting the contrast material may of themselves lead to complications.

A complication common to the intravenous injection of contrast material is hypersensitivity to the dye. Most patients have a sensation of warmth, often unpleasant, as a bolus of dye is injected. Specific hypersensitivity is usually noted promptly and consists of generalized urticaria, which occasionally progresses to angioneurotic edema, respiratory difficulty, respiratory collapse and even death. The incidence of serious hypersensitivity reactions is less than 1% in women not previously sensitized, and minor hypersensitivity occurs in 5 to 10% of such women. Treatment requires the use of epinephrine or an antihistamine together with resuscitative measures (see Chapter 13). Hypersensitivity reactions can be prevented in large part by an accurate history (sensitivity to iodine or eating shellfish), sensitivity testing and antiallergic precautions such as the use of corticosteroids prior to the procedure.

Two special complications of contrast studies are worthy of note. First, intravenous pyelograms, which are commonly performed, are occasionally (less than 1%) followed by oliguria or anuria. Management is covered in Chapter 4. Adequate hydration and a reduction in the dosage of contrast material may prevent this in patients who are elderly or who have diabetes or prior renal insufficiency. Alternatively, the information required may be obtained by ultrasonography of the kidney. Second, in older patients the intestinal preparation required may sometimes induce electrolyte imbalance. This may be avoided by modification of the usual regimen.

Angiography is occasionally used in gynecology to determine the site of persistent hemorrhage or to demonstrate increased blood supply to the uterus, such as occurs in gestational trophoblastic disease. Bleeding from the puncture site and extravasation of dye occur occasionally. Bleeding can usually be prevented by adequate pressure after withdrawal of the needle—at least 10 minutes. Treatment of extravasation is conservative; the drug will eventually be absorbed.

Lymphangiograms are primarily used in gynecology to demonstrate involvement of pelvic and para-aortic lymph nodes by metastatic cancer. The procedure involves identifying lymphatic channels on the dorsum of the feet by subcutaneous injection of a blue dye (vital blue), cannulation of one channel and injection of contrast material. Local complications consist of delayed healing of the skin incision on the foot (stitches should be left in place at least seven days) and persistence of discoloration of the foot and often of the ascending lymphatic vessels for up to two months. General complications (apart from hypersensitivity reactions) include fever and pulmonary embolization of particles of contrast medium that enter the venous circulation through the thoracic duct or through other lymphaticovenous communications. Water-soluble dye is less likely to produce these effects.

They resolve spontaneously with supportive therapy.

Hysterosalpingography is used to diagnose uterine anomalies and as part of the workup of the infertile patient. The procedure involves occluding the cervical os with a rubber acorn cannula or a cup and injecting dye into the uterine cavity and tubes, usually with fluoroscopic observation. Special immediate complications consist of pain as the occlusive device is being inserted and as the uterus is being filled with contrast material. Although premedication is not strictly necessary, the use of diazepam and an antiprostaglandin lessen anxiety, spasm and pain in selected patients. Late complications include pain in 2.7%, pelvic infection in 1.2%, and passage of dye into veins (1.2%) (Measday, 1960). Pelvic pain with or without fever usually occurs within 24 hours. It is commonly associated with distal tubal disease and obstruction. The patient should be examined promptly and appropriate antibiotics (see Table 4–4) should be given if there is clinical evidence of infection, peritonitis or pelvic abscess (Siegler, 1983). Passage of dye into the veins of the pelvis and the development of a granuloma are less common with the use of water-soluble than with oil-soluble contrast material. Prophylactic antibiotics may be appropriate for patients with a history of pelvic inflammation.

Ultrasonography has become a very valuable technique for the diagnosis of pelvic masses as well as in obstretrics (see Chapter 9). The quantities of ultrasound used do not appear to cause any effects on the most sensitive organ of the pelvis, the ovary, except for the possibility of producing sister chromatid exchange (Martin et al, 1984). In pregnant patients no deleterious effects on the offspring were noted by Stark and co-workers (1984) in comparison with matched control patients (see Chapter 9).

Magnetic resonance imaging (MRI) is the latest non-invasive technique for studying pelvic masses. No specific physical complications have been clearly identified as yet. The expense of the machine, the length of time needed for a thorough study (about 1 hour) and the fact that life support systems cannot be placed in the scanning room limit the use of MRI, particularly in critically ill patients.

Miscellaneous Devices and Procedures

MENSTRUAL PROTECTION

Perineal or intravaginal menstrual collectors have been used for generations and have been made of various materials from grass to soft papyrus, wool and cloth. It was not until 1921 that the first commercially successful disposable napkin was introduced in the United States and not until 1960 that internal tampons became widely used, although they had been available since 1936.

Perineal pads cause few complications. If they are worn for many days, the vulvar skin may become irritated, red and even ulcerated. If a deodorant has been added to the pad or deodorant sprays have been used, the patient may occasionally develop a local allergic response with itching, swelling and redness. Pads can be discarded in favor of loose towels (if protection is still needed) or a change made to tampons. Baths and the local use of packs soaked in cold Burow's solution (1 packet of Domeboro powder [aluminum sulfate and calcium acetate] in one pint of water) provide symptomatic relief.

Tampons are commonly used nowadays for menstrual protection. They are made with varying degrees of absorbency, holding from 10 to 20 gm of fluid (Bachmann, 1984). Complications of their use include:

1. Difficulty of insertion. This occurs principally in young girls who are trying this method of protection for the first time. Gentle dilatation of the vaginal opening by the patient with a lubricated finger will overcome the problem unless there is vaginal agenesis or an imperforate hymen.

2. Retention. The string may retract inside the vagina, and the patient may not remember that the tampon is still in place. A foul odor, developing after two to three days, may bring the patient to the gynecologist. Removal and a cleansing douche or bath are all that is needed.

3. Vaginal laceration or ulceration. The vagina is occasionally lacerated as a tampon is inserted. The six cases reported by Gray and co-workers (1981) appeared to have been related to the plastic inserter; one required sutures. Tampons cause exaggeration of the drying and layering of the vaginal mucosa that occurs normally during and even between menstruation. Micro-ulcerations and ulcerations occurred in five of 300 (1.7%) cycles in which tampons were used, being more frequent with super-plus rayon polyacrylate tampons with applicators (Berkeley et al, 1985). Ulcers may cause vaginal bleeding and discharge (Weissberg and Dodson, 1983). Conservative treatment is appropriate unless bleeding requires sutures.

4. Toxic shock syndrome. In some instances, this appears to be related to the prolonged use of high-absorbency tampons, although the connection with *Staphylococcus aureus*, which produces the toxin is not clear. The syndrome is discussed in Chapter 4. Patients who have once had this problem should not use tampons, and tampon users should be advised to leave them in for only four to six hours and not overnight.

5. Urinary tract infections. Foxman and Frerichs (1985) found primary and secondary infection to be moderately associated with the use of tampons.

PESSARIES

Pessaries were used in the past for patients with dysmenorrhea and mobile retroflexed uteri. The uterus was replaced in the anterior position and maintained there by a Smith or a Hodge pessary. Inflated or solid ring pessaries or cubes are occasionally used to support the prolapsed uterus, rectum or vagina in elderly women who cannot withstand or do not wish operative repair. The danger is that they may be forgotten for many months or even years and cause ulceration of the vagina. If ulceration occurs, the pessary must be removed. Ulceration can be prevented or detected early by regular removal and examination of the vaginal wall every two months. Intravaginal estrogens may be helpful.

DOUCHES

Douches are still widely used in the United States, occasionally for medical indications, more often as a cleansing device and as a means of removing odors, particularly after coitus or menstruation. Douches commercially available contain a variety of substances (Kilroy, 1977). Most often water is used either with or without vinegar added in various proportions (1 to 4 Tbsp. per quart). Complications are rare. They include (1) possible trauma to the vaginal wall from the douche nozzle or the use of excessive force (douche bag held too high or solution squeezed in); (2) accidental insertion of the nozzle into the urethra and bladder; (3) burns from hot solutions; (4) air embolism (reported rarely during pregnancy); (5) chemical vaginitis with pain and leukorrhea due to allergic or chemical reaction to a substance in the douche; and (6) alteration in the vaginal flora. All these problems can be managed by discontinuing douches. The possible relationship of douching to ectopic pregnancy has been raised by Wong-Ho Chow and co-workers (1985).

ARTIFICIAL INSEMINATION

Insemination with the husband's (AIH) or donor's sperm (AID) is occasionally used in infertile women. The semen is usually deposited in and around the cervix, and the patient remains on her back with her hips elevated for 15 to 30 minutes to permit additional access of sperm to the cervical canal. Occasionally, semen is injected into the uterus itself. Uterine cramps have been reported to occur in 15% of such patients; in three out of 400 the cramps were severe enough to require admission to the hospital (Barwin, 1974). There is a possibility that infection, including AIDS and the hepatitis virus, may be transmitted by insemination.

PHYSICAL EXERCISE

Increased physical exercise and sports activity by women in the past 20 years has led to concern about possible effects on reproductive function. Three observations are relevant. First, individuals vary greatly in their response to exercise. Second, data are hard to obtain because the amounts of effort and physical stress vary greatly from woman to woman. Third, studies on hormonal changes are conflicting and difficult to interpret. Given the above uncertainties there is currently evidence that:

1. Delayed menarche occurs when female athletes begin training before they start to menstruate (Frisch and Gotz-Welbergen, 1981).

2. There is a high incidence of amenorrhea and oligomenorrhea among athletes (trained or untrained), particularly among runners as opposed to competitors in other sports (Sanborn et al, 1982). This may be related to the menstrual pattern prior to training and to body weight. Although hypoestrogenism and a shortened luteal phase of the menstrual cycle have been implicated, data are by no means consistent (Shangold and Levine, 1982; Galle et al, 1983). Amenorrheic runners are at some risk for exercise-related fractures and decreased mineral density of the lumbar spine (Marcus et al, 1985).

3. Menstruation usually reverts to the original pattern after athletic participation is discontinued, and there does not appear to be any long-term effect on reproductive performance.

4. Concern has been expressed that running or other vigorous exercise may increase pelvic relaxation and therefore increase cystocele, rectocele or prolapse. There is no evidence that this occurs. Women who have slight stress incontinence may find this exaggerated with major physical exertion; emptying the bladder prior to such exercise is helpful.

Contraception

In this section contraceptive devices, vaginal, cervical and intrauterine, will be considered. Systemic oral contraceptives are discussed in Chapter 13.

OCCLUSIVE DEVICES

Throughout recorded history intravaginal substances have been used in attempts to prevent conception. Currently, such methods include diaphragms, sponges, cervical caps and spermicidal foam, jellies and suppositories. From the woman's point of view the main complication of any method is pregnancy. Data vary, but ranges of pregnancy rates are given in Table 12–4. The differences are largely due to the user and less to the device's effectiveness. Specific complications for each method follow.

Diaphragm

PAIN. Pain may occur during insertion or during or after intercourse. It may be associated with inability to void. Pain may be caused by an incorrectly sized device, reluctance to use the diaphragm on the patient's part or dislodgement during intercourse. In any case, a careful history must be taken and the size checked. In general, a smaller diaphragm appears to be equally effective and may cause less discomfort.

Table 12–4. Pregnancy Rates for Vaginal Contraceptives*

Type of Contraceptive	Rate/100 Women-Years of Use
Creams	4.7–9.1
Diaphragms	2.2–33.6
Foam	1.8–35.0
Foaming tablets	2.3–38.3
Jellies	2.7–36.1
Suppositories	0.0–27.0
Cervical caps	7.6–16.9†

*Data from Edelman DA. *Int. J. Gynaecol. Obstet.* 22:11, 1984.

†Data from Johnson JM. *Am. J. Obstet. Gynecol.* 148:604, 1984.

BLEEDING. Bleeding into the diaphragm is quite commonly reported. It may be physiologic, owing to the onset of menstruation, or pathologic, owing to changes in the cervix or endometrium. Investigation of all possible causes is indicated.

INFECTION. Retention of a diaphragm for 24 hours or more causes an increase in the number of bacteria of all types that can be recovered from the vagina (Baehler et al, 1983). In this study there was no evidence of clinical infection; nor is the effect of leaving the diaphragm in the vagina for the more usual time of six to ten hours known. However, vaginal colonization with *E. coli* was found to be increased in users of diaphragms or cervical caps. This is probably related to the higher incidence of urinary tract infection found among diaphragm users (Percival-Smith et al, 1983; Fihn et al, 1985). Voiding before coitus and the use of a single small dose of urinary antibiotics (320 mg trimethoprim with 1200 mg sulfamethoxazole) after intercourse may help to prevent recurrent infections.

Cervical Cap. Cervical caps have been more widely used in Europe than in the United States, although there was some upsurge in interest in them in the U.S. during the late 1970's and early 1980's because of concern about the dangers of oral contraceptives and intrauterine devices. The cap appears to be a less effective contraceptive than the diaphragm. Complications include the difficulty of fitting the cap to the cervix, the length of time taken for instruction of the patient and the possibility of dislodgement during coitus. Also mentioned have been vaginal odor, partner discomfort and deterioration of the cap after one year of use (Cagen, 1986).

Vaginal Sponge. Recently contraceptive sponges incorporating the spermicide nonoxynol 9 have become available. They can be used for multiple coital exposures and left in place for 24 hours. Limited data are available on their use. The pregnancy rate is slightly higher than that for the diaphragm. As compared with diaphragm users, sponge users found insertion easier but expulsion more common and were more likely to discontinue use because of "allergic" reactions or discomfort (itching). Occasional difficulty in removal has been reported because the string disappeared into the vagina (Edelman et al, 1983; Family Planning Perspectives, 1985). Toxic shock syndrome has been reported to occur once per estimated 100,000 users (13 cases) (North and Vorhauer, 1985).

Spermicides. Various spermicides have been used for contraception, either alone or with occlusive devices. No specific ill effects have been detected. Concern that these agents, if used around the time of conception, might increase the incidence of abortions, reduced birthweight infants or congenital malformation has been shown to be unfounded (Mills et al, 1985).

INTRAUTERINE DEVICES

An intrauterine contraceptive device was first described by Grafenberg in 1928, but was not favorably regarded as a method of birth control until the 1960's. Then came a spate of loops, spirals, bows and rings made of steel and plastic material (Tietze, 1965). Later copper and progesterone-containing devices were developed. Although many different types are available worldwide (Population Reports, 1982), the Lippes loop and the Copper 7 were almost exclusively used in the United States until recently. The withdrawal of both these devices from the market has currently deprived American women of an effective method of contraception. However, since it is likely that these IUDs are still in place in a number of women and more devices may be manufactured in the future, it is appropriate to review the complications that can follow their insertion.

Difficulty of Insertion. Insertion is usually painful because of the required dilatation of the cervix and the irritability and contractions of the uterus once the device is in place. The discomfort of insertion can be reduced by performing it at the end of menstruation when the cervix is somewhat open. Local anesthesia, in the form a of paracervical block, can be used, but this lengthens the time required for the procedure and of itself causes some discomfort. Uterine contractions usually last only a few minutes but may continue for one to two days; analgesics and antiprostaglandins are helpful. The length of the endometrial cavity may affect the performance of the IUD. Thus, if the cavity is shorter or longer than the IUD by 2 cm or more, pregnancy, expulsion or the need for medical removal increase significantly (Hasson et al, 1976). The mode of insertion does not seem to be related to the occurrence of complications (Bayad et al, 1981).

Alteration in Menstrual Flow and Pain. Women wearing IUDs have increased blood loss at menstruation, the loss being somewhat more for those with Lippes loops than for those with Copper 7s (Guillebaud et al, 1976). In addition, bleeding often occurs for several days after insertion, and menstruation may be prolonged at least for several months. Women wearing IUDs should be counseled about eating foods rich in iron (see Table 4–2) and should probably receive supplemental iron. Excessive bleeding may be a reason for removing the IUD. Use of the progesterone-containing IUD reduces menstrual blood loss (Hefnawi et al, 1982), but the incidence of intermenstrual spotting is increased, and the device has to be replaced annually, as compared with every three years (present recommendation) for the Copper 7 and for an indefinitely longer time with the Lippes loop.

Some women who wear IUDs report increased dysmenorrhea. This, however, may be related to the patient's history of prior menstrual pain, and it may also signify impending expulsion of the device. In any case, severe pain unrelieved by antiprostaglandins is an indication for removal of the IUD.

Perforation, Expulsion, Disappearance. Normally an IUD remains free in the uterine cavity and can be removed easily. Perforation of the uterine wall by the device is believed to occur in 1 of 350 to 1 of 2600 insertions. The IUD may be inserted initially through the wall or it may be inserted into the wall and work its way through many months later. Also, it may erode the wall and become covered by epithelium and imbedded or incarcerated. Perforation does not seem to be related to the type of IUD used but rather to local anatomic differences. Lactating women appear to be at higher risks of perforation (Heartwell and Schlesselman, 1983).

It is not always possible to avoid perforating the uterus at the time of insertion. However, determination of the position of the uterus, careful sounding of the cavity and gentleness in insertion can reduce the chances of perforation (Walden, 1984). No force should be used. The procedure should be stopped if it becomes difficult or if the patient has excessive pain. If perforation is suspected at the time of insertion, steps should be taken, as outlined later, to identify the position of the IUD. Late perforation may be accompanied by migration of the IUD into the intestine or bladder (Zakin, 1984) or it may become imbedded in the mesentery of the small intestine, occasionally causing intestinal obstruction (Fig. 12–4).

The patient may report disappearance of the IUD either because it has been expelled with-

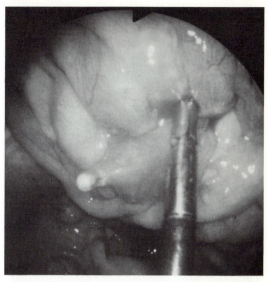

Figure 12–4. IUD in the mesentery of the small intestine.

out her knowledge or because she can no longer feel the string protruding from the cervix. On examination the string may be visible; in this case, reassurance and reinstruction about feeling the string are all that are needed. If the string cannot be seen, a search must be made for it, since it may have retracted up into the uterus or the device may have perforated the uterine wall. The following steps should be taken.

1. Extrauterine location may be suspected on pelvic examination. The possibility of pregnancy with a retained IUD must be kept in mind (see later section).

2. Attempts should be made to grasp the string in the cervical canal with a uterine dressing forceps.

3. Ultrasonography should be performed to determine the presence and site of the IUD. If the ultrasonographic examination is inconclusive, an x-ray examination should be obtained.

4. If the device appears to be in the uterus, it can often be pulled down with a crochet hook or a small Novak's endometrial biopsy curette, using local paracervical block anesthesia. The use of a Karman cannula and suction has also been suggested (Goh, 1978).

5. Hysteroscopy may identify the device in the uterus and permit extraction.

6. If the device appears to be outside the uterus (i.e., to have completely perforated the uterine wall), laparoscopy and possible laparotomy are required for removal.

Infection

PELVIC INFLAMMATORY DISEASE. Many studies have shown an association between the use of IUDs and pelvic inflammatory disease (PID) (Cramer et al, 1985), although not all investigators agree (Larsson et al, 1981). It appears likely that women with a previous history of PID may be more susceptible to infection when the IUD is in place. Younger nulliparous women were thought to be more liable to such infections (Westrom et al, 1976; Booth et al, 1980), but after stratifying for age, O'Brien and co-workers (1983) found PID to be more common in parous than in nulliparous IUD users. The incidence of acute PID decreases with the length of time the IUD has been in place (Vessey et al, 1981). Of the various types of IUDs, the Dalkon shield was associated with the highest incidence of PID.

The reason for the development of pelvic infection with IUDs appears to be the ascent of bacteria from the vagina and cervix along the tail of the device. Cultures from removed IUDs showed more pathogenic bacteria in those from patients with documented PID than in those without such infection (Nilsson et al, 1981). Also, Sparks and co-workers (1981) found bacteria in the endometrium in 15 of 17 women with tailed devices. The persistence of these organisms was noted long after insertion, and colonization of the endometrium was thought to be important, since bacteria were cultured from only four of the devices themselves. Surface alterations in the IUD itself may also contribute to infection (Schmidt, 1982). An increase in the number of sexual partners and in the incidence of sexually transmitted diseases may also add to the occurrence of PID in women who may be more susceptible to infection because they are wearing IUDs (Newton and Keith, 1985). Chlamydia infections may be of special importance (Guderian and Trobough, 1986).

The clinical picture of PID associated with IUDs includes lower abdominal pain and fever. Examination shows tenderness on motion of the cervix and in the region of the tube. Pelvic masses may also be felt. Management is by antibiotics, preferably tetracycline, which should be started as soon as a culture is obtained, although the offending organism is not known immediately. The IUD should be removed, although some authors recommend removal only if the infection is not controlled in 48 hours. Unilateral or bilateral tubo-ovarian abscesses may follow acute salpingitis, as with any type of pelvic infection.

The long-term effects of pelvic inflammation associated with IUDs include infertility and ectopic pregnancy. Cramer and co-workers (1985) and Daling and co-workers (1985) noted increased tubal infertility among women who had used IUDs, although the risk was less with the copper IUD. Data from various sources indicate a higher than expected incidence of ectopic pregnancy among IUD users, but quantitation of the risk is difficult because existing data lack controls (Malhotra and Chaudhury, 1982). Such information as is available suggests that an ectopic pregnancy occurs in about 1 in 30 pregnancies among patients wearing IUDs as compared with 1 in 125 in non-users. Explanations for this increase are that IUDs protect against intrauterine but not against extrauterine pregnancy, or that the IUD may in some way affect the function of the fallopian tube.

ACTINOMYCOSIS. *Actinomyces israelii*, an opportunistic anaerobic organism found in the skin, mucous membranes, oral cavity and gastrointestinal tract, has been reported to be present in the genital tract of IUD users much more frequently than in women not wearing IUDs. Among 6925 women it was found in 1.6%; all were IUD users (Valicenti et al, 1982). Similarly Petitti and co-workers (1983) noted that 104 of 107 women with *Actinomyces*-like organisms in cervicovaginal smears were wearing IUDs. However, the careful studies of Persson and Holmberg (1984) indicate that *A. israelii* may, in fact, be part of the indigenous flora of the genital tract and not related to different contraceptive methods.

The majority of women in whom *Actinomyces* are found are asymptomatic (110 of 112 described by Valicenti et al, 1982). However, endocervicitis, endometritis, salpingitis or pelvic abscess can occur (Yoonessi et al, 1985) and are potential problems whenever actinomycosis is present. Thus, many authors (International Correspondence Society of Obstetricians and Gynecologists, 1982) have recommended removal of the IUD, once the diagnosis has been established by review of the slides or by a second careful cytologic study, but no treatment is advised for the asymptomatic patient. With evidence of infection, high doses of penicillin (20 mil units per day over 4 to 6 weeks) and surgical therapy (unilateral or bilateral removal of tube and ovary) may be necessary.

PREGNANCY. When an intrauterine pregnancy occurs with an IUD in situ, abortion results in 50% of women; this is two to three times the normal rate, with a large proportion of abortions occurring in the second trimester.

Removal of the IUD early in pregnancy reduces the abortion rate by half (Foreman et al, 1981). If, in a pregnant patient, the IUD string cannot be seen, or if a tailless device is present, the IUD must be left in place if the woman wants to continue the pregnancy. In this case, infection may occur later with only mild symptoms. Prompt removal of the IUD and multiple antibiotic therapy is then indicated. Also, premature deliveries, stillbirths and low-birth-weight infants are more common when the IUD remains within the uterus.

REFERENCES

Actinomyces in patients using IUDs, collected letters. *Int. Correspondence Soc. Obstet. Gynecol.* Lakeland, FL. 23(21) November 1982.

Aitken DR, Minton JP: The "Pinch-off sign": a warning of impending problems with permanent subclavian catheters. *Am. J. Surg.* 148:633, 1984.

Anasti J, Buscema J, Genadry R: Rectal serosal hematoma: an unusual complication of culdocentesis. *Obstet. Gynecol.* 65:72S, 1985.

Bachmann GA: Evaluating menstrual hygiene devices. *Contemp. Obstet. Gynecol.* 24:71, 1984.

Badder EM, Nahrwold DL: A selective approach to outpatient breast biopsy under local anesthesia. *J. Reprod. Med.* 19:133, 1977.

Baehler EA, Dillon WP et al: The effects of prolonged retention of diaphragms on colonization by staphylococcus aureus of the lower genital tract. *Fertil. Steril.* 39:162, 1983.

Barwin BM: Intrauterine insemination of husband's sperm. *J. Reprod. Fert.* 36:101, 1974.

Bayad MAB, Osman MI et al: Effect of mode of insertion of IUDs on the occurrence of complications. *Contracept. Del. Syst.* 2:37, 1981.

Belinson JL, Lynn JM et al: Fine-needle aspiration cytology in the management of gynecologic cancer. *Am. J. Obstet. Gynecol.* 139:148, 1981.

Berkeley AS, Micha JP et al: The potential of digitally inserted tampons to induce vaginal lesions. *Obstet. Gynecol.* 66:31, 1985.

Bertario L, Reduzzi D et al: Outpatient biopsy of breast cancer: influence on survival. *Ann. Surg.* 201:64, 1985.

Booth M, Beral V, Guillebaud J: Effect of age on pelvic inflammatory disease in nulliparous women using a copper 7 intrauterine contraceptive device. *Br. Med. J.* 2:114, 1980.

Cagan R: The cervical cap as a barrier contraceptive. *Contraception* 33:487, 1986.

Chow WH, Daling JR et al: Vaginal douching as a potential risk factor for tubal ectopic pregnancy. *Am. J. Obstet. Gynecol.* 153:727, 1985.

Collignon PJ, Munro R, Sorrell TC: Systemic sepsis and intravenous devices: a prospective survey. *Med. J. Aust.* 141:345, 1984.

Cotton DB, Benedetti TJ: Use of the Swan-Ganz catheter in obstetrics and gynecology. *Obstet. Gynecol.* 56:641, 1980.

Cramer DW, Schiff I et al: Tubal infertility and the intrauterine device. *N. Engl. J. Med.* 312:941, 1985.

Daling JR, Weiss NS et al: Primary tubal infertility in relation to the use of an intrauterine device. *N. Engl. J. Med.* 312:937, 1985.

Dodd GD: Mammography: state of the art. *Cancer* 53:652, 1984.

Edelman DA: Vaginal contraception: an overview. *Int. J. Gynaecol. Obstet.* 22:11, 1984.

Edelman DA, Smith SC, McIntyre S: Comparative trial of the contraceptive sponge and diaphragm—a preliminary report. *J. Reprod. Med.* 28:781, 1983.

Failure rates for sponge are higher than for diaphragm: parous sponge users are most likely to conceive, editorial. *Fam. Plann. Perspect.* 17:80, 1985.

Fares LG, Block PH, Feldman SD: Improved house staff results with subclavian cannulation. *Am. Surg.* 52:108, 1986.

Fihn SD, Latham RH et al: Association between diaphragm use and urinary tract infection. *J. Am. Med. Assoc.* 254:240, 1985.

Foreman H, Stadel BV, Schlesselman S: Intrauterine device usage and fetal loss. *Obstet. Gynecol.* 58:669, 1981.

Fortier KJ, Clarke-Pearson DL, Creasman WT: Fine-needle aspiration in gynecology: evaluation of extrapelvic lesions in patients with gynecologic malignancy. *Obstet. Gynecol.* 65:67, 1985.

Foxman B, Frerichs RR: Epidemiology of urinary tract infection: II. Diet, clothing and urination habits. *Am. J. Publ. Hlth.* 75:1314, 1985.

Frisch RE, Gotz-Welbergen AV: Delayed menarche and amenorrhea of college athletes in relation to age of onset of training. *J. Am. Med. Assoc.* 246:1559, 1981.

Galle PC, Freeman EW et al: Physiologic and psychologic profiles in a survey of women runners. *Fertil. Steril.* 39:633, 1983.

Gillies H, Rogers HJ et al: Is repeated flushing of Hickman catheters necessary? *Br. Med. J.* 290:1708, 1985.

Gilligan JE, Phillips PJ et al: Streptokinase and blocked central venous catheter. *Lancet* 2:1189, 1979.

Goh TH: The use of a Karman cannula and suction to manage a retained IUD with a retracted thread. *Int. J. Gynaecol. Obstet.* 16:80, 1978.

Gray MJ, Norton P, Treadwell K: Tampon-induced injuries. *Obstet. Gynecol.* 58:667, 1981.

Guderian AM, Trobough GE: Residues of pelvic inflammatory disease in intrauterine device users: a result of the intrauterine device or chlamydia trachomatis infection? *Am. J. Obstet. Gynecol.* 154:497, 1986.

Guillebaud J, Bonnar J et al: Menstrual blood-loss with intrauterine devices. *Lancet* 1:387, 1976.

Hasson HM, Berger GS, Edelman DA: Factors affecting intrauterine contraceptive device performance. 1. Endometrial cavity length. *Am. J. Obstet. Gynecol.* 126:973, 1976.

Heartwell SF, Schlesselman S: Risk of uterine perforation among users of intrauterine devices. *Obstet. Gynecol.* 61:31, 1983.

Hefnawi F, Hamza A et al: Menstrual pattern and blood loss with U-coil inert progesterone-releasing IUDs. *Contracept. Del. Syst.* 3:91, 1982.

Hindle WH, Navin J: Breast aspiration cytology: a neglected gynecologic procedure. *Am. J. Obstet. Gynecol.* 146:482, 1983.

Holland RB, Levitt MW et al: Intravenous cannulas. Survey of their use in patients undergoing elective surgery. *Med. J. Aust.* 2:86, 1982.

Johnson JM: The cervical cap: a retrospective study of an alternative contraceptive technique. *Am. J. Obstet. Gynecol.* 148:604, 1984.

Kilroy PM: Feminine hygiene products: issues and answers. *J. Obstet. Gynecol. Neonat. Nurs.* 6:37, 1977.

Lambert MJ: Air embolism in central venous catheterization—diagnosis, treatment, and prevention. *South. Med. J.* 75:1189, 1982.

Larsson B, Rodau S, Patek E: Pelvic inflammatory disease among women using copper IUDs, progesta-sert, oral contraceptive pills or vaginal contraceptive pills—a 4-year prospective investigation. *Contracept. Del. Syst.* 2:237, 1981.

Livraghi T, Damascelli B et al: Risk in the fine-needle abdominal biopsy. *JCU* 11:77, 1983.

Lokich JJ, Becker B: Subclavian vein thrombosis in patients treated with infusion chemotherapy for advanced malignancy. *Cancer* 52:1586, 1983.

Malhotra N, Chaudhury RR: Current status of intrauterine devices. II. Intrauterine devices and pelvic inflammatory disease and ectopic pregnancy. *Obstet. Gynecol. Surv.* 37:1, 1982.

Marcus R, Cann C et al: Menstrual function and bone mass in elite women distance runners: endocrine and metabolic features. *Ann. Intern. Med.* 102:158, 1985.

Martin AO, Simpson JL et al: Sister chromatid exchanges after exposure to ultrasound and mitomycin C. *Am. J. Obstet. Gynecol.* 148:991, 1984.

McDonald TW, Morley GW et al: Fine needle aspiration of para-aortic and pelvic lymph nodes showing lymphangiographic abnormalities. *Obstet. Gynecol.* 61:383, 1983.

Measday B: An analysis of the complications of hysterosalpingography. *J. Obstet. Gynaecol. Br. Commonwlth.* 67:663, 1960.

Miller JDB, Broom J: Early non-radiological recognition of misplacment of central venous catheter. *Br. Med. J.* 287:95, 1983.

Mills JL, Reed GF et al: Are there adverse effects of periconceptional spermicide use? *Fertil. Steril.* 43:442, 1985.

Minkowitz S, Moskowitz R et al: Tru-Cut needle biopsy of the breast. An analysis of its specificity and sensitivity. *Cancer* 57:320, 1986.

Mitchell GW, Homer MJ: Outpatient breast biopsies on a gynecologic service. *Am. J. Obstet. Gynecol.* 144:127, 1982.

Newton W, Keith LG: Role of sexual behavior in the development of pelvic inflammatory disease. *J. Reprod. Med.* 30:82, 1985.

Nilsson CG, Vartiainen E, Widholm O: Bacterial cultures from intrauterine devices removed from patients with pelvic inflammatory disease. *Acta Obstet. Gynecol. Scand.* 60:563, 1981.

North BB, Vorhauer BW: Use of the Today contraceptive sponge in the United States. *Int. J. Fertil.* 30:81, 1985.

O'Brien FB, Stewart WC, Sturtevant FM: Incidence of pelvic inflammatory disease in clinical trials with Cu-7 (intrauterine copper contraceptive): a statistical analysis. *Contraception* 27:111, 1983.

Parsa MH, Tabora F: Establishment of intravenous lines for long-term intravenous therapy and monitoring. *Surg. Clin. North Am.* 65:835, 1985.

Percival-Smith R, Bartlett KH, Chow AW: Vaginal colonization of Escherichia coli and its relation to contraceptive methods. *Contraception* 28:497, 1983.

Persson E, Holmberg K: A longitudinal study of *Actinomyces israelii* in the female genital tract. *Acta Obstet. Gynecol. Scand.* 63:207, 1984.

Pessa ME, Howard RJ: Complications of Hickman-Broviac catheters. *Surg. Gynecol. Obstet.* 161:257, 1985.

Peters JL (Ed.): *A Manual of Central Venous Catheterization and Parenteral Nutrition.* Bristol, John Wright & Sons, 1983.

Petitti DB, Yamamoto D, Morgenstern N: Factors associated with actinomyces-like organisms on Papanicolaou smear in users of intrauterine contraceptive devices. *Am. J. Obstet. Gynecol.* 145:338, 1983.

Population Reports: Series B No. 4, Baltimore, *Population Information Program,* July 1982.

Press OW, Ramsey PG et al: Hickman catheter infection in patients with malignancies. *Medicine* 63:189, 1984.

Rapp RP, Bivins B: Lowering costs and complications with in-line filters. *Infect. Surg.* 4:400, 1985.

Sanborn CF, Martin BJ et al: Is athletic amenorrhea specific to runners? *Am. J. Obstet. Gynecol.* 143:859, 1982.

Schmidt WA: IUDs, inflammation, and infection: assessment after two decades of IUD use. *Hum. Pathol.* 13:878, 1982.

Selim MA, Beck D: Parametrial needle biopsy: follow-up of pelvic malignancies. *Cancer Detect. Prev.* 7:269, 1984.

Shangold MM, Levine HS: The effect of marathon training upon menstrual function. *Am. J. Obstet. Gynecol.* 143:862, 1982.

Siegler AM: Hysterosalpingography. *Fertil. Steril.* 40:139, 1983.

Smith VC, Hallett JW: Subclavian vein thrombosis during prolonged catheterization for parenteral nutrition. *South. Med. J.* 76:603, 1983.

Somers RG, Young GP et al: Fine-needle aspiration biopsy in the management of solid breast tumors. *Arch. Surg.* 120:673, 1985.

Sparks RA, Purrier BGA et al: Bacteriological colonisation of uterine cavity: role of tailed intrauterine contraceptive device. *Br. Med. J.* 282:1189, 1981.

Stark CR, Orleans M et al: Short- and long-term risks after exposure to diagnostic ultrasound in utero. *Obstet. Gynecol.* 63:194, 1984.

Swartz HM, Reichling BA: The risks of mammograms. *J. Am. Med. Assoc.* 237:965, 1977.

Swartz HM, Reichling BA: Hazards of radiation exposure for pregnant women. *J. Am. Med. Assoc.* 239:1907, 1978.

Tietze C: History and statistical evaluation of intrauterine contraceptive devices. *J. Chron. Dis.* 18:1147, 1965.

Valicenti JF, Pappas AA et al: Detection and prevalence of IUD-associated actinomyces colonization and related morbidity: a prospective study of 69,925 cervical smears. *J. Am. Med. Assoc.* 247:1149, 1982.

Vasquez RM, Jarrard MM: Care of the central venous catheterization site: the use of a transparent polyurethane film. *JPEN* 8:181, 1984.

Vessey MP, Yeates D et al: Pelvic inflammatory disease and the intrauterine device: findings in a large cohort study. *Br. Med. J.* 282:855, 1981.

Walden WD: Uterine perforation: management and prevention. *Infect. Surg.* 3:914, 1984.

Weissberg SM, Dodson MG: Recurrent vaginal and cervical ulcers associated with tampon use. *J. Am. Med. Assoc.* 250:1430, 1983.

Westrom L, Bengtsson LP, Mårdh P-A: The risk of pelvic inflammatory disease in women using intrauterine contraceptive devices as compared to non-users. *Lancet* 2:221, 1976.

Yoonessi M, Crickard K et al: Association of actinomyces and intrauterine contraceptive devices. *J. Reprod. Med.* 30:48, 1985.

Zakin D: Perforation of the bladder by the intrauterine device. *Obstet. Gynecol. Surv.* 39:59, 1984.

Zakin D, Stern WZ, Rosenblatt R: Perforated and embedded intrauterine devices. *J. Am. Med. Assoc.* 247:2144, 1982.

COMPLICATIONS OF DRUG THERAPY IN GYNECOLOGY AND OBSTETRICS

13

MICHAEL NEWTON
EDWARD R. NEWTON

In this chapter, the main side effects of drugs commonly used for gynecologic and obstetric conditions will be considered. In the discussion of the gynecologic patient, drugs used for disorders of other organ systems will not be included unless they have a specific effect on reproductive function. For the obstetric patient, a different approach to drug complications is needed because of the possible effects of drugs on the fetus or, in the case of lactation, on the newborn. In general, categories rather than individual drugs will be covered. Over-the-counter (OTC) drugs will be included insofar as they are likely to cause complications.

The incidence of drug complications is hard to determine for several reasons. First, data obtained from introductory studies are often reliable but include relatively few cases; greater use results in the discovery of unexpected effects, and reports on these tend, at least at first, to be anecdotal rather than statistical. Second, the drug itself may be responsible for the complication, or the complication may result from a combination of the drug in question with other drugs that the patient is receiving. Third, the supposed effects may be caused by some entirely unrelated condition or event. Fourth, individuals respond to drugs in different manners, depending upon genetic, racial, ethnic and familial factors and environmental and personal factors such as climate, temperature, food, alcohol use, or smoking. What may be a minor and temporary inconvenience to some may be catastrophic for others. When accurate data are not available or there is confusion in the results, qualitative terms will be used. Thus, in this chapter, "rarely" means less than 1%, "sometimes" or "occasionally," 1 to 9%, "commonly" or "frequently," 10 to 49%, and "usually," 50% or more.

PREVENTION OF COMPLICATIONS

The principles of preventing complications of drug therapy apply to all classes of drugs. They include the following:

1. A history of allergy or sensitivity to the proposed medication or related compounds should always be obtained. Even if the patient has given a negative history in the past, the history should be checked again, because changes develop over the years, or the patient may have reacted to the planned drugs since the negative history was obtained.

2. Age and sex differences must be considered. For example, 70-year-old women tolerate postoperative pain medication less well than those who are 30. Doses must generally be larger in women weighing 100 kg than in those weighing 50 kg. Any other drugs that the patient is taking must be reviewed to avoid antagonistic or cumulative action.

3. Informed consent is just as important prior to drug therapy as it is before operations. The same dilemma occurs in regard to the number of possible complications that should be described to the patient. Although there is no hard and fast rule, complications that are especially important (i.e., hypertension or thrombosis with oral contraceptives) or those that are likely to occur in 1% or more of patients (i.e., vasomotor symptoms with danazol) should be discussed.

4. Care must be taken in prescribing. This means providing legible and specific instructions that are to be written on the bottle or container. The number of doses should be limited to those necessary to obtain the desired effect. The number of refills should be clearly identified and the possibility of drug dependency always kept in mind. The use of generic or brand names is a matter of individual preference. Expense to the patient must always be considered. Prescribing by telephone is acceptable if the patient and her problem are well known, but it is to be avoided for unknown (or known) patients with undiagnosed disease; the potential medicolegal problems are considerable.

5. Instructions to the patient must be clear. It is best to write down the essential ones; if a printed form is available for a particular medication, it is important to be sure that it fits one's practice, and, if not, to change it. It is wise to be familiar with package inserts used by the manufacturer or required by the U.S. government. Instructions must include what to do if the medication does not help or if the patient is sensitive to it. A major part of drug therapy is persuading the patient to take the medication at the recommended time and for the recommended duration. Health professionals tend to refer to this process as "patient compliance," but it is better to think of it as the implementation of an agreement between patient and physician to treat the patient's complaint or prevent further disease. Methods used to improve "compliance" include one-to-one counseling, group education, written materials, labels, audio-visual materials, memory aids and package inserts. The first is the most important, especially when combined with other techniques.

DRUGS USED IN GYNECOLOGY

Analgesics

The complications of analgesia can be classified according to the class of drug and to individual medications.

ANALGESICS FOR MILD TO MODERATE PAIN

These include a large number of single and combined drugs. They are primarily given by mouth. Aspirin and acetaminophen (650 mg every 3 to 4 hours) frequently serve as standards.

Aspirin. Aspirin is a weak anti-inflammatory agent and is useful for rheumatic disease and as an antipyretic and pain-reliever. Complications usually follow large doses, but occur occasionally with small ones. They include gastrointestinal symptoms of epigastric distress, nausea, vomiting and anorexia. Small mucosal ulcers may lead to severe intestinal bleeding; bleeding from various sites due to prolongation of clotting time may also occur (inhibition of platelet aggregation). Headaches, dizziness and tinnitus and hypersensitivity (rare) are other complications.

Acetaminophen. Acetaminophen has actions similar to those of aspirin, but does not have anti-inflammatory properties. Complications are rare although skin rashes, drug fever, myelosuppression and, with large doses over prolonged periods, methemoglobinemia or renal and liver toxicity may occur.

Proproxyphene. Propoxyphene (Darvon), in doses of 65 mg, is less potent than aspirin or codeine (see later section), but its analgesic effect is increased by combination with acetaminophen. Blood levels are cumulative, reaching a steady state in plasma in one to two days after doses given every six hours. Complications, which rarely accompany the usual therapeutic doses, include dizziness, sedation, nausea and vomiting and respiratory depression.

Antiprostaglandins. Antiprostaglandins include a variety of drugs such as indomethacin (Indocin), sulindac (Clinoril), mefenamic acid (Ponstel), ibuprofen (Motrin) and naproxen (Naprosyn, Anaprox). These drugs have anti-inflammatory properties but also relieve pain and reduce fever. They are especially useful for dysmenorrhea, being effective in 70 to 80% of women. The chief complications of all these agents are gastrointestinal and consist of anorexia, nausea and abdominal pain with, rarely, development of ulcers leading to hemorrhage and anemia. Complications are commonest with indomethacin (35 to 50%) and occur somewhat less commonly (25%) with the other agents. Neutropenia, thrombocytopenia, increased bleeding time (inhibition of platelet aggregation) and aplastic anemia occur rarely; hypersensitivity reactions have also been reported. The gastrointestinal side-effects may necessitate discontinuation of the drug in up to 25% of patients. However, another product of the same class can be tried, since the same side effect may not be observed.

OPIOID ANALGESICS FOR MILD TO MODERATE PAIN

Opioid analgesics are usually given by mouth. There are two main types: codeine and oxycodone (Percodan).

Codeine. Codeine is commonly used in combination with acetamenophen or aspirin in doses of 30 to 60 mg. The side effects of codeine are similar to those of other opioids given for severe pain (see later section), including the potential for addiction. Since codeine is effective by mouth (60% as potent as when it is given intramuscularly) and many oral preparations of codeine in combination with other drugs are available, nausea and vomiting are important reactions especially because they may lead to discontinuation of the drug.

Oxycodone. Oxycodone with or without acetamenophen serves as an alternative to codeine. Gastrointestinal effects are less common, but otherwise it shares the complications of other opioids. It has considerable potential for drug dependency.

OPIOID ANALGESICS FOR SEVERE PAIN

Opioid analgesics may be given for acute episodes of pelvic pain, for postoperative pain or for the pain of malignant disease. The management of postoperative pain is discussed in Chapter 4. Analgesics are usually given subcutaneously or intramuscularly, or, rarely, intravenously in these situations. The treatment of cancer pain is covered in Chapter 7. For these patients the oral route of administration is often preferable.

Morphine. Morphine serves as a standard against which these analgesic opioids are judged, and equivalent doses of other agents (oral and parenteral) are shown in Table 13–1. All opioid analgesics have similar complications, although they vary somewhat from drug to drug. Complications include:

1. Respiratory depression. This is common and similar for all opioids. It is of importance primarily in elderly or debilitated women or in those with decreased respiratory reserve. Lower doses should be given to these patients.

2. Nausea occurs in 40% and vomiting in 15% of ambulatory patients, but only occasionally in those who remain recumbent. These complications may be alleviated by concomitant use of dimenhydrinate, promethazine or diazepam.

3. Constipation is common in patients taking opioids for more than a few doses. Meperidine is somewhat less likely than morphine to cause constipation.

4. Increase in sphincter tone occasionally affects the biliary system and urinary tract, making obstruction (biliary colic or urinary retention) more likely in those patients with biliary disease or any persisting urinary tract obstruction. These complications are somewhat less likely to occur with meperidine.

Table 13–1. Comparison of Analgesics

Analgesic	Dose (mg) Equivalent to 10 mg Morphine I.M.	
	I.M.	P.O.
Morphine	10	60
Meperidine (Demerol)	75	300
Codeine	130	200
Methadone (Dolophine)	10	20
Oxymorphone (Numorphan)	1	6
Hydromorphone (Dilaudid)	1.5	7.5
Levorphanol (Levo-Dromoran)	2	4
Oxycodone	15	30

5. Mood alteration. Euphoria usually comes with relief of pain, but if opioids are given regularly, depression is noted for the first 48 to 72 hours. Later, affect becomes relatively normal in spite of high doses, but creative ability is impaired.

6. Acute toxicity. This is rarely seen in the average gynecologic patient. Coma, pinpoint pupils and depressed respiration are characteristic. The primary management is to establish an airway, ventilate the patient and continue careful monitoring as described in Chapter 4. A narcotic antagonist such as naloxone (Narcan), in doses of 0.4 mg intravenously every two to three minutes in acute situations, should be given as necessary.

7. Addiction (drug dependency) is a concern when patients require regular use of opioid analgesics by injection (and also by mouth) over a prolonged period. Under acute circumstances, as seen in gynecologic patients, dependence is rare; when pain subsides most patients prefer to discontinue the use of analgesics. If a patient seems to be dependent, it is important to be sure that no reason for pain exists. If there is no demonstrable reason for the pain, a change to oral medication and the use of tranquilizers (phenothiazines) with decreasing doses of opioids should be attempted. If this technique fails, consultation with a psychiatrist, especially one experienced in drug dependency, is advisable.

Antibiotics

GENERAL

Indications for the preoperative and prophylactic use of antibiotics in gynecology and obstetrics are given in Chapter 2; indications for antibiotics use in postoperative infections are discussed in Chapter 4. The latter also includes tables of antibiotics appropriate for specific organisms (see Tables 4–5, 4–6, 4–7).

The complications of antibiotic therapy are important because these drugs are widely used. It is estimated that in the United States 30% of hospitalized patients receive antibiotics. Very many more receive them as outpatients. The side-effects of antibiotics may be divided into those common to many different classes of antibiotics and those specific to one class of drugs or to one drug within a class.

Two significant general complications are the development of resistance and superinfection. Resistance varies from drug to drug and is largely unpredictable. Hospital-acquired bacteria are characteristically more resistant to antibiotics, but in the case of *Staphylococcus aureus*, for example, community-acquired strains are often insensitive to penicillin G. Strains of gonococci and pneumococci have also developed resistance to the once effective agent, pencillin G. Prevention of this complication lies in the use of appropriate sensitivity testing of bacteria as soon as antibiotics are started (if used empirically) and repeated sensitivity testing if the apparently correct antibiotic is not effective and there is no other obvious reason for continued infection, such as an abscess.

Superinfection occurs when a new infection emerges during treatment of a primary one. The normal bacteria of the upper respiratory, gastrointestinal and genitourinary tracts are altered by antibiotics, and one or more organisms may become predominant, invade the host and cause an infection. In the respiratory tract, for example, *Staphylococcus*, *Candida* and *Proteus* strains can cause oropharyngeal infections or pneumonia. The original antibiotics should be stopped and appropriate alternates used. In the intestinal tract diarrhea occurs frequently after antibiotic use. Immediate discontinuation of antibiotics is appropriate. The use of plain yogurt, sweetened by added natural fruit, may help to restore intestinal bacteria to normal. A more serious complication is (pseudomembranous) enterocolitis due to *Clostridium difficile*. This is reported to occur in 1 in 10 to 1 in 10,000 patients receiving antibiotics. It is more common in older women, those with cancer and patients in intensive care units. Although almost every antibiotic has been found to be responsible, it is most commonly caused by clindamycin. Pathologically, inflammation and ulceration are found, and a pseudomembrane may be formed. Clinically, symptoms begin four to nine days after antibiotics are started, although they may occur after the antibiotics have been stopped. Symptoms consist of watery, often bloody diarrhea, fever, abdominal tenderness and leukocytosis. In untreated cases, they may progress to electrolyte imbalance, toxic megacolon, perforation and hemorrhage, occasionally leading to death. The diagnosis is made by the presence of leukocytes in the stool, demonstration of specific cytotoxin and positive cultures for *C. difficile*. In mild cases, diarrhea subsides in seven to 10 days with discontinuation of the responsible antibiotics and supportive therapy. Antidiarrheal agents are not indicated, since they slow the excretion of the toxin. Vancomycin is the treatment of choice and is given in a dose of 500 mg by mouth (or nasogastric tube) every six hours for at least five days. *C. difficile* is also susceptible to metronidazole and rifampin. Recurrence occurs in 10 to 12% of patients treated with vancomycin. Retreatment with vancomycin for seven to 10 days is indicated (Fekety, 1982). In the genitourinary tract *Pseudomonas* infection may be superimposed when the original infection has been successfully treated by broad spectrum antibiotics. A change to an antibiotic to which the organisms are sensitive is necessary. *Candida* infection of the vagina, urine, mouth and other organs commonly follows the use of parenteral broad spectrum antibiotics. Recognition of this possibility should prompt the prophylactic use of vaginal antifungal agents (see later section) in susceptible individuals, i.e., those who have had this complication previously. Mycostatin mouthwash is helpful for those who have oral candidiasis.

COMPLICATIONS OF SPECIFIC ANTIBIOTIC DRUGS

For the purposes of this chapter the term "antibiotics" refers to antimicrobial agents, antifungal agents, antiviral agents and miscellaneous antiinfective agents used in gynecology and obstetrics. The development of new antibiotics has proceeded rapidly and is continuing to do so. It is not possible in a review such as this to describe the complications of the latest additions, but only to review those that have been in use sufficiently long for information on their side-effects to be well documented.

Antimicrobial Agents. Sulfonamides prevent normal bacterial utilization of PABA for the synthesis of folate. *Trimethoprim* inhibits the reduction of trihydrofolate to tetrahydrofolate. Both are bacteriostatic; cellular and hormonal mechanisms of the host are required to eliminate infection. The overall incidence of complications is about 5%. Hypersensitivity reactions occur in 1 to 2% of patients. They are characterized by a variety of skin rashes, including exfoliative dermatitis (Stevens-Johnson syndrome); fever may also be present. Blood dyscrasias, acute hemolytic anemia, agranulocytosis, thrombocytopenia and aplastic anemia occur rarely. A variety of other reactions involving most organ systems have been reported. Sulfonamides may enhance the effect of anticoagulants and methotrexate.

Penicillins, cephalosporins, vancomycin and *bacitracin* inhibit synthesis of bacteria or activate enzymes that disrupt bacterial cell walls (lysis). Penicillins and cephalosporins are probably the most widely used antibiotics and their side-effects are therefore of great importance. Many derivatives of both, with a variety of antibacterial activities, have been developed (see Table 4–6).

Hypersensitivity reactions are the commonest adverse effect of the *penicillins*, occurring in 0.7 to 10% of patients. They may follow the use of any of the penicillins and any dose of them. Severe reactions, such as angioedema and anaphylaxis occur in 0.01 to 0.04% of patients. They are characterized by swelling of the face and tongue, respiratory difficulty and giant hives and may be life-threatening, with death occurring in 1 of 200 such patients. Treatment is similar to that used in any kind of acute allergic or anaphylactoid response to medication or insect stings. It consists primarily of epinephrine, 0.25 to 0.5 ml of a 1:1000 solution in 10 ml saline, given intravenously and repeated every 5 to 10 minutes with maintenance of an adequate airway. In profound hypotension epinephrine may be given through the endotracheal tube. Although epinephrine is generally effective, the possibility of hypertension and cardiac ischemia must be kept in mind (Barach et al, 1984). Persisting bronchospasm may be managed by aminophylline (500 mg) infused intravenously at a rate of no more than 20 mg/minute, or an antihistamine such as diphenhydramine (10 to 30 mg intravenously).

Less serious but still troublesome hypersensitivity reactions include skin rashes, serum sickness and fever. Skin rashes may take any form, the most severe being a generalized exfoliative dermatitis. They occur at varying times after the administration of the penicillin. They are more common 7 to 10 days after the use of ampicillin, occurring in about 9% of cases. Symptoms may be relieved by oral antihistamines (diphenhydramine 50 mg 3 or 4 times daily), wet compresses or local application of a low-strength cortisone preparation such as 1% hydrocortisone. Serum sickness occurs one to two weeks after the administration of penicillin and may last for several days. It is accompanied by varying degrees of fever, arthritis or leukopenia. Treatment is by antihistaminics and symptomatic medication for pain. Fever may occur without other symptoms and may be difficult to distinguish from that due to other causes. Eosinophilia, as high as 10 to 20%, may be present. Other toxic reactions to the penicillins are rare. For example, interstitial nephritis may rarely be seen, especially with methicillin.

If the use of penicillin is indicated and the patient's history suggests that she might be sensitive, more detailed information is needed; questions that should be asked include:

1. If a rash was present, was it accompanied by itching? Itching suggests an allergic response.

2. To what kind of penicillin was the patient supposedly sensitive? For example, 90% of patients with mononucleosis who receive ampicillin develop a rash, but this does not necessarily indicate future sensitivity.

3. How recent was the allergic response? Both reactivity and memory fade with time.

4. Has the patient received other antibiotics, particularly other penicillins, without reaction subsequent to the "allergic" incident?

In general, caution is indicated in using penicillin for a patient whose history is suggestive of sensitivity, and other antibiotics, except possibly a cephalosporin (see following discussion), should be used. If a penicillin is really indicated, however, the question of allergy can be settled by a skin test. This is done with penicilloyl-polylysine (PPL) and minor determinant mixture (MDM). If the test is positive, desensitization by the oral or parenteral route can be performed according to the protocol suggested by Levitz and Mendelson (1982).

Cephalosporins have been available since 1962, and many varieties have been developed. First, second, third and even fourth generation cephalosporins have an increasingly wide range of antibacterial action. All cephalosporins are active against most gram negative bacilli, e.g., *E. coli*. First generation drugs are more effective against gram positive organisms. Among the second generation drugs cefamandole is effective against Enterobacter species and cefoxitin against beta-lactamase–producing bacteroides as well. Of the third generation cephalosporins, moxalactam is active against *Pseudomonas aeruginosa* and *Bacteriodes fragilis* and has a longer half-life and better penetration of the central nervous system.

Allergic or hypersensitivity reactions to cephalosporins are similar to those of the penicillins, probably because of their similar structures. Cross-reactivity with penicillin may occur in 5 to 20% of patients. Reactions usually subside promptly on discontinuation of the drug. A history of a recent severe reaction to penicillin is a contraindication to the use of a cephalosporin, but a patient who has had a mild reaction or one that occurred in the distant past can probably be given a cephalosporin with safety if its use is indicated. Potential toxicity to the kidneys has been shown with very large doses of cephalosporins. Moxalactam has been associated with mild reversible hepatic dysfunction and elevation of the prothrombin time, which is reversible with vitamin K. The development of resistance by gram negative bacteria must always be considered when cephalosporins are used (Thompson and Wright, 1983).

Vancomycin is used for penicillin resistant staphylococcal infections and in enterocolitis due to *C. difficile* or *Staphylococcus aureus*. When it is given rapidly by intravenous injection hypotension occasionally occurs. Ototoxicity (primarily hearing loss) occurs occasionally with concentrations above 30 micrograms/ml and is usually not reversible. Nephrotoxicity is a possibility when renal function is already compromised, unless care is taken to reduce the dose (Geraci and Hermans, 1983).

Bacitracin is occasionally used locally. Hypersensitivity reactions are rare.

Aminoglycosides include streptomycin, kanamycin, gentamicin, tobramycin, amikacin and neomycin. They act by binding to the 30S bacterial ribosome, inhibiting protein synthesis and causing cell death. They must be given intravenously or intramuscularly, except for neomycin, which is used topically or for intestinal sterilization. The main use of the aminoglycosides is in serious infections due to gram negative bacteria.

The chief complications of all the aminoglycosides are ototoxicity and nephrotoxicity. Ototoxicity includes both vestibular and auditory effects. The former are more common with streptomycin and gentamicin and the latter with kanamycin, amikacin and neomycin, whereas tobramycin may involve both vestibular and auditory complications. It is estimated that overt ototoxicity occurs in about 2% of patients receiving amikacin, 2% of those receiving gentamicin and 1% of those receiving tobramycin, streptomycin and kanamycin when treatment is given for two weeks or less. Subclinical changes may be more common than this. Prolonged use, high doses and previously impaired renal function increase the chance of ototoxicity. It is potentiated by diuretics such as furosemide. The vestibular changes are likely to improve and be compensated, but hearing loss tends to be permanent. Nephrotoxicity, as defined by an increase in serum creatinine of at least 0.4

mg/dl or the onset of acute renal failure, has been estimated to occur in 2 to 10% of patients receiving aminoglycosides (Appel and Neu, 1977). It is more likely to occur with higher doses of aminoglycosides and after 5 to 7 days of therapy. Advanced age, previous renal disease, acidosis and concomitant therapy with furosemide are predisposing factors (Francke and Neu, 1983). Damage occurs primarily in the proximal tubular epithelial cells with inability of the kidney to concentrate urine. No treatment is known except to discontinue the drug. Slow recovery may be expected, but the long-term effect on renal function is uncertain. General principles of management are covered in Chapter 4. It is important to obtain blood levels when aminoglycosides are used in pregnancy and in patients who are at high risk for complications.

Minor and rare complications with aminoglyosides include skin rashes and drug-induced fever. These usually disappear promptly after the drug is discontinued. A serious problem with all these drugs has been the emergence of resistant organisms. This was particularly true of streptomycin, the first drug of this group, which is now rarely used.

Tetracyclines, chloramphenicol, erythromycin and clindamycin all act by inhibiting bacterial protein synthesis. They are rapidly absorbed from the gastrointestinal tract, metabolized by the liver and excreted by the kidney. However, they vary in their indications for use (Table 13–2) and toxic effects (Wilson and Cockerill, 1983).

The tetracyclines have gastrointestinal, skin, liver and renal toxicity and occasionally hypersensitivity. Given to pregnant women, neonates or children under 12 years of age tetracycline may cause hypoplasia of tooth enamel and darkening of both primary and permanent teeth (see later section). Gastrointestinal complications include epigastric distress, nausea and vomiting. These may be decreased by administering the drug with meals (not with milk or other dairy products) or with an antacid (those not containing aluminum, magnesium or calcium). Diarrhea may occur and may be benign, or it may be caused by C. difficile. Skin changes consist of redness on exposure to strong sunlight (photosensitivity), which occurs in 1 to 2% of patients. Destruction and pigmentation of the nails may also occur simultaneously. Hepatic toxicity occurs rarely in patients receiving over 2 gm per day; jaundice with evidence of hepatic damage may be followed by liver failure. Nephrotoxicity is rare but similar to that occurring with aminoglycosides. Hypersensitivity reactions (see discussion in section on penicillins) are rare. However, superinfection (enterocolitis or candidiasis) is common with prolonged use. Also, there is marked cross-sensitization between the members of this group of drugs.

Chloramphenicol shares the gastrointestinal and hypersensitivity complications of the tetracyclines to some extent. However, its most important complication is myelosuppression. This takes two forms, pancytopenia that is related to dose and occurs when plasma concentrations are 25 micrograms/ml or higher and after prolonged therapy, and aplastic anemia that is not related to dose. In the former, recovery usually occurs within three weeks after the drug has been discontinued. The latter is thought to occur in about 1 in 30,000 to 1 in 40,000 courses of chloramphenicol. The fatality rate is high, and death is more likely when there has been a longer interval between the last day on which the drug was given and the first sign of the blood dyscrasia. During therapy with chloramphenicol the hematopoietic system must be monitored by complete blood counts every two to three days. The seriousness of these side-effects should not prevent the use of the drug when specifically indicated, in S. typhi or in other gram negative infections not responding to other antibiotics. Its use in neonates is generally contraindicated because of the possibility of the rare case of fatal toxicity with cardiovascular collapse, the "gray baby" syndrome.

Erythromycin has relatively few complica-

Table 13–2. Some Indications for the Use of the Tetracyclines, Chloramphenicol, Erythromycin and Clindamycin

Agent	Indication
Tetracyclines	Urinary tract infections
	Chlamydia
	Gonorrhea and syphilis in patients allergic to penicillin
Chloramphenicol	S. typhi, Anaerobic infections, especially B. fragilis and H. influenzae, rickettsial infections
Erythromycin	S. aureus, B hemolytic streptococcus, S. pneumoniae, M. pneumoniae and Legionella infection
	In patients allergic to penicillin for gonorrhea and syphilis and as prophylaxis for subacute bacterial endocarditis
Clindamycin	Anaerobic infections, especially B. fragilis

tions. Gastrointestinal irritation occurs occasionally and an allergic hepatitis is observed rarely with erythomycin estolate.

Clindamycin use is complicated by diarrhea in 6 to 8% of cases, associated with the overgrowth of clindamycin-resistant strains of *C. difficile*. Treatment is by the use of vancomycin (see earlier discussion).

Antifungal Antibiotics. Antifungal antibiotics are used frequently in gynecology and obstetrics to treat *Candida* infections of the vagina, mouth and skin. They are rarely used for systemic infections and then only in seriously ill patients with multiple medical problems. These drugs act directly on the cell membrane, affecting permeability and leading to leakage of intracellular compounds.

Nystatin is commonly used. Complications are rare except for mild gastrointestinal effects when it is taken orally to reduce the intestinal source of *Candida*.

Miconazole causes burning, itching, urticaria, rash, headache and pelvic cramps in about 7% of patients during the first week of intravaginal therapy.

Clotrimazole therapy is occasionally accompanied by similar skin reactions, and about 1.5% of patients report a burning sensation after intravaginal application.

The use of candicidin and chloradantoin has rarely been accompanied by side-effects, except for occasional local irritation and hypersensitivity.

Gentian violet applied to the vaginal surfaces or as a suppository has minimal side-effects, except for the stains produced on clothing.

Amphotericin B is used intravenously for systemic fungal infections. It is accompanied by many side-effects. Initial injections are associated with chills in 50% of patients, vomiting in 20% and fever in most. Renal toxicity, in both glomeruli and in tubules, occurs in over 80% of patients, and some permanent damage may result.

Antiviral Agents. The development of antiviral agents is in its infancy. Acyclovir, used locally or by mouth, has been found to be clinically effective in first episodes of genital infection due to herpes simplex type 2 (HSV-2) and, used by mouth, in reducing the number of recurrences but not preventing them. Significant side-effects have not been reported so far (Douglas et al, 1984; Strauss et al, 1984).

Miscellaneous Anti-infective Agents. Metronidazole is effective orally against *Trichomonas vaginalis*, and is a useful agent orally and intravenously against anerobic bacteria. Side-effects

are relatively uncommon and include gastrointestinal symptoms such as nausea, epigastric distress and abdominal cramping and diarrhea. A metallic taste, glossitis and stomatitis have been reported. Patients who drink alcoholic beverages during or within one day after taking metronidazole may occasionally experience abdominal distress, vomiting, flushing and headaches (disulfuram-like effect). It should be used with caution in patients with abnormal liver function. Leukopenia and CNS symptoms may occur rarely. There is a possibility of teratogenetic effects if the drug is given during the first trimester of pregnancy (Robbie and Sweet, 1983; Charles, 1984).

Chemotherapeutic Agents

The use of chemotherapeutic agents in the management of cancers of the female genital tract has increased greatly in the last 30 years, starting with the successful treatment of disseminated trophoblastic disease by Hertz and co-workers (1961). Currently, chemotherapy has also been proved to be of value for early and advanced or recurrent cancer of the ovary, and of possible value in advanced or recurrent epithelial or mesodermal tumors of the uterine corpus and cervix. Agents presently in use in gynecology and obstetrics, either singly or in combinations, include antimetabolites (methotrexate and 5 fluorouracil), alkylating agents (melphalan, cyclophosphamide, dacarbazine [DTIC]), antibiotics (actinomycin D, doxorubicin, mitomycin C, mithramycin), vinca alkaloids (vinblastine and vincristine) and those agents with uncertain actions such as cisplatin, hexamethylmelamine and etoposide.

The attitude of physicians and patients toward the complications of chemotherapy has been different from that in regard to most other drugs. Up to the present, chemotherapy has represented a patient's only chance of survival, often a limited one. Therefore, in view of the alternative, progression of the disease and death, severe complications have been acceptable. More recently, with long-term survival likely, for example, in trophoblastic disease and ovarian cancer, attention is being paid to the less serious complications of chemotherapy and the quality of life for patients receiving it.

Chemotherapeutic agents are most commonly given intravenously, less frequently by mouth or intramuscularly. More recently the intraperitoneal route has been used, for example, with cisplatin for ovarian cancer. Prevention and management of complications are best handled by a team of physicians and nurses who are familiar with and can assess the course of the disease. In gynecologic cancer, experience in detecting the changing findings on pelvic examination is essential. This can usually best be done by the gynecologic oncologist.

Complications of chemotherapy will be covered under two headings, those common to several agents and those specific to individual drugs. Because of the widespread effect of these agents upon body cells, a great variety of complications is possible.

GENERAL COMPLICATIONS

Hypersensitivity. Hypersensitivity reactions, consisting of anaphylaxis, skin rash, fever and chills, occasionally occur with most agents. Anaphylaxis has been noted especially with cisplatin, skin rashes with methotrexate, doxorubicin and cisplatin and chills and fever with actinomycin D, doxorubicin, dacarbazine and bleomycin. Local hypersensitivity may occur in as many as 3% of patients receiving doxorubicin. A hypersensitivity reaction presents as a dull ache over the vein, erythema along its course, local urticaria and pruritus. It may be difficult to distinguish from extravasation (see following section), but usually subsides in less than 30 minutes. The injection should be stopped, the needle removed and ice applied locally. The same reaction may not recur if the injection is then started in another vein. Antihistaminic agents are of little value.

Extravasation. Extravasation can be a serious problem when it occurs with vesicant drugs such as doxorubicin, actinomycin D, vinblastine, vincristine, mitomycin C and mithramycin. Most of the studies on extravasation have been reported with doxorubicin (Harwood and Aisner, 1984). The patient may immediately experience pain, redness or swelling at the site of the injection, or the only sign may be a decrease in the rate of the intravenous flow or a lack of blood return. These reactions may progress over hours and even weeks, and they range from minor skin or vein discoloration to severe necrosis of the skin and underlying tissues.

Factors affecting the severity of extravasation include:

1. The site of injection. Extravasation is more likely to occur if the chemotherapy is given in the arm of a patient who has had a mastectomy on the same side. Also, in the antecubital fossa the extravasation may not be noticed early because of the depth of the injection. On the dorsum of the hand extravasation is likely to involve the extensor tendons and this area is difficult to cover later with a skin graft.

2. Concentration of the drug. More dilute solutions are likely to produce less severe reactions. Also, the longer the time taken for infusion, the greater is the risk of the drug diffusing outside the vein.

3. Previous radiation therapy. Injection given in a radiated area may result in a "recall phenomenon," with a worse local reaction. This is unlikely to happen during the usual administration of chemotherapy, since the arm has seldom been irradiated.

4. Technique of injection. Multiple punctures in the same vein may permit extravasation even if the drug appears to have been injected satisfactorily into the vein.

The immediate treatment of extravasation is largely empirical.

1. The infusion should be stopped. Three to 5 ml of blood is withdrawn from the vein, and the subcutaneous swelling is aspirated with a No. 27 needle. The purpose is to remove as much of the agent as possible from the local area.

2. Various antidotes have been suggested such as 8.4% bicarbonate (5 ml) for doxorubicin, vinblastine or vincristine: 10% sodium thiosulfate (4 ml plus 6 ml sterile water) for actinomycin D, mitomycin C or mithramycin; hyaluronidase (150 mg in 1 ml) for vinblastine and vincristine, or dexamethasone (4 mg in 1 ml) for doxorubicin. These antidotes are injected locally around the vein.

3. Heat or cold may be applied locally (Ignoffo and Friedman, 1980).

In the absence of good evidence supporting the effectiveness of any of the listed antidotes, the author's preference is to carry out Step 1 and then apply cold compresses for 30 minutes and subsequently for 10 minutes four times daily for two to three days, depending on symptoms. Minor degrees of extravastion may resolve with this regimen. However, later onset of damage is to be expected and frequent reexamination is desirable. If the patient remains symptomatic (i.e., has pain after two weeks and redness or induration is marked), the patient should be seen by a plastic surgeon. Early debridement and skin grafting may then be desirable (Larson, 1982).

Extravasation can be minimized by
1. Experience in the use of chemotherapy.
2. Proper selection of the injection site, the order of preference being forearm, dorsum of

hand, wrist and antecubital veins. In patients with poor veins who are receiving many courses of chemotherapy, a central venous line may be utilized.

3. Use of a butterfly needle (25 gauge), which should be taped in place with the site of entry visible.

4. Checking blood return before, during and after administration of the drug.

5. Repeated monitoring of flow, intravenous site and the patient's discomfort.

6. Flushing the line with fluid before removal to eliminate backspill of the drug.

Risks to Personnel. Medical personnel who handle antineoplastic agents can be exposed to low doses of drugs by direct contact, inhalation and ingestion. This may be especially important for those who are pregnant. Mutagenic activity or chromosomal damage are theoretically possible. The findings of Selevan and co-workers (1985) indicated that nurses handling antineoplastic drugs in the first trimester of pregnancy had a greater risk of fetal loss than those in a control group. However, as Mattia and Blake (1983) pointed out, data on the extent of the danger are difficult to obtain because of the many possibilities of bias. Long-term risks are particularly hard to evaluate. A possible immediate effect is irritation of the skin and mucous membranes, especially from the vesicant drugs. Guidelines for safe handling of parenteral antineoplastic drugs during preparation and administration are summarized by the AMA Council on Scientific Affairs (1985). Drugs should be reconstituted by pharmacy personnel in a Class II laminar-flow biology safety cabinet with appropriate precautions to prevent contact with the drug and to dispose of contaminated material. Whoever administers the drug should use protective clothing with gown and gloves, and a protocol for disposal of supplies should be followed.

Gastointestinal Complications

NAUSEA AND VOMITING. These occur usually after administrations of cisplatin, frequently after administration of doxorubicin, cyclophosphamide and dacarbazine and occasionally after administration of methotrexate, 5FU, bleomycin, melphalan, vinblastine and vincristine. The onset may be delayed until several hours after therapy, especially following use of doxorubicin, cyclophosphamide or cisplatin. Apart from the immediate discomfort and the possible effects on nutritional status, the fear and anticipation of nausea and vomiting recurring during each course of chemotherapy are severe stresses to the patient and her family and adversely affects her quality of life and ability to continue treatment.

Treatment is both therapeutic and preventive. Many studies of therapy suffer from methodologic problems (Pater and Willan, 1984). Some of these problems are

1. Including patients who have received a variety of agents with different emetogenic properties or other concomitant medication.

2. Lack of randomization.

3. Variations in assessment of outcome, such as quantitation of nausea and vomiting and differing criteria for response.

4. The toxic effects of antiemetic drugs.

Until recently the only available agents for antiemetic use were phenothiazines and sedatives such as barbiturates. However, these are ineffective against high doses and combinations of alkylating agents, doxorubicin, dacarbazine and cisplatin. Further, since a poor first experience with nausea and vomiting engenders subsequent poor responses, the initial antiemetic therapy must be as effective as possible.

Phenothiazines such as perchlorperazine are useful against mildly emetogenic drugs such as cyclophosphamide, doxorubicin or dacarbazine given in moderate doses. Pretreatment with oral (10 mg) or intramuscular (10 mg) prochloperazine is followed by a similar dose every four to six hours for 12 to 24 hours. Rectal suppositories of perchlorperazine (25 mg) every six hours may also be used. Other phenothiazines such as chlorpromazine may be tried if perchlorperazine does not seem to be effective. The side-effects of phenothiazines, especially in large doses, include hypotension and sedation and extrapyramidal symptoms. The last consist of rigidity and tremor (Parkinsonism syndrome), akathisia (need for constant motion), dystonic reactions (grimaces or seizure-like events) or tardive dyskinesia (purposeless repetitive movements). Treatment is by the use of diazepam or benztropine (Cogentin).

Tetrahydrocannabinol (THC) and synthetic cannabinols (nabilone) have been found to be useful antiemetic agents. In several well controlled studies, orally administered THC was shown to be superior to placebo or standard antiemetic agents such as perchloperazine (Poster et al, 1981). Mood changes (dysphoria) occurred in up to 81% of patients in these studies but were not necessarily deleterious. They were severe in only 9%. Somnolence was frequent. These effects appear to be temporary. The disadvantage of these agents is that, in addition to their usual unavailability, they can only be given by mouth.

With large doses of single chemotherapeutic agents or with combinations of agents, more potent antiemetics are needed. This is especially true when cisplatin is used alone or in combination with drugs such as cyclophosphamide and doxorubicin. Various combinations of drugs have been suggested with metoclopramide as an important component. On the author's service, 100 mg of metoclopramide (Reglan) in 50 ml 5% dextrose and water, repeated every two hours for five doses is given with a steroid (Decadron; 20 mg intramuscularly, one dose), an antihistamine (Benadryl; 25 mg intramuscularly, one dose), and an antianxiety and sedative agent (Ativan; 2 mg intravenously, repeated in four hours as needed). The effectiveness of a similiar combination has been shown by Kris and co-workers (1985a). Side-effects related to the use of these antiemetic drugs include persistent sedation and occasional post-treatment restlessness. With metachlopramide alone or in combination with other drugs the risk of dystonia or dyskinesia was estimated to be 0.3% (Bateman et al, 1985).

MUCOSITIS AND ULCERATION. The mucous membranes of the gastrointestinal tract are commonly involved in chemotherapy, leading to stomatitis, glossitis, esophagitis and mucositis of the small and possibly the large intestine. These conditions occur seven to 14 days after a course of treatment. Oral ulceration is most obvious and can be so bad as to prevent swallowing even of liquids. Actinomycin D, methotrexate, doxorubicin and 5FU are most likely to cause these complications, whereas cyclophosphamide, vinblastine and bleomycin may sometimes cause them. Pain can be partially relieved by an anesthetic mouthwash such as viscous lidocaine, and secondary infection can be lessened with an antibacterial and antifungal mouthwash. The mucosal complications improve within 7 to 14 days. There is no way to prevent them and their extent is unpredictable. When possible, oral hygiene and major dental problems should receive attention prior to chemotherapy (Carl, 1983; Barrett, 1984).

NUTRITIONAL STATUS. Chemotherapy produces intermittent (or occasionally continuous) anorexia. Even if the cancer is not growing actively, weight loss and possible nutritional deficiencies may occur. Dietary advice is important for most patients undergoing chemotherapy. It should emphasize adequate intake, in small amounts, of palatable food containing sufficient protein. Supplemental protein drinks may be advisable. Multivitamins should be regularly prescribed, especially vitamin C in doses of 500 mg every six to eight hours. Parenteral or enteral feeding may occasionally be useful if it is likely to assist the chemotherapy and not merely feed the cancer.

Dermatologic Complications. Alopecia follows the administration of doxorubicin, cyclophosphamide or vincristine in almost 100% of cases. It begins two to three weeks after the first course and is usually complete after the second. It may also follow (at least in part) the use of bleomycin, 5FU, methotrexate and vinblastine. Scalp cooling with a venous tourniquet and an ice pack, used before, during and after treatment with low doses of doxorubicin (used alone) can decrease the amount and retard the onset of hair loss. This technique is not effective when large doses of doxorubicin or combinations of drugs are being administered (Middleton et al, 1985). Hair will grow again after chemotherapy is completed.

Erythemathous rashes and allergic skin responses commonly follow chemotherapy. If the patient has previously received radiation therapy, a "radiation recall" reaction may occur in the radiated skin after the administration of actinomycin D, doxorubicin or 5FU. Similarly, an area of previous sunburn may be reactivated by methotrexate and 5FU, whereas vinblastine, if present at the time of exposure to ultraviolet light, may cause an exaggerated skin reaction. Patients receiving these drugs should not expose themselves to sunlight. Hyperpigmentation often follows these skin reactions and may also occur in the nails and at the metacarpophangeal joints after the administration of doxorubicin or 5FU (Dunagin, 1984).

Hematopoetic Complications. The bone marrow is depressed in varying degrees by most chemotherapeutic agents, with the exception (usually) of bleomycin, cisplatin, vincristine and the steroidal hormones. The depression is in part dose-dependent. The greatest effect (nadir) occurs at seven to 14 days with most agents but later with dacarbazine (21 to 28 days) and mitomycin C (28 to 42 days). Patients who are in poor nutritional status or have previously received chemotherapy or radiation therapy are likely to have more marked effects. Neutropenia usually occurs first, followed by thrombocytopenia. In most instances recovery occurs in 21 to 28 days from the time the drug was given but may be prolonged. Depression of red cell elements with anemia is common after repeated courses of chemotherapy.

NEUTROPENIA. Infection is the most serious danger when leukopenia is present. Practically speaking one should be concerned when the total white blood count is less than 1000/mm³ or the granulocyte count is less than 500/mm³. If such patients have a fever of over 38.5 degrees C (101.3 degrees F) taken on two consecutive occasions four hours or more apart, a search should be made for a possible site of infection by cultures of blood and appropriate orifices. Then broad spectrum antibiotic therapy should be promptly instituted. An aminoglycoside such as gentamicin or tobramycin with a penicillinase-resistant penicillin such as ticarcillin and either clindamycin or metronidazole (see Chapter 4) provide the broadest coverage. Another possible combination consists of an aminoglycoside and a broad spectrum semisynthetic penicillin such as piperacillin. Antibiotics are changed according to culture reports. With prolonged fever and persistent granulocytopenia, the possibility of superinfection with fungi must always be considered. If the granulocytes recover and the patient defervesces, antibiotics should be stopped 24 hours after the temperature has reached normal. How long antibiotic administration should be continued in the presence of defervescence but persistent agranulocytosis is very difficult to decide, since up to 50% of such patients have relapses with recurrent fever (Pizzo, 1984). At least three days seems reasonable. Granulocyte transfusions are of possible value in such patients.

Table 13–3 illustrates methods of preventing infection in immunosuppressed or myelosuppressed patients (Pizzo and Schimpff, 1983). Some amelioration of leukopenia may be obtained by the use of lithium carbonate at a dose of 300 to 400 mg three times daily, modified to maintain a serum lithium level of 0.6 to 1.3 mEq/liter (Stein et al, 1981). This dose of lithium may also increase the number of platelets (Richman et al, 1984).

THROMBOCYTOPENIA. Petechiae and easy bruising are the first manifestations of thrombocytopenia. Overt bleeding does not usually occur until the platelet levels are very low (usually less than 20,000/mm³) or there is major trauma such as a surgical procedure. Treatment is not usually indicated unless bleeding occurs, except for the possible use of small doses of corticosteriods. Significant bleeding may be treated by random donor platelet transfusions (ABO and Rh compatible). If the patient becomes refractory to random donor platelets, the use of group-specific HLA-identical single donor platelets may be indicated.

ANEMIA. This is managed in the usual manner by diet, iron, vitamins and, if necessary, by transfusions.

LEUKEMIA. Leukemia may develop as a late complication of chemotherapy. It appears to be associated primarily with the use of alkylating agents, chiefly melphalan because of the frequency of its use. It occurs three or more years after chemotherapy in 1 to 2% of patients, especially in those who have received larger total doses (i.e., more than 800 mg) of melphalan. Diagnosis and management are both difficult. Unexpected pancytopenia was found in nine patients at a median duration of six months before a bone marrow diagnosis was made. Survival after diagnosis was short (Reimer et al, 1977).

Complications of Reproductive Function. The reproductive consequences of chemotherapy for gynecologic cancers have become important in the treatment of trophoblastic disease and of germ cell and stromal cell tumors of the ovary in children and young women. Ovarian cancer of epithelial origin appearing in women of reproductive age usually requires an extirpative operation, so the reproductive effect of subsequent chemotherapy is not of concern.

After single drug chemotherapy with methotrexate for trophoblastic disease resumption of normal menstrual cycles is the rule. Rustin and co-workers (1984) found that among 445 long-term survivors after methotrexate treatment, 97% of those who wished for a pregnancy did in fact conceive and 86% had at least one living child. Women who had received three or more drugs were less likely to have living children. There was no statistically significant excess of congenital malformations among those who had received methotrexate. These findings have been confirmed by data from the Brewer Trophoblastic Disease Center (Lurain, 1984).

Recent work by Choo and co-workers (1985) suggests that etoposide given for trophoblastic disease may produce ovarian failure that is transient in younger women and permanent in older women. On the other hand, following removal only of the ovary containing the tumor,

Table 13–3. Prevention of Infection in Myelosuppressed Patients

1. Improve host defense mechanisms: nutrition, vaccines, lithium.
2. Reduce damage to natural body barriers: care with venipuncture.
3. Avoid invasive procedures when possible: central venous or urinary catheters.
4. Reduce acquisition of organisms from environment: handwashing, housekeeping, reducing contamination of food and water.
5. Suppress colonizing organisms: antisepsis and antibiotics.

young women with germ cell tumors of the ovary have been reported to be able to menstruate and conceive after multiple-agent chemotherapy.

Teratogenic effects are possible with the use of any chemotherapeutic agent in the first trimester of pregnancy, but are uncommon in the last two trimesters. Data are scanty and treatment must be individualized. Chemotherapy during lactation is usually inadvisable. Information on the effect of prior chemotherapy has been obtained largely from the study of patients with Hodgkin's disease, treated with a variety of agents, and to a lesser extent from the study of patients treated for other cancers. Autopsy data from 21 girls (11 less than 10 years of age and ten 10 years of age or over) who died one to two months after the cessation of chemotherapy for extragonadal solid tumors showed impaired follicle maturation (Nicosia et al, 1985). Their future reproductive capacity would probably have been reduced. This likelihood is confirmed by follow-up data after treatment for Hodgkin's disease. However, patients often receive both chemotherapy and radiation therapy, making the effect of each difficult to discern. After MOPP chemotherapy (methylchlorethamine, vincristine, procarbazine and prednisone), oligomenorrhea or amenorrhea occurred in about one quarter of patients, significantly more frequently in those over than in those under 30 years of age. Women who continue to menstruate appear to be fertile and to have relatively normal pregnancies and offspring (Andrieu and Ochoa-Molina, 1983). Amenorrhea may not occur until several months after chemotherapy, and premature menopause is a possibility. Patients with amenorrhea are unlikely to resume menses. The total dose of the drug (e.g., cyclophosphamide) may be an important factor, as well as the patient's age (Damewood and Grochow, 1986). Menopausal changes, including hot flashes, irritability, insomnia and dyspareunia, accompany the amenorrhea. Hormone replacement therapy, nutritional advice and counseling are especially important for these women.

Psychologic Complications. Chemotherapy poses a major stress. The patient knows that she has cancer, which may or may not have been eradicated by the operation or radiation therapy. Repeated courses of chemotherapy prolong the uncertainty of cure. In addition, nausea, vomiting and other symptoms that accompany the treatment are very difficult to tolerate. This may result in the patient's concluding that life with chemotherapy is not worth living and lead her to refuse further courses of treatment. She may become severely depressed or may act in a hostile manner toward her caregivers. When the initial courses of chemotherapy are associated with nausea and vomiting, anticipatory nausea and vomiting may occur as the patient leaves for the hospital for subsequent treatments or at any time before she actually receives the medication. It is important to be alert to these emotional reactions throughout a patient's treatment. Methods of helping her include the time-honored method of reassurance with empathetic understanding, appropriate antinausea medication given well in advance of the treatment and a variety of psychologic techniques such as guided imagery and desensitization (Morrow and Morrell, 1982). Hypnosis or possibly group therapy can help (see Chapter 7).

Specific Chemotherapeutic Agents

Only those agents that have specific complications not discussed in the preceding general section are included.

Bleomycin. Bleomycin is given intravenously in a dose of 10 to 20 units/M^2. Fever occurs occasionally (8%) during administration. The effects of bleomycin on respiratory function are important and limit its use. Toxicity occurs sporadically at all doses, but increases sharply when the total dose is over 400 units. The chief change is pulmonary fibrosis. Symptoms consist of dry cough and dyspnea with fine and coarse rales at the lung bases and radiologic findings of basilar infiltrates which may progress to lobar consolidaton. These changes may not appear until one to three months after the conclusion of bleomycin therapy. They may occasionally progress to respiratory failure (see Chapter 4). Abnormal pulmonary function tests may precede clinical toxicity. The most useful test is that of carbon monoxide diffusing capacity. This test should be performed before each course of bleomycin therapy; if the diffusing capacity it falls to less than 40% of the pretreatment value, further therapy should be withheld. Most patients with minimal x-ray and lung function changes and a normal PO_2 at rest will not show progression if the drug is stopped. There is no known treatment except supportive measures.

Cisplatin (Platinol). Cisplatin is currently used alone or in combination with other agents primarily for the treatment of advanced epithelial cancer of the ovary and less commonly for other ovarian tumors and recurrent or advanced carcinoma of the cervix. It is given intravenously in doses of 50 to 100 mg/M^2 when given alone or less when given in combination with other drugs. Cisplatin differs from other agents in that it is ototoxic, nephrotoxic and neurotoxic as well as having the other general toxicities described previously. Early nausea and vomiting are almost always present, and delayed nausea and vomiting (24 to 120 hours after treatment) occurred in 93% of patients studied by Kris and co-workers (1985b).

Ototoxicity includes tinnitus, which is reported to occur in 9% of patients, and hearing loss that is clinically apparent in 6% of patients, although it is detectable in high frequency tone by audiograms in 24%. The hearing loss is bilateral and symmetrical. Tinnitus is commonly reversible, but hearing loss is not (Von Hoff et al, 1979). Hearing loss is more likely to occur in patients with a baseline abnormal audiogram and in older women. It may be potentiated by other drugs that have ototoxic properties, for example, aminoglycoside antibiotics or aspirin. There is no known way of preventing the ototoxic effects. A pretreatment audiogram is probably advisable. Patients should be warned of the possibility of tinnitus and hearing loss. Retinal toxicity has been reported after high-dose cisplatin therapy. Visual acuity improved when the patient was taken off therapy, but color vision abnormalities persisted for as long as 16 months after treatment had been completed (Wilding et al, 1985).

Nephrotoxicity is the main dose-limiting effect of cisplatin. Pathologic studies of patients with cisplatin-induced kidney damage have shown extensive necrosis of the proximal and distal tubules without glomerular injury (Schilsky, 1984). Clinical effects include a rise in BUN and creatinine levels and a fall in creatinine clearance. Hypomagnesemia (less than 1.5 mEq/liter), occasionally accompanied by hypocalcemia and tetany, is also likely to occur as a result of the damaged kidney's inability to reabsorb magnesium. This was present in 41 of 69 patients (59%) studied by Ashraf and co-workers (1983) and was associated with neurotoxicity in 31 of the 41 patients (76%). Hypomagnesemic patients show marked lassitude and weakness.

The renal effects of cisplatin appear to be related to dose and the patient's hydration. Diuresis before, during and after administration, producing a urine output of at least 100 ml/hr, decreases the toxicity to very low levels and is essential whether the patient is treated as an inpatient or as an outpatient. A protocol for hydration during the in-patient administra-

tion of cisplatin is shown in Table 13–4. Creatinine levels and BUN are obtained before each treatment. If they are below 2.0 and 25 mg per cent respectively, treatment is given. Creatinine clearances (60% or higher) may also be used as a guide. If the levels of BUN and creatinine are above the acceptable limits, cisplatin should not be given because of the danger of permanent renal damage. Hypomagnesemia may be treated with oral magnesium oxide (600 mg twice daily) and calcium. Intravenous magnesium sulfate ($MgSO_4$) is occasionally necessary.

Neurotoxicity from cisplatin (other than auditory toxicity) takes the form of peripheral neuropathy in 4 to 5% of patients. Symmetrical foot and hand distribution of sensory changes, including paresthesias and dysesthesias, is most common. These sensory changes may lead to disturbances of gait. Some improvement is noticed after discontinuation of the drug.

Intraperitoneal administration of cisplatin has recently been proposed as a better method of direct treatment of intraperitoneal disease. It appears to have similar, but less toxic effects. When cisplatin was given by the intraperitoneal route in combination with cytosine arabinose, Markman and co-workers (1985) noted bacterial peritonitis in 5% of patients, abdominal pain in 10% and fever in 20%. When a temporary single-use catheter was used, 19% of patients were found by Runowicz and co-workers (1986) to have usage complications compared with 67% who had complications with a permanent (Tenckhoff) catheter.

Cyclophosphamide (Cytoxan). Cyclophosphamide, one of the most commonly used alkylating agents, produces the same general side-effects as the others. It is usually given intravenously in a dose of 500 to 1000 mg/M^2, depending on whether it is used alone or in combination with other drugs. Special complications affect respiratory and urinary tract function. Interstitial pneumonitis has rarely been

Table 13–4. Protocol to Lessen Cisplatin Nephrotoxicity

1. 1000 ml D_5/½NS* + 20 mEq KCl over 4 hours
2. Furosemide 40 mg intravenously
3. 1000 ml D_5½NS + 18.75 gm mannitol + ½ total cisplatin dose over 3 hours
4. Repeat step 3
5. 1000 ml D_5/½NS + 20 mEq KCl over 6 hours
6. Repeat step 4

*5% dextrose in 0.45% normal saline.

reported in patients receiving cyclophosphamide for gynecologic cancer (Tsukamoto et al, 1984). Other than a possible benefit from corticosteroids, there is no known effective treatment. Sterile hemorrhagic cystitis occurs in 5 to 10% of patients receiving cyclophosphamide. It can usually be prevented and treated by insuring adequate fluid intake and diuresis. When preceded or followed by pelvic radiation, cyclophosphamide use can cause hematuria, which may be life-threatening. For management of hematuria see Chapter 4. Bladder cancer has also been reported following the use of cyclophosphamide.

Doxorubicin (Adriamycin). The chief special side-effect of doxorubicin is cardiac toxicity. Doxorubicin is usually given intravenously at a dose of 30 to 100 mg/M^2. The most important changes are alterations in the electrocardiogram and the more serious change, cardiomyopathy. Various electrocardiographic changes have been reported, including ST-T changes, sinus tachycardia, premature atrial and ventricular contractions and low voltage QRS complexes. All except possibly the last appear to be reversible. They may be more common in women with abnormal baseline electrocardiograms, but do not seem to be clearly related to the later development of cardiomyopathy.

Cardiomyopathy leading to cardiac failure may occur during therapy, but commonly appears one week to two and a half months after the final dose of doxorubicin. Risk factors include age (over 70), preexisting cardiac disease and, possibly, concurrent administration of other chemotherapeutic drugs. The total dose of doxorubicin is the most important risk factor. The incidence appears to be about 1% at a dose between 450 and 550 mg/M^2. Above 550 mg/ M^2 the risk may rise to 30% or higher (Saltiel and McGuire, 1983). Clinically, the patient with doxorubicin-induced cardiac toxicity presents with symptoms and signs of congestive heart failure. Unfortunately, there is no standard method of predicting this complication. The most widely accepted method of monitoring cardiac status is measurement of the ejection fraction (left ventricular function) by radionuclide angiography. A normal value has been set at 50%. An ejection fraction of less than 30% was present in all five patients with cardiac failure studied by Alexander and co-workers (1979). The same authors describe a value of less than 45% with a drop of at least 15% from the baseline as indicative of moderate cardiomyopathy. The more invasive technique of endomyocardial biopsy has also been found to be of value (Druck et al, 1984).

High doses of doxorubicin are not generally used in the treatment of gynecologic cancer. Common combinations of doxorubicin with other drugs usually require limiting the total doxorubicin dose to 400 mg/M^2. It is appropriate to evaluate cardiac status and obtain an electrocardiogram and the results of an ejection fraction test before beginning therapy, to repeat the electrocardiogram when a dose of about 250 mg/M^2 has been given and to obtain more detailed studies if there are clinical or electrocardiographic indications. If doses of more than 400 mg/M^2 are planned, ejection fraction tests should be repeated every 100 mg/M^2. Major electrocardiographic changes and moderate cardiomyopathy, as described previously, indicate that the drug should be stopped.

Etoposide. Etoposide has been found of value in gestational trophoblastic disease and possibly in ovarian cancer, especially of the germ cell type. It is usually given intravenously in a dose of 50 to 150 mg/M^2 for three to five days at intervals of 21 days, alone or in combination with other drugs. Special toxicities have not yet been identified (O'Dwyer et al, 1985).

Fluorouracil. Fluorouracil (5FU) is seldom used alone in gynecologic oncology except as a topical agent applied for treatment of intraepithelial carcinoma of the vulva or vagina. It is also part of some drug combinations used for ovarian cancer. Used locally it produces irritation and pain; this limits the dose used for vulvar lesions and necessitates protecting the vulva with an ointment such as zinc oxide when 5FU is used inside the vagina (Sillman et al, 1985). Used systemically 5FU has the general side-effects noted earlier. In addition, excessive lacrimation occurs in up to one third of patients. Conjunctivitis has also been noted. Both appear to improve and disappear gradually after 5FU has been discontinued (Oster, 1984).

Hexamethylmelamine. Hexamethylmelamine is used alone or in combination with other agents for advanced or recurrent ovarian cancer and occasionally for other recurrent gynecologic cancers. Apart from myelosuppression, its chief toxic effects are nausea and vomiting and neurotoxicity. The former complications may limit its effectiveness, since the drug has to be given by mouth. Nausea and vomiting occurred in 21% of 24 patients given hexamethylmelamine as second line chemotherapy for advanced ovarian cancer (Rosen et al, 1987), but these effects did not necessitate discontinuing therapy. Peripheral neuropathy is the chief manifestation of neurotoxicity. The patient experiences numbness and tingling in the fingers and toes with loss of deep tendon reflexes, leading to difficulty in walking and in performing fine movements with the fingers. When these symptoms and signs are definite hexamethylmelamine should be discontinued. Recovery is usually incomplete. Pyridoxine (300 mg/day) given with hexamethylmelamine may prevent or lessen some of the neurotoxic consequences (Weiss, 1981). Neuropathy occurred in 21% of patients in the study discussed earlier, and it was responsible for stopping therapy in 8% (Rosen et al, 1987).

Methotrexate. The primary use of methotrexate in gynecologic oncology is for the management of trophoblastic disease. It has also been used in combination with other agents for ovarian cancer and in high doses (500 mg/M^2 or more with leukovorin rescue) for recurrent ovarian and other cancers. Side-effects not described in the general section include ocular symptoms, inflammation of serous membranes and neurologic, renal and hepatic effects. Conjunctivitis, excessive tearing, photophobia and eye pain occur rarely with standard doses. With high doses ocular symptoms are more common. When methotrexate is combined with 5FU excessive tearing is frequent. Pleural or peritoneal irritation was reported in 8.5% of 210 patients receiving high-dose methotrexate therapy (Urban et al, 1983). These complications occur occasionally in patients receiving conventional doses of methotrexate. The symptoms of chest and abdominal pain are often acute and quite severe but subside without treatment in a few days. Jaffe and co-workers (1985) noted neurologic symptoms in 15% of 60 patients treated with high doses of methotrexate. There were no permanent neurologic deficits. Renal complications are rare with ordinary doses of methotrexate but may occur with high doses. They can be minimized by hydration and alkalinization of the urine. Liver damage (fibrosis/cirrhosis) from methotrexate is unusual when the drug is given intermittently by the parenteral route. In high doses given at intervals of greater than 11 days hepatocellular damage may occur.

Vincristine, Vinblastine. The chief special complication of the vinca alkaloids is neuropathy. Most often the neuropathy is peripheral and autonomic but it may also involve the cranial nerves. It is more common with use of vincristine than with vinblastine. Peripheral neuropathy occurs in about 50% of patients receiving vincristine. It occurs after single or more commonly after multiple doses and is dose related. Initially patients are asymptomatic but the Achilles tendon reflexes are lost. Paresthesias of the hands and feet may then develop and may progress to pain, weakness, gait disturbance and sensory impairment. The dorsiflexors of the foot (and hand) are most affected, giving the patient foot-drop and a slapping gait. If vincristine therapy is stopped at the onset of symptoms, recovery will usually occur but may take several months. Autonomic neuropathy leads to constipation and colicky abdominal pain, which occur in 30 to 40% of patients. Bladder atony and orthostatic hypotension have also been reported.

Combination Chemotherapy. The objective of using more than one chemotherapeutic agent is to employ drugs that act on different parts of the cell cycle but whose toxicity affects different organs or systems. This means that the patient has to cope with multiple side-effects, and in some instances these may be cumulative. For instance, with the combination of cyclophosphamide, doxorubicin and cisplatin, often used for ovarian cancer, the hematologic toxicity of cyclophosphamide and doxorubicin makes myelosuppression more common and more severe than that occurring with either drug alone. Also, the relatively minor nausea and vomiting resulting from cyclophosphamide and doxorubicin use is augmented by the major emetogenic action of cisplatin. In general, the complications of combination chemotherapy can be ascertained by knowing those of the individual drugs.

Hormones and Related Compounds

ESTROGENS

Estrogens are available as steroidal (e.g., estradiol) and non-steroidal (e.g., diethystilbestrol) compounds. They may be given as single substances or as a combination of naturally occurring estrogens (conjugated estrogens). Indications for their use in women of reproductive age include (1) promotion of growth of secondary sexual organs in young women with ovarian dysgenesis; (2) control of excessive menstrual bleeding; (3) postcoital contraception and (4) occasionally to promote adequate endometrial growth and improve fertility. In perimenopausal and postmenopausal women estrogens are commonly used to prevent or treat postmenopausal vaginitis, emotional disturbances and osteoporosis. Their use in women whose ovaries have been removed has been discussed in Chapter 6. Estrogens may also be used in the management of advanced breast cancer. In general, estrogens are given by mouth, occasionally by injection or by inunction and, in postmenopausal women, vaginally. Estrogens may also be given in combination with progestins either for contraception or for perimenopausal symptoms (see later discussion).

The side-effects of estrogens depend upon the age of the patient to whom they are given, the dose used and the route of administration. They are best considered in relation to the organ systems involved.

Genital Tract. The deleterious effects of estrogens (DES) given to pregnant women to improve fetal outcome have been well established. Since estrogens are no longer used for this purpose the ill effects will eventually be self-limited. In the meantime, they present, for the exposed young women, abnormalities of the vagina, cervix, uterus and possibly tubes and affect reproductive functions to a varying extent. These changes have been described by Herbst and Bern (1981) and summarized by Stillman (1982). Of recent interest are the possible increase in cervical dysplasia in these women (Robboy et al, 1984) and the decrease in sexual activity and functioning (Meyer-Bahlburg et al, 1985).

UTERUS. The effect of exogenous estrogen on the endometrium is to cause stimulation and proliferation. Prolonged use results in endometrial hyperplasia in about 12% of patients. Endometrial hyperplasia is potentially malignant, since in up to 25% of cases it may progress to adenocarcinoma, the frequency being greatest when cellular and nuclear atypicalities are present, intermediate in adenomatous hyperplasia and least in cystic hyperplasia (Fig. 13–1). Thus, patients on intermittent or continous estrogen replacement therapy (ERT) have an increased relative risk of developing endometrial adenocarcinoma estimated to range from 1.7 to 12.5. This risk appears to depend on the dose and length of therapy. With the usual dose of 0.3 to 1.25 mg of conjugated estrogens, at least one year of therapy and possibly longer is needed to increase the risk at all, but it increases progressively with further use. Since the majority of women who receive ERT are peri- or postmenopausal, the greatest risk is in women over 50 years of age. However, risk is also present in young women receiving this therapy for various forms of ovarian dysgenesis.

In recent years it has become clear that the addition of a progestin, such as Provera 10 mg for the last 10 to 14 days of estrogen administration (days 12 to 16 through 25 of each month), significantly reduces the risk of endometrial cancer (Gambrell, 1982). Such a combination of hormones should be used if the uterus is present.

Cyclical bleeding is likely to occur with any regimen of hormone replacement. Therefore, some authorities have recommended sampling the endometrium prior to starting therapy. For many women this is an uncomfortable procedure. It can be omitted if there has been no abnormal bleeding or, after therapy has been started, if the withdrawal bleeding is regular, neither excessive nor prolonged. It should be noted that withdrawal bleeding may cease after continued use of hormonal therapy. Also, the use of hormones on a rigorous schedule taxes the patience of many women and irregular use or sudden discontinuation may be accompanied by vaginal bleeding. In any case, if there is doubt about the nature of the bleeding, an endometrial sample should be obtained. This can preferably be done in the office using a Vabra aspirator or similar instrument, with or without local anesthesia by paracervical block. If this approach is not feasible, a dilatation and curettage procedure under local or general anesthesia is necessary.

The further management of a patient who has irregular vaginal bleeding during estrogen therapy depends on the endometrial findings. Adenocarcinoma clearly requires definitive therapy—hysterectomy. Hyperplasia, whether atypical, adenomatous or cystic, indicates discontinuation of replacement therapy. Atypical hyperplasia may indicate hysterectomy in certain cases. However, both it and adenomatous and cystic hyperplasia may be treated by continuous administration of a progestin (e.g., megestrol 40 mg twice daily for eight weeks) or cyclical progestin, if it has not been used previously (e.g., 10 mg Provera by mouth) from days 12 to 25 of each month. Follow-up endometrial sampling is necessary after a period of therapy and six months later. Recurrence of irregular bleeding or hyperplasia may be an indication for hysterectomy. If the initial endometrial sampling shows no more than proliferative changes, discontinuation of replacement therapy should be sufficient treatment. If such a patient continues to have severe menopausal symptoms, Depo-Provera (150 mg) may be given intramuscularly every two to three months. Resumption of estrogen therapy, per-

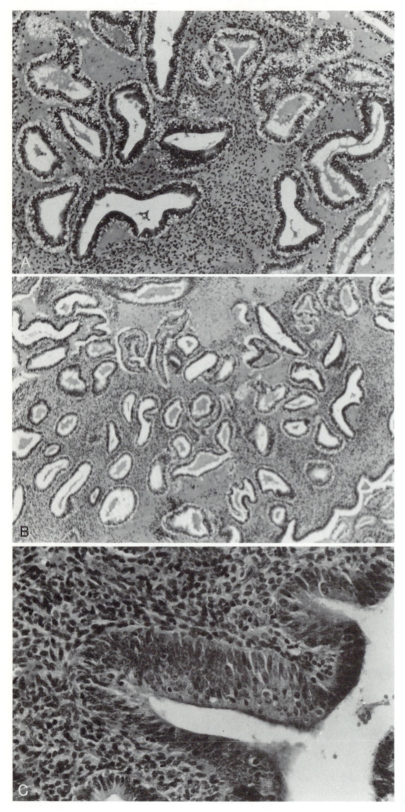

Figure 13–1. A, Cystic, Adenomatous (B), Atypical (C) hyperplasia of the endometrium.

haps desirable to lessen the chance of osteoporosis, should be undertaken only with regular endometrial sampling (before treatment and at six to 12 month intervals). Equally important in prevention of osteoporosis are adequate diet, supplemental calcium and appropriate exercise.

The effect of estrogen on the growth of leiomyomata is uncertain. In younger women, and particularly those taking estrogens as part of birth control pills, there is some evidence of increased growth of these tumors. However, in postmenopausal women receiving the usual dose of 0.3 to 1.25 mg of conjugated estrogens intermittently (with or without a progestin), these tumors do not seem to grow, although their regression may be delayed. The risk of endometrial changes is theoretically the same after prolonged use of intravaginal estrogens since they are readily absorbed by this route. Horwitz and Feinstein (1979) did not find this. However, they did not report the frequency or the duration of vaginal use.

Cardiovascular System. Estrogens given postmenopausally, in contrast to those given as part of oral contraceptives (see later discussion), do not seem to cause an increase in coronary or cerebral vascular disease, hypertension or thromboembolism (Hammond et al, 1979).

Gastrointestinal Tract. When estrogens were used in large doses (5 mg ethinyl estradiol or 25 mg DES daily) postcoitally to intercept pregnancy, nausea occurred in at least half the recipients, and vomiting occurred in a quarter of them (Haspels and Andriesse, 1973). Concurrent use of an antiemetic such as prochlorperazine is advisable. Nausea is occasionally noted after the usual doses of conjugated estrogens in postmenopausal women. For this reason estrogen should be taken at night. Antiemetics are rarely necessary; in fact, if they are needed, other causes for nausea and vomiting should be sought, and, if none are present, the continued use of estrogen is to be questioned. Gallbladder disease with stones may be increased in postmenopausal women taking estrogens. Customary medical or surgical management is necessary (Honore, 1980). Conjugated estrogens taken by mouth produced significant alteration in some markers of hepatic function, e.g., total cholesterol and LDL cholesterol levels fall and HDL cholesterol levels rise. These changes do not seem to occur when estrogen is administered transdermally (Chetkowski et al, 1986).

Breast. Estrogens cause cyclical swelling of breast tissue at the end of the cycle of administration. This is usually minor and rarely re-

quires discontinuation of the medication. It is usually relieved by adding a progestin to the last 10 to 14 days of the estrogen therapy cycle. Currently there is no indication that postmenopausal estrogen use increases the risk of breast cancer (Kaufman et al, 1984). The incidence of breast cancer may possibly be increased in mothers given DES during pregnancy (Greenberg et al, 1984), but this finding needs confirmation.

PROGESTINS

Various progestins are available for use; they are primarily given by mouth (e.g., Provera), as vaginal suppositories or intramuscularly. Progestins are used for the diagnosis of amenorrhea and for the treatment of anovulatory bleeding (with or without endometrial hyperplasia), endometriosis or (in large doses) widespread or recurrent adenocarcinoma of the corpus uteri. They are also an essential part of combined oral contraceptives and are used alone for birth control. When used alone, progestins do not seem to produce a greater risk of cardiovascular disease, including hypertension. Weight gain with water retention is occasionally seen, especially in those patients receiving over 100 mg per day of Provera or equivalent doses of other preparations. When used alone as a contraceptive agent, progesterone is frequently accompanied by irregular bleeding. A recently reported complication is the development of functional ovarian cysts (detected by ultrasonography). Cysts developed in 8 of 21 patients (38%) studied by Tayob and co-workers (1985), but they disappeared by the second cycle after the progesterone was discontinued.

COMBINED ESTROGEN-PROGESTIN COMPOUNDS

The introduction in 1960 of combined estrogen-progestin preparations for use in preventing pregnancy was one of the most important recent pharmaceutical advances. In the last 26 years the number of these compounds has multiplied greatly. Their efficacy has remained relatively constant, but it took 20 years for complications, many of them unsuspected at first, to be recognized and categorized. It is likely that complications will continue to be discovered at least until women who have taken the medication over many years reach the end of their lives.

Oral contraceptives (OC) affect virtually all organ systems. Some effects are minor and appear at present to be inconsequential, although with long-term follow-up they may not be so. Many important side-effects are due in large part to the estrogen fraction, although the combination of the two agents produces effects quantitatively if not qualitatively different from those of each of the two components. For example, in the 1970's attention was focused on the estrogen component, since it was recognized that a larger amount of estrogen increased the risk of thromboembolism. However, certain progestins (particularly those with androgenic properties) decrease serum high density lipoprotein levels, a finding associated with an increased risk of myocardial infarction or stroke (Wynn and Niththyananthan, 1982). Moreover, evidence from the Royal College of General Practitioners study indicates that the greater the amount of progestin in a contraceptive pill, the greater is the risk of arterial disease (Kay, 1982). Ultimately, however, the risks of OC must be weighed against the risks of pregnancy (i.e., reproductive mortality).

Metabolic Changes. As is illustrated in Table 13–5 changes occur in serum and plasma levels of many substances, including vitamins. Decreases in serum albumin and increases in synthesis of carrier proteins are responsible for many additional changes. Few clinical effects are noted from these changes; their significance lies in their possible long-term effects and their influence on possible contraindications to the use of OC and precautions in prescribing them.

Hematopoietic System Complications. Various changes have been reported. Consistent increases in plasma fibrinogen, plasma prothrombin time and factors VII and X have been noted. Platelet numbers appear to be unaltered, while platelet aggregation may be less inhibited. Changes in fibrinolytic systems, antiplasmin activity and antithrombin activity are inconsistently reported. Much of the confusion in the findings is thought by Beller and Ebert (1985) to be caused by methodologic errors. The importance of the changes described is that the woman taking oral contraceptives is likely to be in a hypercoagulable state and therefore more prone to thromboembolic episodes.

Cardiovascular System Complications. Much has been written about the possible increased risk of thromboembolism, myocardial infarction and stroke among users of oral contraceptives (OC). There are three major problems in evaluating the reports. First, as pointed out by Relini and Goldzeiher (1985), many methodologic weaknesses in the case control, cohort and mortality studies are discovered if rigid stand-

ards of evaluation are used. Second, at least in the United States, there has recently been a sharp increase in the prescription of OC containing less than 50 micrograms of estrogen, compared with those containing 50 micrograms or more; much of the data has been obtained from studies of the high estrogen compounds. Third, the amount of progestin combined with estrogen may be important.

If OC with a low estrogen and a low progestin content are given to healthy women aged 15 to 44 who are without risk factors (i.e., hypertension, diabetes, thromboembolism, stroke, myocardial infarction, pregnancy or serious predisposing illness), it seems likely that there is a slightly increased risk of thromboembolism among OC users. Although this complication is rare, Porter and co-workers (1985) found that the relative risk of thromboembolism was 2.8 in OC used as compared with non-users. However, the association between these doses of OC and other cardiovascular events such as myocardial infarction is less clear. Moreover, smoking appears to be an important factor adding to the risk of cardiovascular events, especially in women 35 years of age or over.

Management of the cardiovascular complications of oral contraceptives is primarily medical and is not discussed here. However, since these complications are potentially serious, they deserve consideration in women of any age who are contemplating the use of this method of birth control. The risk is clearly less, although still present, in women who do not smoke, do not have risk factors and are under 35 years of age.

Gastrointestinal System Complications. Nau-

Table 13–5. Some Metabolic Effects of Oral Contraceptives

Metabolite	Increased	Decreased
Total thyroxine	x	
Resin uptake of triiodothyronine (T_3)		x
Cortisol binding globulin	x	
Total serum cortisol	x	
Glucose tolerance		(x)*
Low density lipoprotein	x	
High density lipoprotein		x
Triglycerides	x	
Cholesterol	(x)	
Riboflavin		x
Pyridoxine (Vitamin B_6)		x
Folic acid (Vitamin B_{12})		x
Vitamin C		x
Copper (ceruloplasmin)	x	
Zinc		x
Vitamin A	x	

*(x) = possible effect.

sea, vomiting (rarely) and epigastric distress are occasionally reported by OC users, most frequently in the early weeks. The symptoms are similar to but usually less marked than those of early pregnancy. Taking the pills at night or adding 50 mg of supplementary pyridoxine (vitamin B_6) three times daily may help. If the symptoms are severe enough to need specific antiemetics, a change in the method of birth control should be strongly considered.

Cholecystitis and cholelithiasis have been reported to occur more frequently in the early years of OC use than in controls. More recent data on continued use show a lower incidence (Kay, 1984). This suggests that OC may accelerate the development of gallbladder disease in susceptible women.

Genital Tract Complications

CERVIX. There is at present no clear evidence that OC predispose to or are associated with an increased incidence of cervical carcinoma. However, epidemiologic studies of this question are extremely difficult to evaluate because of the many possibilities of bias. Women using oral contraceptives may show increased vascularity and overgrowth of the columnar epithelium either on the ectocervix or within the cervical canal (Fig. 13–2). This overgrowth is usually asymptomatic, but its possible occurrence emphasizes the importance of at least an annual inspection of the cervix, cytologic studies with colposcopic evaluation if indicated and treatment of symptomatic patients by cryotherapy or laser therapy.

UTERUS. Breakthrough bleeding (intermenstrual bleeding) commonly occurs in the first few cycles of OC use. It can usually be managed expectantly, because it disappears. A common cause is omission or irregular ingestion of the daily pill. If bleeding is persistent or severe it

Figure 13–2. Pseudoadenomatous changes in the cervix following oral contraceptive use. A, Low power view. B, High power view.

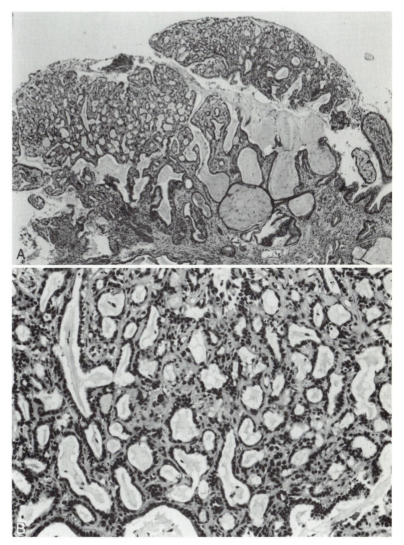

Table 13–6. Estrogen and Progestin Content of Representative Oral Contraceptives

Contraceptive	Estrogen Content*	Progestin Content
Brevicon	L	L
Demulen	M	H
Loestrin 1.5/30	L	M
Loestrin 1/20	L	M
LoOvral	L	H
Modicon	L	L
Nordette	M	M
Norinyl 1 + 80	H	L
Norinyl 1 + 50	M	L
Norlestrin 1 mg	M	M
Ortho-Novum 1 + 80	H	L
Ortho-Novum 1 + 50	M	L
Ortho-Novum 1 + 35	L	L
Ovcon-50	M	L
Ovcon-35	L	L
Ovral	M	H
Ovulen	H	H
Zorane 1/50	M	M
Zorane 1.5/30	L	M
Zorane 1/20	L	M

*L = low; M = moderate; H = high.

is usually due to insufficient estrogen. Additional estrogen can be given for the current cycle or a preparation with a higher estrogen content can be substituted (Table 13–6). A common practice is to advise the patient to take two OC pills instead of one for the rest of the involved cycle. This method is frequently successful but may not resolve the estrogen-progesterone imbalance. A common effect of OC is to decrease menstrual flow and lessen dysmenorrhea. Occasionally, menstruation does not take place. If amenorrhea or marked oligomenorrhea persists, temporary discontinuation of OC use or a change to a lower dose preparation should be considered. Pregnancy must always be ruled out.

When OC are stopped there is commonly slight delay in the return of menstruation; the length of the first cycle averages 36 days. Resumption of flow usually occurs in less than 180 days, but is later than this in 1 to 3% of women. If menstruation has not returned by that time, a workup for all possible causes of amenorrhea should be undertaken. Among women who had six or more months of amenorrhea spontaneous resumption of menses occurred in 25 of 45 (58%) women who had regular cycles prior to taking OC but in only 19 of the 51 (37%) who had irregular menses previously (Soltan and Hancock, 1982). In this series 28% of those desiring pregnancy conceived spontaneously

while a further 55% conceived after induction of ovulation. When pregnant women have used OC in the three months prior to the last menstrual period, the likelihood of uncertain dates is increased. Oral contraceptive users in South Glamorgan, Wales were found by Kasan and Andrews (1986) to have had a higher incidence of neural tube defects among their offspring than non-users. However, there was no overall difference in congenital anomalies or in the sex distribution of the offspring.

Blood Pressure Changes. Oral contraceptives consistently raise blood pressure. In a small study, Weir and co-workers (1974) showed a mean rise of 9.2 mmHg in systolic blood pressure and a rise of 5.0 mmHg in diastolic pressure during a three year prospective trial. These results have been confirmed by studies of women taking lower dose OC compounds. The estrogen moiety appears to be primarily responsible, although the exact mechanism of action has not been elucidated. Blood pressure usually returns to normal after discontinuation of OC use. The incidence of severe and acute hypertensive episodes appears to be low, but remains a matter of concern. Patients with established hypertension should be considered at higher than normal risk for the complications of OC use. Regular blood pressure determinations should be made on women receiving OC (3 months or less after beginning OC use and then every 6 months). If a significant elevation of blood pressure is found, OC use should be stopped. With a slight elevation of blood pressure, long-term risks are uncertain, but they must be evaluated in terms of overall birth control management.

Breast Changes. There is considerable evidence that OC use reduces the incidence of fibrocystic and other benign diseases of the breast (Lyle, 1980). Similarly, OC do not appear to increase the risk of breast cancer (Lipnick et al, 1986), although Pike and co-workers (1983) in a case control study reported a higher incidence in women taking OC with a high progestin content for a long period (5 years or more) before the age of 25. These findings did not hold true in another case control study reported by Stadel and co-workers (1985).

Skin Complications. Discoloration (darkening or melasma) of facial skin occurs in some women, especially Caucasians, taking OC. With high dose pills the incidence was reported to be 29% (Resnick, 1967), but it is much lower with the more recent lower dose OC use. Melasma does not completely regress after discontinuing OC. Increased acne is sometimes noted with OC. Estrogens decrease sebum excretion, but androgens may increase it. Therefore, in acne-prone women, OC containing a progestin with a relatively high androgenic content, e.g., norgestrol, should be used with caution.

Psychosocial and Sexual Complications. The psychologic complications of oral contraceptives are difficult to ascertain for several reasons. First, background emotional factors may be important. Second, many studies suffer from methodologic faults, e.g., lack of control subjects, poor assessment of pretherapeutic mood states or failure to define such terms as depression. Third, different contraceptive pills may have different effects. Fourth, there has been a considerable change in the formulation of oral contraceptives in the past 15 years; many current preparations contain much smaller amounts of both estrogen and progesterone. Fifth, concern has increased among women during the past 10 years about the overall effect of oral contraceptives upon their bodies and about the widespread reports in the media regarding untoward side-effects.

In the late 1960's and early 1970's depression was often thought to be associated with oral contraceptive use. However, Goldzieher and co-workers (1971), in a placebo-controlled, double-blind trial of four oral contraceptive agents, concluded that most of the nervousness, depression and weight gain noted in oral contraceptive users is either coincidental or associated with the psychologic impact of taking these agents rather than with any pharmacologic effect. Nevertheless, Slap (1981) found that in nine of 12 clinical studies that he reviewed depression was reported in 16 to 56% of women using oral contraceptives. Some support for the occurrence of depression comes from the observation that increased tryptophane and decreased tyrosine levels accompany the use of oral contraceptives. Miller (1981) suggests that because of a decreased brain tyrosine concentration, a substrate-limited brain norepinephrine synthesis may contribute to depressive symptoms in susceptible women. An interesting related observation was made by Morris and Udry (1969); they found that the use of oral contraceptives was associated with lessened physical activity in some women. This change of itself might contribute to depression and also to weight gain. As far as other mood changes are concerned, the smoothing-out of the normal pattern during the menstrual cycle may be of benefit in the management of marked mood changes, especially the premenstrual tension syndrome.

The sexual complications of oral contraceptive use are also difficult to determine. Decreased libido has been described by some authors, but equally important is the sense of security that comes from using an effective contraceptive (Gambrell, 1976). The physiologic alterations in cervical mucus that occur with oral contraceptive use (i.e., thick and more scanty mucus) do not seem to affect coital response since the main source of lubrication is transudation of fluid through the vaginal wall.

Miscellaneous Complications. Prolonged OC use is associated with an increased incidence of hepatoma, as compared with that in the population at large. Rarely, this tumor may become malignant (hepatocellular carcinoma) (Gala and Griffin, 1983). Because of its rarity routine liver screening tests are impractical and indeed may not be helpful. Regular physical examinations and prompt diagnosis of the cause of an enlarged liver are appropriate. Surgical excision is possible in most cases. Many other side-effects have been reported, but in the absence of control studies their frequency is difficult to determine. Of interest is the rare occurrence of carpal tunnel syndrome, which is improved by discontinuing the medication (Sabour and Fadel, 1970).

Prevention of Complications. Many but not all the complications of oral contraceptives can be avoided by care in prescribing. The following measures are helpful:

1. The presence of risk factors should be determined for each patient (Table 13-7).

2. A thorough general physical and pelvic

Table 13–7. Contraindications to Oral Contraceptives

Absolute
  Thrombotic disorders
  Estrogen dependent tumors
  Pregnancy
  Abnormal uterine bleeding
  Impaired liver function

Relative
  Age over 35 (especially smokers)
  Hypertension
  Gestational diabetes
  Migraine headaches
  Epilepsy
  Varicose veins
  Prior amenorrhea
  History of depression

examination should be performed and a Pap smear obtained.

3. Alternative methods of contraception and possible complications of oral contraceptives should be discussed in detail with the patient so that she understands and accepts therapy.

4. Oral contraceptive pills containing low doses of both estrogen and progestin should be prescribed at first. Persistent break-through bleeding or other complications may necessitate the addition of estrogen or a change to pills of a different composition.

5. Initial follow-up should be in less than three months, with particular reference to checking the blood pressure. Later follow-ups should be at six to 12 months, depending on circumstances.

6. Oral contraceptives should be discontinued if hypertension persists or thrombotic episodes, persistent headaches or other significant complications occur.

7. If an elective operation that is likely to increase the risk of thrombosis is contemplated, oral contraceptives should preferably be stopped at least four weeks prior to the procedure (Guillebaud, 1985).

8. Women taking oral contraceptives should be advised to take a multivitamin tablet daily or an adequate amount of vitamin B_6 (pyridoxine 10 mg three times daily), vitamin C (at least 100 mg daily) and folic acid (0.4 mg twice daily). Vitamin B_2 (riboflavin) and zinc may also be advisable.

Testosterone

The gynecologic uses of testosterone include (1) suppression of lactation after delivery (testosterone enanthate with estradiol valerate, Deladumone 2 mg); (2) topical application in white petrolatum (2%) for lichen sclerosus of the vulva; (3) management of the symptoms of mild endometriosis (rarely); (4) therapy of osteoporosis in combination with an estrogen; and (5) treatment of advanced or recurrent breast carcinoma. Symptoms of masculinization are the chief side-effects. They include acne, growth of hair on the face and body, increased libido and hoarseness. At the same time there is defeminization, i.e., oligomenorrhea or amenorrhea and atrophy of breast tissue. Later, enlargement of the clitoris, prominent musculature and baldness may occur. The incidence of these side-effects depends largely upon the dose and duration. In the amounts commonly used with estrogen for suppression of lactation they do not occur. In the second category of usage, virilization is seldom a problem, but the increased libido may be of concern among older women. In the third category there are individual variations in response. A total dose of 150 mg per month has a 25% chance of causing masculinization, whereas this chance is very small with 100 mg per month or less. When testosterone is given with estrogens for osteoporosis, masculinization is rare, but masculinization is common with the large doses sometimes used for breast carcinoma.

Corticosteroids

Corticosteroids are widely used in gynecology by inunction as anti-inflammatory and antipruritic agents. Specifically their use is appropriate for hypertrophic vulvitis or alternated with testosterone in petrolatum for lichen sclerosus of the vulva. They may be used orally or parenterally for a few gynecologic conditions such as allergic reactions or toxic shock. More important to the gynecologist-obstetrician is the management of patients already receiving corticosteroids for other disorders, since the presence of side-effects and the prior duration of therapy affect many operative procedures and treatments. The chief early complications of any cortisone or cortisone-derived compound are fluid retention, typically facial edema, and hypertension. Later complications (usually after prolonged use) include electrolyte changes, glycosuria, increased susceptibility to infections, peptic ulceration, myopathy, behavioral changes, cataracts and osteoporosis leading to vertebral compression fractures. Adrenal failure may follow withdrawal of cortisone, especially if it has been used for a long time. Therefore, in patients already taking cortisone additional cortisone must be given during and for the first few days after any major operation (see Chapter 2).

Fertility Agents

Clomiphene. Clomiphene is the chief agent used to induce ovulation. It is a weak antiestrogen that has a central effect on the hypothalamus. Given for five days, beginning on the fifth day of the menstrual cycle, to a woman with endogenous estrogen production, it causes an increased secretion of gonadotrophins (luteinizing hormone [LH] and follicle stimulating hormone [FSH]. These hormones cause maturation of quiescent follicles, and ovulation occurs five to 11 days later. Luteal phase deficiency (LPD) is a possible result of this type of ovulation induction. The usual initial dose of clomiphene is 50 mg per day, but this may be increased to as much as 200 mg per day. The most common immediate side-effects include vasomotor flushes (10%), abdominal and pelvic discomfort (6%), nausea and vomiting (2%), breast discomfort (2%), visual symptoms of various sorts (1.5%) and headache (1.3%) (Speroff et al, 1983). Many other symptoms have been reported to occur but in less than 1% of patients. Ovarian enlargement (ovarian hyperstimulation syndrome or OHSS) occurs in about 5% of patients. It is usually mild but the ovaries may reach a diameter of 12 cm or more and the patient may present with severe pain, abdominal distension, ascites and circulatory and electrolyte disturbances. The enlarged ovary may twist or rupture. Management of OHSS is usually conservative with observation and hydration, unless an acute accident is suspected. Multiple gestation occurs in about 5% of patients receiving clomiphene, and this, in itself, causes problems in pregnancy. However, in single pregnancies there is no evidence of adverse outcomes in women who receive clomiphene, and fetal growth and development appear to be normal (Scialli, 1986).

Human Menopausal Gonadotrophin (HMG). Human menopausal gonadotrophin (HMG or Pergonal) contains an equal mixture of LH and FSH. Given by intramuscular injection of 1 to 2 ampules per day for seven to 14 days, it causes follicle development and estrogen production. Because of its high cost and the difficulty of monitoring its effect, it is usually given when clomiphene has been ineffective or in sequence after the use of clomiphene. The major complications of HMG therapy are similar to those of clomiphene—OHSS and multiple gestation. The latter has an incidence of about 25%. The number of follicles maturing and likely to result in gestation can be monitored somewhat by tailoring the dose of HMG to the rise in serum estrogen levels, determined every one to two days, and by ultrasonography.

Bromocriptine. Bromocriptine is a dopamine agonist. It inhibits pituitary secretion of prolactin and, in amenorrheic women, permits the resumption of ovulation and of menstruation. It has also been used for severely symptomatic fibrocystic breast disease. During initial therapy side-effects are relatively common and consist of nausea (50%), headaches (18%), dizziness (16%), orthostatic hypotension (6%) and vomiting (5%) (Cuellar, 1980). Persistence in treatment, taking the medication at night and increasing the dose slowly, starting with 2.5 mg and increasing 2.5 mg every four weeks, help to reduce side-effects. If pregnancy occurs during treatment with bromocryptine, adverse effects on the fetus have not been shown.

MISCELLANEOUS AGENTS

Danazol. Danazol is primarily used in the management of endometriosis; it may also be effective in fibrocystic breast disease with marked symptoms. Its action is complex, but in effect danazol is an anti-estrogen with some androgenic properties. Anovulation and amenorrhea occur with a dose of 800 mg per day. When this dose is given for six months, side-effects are very common (Table 13–8). They are less frequent with a dose of 400 mg per day, although there may be some doubt about the effectiveness of the drug at this dose. When 200 mg per day is given, irregular uterine bleeding occurs frequently and a small percentage of women ovulate. Symptoms and signs with the possible exception of hirsutism generally disappear when danazol is discontinued.

Other Drugs Used for Gynecologic Disorders

VULVA AND VAGINA

Anti-infective, anti-fungal, anti-viral and chemotherapeutic agents used for vaginal and vulvar disease have been described earlier. Local

Table 13–8. Complications of Danazol Therapy

Complication	Buttram et al (1982) 71 Patients	Barbieri et al (1982) 100 Patients
	%	%
Weight gain	85	55
Muscle cramps	52	—
Decreased breast size	48	34
Flushing	42	—
Mood change	38	—
Oily skin	37	11
Depression	32	—
Sweating	32	—
Edema	28	55
Change in appetite	28	—
Acne	27	—
Fatigue	25	—
Hirsutism	21	17
Deepening of voice	7	8

spermicides and cleansing agents are covered in Chapter 11. Many over-the-counter medications are available for minor problems. Most contain small amounts of antipruritic, antiinfective and local anesthetic agents. Their use is not accompanied by side-effects except, rarely, hypersensitivity and local irritation.

The absorption of substances used to cleanse the vagina before surgical procedures may occasionally be significant. For example, serum iodine levels were found to be elevated for 15 to 60 minutes after the use of povidone-iodine in disinfecting the vagina (Vorherr et al, 1980). Hexachlorophene may also be absorbed when used in a similar manner (Strickland et al, 1983). Consideration of these findings may be important when therapy for the pregnant woman and her fetus are evaluated.

Podophyllin. Podophyllin (25% in ticture of benzoin) is commonly used for treatment of small condylomata acuminata of the vulva. It is contraindicated in pregnancy. The condylomata are painted with the solution and the treatment may be repeated. Podophyllin is very irritating to normal skin and a marked local inflammatory reaction results. To prevent this reaction, the area treated must be washed by bathing and the use of mild soap within six hours of the treatment. If local reaction does occur, it is best managed by repeated applications (15 minutes every two to three hours) of cold Burow's solution (1:40 or 1:20 solution of aluminum sulfate and calcium acetate) and systemic analgesics.

URINARY TRACT

Urinary tract antibiotics were covered earlier in this chapter and in Chapter 4. In addition, anti-infective agents specific for the urinary tract are in common use. These include nitrofurantoin, nalidixic acid, methenamine compounds and vitamin C. A number of side-effects have been reported with the nitrofurantoins, initially hypersensitivity reactions, especially dermatitis, and anorexia, nausa and vomiting. Later, peripheral neuropathy or chronic pulmonary symptoms with interstitial pneumonitis, pulmonary fibrosis and decreased pulmonary function may occur. Naladixic acid is occasionally associated with hypersensitivity reactions or central nervous system symptoms. Methenamine (1.0 gm four times daily) and vitamin C (500 mg three or four times daily) are rarely associated with side-effects.

Drugs that affect the motility of the urinary tract, especially the bladder, are widely used.

Bethanechol (Urecholine) stimulates the parasymphathetic nervous system and causes the bladder to contract and expel urine. Even in the usual dose of 10 to 50 mg three or four times daily, bethanechol may produce abdominal discomfort, salivation, flushing and sweating. Atropine 0.6 mg, given subcutaneously, is a specific antidote. Several drugs inhibit the parasympathetic system and thus expulsion of urine. Among the most commonly used and effective are banthine, probanthine and Bentyl. All may be accompanied by dryness of the mouth, blurred vision, constipation and tachycardia. The presence of these symptoms indicates the need for a reduction in dose or discontinuation of the drug.

Many urinary tract medications contain two or more agents with complementary actions. Side-effects are often less pronounced since the dose of each is smaller than usual. In some formulations pyridium is added as a mild urinary tract analgesic. This colors the urine orange. The coloration is of no clinical significance but concerns the patient if she is not aware of the possibility of it occurring.

DRUGS USED IN OBSTETRICS

Seventy to 80% of women are exposed to a wide variety of prescription and non-prescription drugs during conception, pregnancy, labor, delivery and lactation (Brocklebank et al, 1978; Doering and Stewart, 1978; and Rayburn et al, 1982). The average first trimester exposure is to one to five drugs, excluding dietary supplements. Many of these drugs can be obtained without physician consultation. For example, mild analgesics such as aspirin or acetaminophen are used by as many as 75% of gravidas. In addition, exposure to illicit drugs and environmental toxins is widespread. Between 30 to 40% of women smoke, drink 1 to 2 ounces of ethanol a week or have more than seven cups of coffee a week.

The adverse outcomes of pregnancy include first trimester loss (20%), perinatal loss (1 to 2%), major birth defects (2 to 5%), intrauterine growth retardation (10%), prematurity (6%), and long-term neurologic abnormalities (1 to 3%). The relationship of drug exposure during pregnancy to these outcomes is not clear. Many questions remain concerning maternal and fetal pharmacokinetics and susceptibility to drugs. Animal studies on the fetal effects of drugs are limited in their reference to humans (Brown and Fabro, 1983). Yet, human research is restricted by ethical, medicolegal and governmental restrictions, The United States Food and Drug Administration (FDA) is given the responsibility of monitoring the safety of current and new drugs. This task is enormous; 1,000 to 3,000 new drugs or chemicals are introduced into the market each year.

The provider of care to any pregnant woman has the responsibility of educating her about the possible consequences of drug therapy during pregnancy. This informed consent should be no less complete nor have less documentation than that for a surgical procedure. The essentials of informed consent involve a two way discussion of the benefits, risks, alternative therapy, and consequences of no therapy. The patient should be allowed to ask questions and seek other opinions if she wishes.

Discussion of the fetal and maternal risks of non-obstetric drugs is beyond the scope of this book. The reader is referred to a more detailed discussion in any one of several reference books (Berkowitz et al, 1981; Briggs and Bodendorfer, 1986; Lawrence, 1984; Rayburn and Zuspan, 1982).

The FDA and most authors rank drugs by five categories of fetal risk.

Category A. Controlled studies in women fail to demonstrate a risk to the fetus in the first trimester (and there is no evidence of risk in later trimesters) and the possibility of such risk appears remote.

Category B. Either animal reproduction studies have not demonstrated a fetal risk but there are no controlled studies in pregnant women, or animal reproduction studies have shown an adverse effect (other than a decrease in fertility) that was not confirmed in controlled studies in women in the first trimester (and there is no evidence of risk in later trimesters).

Category C. Either studies in animals have revealed adverse effects on the fetus (teratogenic, embryocidal or other) and there are no controlled studies in women, or studies in women and animals are not available. Drugs should be given only if the potential benefit justifies the potential risk to the fetus.

Category D. There is positive evidence of fetal risk but the benefits from use in pregnant women may be acceptable despite the risk, for example, if the drug is needed in a life-threatening situation or for a serious disease for which safer drugs cannot be used or are ineffective.

Category X. Studies in animals and humans have demonstrated fetal abnormalities, or there is evidence of fetal risk on human experience or both, and the risk of the use of the drug in pregnant women clearly outweighs any possible benefit. The drug is contraindicated in women who are or may become pregnant.

The vast majority of drugs are classified as Category B, C or D. Only electrolytes and vitamins in normal doses can be classified as Category A. There are also relatively few category X drugs; aminopterin, paramethadione, trimethadione, thalidomide, diethylstilbestrol, clomiphene, disulfiram, phencyclidine and valproic acid are among them.

The health care provider must perform a risk-benefit evaluation prior to prescribing a drug. The evaluation is facilitated by asking a series of questions. The first category of questions relates to the maternal parameters. How serious is the mother's condition that requires the drug? For example, the use of diuretics to reduce pedal edema of pregnancy is very different than their use in treating pulmonary edema. What is the efficacy of the drug therapy? Are there changes in maternal pharmacokinetics that will affect drug transfer? For example, low albumin in preeclampsia may increase the free drug concentration. Are there indirect fetal effects caused by drug-mediated changes in physiology? Uteroplacental perfusion is a common focus in the study of antihypertensive drugs during pregnancy. Do these drugs affect the absorption or metabolism of essential vitamins or minerals? Hydralazine, isoniazid, and penicillamine increase the excretion of vitamin B_6. Antacids block the absorption of calcium (Ovesen, 1979). Will drug therapy mask the development of perinatal disease? For example, use of steroids may mask the development of chorioamnionitis after premature rupture of membranes.

The second category of questions relates to the specific drug pharmacokinetics. These questions focus on the route of administration, absorption, ionization, protein-binding of competitive drugs or compounds, mode of transport to the tissues, metabolism, excretion, and the pharmacologic and biologic properties of the metabolites. Knowledge of the mechanism of action allows anticipation of the direct and indirect fetal effects.

The third category of questions relates to the fetus or neonate. What is the gestational age? Is there a familial risk of developmental defects? Do current perinatal problems affect placental transport? How does the fetus metabolize the drug? Is there a toxic risk from the drug's metabolites? How does delivery affect the metabolism or distribution of the drug in the neonate? After delivery or during lactation does the drug or its metabolites affect intrapersonal relationships (bonding)? Is the drug used in neonates, and if so, what precautions are needed?

Pharmacology of Pregnancy

MATERNAL

Pharmacokinetics deals with the rates of four basic processes that can be fundamental determinants of drug action:absorption, distribution, biotransformation and excretion. The study of the pharmacokinetics of pregnancy requires a separate focus on the mother, placenta and fetus. Each has its own unique problems, which are different from those in the pharmacokinetics of non-pregnant adults.

Maternal drug absorption is most changed by oral and ventilatory routes of administration. Nausea and vomiting can markedly reduce absorption. During antibiotic therapy a vomited dose is equivalent to a missed dose, thus increasing the potential for inadequate plasma concentrations and the emergence of resistant strains. Pregnancy also reduces gastric hydrochloric acid secretion and decreases motility. Weak bases (aspirin) are more poorly absorbed and weak acids (narcotic analgesics) are more rapidly absorbed. Slowed motility may increase bacterial transformation or inactivation in the gut. During pregnancy the increase in minute ventilation enhances the absorption of inhalation anesthetics.

The distribution of drugs in women is markedly altered by pregnancy. Two major factors are an increase in circulating blood volume and a relative decrease in the serum albumin level. Volume dilution decreases the serum concentration of the drug and decreases clearance by increasing the volume to be cleared by the organs of metabolism, the liver and kidneys. A relative decrease in albumin concentration affects drugs that bind exclusively to plasma albumin (warfarin, salicylates). Competitive displacement by other drugs further increases the concentrations of free drugs. In addition, there seems to be a decrease in affinity to albumin, thus increasing the available free drug (Juchau and Faustman-Watts, 1983). An increase in the availability of free drug will increase its metab-

olism and placental transfer and mitigate the decrease in clearance by volume dilution.

The role of biotransformation of a drug or chemical is related to the levels of the enzyme systems specifically capable of drug metabolism. This is most true of slowly metabolized drugs. Pregnancy generally slows those systems. On the other hand, the rate of blood flow through the principal organs of biotransformation (liver, kidneys, adrenal glands) will determine the clearance of rapidly metabolized drugs. The increases in blood flow during pregnancy will increase the clearance of these drugs.

The disappearance of drugs from the circulating blood relates to sites of accumulation (fat), rates of biotransformation and the rate of excretion. Clearance of a drug or chemical is not equivalent to the termination of its biological effects. The drug may only induce changes in a biologic system (steroids and respiratory distress), or its metabolites may have therapeutic effects (normeperidine) or toxic effects (diphenylhydantoin). The accumulation of lipophilic drugs and increased renal excretion during pregnancy reduce the concentration of free drug. Increased biotransformation of rapidly metabolized water soluble drugs will reduce the fetal dose. However, hepatic excretion may be reduced during pregnancy. Pregnancy induces a delay in the excretion of bromsulfalein into the bile. Whether this is also true of other foreign chemicals is not known.

PLACENTA

Many different factors affect the placental transfer of chemicals to the fetus. These factors include maternal/fetal plasma concentrations, lipid solubility, maternal/fetal cardiac output, maternal/fetal blood protein concentrations, maternal/fetal drug-to-protein affinity, maternal/fetal acid-base differences, the physical characteristics of the placental/maternal interface (diffusion distance, surface area), placental blood flow, placental clearance, placental metabolism and active transport mechanisms. There are many gaps in our knowledge about these characteristics and their impact is beyond the scope of this book. However, several general observations can be made. During most of gestation, the placenta acts as a lipoidal impedence to the translocation of water soluble, foreign organic chemicals. Transfer of small lipid soluble chemicals proceeds readily by way of simple diffusion along a concentration gradient.

Larger ionized molecules are transferred less well.

The status of physical and physiologic characteristics affects placental transfer. Maternal vasoactive chemicals can change the rate of placental blood flow and thus transfer. Normal anatomic maturation of the placenta favors transfer in late gestation. The absorptive surface of the villi multiplies, and the diffusion distance decreases from 25,000 Å in the first trimester to 2,000 Å near term. There are major gaps in our knowledge about the physiology of the placenta. For example, control of placental blood flow and the role of placental clearance and metabolism must still be studied. These gaps in knowledge are illustrated by the problem of accumulation of toxic heavy metals such as cadmium and mercury in the placenta. Another question is why and how "physiologic" compounds preferentially accumulate in the fetus.

Pathologic states of the placenta, fetus and mother can affect the rate of transfer. Preeclampsia may alter uteroplacental blood flow and affect maternal serum concentrations. Placental infarcts reduce the absorption area. Villous edema increases the diffusion distance, and fetal acidosis favors the placental transfer of weak bases.

FETAL

The distribution and biotransformation of chemicals in the fetus are quite different from that in the adult or neonate. These processes are affected by decreased concentration and affinity of binding proteins, decreased metabolic activity, differences in regional blood flow and a porous blood-brain barrier. Thus, many chemicals accumulate to a higher extent in the fetal brain and adrenal gland than in maternal organs.

The biotransformation of chemicals is markedly different in the fetus. Research on fetal drug transformation is in an early stage. However, a number of observations have been made: (1) the activity of most enzyme systems involved with the biotransformation of xenobiotic chemicals is lower than in adults; (2) the developmental pattern of such enzyme systems is dependent on species, strain, substrate, specific metabolic pathway exposure to "impurities," chemicals and other factors; (3) activities increase with gestational age and environmental exposure; (4) primate fetuses appear to possess higher levels of many drug-transforming enzymes than fetuses of other species; the liver and adrenals seem to be most active in biotransformation; (5) if the fetus metabolizes a lipid soluble chemical to a water soluble toxic metabolite, the metabolite will accumulate because the lipoidal impediment of the placenta is maintained.

Fetal Drug Effects

The effect of a drug upon a fetus may be manifested by abortion, teratogenesis, carcinogenesis, growth retardation or adverse fetal physiology. The fetus may also be influenced by adverse maternal physiologic changes such as hypotension or preterm labor. These effects depend on the dose reaching the developing organism, the gestational age at the time of the exposure, the duration of exposure, the genotypes of the mother and fetus, and coexisting enviromental toxins and influences. The gestational age and duration of exposure are crucial. The most common divisions of fetal development are the fertilization period (conception to day 15 to 20), the embryonic period (day 17 to 56) and the fetal period (day 57 to birth). The neonatal period is also a critical period.

The effects of drug exposure are generally worse the earlier the exposure occurs. An isolated exposure in the fertilization period has an all (abortion) or nothing effect. Exposure in the embryonic period can have all the adverse outcomes. For example, first trimester diethylstilbestrol exposure causes teratogenic effects (adenosis and upper reproductive tract changes) and carcinogenic effects (vaginal clear cell carcinoma). Drug exposure in the fetal period can result in abnormal fetal growth or changes in fetal physiology. However, the immune and central nervous systems are still developing through the fetal and neonatal periods, and the reproductive tract is developing until 20 to 22 weeks. Drug exposure in the neonatal period results primarily in physiologic effects. The neonate is at greater risk for a drug reaction because of more free drug availability, greater cellular permeability, reduced hepatic capacity and delayed renal excretion.

The flood of lawsuits against physicians and pharmaceutical companies seriously threatens the quality of medical care in the United States. The "theoretical" relationship between drug exposure and birth defects is one major issue.

Aside from legislative reform, the best ways to prevent this legal complication are (1) public awareness, and caretaker and patient education as to the sources and reliability of data concerning birth defects; (2) precise selection of patients for drug therapy; (3) informed consent and (4) documentation.

The causes of human malformations are traditionally listed as known genetic transmission (20%), chromosomal abnormalities (5%), environmental factors (10%) and multifactorial or unknown causes (65%). Environmental factors include infections such as rubella (2 to 3%), maternal disorders such as diabetes or seizure disorder (2 to 4%) and drugs or chemicals, such as mercury and Category X drugs (4 to 5%).

A genetic component contributes to the development of multifactorial defects. Some family histories reveal a legacy of developmental defects, usually, but not necessarily, of the same organ system. When one or more environmental factors insult a conceptus of this family, there is a higher likelihood of defect. The familial risk is exposed by a family history positive for birth defects, perinatal deaths, childhood deaths and non-traumatic or non-infectious deaths in young adults or children. The risk of developmental defects increases with the frequency of defects and the percentage of shared genes (cleft palate). In some cases the sex of the proband is a factor in risk determination (pyloric stenosis). The genotypic risk or protection helps explain why even a strong teratogen such as rubella infection at 5 to 6 weeks' gestation will only affect 50 to 60% of exposed fetuses.

Data relating a drug to a birth defect are usually poor. The best information results from a prospective randomized human trial with complete long-term follow-up. The subjects must be controlled for familial risk and coexisting environmental factors. Unfortunately, this type of study has never been performed. Therefore, the relationship between new drugs and birth defects rests upon epidemiologic studies, case reports and animal studies. All these studies have their weaknesses.

Epidemiologic studies suffer from selection bias and confounding variables. Case reports may be very helpful in directing further research if the defect is rare and recurrent (i.e., limb reduction). However, when the defect is more common, such as congenital heart disease or cleft palate, statistical analysis requires accurate assessment of confounding variables and large numbers. Animal study provides great control over confounding variables. Unfortunately, animals have proved to be much different from humans in their responses to teratogens (Brown and Fabro, 1983). For example, when a known human teratogen is used in studies with rat or hamster models, the percentage of studies with a positive response (i.e., teratogenicity in that species) is 80% for rat models and 45% for hamsters. The likelihood is 97% that if all species were tested, one other species would confirm human teratogenetics. On the other hand, if different species are treated with a drug commonly felt to be a non-teratogenic in humans, rat model studies would demonstrate teratogenicity in 50% and hamster models in 35%. When all species models are used only 28% agree that a given drug is non-teratogenic.

Specific Obstetric Drugs

NUTRITIONAL SUPPLEMENTS

Iron. The iron storage of American women is notoriously poor and pregnancy demands a minimum of 800 to 900 mg of additional usable iron to meet maternal and fetal requirements. Only 10% of dietary sources and supplements of iron is absorbed in early pregnancy, although as much as 20% is absorbed in late pregnancy and in iron deficiency states. Vegetable sources and the use of antacids reduce absorption. Vitamin C (500 mg) improves absorption. The usual oral preparations are ferrous gluconate or ferrous sulfate 325 mg t.i.d. Sustained release iron preparations are sometimes used to avoid gastric irritation. However, they are transported to the duodenum and proximal jejunum where the alkalinity inhibits absorption. When anemia is severe and oral therapy is not successful, parenteral administration of iron may be necessary. The rate of hemoglobulin production is essentially the same whether iron is administered orally, intramuscularly or intravenously.

The complications of oral therapy relate to irritation of the gastrointestinal tract, including nausea, vomiting, intestinal cramps, diarrhea and constipation. Taking iron preparations with meals reduces the symptoms but also reduces absorption. Constipation is treated with an increase in dietary fiber and fluids, or occasionally by adding 100 mg of docusate sodium daily.

Intramuscular injection of iron solutions requires large bore needles, large volumes and multiple injections. The complications include pain, hematoma, sterile abscess formation and skin discoloration. Systemic allergic reaction occurs most commonly with the intravenous route and in less than 1% of cases. The allergic reaction is usually manifest within 10 minutes. A 0.5 ml test dose is recommended at the initiation of therapy. Bronchospasm and hypotension are treated with epinephrine and fluids. Local skin discoloration is limited by a Z track technique of injection.

Vitamins. In general, dietary sources and the usual therapeutic doses are safe (Category A) in pregnancy. Teratogenesis has been associated with megadoses of Vitamin A (100,000 units) and Vitamin D (50,000 units). Excess water soluble vitamins are rapidly excreted, and there is little known fetal risk.

ANTIEMETICS

Nausea and vomiting are common complaints in early pregnancy. They may be related to elevated hormonal levels, although this has not been confirmed. Other causes of persistent nausea and vomiting must be ruled out. The complications are severe dehydration and ketonuria. These complications have known fetal risks, but unfortunately, drug therapy is limited for the treatment of nausea and vomiting. Promethazine and prochlorperazine have been used, but they have the significant side-effects of phenothiazines. These include hypotension, extrapyramidal effects, dyskinesia, dry mouth, skin reaction, jaundice and blood dyscrasia. The fetal effects are unknown.

DRUGS TO INHIBIT LABOR

Beta-Sympathomimetics (Beta-Agonists). At least 100,000 pregnant women per year receive a beta-sympathomimetic agent to inhibit their premature labor. The most common drugs of this class are ritodrine hydrochloride, terbutaline and hexaprenaline; only ritodrine hydrochloride has been approved by the FDA for the treatment of premature labor. The toxicity of these agents is related to their non-specific stimulation of beta receptors in the heart, kidney and pancreas. Stimulation of cardiac beta receptors can triple the cardiac output and result in chest pain, myocardial ischemia and pulmonary edema. Stimulation of beta$_2$ receptors of the pancreas releases glucagon, which in turn stimulates gluconeogenesis, glycogenolysis

and an acute rise in the plasma glucose level. In most non-diabetics glucose concentration peaks in three hours and falls to preinfusion levels after 24 hours. The glucose level rarely rises above 200 mg/dl. Insulin levels and lactic acid levels rise and fall in response to the serum glucose (Richards et al, 1983). Beta sympathomimetics should be used with caution in patients who are diabetic. Serial glucose determinations and intravenous insulin administration for blood sugar levels greater than 200 mg/dl are recommended for these patients.

Both humans and animals experience falls in serum potassium levels between 0.6 and 1.0 mg/dl below preinfusion level. The levels correspond to insulin-mediated intracellular transport of glucose and, like the glucose levels, normalize with time. This theory is supported by a decrease in urinary potassium excretion. If the serum potassium level drops below 2.5 mg/dl, then potassium 20 mEq/l, is given. In theory, this treatment limits the potential for cardiac arrhythmias associated with hypokalemia.

Beta-receptor stimulation leads to activation of the renin-angiotension system and subsequent tubular sodium reabsorption and obligate water absorption. Through a separate mechanism the antidiuretic hormone arginine vasopressin is released. Free water is reabsorbed by the kidneys. The excess fluid and electrolyte resorption can lead to pulmonary edema especially in patients with an expanded fluid volume (patients with multiple gestations or excess fluid infusion). The risk of pulmonary edema can be decreased by limiting fluid intake to 2 l/24 hr, measuring intake and output strictly and using 5% dextrose in water in 1/4 normal saline rather than normal electrolyte solutions.

Pulmonary edema is the most common life-threatening complication of therapy with sympathomimetic agents. The incidence can be as high as 5%. The complication relates to fluid retention and excess increases in cardiac demand resulting from beta receptor stimulation. Increased pulmonary capillary permeability is not felt to play a role unless infection is present. Steroids were initially implicated in the development of pulmonary edema, but it has occurred without the use of steroids and the mineralocorticoid effects of these drugs do not contribute significantly to the fluid overload. Management includes discontinuing tocolytic therapy, administering oxygen, elevating the patient's head and giving diuretics (furosemide 20 mg intravenously).

Pregnancy, premature labor, use of beta-sympathomimetics and fluid overload combine to increase cardiac output and myocardial oxygen demands. Beta-sympathomimetics increase oxygen demand by increasing heart rate and contractility; at the same time they decrease the oxygen supply by lowering mean arterial pressure and shortening diastolic filling time. Preexisting cardiac disease severely compromises compensation and is a contraindication to beta-sympathomimetic therapy. Ten to 15% of patients on intravenous ritodrine therapy will develop chest pain and one third to one half of these will have electrocardiographic changes that are consistent with ischemia. Because of the frequency of these changes some authors advocate a pretreatment ECG (Benedetti, 1983). If ECG changes appear with chest pain, the medication is discontinued and a follow-up ECG is performed. If there are no ECG changes, the medication is discontinued until the pain disappears, and then is restarted at a much lower dosage. Recurrence of chest pain is a contraindication to continued beta-symphathomimetic therapy. Ingemarsson and Bengtsson (1985) reported much lower rates of cardiovascular side-effects with the use of intravenous terbutaline. Only 6 of 330 patients had significant cardiovascular side-effects.

Hyperthyroidism is associated with excessive sympathetic stimulation and therefore contraindicates therapy with beta-sympathomimetics. Cerebral ischemia has also been associated with the use of beta-sympathomimetic agents in a patient with migraine headaches (Rosene et al, 1982). This reaction is understandable since propanolol, a beta blocker, is useful in the management of migraine. Propranolol, 1 mg given by slow intravenous infusion, can be used as an antidote to acute beta-sympathomimetic overdose.

The fetal effects of maternal beta-sympathomimetic therapy are direct and indirect. The direct effects are the transplacental transfer of the drug. The fetal/maternal plasma ratio of ritodrine is 1.7 ± 0.48 and varies inversely with the length of time the drug was discontinued prior to delivery (Gross et al, 1985). Theoretically, beta-sympathomimetics will cause an increase in fetal cardiac output, hyperglycemia and fluid retention. These changes might limit the fetal cardiac response to stress and induce macrosomia with prolonged therapy. Fetal and neonatal tachycardia and transient neonatal hypoglycemia have been noted. The indirect adverse effects may reflect maternal abnormalities. Glucose and lactic acid can pass to the fetus. While hyperlactacidemia tends to improve with time in the mother, elevated fetal lactic acid levels persist (Bassett et al, 1985). The pathologic implication and consequences in the fetus are not understood.

Magnesium Sulphate. Magnesium sulfate ($MgSO_4$) is one of the most widely used obstetric drugs. Currently $MgSO_4$ is the therapy of choice for preeclampsia, and it is a second line tocolytic in the treatment of premature labor. Magnesium sulfate is a useful tocolytic agent in cases in which beta-sympathomimetics are contraindicated. The only absolute contraindications to $MgSO_4$ are maternal or fetal myasthenia gravis and complete heart block. Relative contraindications are impaired renal function and recent myocardial infarction. Magnesium in pharmacologic dosages has a curariform action on the neuromuscular junction, presumably interfering with the release of acetylcholine from motor nerve terminals. Neuromuscular blockade during general anesthesia or aminoglycoside therapy may potentiate this effect. Another theory is that the nerve cell membrane is changed by the replacement of calcium with magnesium, thus altering neuromuscular transmission and the excitability of the motor terminal. These theories explain the actions of $MgSO_4$ as an antiepileptic and tocolytic.

In patients with normal renal function the intravenous starting dose is 4 gm given over 10 to 15 minutes, followed by 2 gm per hour. In preterm labor the dose should be the minimum needed to halt cervical changes. Serum magnesium levels are used to adjust the dose in patients with preeclampsia and to monitor toxicity in both preeclampsia and preterm labor. The usual therapeutic level is 5.0 to 8.0 mEq/l. During the initial intravenous bolus injection the patient will feel peripheral vasodilatation as a transient flush. Too rapid an infusion will cause nausea, vomiting and hypotension. A mild sedative effect is often noted. Magnesium toxicity is monitored by serial measurements of magnesium levels and evaluation of reflexes, respiratory rate, urine output and state of consciousness. Magnesium excess is manifest by hypoactive deep tendon relfexes with a serum concentration of 8 to 10 mEq/l. Respiratory paralysis occurs when the concentration exceeds 13 to 15 mEq/l and cardiac conduction is impaired at levels greater than 15 mEq/l. Cardiac arrest can occur with concentrations greater than 25 mEq/l. The antidote is intravenous calcium gluconate or calcium chloride in a 10% solution; 10 ml (1 gm) is injected slowly.

Magnesium is freely transported to the fetus.

In term infants fetal cord magnesium levels are elevated but less than maternal levels and remain elevated for 24 to 72 hours after delivery. Cord levels in premature infants have not been studied. The neonatal effects are hypotonia and lethargy, but these are usually mild and transient.

The fetal effects of prenatal $MgSO_4$ therapy are difficult to assess. One could predict a decrease in fetal activity and perhaps a fetal heart tracing corresponding to a fetal sleep cycle. This theory is in agreement with the anecdotal clinical experience of decreased long-term variability. Stallworth and co-workers (1981) demonstrated no pathologic decrease in the short-term variability of term fetuses in the first 75 minutes after administration of $MgSO_4$.

Although used as a tocolytic in preterm labor, the effect of $MgSO_4$ on term labor remains controversial. Hall and co-workers (1959) demonstrated in vitro and in vivo inhibition of contractions by magnesium. The length of term labor was doubled in patients receiving $MgSO_4$. Zuspan and co-workers (1968) and Pritchard (1959) failed to demonstrate a decrease in uterine activity with $MgSO_4$. However, these studies represented patients at term with significant hypertensive disease. Oxytocin augmentation will correct a $MgSO_4$ induced decrease in uterine activity.

Other Tocolytic Agents. Ethanol was one of the first tocolytic agents to be used widely. Ethanol acts to block oxytocin release in the posterior pituitary and has a direct suppressive action on the myometrium through the inhibition of prostaglandins or possibly stimulation of $beta_2$ receptors. Although it is reasonably effective, prospective studies have shown it to be less effective than ritodrine or $MgSO_4$ (Lauerson et al, 1977; Steir and Petrie, 1970). In addition, the maternal and fetal effects are considerable. The maternal effects include intoxication, aspiration, hypoglycemia, lactic acidosis and diuresis with dehydration. Serum levels over 300 mg percent can lead to coma and death. The fetal effects include intoxication, lactic acidosis and neonatal depression.

The significant side-effects of beta-sympathomimetics have led to a search for safer tocolytic therapy. Prostaglandin inhibitors and calcium channel blockers are attractive options. Neither of these classes of drugs is approved for tocolytic therapy. Prostaglandin inhibitors have the side-effects of gastrointestinal bleeding, coagulopathy, allergic rashes and bone marrow depression. The neonatal effects include coagulopathy and premature closure of the ductus arteriosus.

Premature closure of the ductus has been associated with the prenatal use of indomethacin in case reports relating to term or near-term infants. Animal and human studies of neonates born at less than 34 weeks suggest that indomethacin does not cross the placenta until term and the ductus arteriosus of the immature fetus is insensitive to the effects of indomethacin (Dudley and Hardie, 1985).

Calcium channel blockers have been the focus of recent research on tocolysis. These agents have potential as tocolytic agents because of their safety, efficacy, and oral mode of therapy. Their mechanism of action relates to the disruption of intracellular calcium dynamics. In one small non-randomized study nifedipine was highly effective after failed ritodrine or $MgSO_4$ in very premature gestations (Dalton et al, 1986). However, much more research needs to be done prior to its widespread use.

FETAL THERAPY

Glucocorticoids. In the late 1960's Liggins (1969) observed increased survival in lambs injected with dexamethasone used to stimulate premature labor. The lambs seemed to have less respiratory distress. The exact mechanism of action is unknown but may be related to increased lung compliance or facilitated degranulation and release of surfactant from the lamellar bodies of Type II pneumocytes. The usual human indication is threatened preterm delivery. The benefits occur after 24 hours and within one week of the first dose. Absolute contraindications include maternal or fetal infection or studies showing mature fetal lungs. Relative contraindications include hypertensive disorders, diabetes, uteroplacental insufficiency, peptic ulcer, hyperthyroidism and premature rupture of the membranes. The most common drugs and dosages are betamethasone 12 mg I.M. Q 24 hours for 2 doses, dexamethasone 4 gm I.M. Q 8 hours for 6 doses or hydrocortisone 500 mg I.V. Q 8 hours for 4 doses. Dexamethasone and betamethasone are the best studied medications, but they require 24 hours to take effect and they have a moderately strong anti-inflammatory action. Hydrocortisone has the advantage of a more rapid effect and less of an anti-inflammatory action, but has the disadvantages of significant mineralocorticoid effects when compared with betamethasone or dexamethasone.

Multiple blinded and randomized prospective studies have shown a significant reduction in the incidence of respiratory distress, hospital costs and neonatal deaths in the treated groups (Zuspan et al, 1982; Collaborative Group on Antenatal Steroid Therapy, 1981; Johnson et al, 1981). Although animal studies have suggested a decrease in growth after exposure to steroids (Johnson et al, 1981), long-term studies in humans have not shown any changes in school or cognitive development in steroid exposed fetuses (MacArthur et al, 1982).

The complications of a short course of steroid therapy are relatively few. Intramuscular injection of steroids is uncomfortable and intravenous therapy is preferred. Dexamethasone and betamethasone have an anti-inflammatory effect for two to three days. During this period infection may be masked. White blood cell counts and fever may be unreliable markers of infection. Glucocorticoids are insulin antagonists and will result in hyperglycemia in patients with glucose intolerance. The use of glucocorticoids in diabetic patients requires frequent glucose determinations and occasionally intravenous insulin. Steroid therapy will depress adrenal secretion of glucocorticoids in the mother and fetus, but does not hinder glucocorticoid responses to stress.

RhoGAM. The efficacy of RhoGAM in the prevention of rhesus isoimmunization has been clear and dramatic. The incidence of isoimmunization has fallen fourfold in the United States since the late 1960's. The mechanism of action involves the administration of pooled gamma globulin directed against the D antigen on fetal red cells circulating in the maternal blood. This allows removal of the antigen prior to maternal sensitization.

In the United States the immune globulin is prepared by the Cohn cold ethanol fractionization method from the pooled raw plasma from at least 20 different human donors. Although immune globulins cannot be pasteurized, infectious diseases such as hepatitis or autoimmune deficiency syndrome have not been reported following its administration. The standard dose is 300 micrograms given intramuscularly prior to the third postpartum day in non-sensitized Rhesus negative women. This dose will control a 30 ml fetal to maternal transfusion. A larger transfusion, determined by a Kleihauer-Betke test, will require additional doses. After first trimester loss (abortion or ectopic pregnancy) a 50 microgram dose is sufficient.

Despite the controversy surrounding routine antepartum prophylaxis (Tovey, 1980; Nusbacher and Bove, 1980; Hensleigh, 1983), the American College of Obstetricians and Gynecologists (Technical Bulletin No. 79) now recommends that 300 micrograms of RhoGAM be given at 28 weeks to all eligible women. Antepartum prophylaxis is indicated in cases in which the pregnancy has been complicated by amniocentesis, external version, fetoscopy or uterine bleeding. However, the following concerns remain about the antepartum use of RhoGAM:

1. The fetal risks are undefined; RhoGAM may induce anemia or the pooled gamma globulin may have an impact on the developing immune system.

2. The economic costs and medical risks of plasmaphoresis in the donors.

3. The potential for epidemic spread of hepatitis or autoimmune deficiency syndrome from the pooled gamma globulin.

4. The development of better techniques for diagnosis of fetal-maternal transfusion and improved identification of patients at risk will reduce the need and subsequently the cost effectiveness of the therapy.

UTERINE STIMULANTS

Oxytocin. Oxytocin is an octapeptide hormone that is synthesized in the supraoptic and paraventricular nuclei of the hypothalmus. Oxytocin is transported to the posterior pituitary gland by carrier proteins where it is released. Oxytocin is an essential hormone closely associated with the reproductive acts of coitus, labor and lactation. Oxytocin stimulates myometrial contractions by binding with myometrial membrane receptors. Ultimately, through a prostaglandin-mediated action, intracellular calcium is increased and muscle excitation occurs. Uterine sensitivity to oxytocin stimulation increases during gestation in response to increased receptor sites stimulated by sex steroid levels.

The three major indications for oxytocin use are augmentation of labor, control of postpartum bleeding and improvement of the let-down (ejection) reflex during lactation. In the presence of a live fetus the dosage of intravenous oxytocin should be monitored by means of an electronic or mechanical pump. Adequate labor usually occurs with dosages between 4 and 8 milliunits/min. Intramuscular injection, intravenous bolus, hand controlled infusion and buccal or nasal administration are to be strongly discouraged as the dosage cannot be adequately controlled (see Chapter 11). When oxytocin is used to control bleeding or improve lactation any route of therapy except oral is effective.

The complications of oxytocin are easily predicted. During induction or augmentation of labor, overdosage is reflected by uterine hyperstimulation and increasing uterine tone (greater than 15 mmHg). The results are uteroplacental perfusion defects and fetal hypoxia. In extreme cases of hyperstimulation or in the presence of structural abnormalities of the pelvis or fetus uterine rupture is a risk. Hyperstimulation can be treated with an intravenous bolus of ritodrine (3 to 6 mg) or terbutaline (0.25 mg) (Caritis et al, 1985; Lipshitz and Klose, 1985), oxygen administration of 4 to 6 liters/min by mask and position change.

The pharmacologic side-effects involve the cardiovascular system and fluid retention. A bolus injection of one or more units of oxytocin can initiate premature ventricular contractions, and direct peripheral dilatation may cause hypotension. This side-effect may be more pronounced if associated with general anesthesia (Hendricks and Brenner, 1970). The adverse cardiovascular symptoms are short-lived once the oxytocin infusion is stopped, as the half-life of oxytocin is 4 to 8 minutes. Free water retention can be a problem with the infusion of high concentrations of oxytocin. Natural and synthetic oxytocin are structurally similar to antidiuretic hormone (ADH). At infusion rates above 20 milliunits/min urine output begins to decrease. If excessive fluid is already present, for example in multiple gestations or in patients undergoing beta-agonist therapy, and 20 units are run in rapidly as prophylaxis for postpartum bleeding, there is potential for fluid overload, hyponatremia, and subsequent convulsions (Abdul-Karin and Assali, 1961). Hypoglycemia and rising triglyceride levels are also associated with prolonged oxytocin use (Burt et al, 1983).

The fetal effects of oxytocin are primarily indirect since oxytocin does not cross the placenta. Iatrogenic prematurity can be caused by non-judicious selection of patients for elective induction. Hyperstimulation leads to acute uteroplacental insufficiency and precipitous delivery; neonatal depression, trauma and hyperbilirubinemia can result (D'Souza et al, 1979).

Ergot Alkaloids. Ergot alkaloids are vasospastic chemicals derived from the fungus *Claviceps purpura*. Vasoconstriction occurs as a result of non-reversible tetanic stimulation of smooth muscle. The uterus is uniquely sensitive. The pattern of contraction is primarily hypertonicity. However, at term, hypercontractility is also noted. This hypercontractility and the irreversible nature of the smooth muscle stimulation directly contraindicate the use of ergot derivatives for any purpose prior to delivery. The vasoconstrictive properties also contraindicate the use of ergot derivatives in patients in whom hypertension, coronary artery disease or peripheral vascular disease (Raynaud's disease) is present. Otherwise, ergot derivatives are very useful for controlling postpartum hemorrhage. The two ergot derivatives most commonly used are ergonovine maleate (Ergotrate) and methylergonovine maleate (Methergine). The usual dosage is 0.2 mg I.M. or P.O. Intravenous doses (0.1 mg) should be reserved for life-threatening situations. The onset of action is about 40 seconds with intravenous infusion and 7 minutes with intramuscular injection.

Ergonovine and methylergonovine have been manufactured to reduce the vasoconstrictive properties. However, even this weak property is utilized in provocative testing for coronary arterial spasms (Fester, 1980). Acute hypertensive episodes and myocardial infarction have been reported with use of these drugs (Taylor and Cohen, 1985). Acute chest pain after treatment with ergot derivatives should be treated promptly with nitroglycerine (0.2 mg) or nifedipine (10 mg sublingually).

Prostaglandins. Prostaglandins are critically important in the intracellular and intercellular function of most organ systems. Their discovery and and the identification of their function have generated extensive research in most branches of medicine. In obstetrics and gynecology prostaglandins E_2 and F_2 alpha are used for pregnancy termination, cervical ripening and control of postpartum hemorrhage. Their use derives from their unique ability to stimulate rhythmic uterine contractions and to aid in the biochemical maturation of the cervical matrix. Their efficacy suggests that they play an integral role in the onset and progression of normal and abnormal labor. This effect is quite local in character, i.e., cervical maturation. Contraindications to prostaglandin use include hypersensitivity, prior classic uterine scar, unfavorable fetal lie, pelvic inflammatory disease and placenta previa. Caution should be exercised in patients with a prior low transverse uterine scar, asthma, seizure disorder, cardiovascular disease, peptic ulcer disease, renal disease and hypertension.

When prostaglandins are given systemically, widespread effects on many organ systems are seen because of the ubiquitous nature of these drugs. Table 13–9 depicts the common side-effects of prostaglandin E_2 and F_2 alpha. Most

*Table 13–9. Adverse Reactions to Prostaglandins**

Adverse Reaction	Prostaglandin $F_2\alpha$	Prostaglandin E_2
Nausea	25	33
Vomiting	50	67
Diarrhea	20	40
Temperature rise ($> 1.1°$ C)	3	50
Headache	3	10
Hypotension (> 20 mmHg)	3	10
Shivering	3	3
Bronchospasm	3	3
Bradycardia	3	3

*From Russ JS, Rayburn WF, Samuel MJ: Uterine stimulants. In Rayburn WF, Zuspan FP (Eds.): *Drug Therapy in Obstetrics and Gynecology*, Ed. 2. Norwalk, Conn., Appleton-Century-Crofts, 1986. Reprinted with permission.

patients will have at least one of these effects. In second trimester terminations the additional instillation of urea (40 mg) or hypertonic saline can reduce the dosage of prostaglandin needed and decrease the likelihood of delivery of a living infant. One half hour prior to the elective use of prostaglandins, the patient should be medicated to reduce the likelihood of adverse reactions. The medication should include a antinauseant (prochlorperazine, 10 mg I.M.), an antidiarrheal agent (Lomotil, 10 mg P.O.), a narcotic (meperidine, 50 to 100 mg I.M.) and an antipyretic (acetaminophen, 325 mg rectal suppository). Potentially life-threatening complications include amniotic fluid embolism and uterine rupture. These are more common with concomitant use of oxytocin, prior uterine surgery, transverse lie and uterine distention (twins, polyhydramnios and uterine size greater than 28 cm). Hyperstimulation is treated with an intravenous dose of a beta-sympathomimetic agent.

PERIPARTUM PAIN: ANESTHESIA AND ANALGESIA

Few subjects have caused as much controversy as pain relief during labor. All too often the argument places the neonatologist against the obstetrician, the obstetrician against the anesthesiologist, and the lawyers and consumer advocates against the physicians. Unfortunately, the mother and fetus often get caught in the middle. Despite the statements by any one adversarial group, there are a number of realities about labor and pain.

Labor is painful. Lack of knowledge, fear and anxiety increase the discomfort. Education with the subsequent reduction in fear and anxiety is not just the responsibility of the childbirth educator. The physician or certified midwife is in a unique position to supply superior educational and psychologic care. Analgesia and anesthesia can be avoided or lessened by this support.

Pain, fear and anxiety have an adverse effect on maternal and fetal physiology. Uterine blood flow (Shnider and Wright, 1979) and progression of labor (Newton et al, 1966; Ledermann et al, 1985) are adversely affected by pain. These adverse effects have the potential of causing fetal acidosis.

All analgesics can have a direct adverse effect on the mother. Narcotic side-effects are those of sedation and allergy. Phenothiazines (Phenergan, Largon) and hydroxyine (Vistaril) are sometimes used to potentiate the narcotic agents. The adverse reactions of phenothiazines include lowered seizure threshold, extrapyramidal effects, direct depression of the myocardium and adrenergic blockage. Severe hypotension is treated with left side positioning, fluid bolus and ephedrine (10 to 20 mg I.V.).

All analgesics cross the placenta and can significantly depress the neonate at birth and change neurobehavior for two to three days. In some cases the metabolite is the culprit, e.g., normeperidine. The peak fetal effect occurs usually less than one and a half to two hours after an intramuscular dose. The treatment of choice is the narcotic antagonist, naloxone. Naloxone (0.4 mg I.V.) can be given to the mother 10 to 15 minutes prior to birth or as an immediate neonatal dose (0.01 mg/Kg I.V.).

Most pregnant women and fetuses are exposed to local anesthestics during delivery. Significant levels in the fetus have been reported after perineal infiltration for episiotomy (Phillipson et al, 1984) and after paracervical (Petrie et al, 1974) or conduction anesthesia (Ralston and Shnider, 1978). Phillipson and co-workers (1984) reviewed lidocaine pharmacodynamics after local infiltration of the perineum. Peak maternal concentrations occurred within 3 to 12 minutes with rapid transfer to the fetus. The mean neonatal/maternal ratio was 1.32 and reflects the effect of acid-base differences between the mother and fetus. Lidocaine accumulation will be higher with fetal acidosis.

The adverse reactions of local anesthetics are either direct or indirect. Corke and Spielman (1985) have reviewed the acute (direct) maternal toxicity of conduction anesthesia. Permanent neurologic damage has been reported as the result of subarachnoid block or venous infiltration. The adverse effects on the neonate have been reviewed by many authors. Scanlon (1981) provides a bibliography and cautions about the methodologic deficiencies of most studies. In general, investigations are weakened by observer subjectivity, sample size, confounding variables and data analysis. However, most studies have demonstrated neurobehavioral changes related to local anesthestic that last for several days after birth.

An acute overdose of a local anesthetic can be a crisis of life-threatening proportions. The maximum dosage and duration of action depend on the chemical and its metabolism. Anesthetics in the ester class are procaine, chloroprocaine and tetracaine. These agents are rapidly metabolized by plasma pseudocholinesterases. The amide anesthestics, lidocaine, mepivacaine and bupivacaine, are metabolized more slowly by the liver. The maximum doses are 1,000 mg for procaine and chloroprocaine and 500 mg for lidocaine. Tetracaine and bupivacaine are longer acting and have maximum doses of 200 and 300 mg, respectively. These drugs are eight times more potent than procaine. The signs of overdose rapidly progress from tinnitus, drowsiness, or slurred speech to convulsions or cardiopulmonary arrest. Tinnitus after the injection of local anesthetic should be a clear warning.

Convulsions should be treated aggressively to prevent asphyxia. Oxygen, under positive pressure, is administered promptly. Muscular activity should be controlled with 0.8 mg/kg succinylcholine. Cerebral cortex seizure activity is controlled with 50 to 100 mg of thiopental. Endotracheal intubation is performed with a cuffed tube to maintain adequate ventilation. The respiratory acidosis that accompanies seizure activity further exacerbates the toxic myocardial depression. Hypotension is treated with fluids and vasopressors (dopamine).

The indirect consequences of obstetric anesthesia and analgesia are more difficult to prove. Those most discussed are slow progress in labor, neonatal depression and disruption of mother-infant bonding (see Chapter 11). No randomized studies have been performed to compare epidural anesthesia versus no epidural anesthesia on the progress of labor. Clinical anesthesiologists agree that a properly administered epidural given to a properly selected patient will not delay labor. Unfortunately, in clinical practice, labor is delayed. A study by Studd and Crawford (1980) is probably representative of those examining this issue. The labors of 282 patients with epidural anesthesia were compared to those of 1,673 patients without epidurals. In this study the use of epidurals seemed to increase the duration of the first and second stages and increase the incidence of forceps rotation. The incidence of cesarean section was not increased.

Datta and Ostheimer (1981) studied the neonatal effect of prolonged induction for elective repeat cesarean section. All patients had prehydration and patients experiencing hypotension with the spinal block were eliminated. In the remaining patients general and spinal anesthesia were examined, using low Apgar scores and low umbilical artery pHs as criteria. During general anesthesia, induction to delivery time greater than eight minutes and a uterine incision time greater than three minutes were associated with significantly more low one minute Apgar scores (less than 7) than faster times (73% versus 4%). Slow induction and uterine incision times were also associated with lower umbilical artery pHs (7.22 vs. 7.31). In groups receiving spinal anesthesia prolongation of the uterine incision to delivery time greater than three minutes was found to be the only important factor influencing fetal outcome as determined by increased acidosis (pH 7.18 vs. 7.30) and by depressed Apgar scores (62% versus 0%).

LACTATION

Physiology of Lactation. During pregnancy estrogen stimulates the maturation and preparation of the mammary ductal system and progesterone supports alveolar growth and function. Despite the high levels of prolactin, milk production is absent, except for a small amount of colostrum. Estrogen and progesterone are felt to block the local effect of prolactin on milk production. After parturition estrogens and progesterone levels fall precipitously and prolactin begins to effect milk production. Breast engorgement and milk secretion occur on the second to the fourth postpartum day. Engorgement is a painful but self-limiting process that lasts 48 to 72 hours and is manifested by swollen, firm, tender breasts. Early breastfeeding and relaxed, demand feeding schedules reduce or eliminate the symptoms. If breastfeeding is not selected, engorgement, breast pain and excessive lactation occur in about 35%, 25% and 20% of patients, respectively.

Lactation is a complex process involving continued tactile stimulation and hormonal support. The reader is referred to Lawrence (1984) for more details. From the point of view of drug therapy during lactation the following points are important.

1. Human milk is an emulsion of lipid and protein-rich fluid. It has 3.8 grams/dl of fat and has a pH around 7.1, with a range of 6.7 to 7.4. These characteristics favor the transfer of lipid soluble drugs and weak bases.

2. The volume varies with the frequency of feeding and the intensity of the stimulation. The stimulation of one breast by a five-week-old infant produced 80 ml of breast milk from the opposite breast in 20 minutes of stimulation (Hall, 1975). Although a large volume is released at the time of the feeding, some is produced and stored in the ducts between feedings. The amount of lipids tends to increase during a feeding while the protein content remains the same.

3. The alveolar epithelium represents a lipid barrier with water-filled pores and is most permeable to drugs during the colostral phase of milk production.

4. Drugs have less affinity to milk proteins than to plasma proteins.

5. Water soluble drugs of a molecular weight below 200 pass through membranal pores into the milk.

6. The metabolic capacity of the alveolar or ductal epithelium is unknown.

7. The amount of drug available per feed is the amount of unbound drug present in the maternal blood that can pass through the alveolar epithelium during a feed. For example, if we make the assumptions that the free drug is completely extracted by the mammary epithelium, the concentration of free drug in the maternal blood is 1 microgram/dl, the mammary blood flow is 500 ml/minute and the feeding time is 10 minutes, the calculated neonatal dose is a maximum of 500 micrograms. In general this translates to a neonatal dose much less than 1% of the maternal dose.

Lactation Suppression. Although uncomfortable, breast engorgement is not life-threatening. Thus, the drugs used for lactation suppression must be virtually free of side-effects. Suppressant drugs must be given prior to prolactin induction of the alveolar epithelium. If a suppressant drug is given at the time of engorgement, improvement is a reflection of the natural resolution of the process rather than a drug effect. Lactation suppressants are of two types: sex hormones (estrogen analogs or a combination of estrogen and testosterone) or bromocriptine mesylate. Sex steroids block pro-

lactin induction of alveolar epithelium; whereas, bromocriptine inhibits prolactin secretion by stimulating dopamine release in the hypothalamus. Both classes of drugs have been shown to be efficacious in reducing severe symptoms of breast engorgement to less than 5% (Nilsen et al, 1976).

Epidemiologic studies of puerperal thromboembolism have implicated hormonal lactational suppressants as well as advanced maternal age (over 35) and cesarean section as risk factors (Turnbull, 1968; Tindal, 1968; Jeffcoate et al, 1968; Nilsen et al, 1975). There is an increase from a baseline of one or two cases of thromboembolism per 1,000 deliveries of lactating mothers to 6 to 10 thromboembolic events per 1,000 deliveries in those treated with estrogens for lactational suppression. Given the benign character of breast engorgement, hormones should only be used selectively.

Bromocriptine is an ergot derivative with potent dopamine agonist activity. Prolactin levels are significantly reduced and lactation is suppressed. The usual postpartum dose is one tablet (2.5 mg) twice a day for 14 days. After therapy 18 to 40% of patients will have rebound breast engorgement. Rebound breast engorgement is treated with an additional seven days of therapy. Unfortunately, bromocriptine has a high frequency of side-effects. Twenty-eight percent of patients given the recommended lactational suppressant dosages have at least one episode of orthostatic hypotension. Twenty-three percent of patients have one or more of the following symptoms: headache, dizziness, nausea, vomiting or syncope. These side effects are reduced by halving the dose for the first day and introducing a 1.5 mg dose at night before sleep. Patient selection may reduce the frequency of side-effects. Bromocriptine should be used with caution in patients with anemia or hypertensive disease and in those taking large doses of parenteral narcotics, recovering from prolonged bedrest or who have a history of syncopal episodes.

Specific Drugs in Breast Milk. The pharmacokinetics of individual drugs in breast milk is beyond the scope of this book. The reader is referred to Lawrence (1984) as a reference source for the specific drugs. All drugs will appear in breast milk to some degree although most often in very small amounts. Most drugs have not been studied in this regard, and the care provider must rely on a derived judgment of safety. Breastfeeding has many physical and psychologic benefits; rarely should breastfeeding be discontinued so that the mother can take the medication. The answers to a series of questions help the care provider define the risks of an unknown drug.

1. Is the agent absorbable to any extent by the gastrointestinal tract?

2. The neonatal liver has a decreased ability to detoxify foreign chemicals or bilirubin if it is displaced by the chemical (e.g., sulfa drugs). Does the drug displace bilirubin? Does the drug require the liver for metabolism?

3. How old is the infant? If the neonate is less than a month old or is premature, its ability to detoxify drugs is decreased. Age is also important in that the older child will drink more milk. On the other hand, the diet of an older child becomes less dependent on human milk.

4. Is the drug fat soluble?

5. Is this a drug that can be given to the infant if necessary? What are the pediatric precautions associated with the use of the drug in infants?

6. Is there a risk of drug sensitization even with the small amount that may be present in milk?

7. Is the drug used in pregnancy? A drug that is safe in pregnancy may not be safe in lactation. On the other hand, if the drug has a significant fetal risk, there is often a neonatal risk as well.

8. Are there laboratory tests with which to follow the neonate for toxicity? For example, prothrombin time is tested when the mother is taking warfarin.

9. Are there alternatives for maternal therapy so that drugs are not needed or another better known drug can be used?

10. Are there any nutritional effects of the drug?

11. Does the drug have an active metabolite?

If a mother needs a specific medication and the hazards to the infant are minimal, the following adjustments can be used to reduce the exposure.

1. Avoid using long-acting forms of the drug. Usually these drugs are detoxified by the liver or are extensively bound to protein.

2. Schedule doses so that the least amount of drug gets into the milk. Determining the rate of absorption and the peak of maternal serum concentrations is helpful in scheduling. Usually, it is best for the mother to take the medication immediately after a feeding.

3. Evaluate the infant frequently. Note behavior changes.

4. When possible, choose the drug that has the lowest milk/plasma ratio.

REFERENCES

Abdul-Karin R, Assali NS: Effects of oxytocin on renal hemodynamics and water and electrolyte excretion. *J. Lab. Clin. Med.* 57:522, 1961.

Alexander J, Dainiak N et al: Serial assessment of doxorubicin cardiotoxicity with quantitative radionuclide angiocardiography. *New Engl. J. Med.* 300:278, 1979.

AMA Council on Scientific Affairs: Guidelines for handling parenteral antineoplastics. *J. Am. Med. Assoc.* 263:1590, 1985.

Andrieu JM, Ochoa-Molina ME: Menstrual cycle, pregnancies and offspring before and after MOPP therapy for Hodgkin's disease. *Cancer* 52:435, 1983.

Appel GB, Neu HC: The nephroxicity of antimicrobial agents. *N. Eng. J. Med.* 296:722, 1977.

Ashraf M, Scotchel PL et al: Cis-platinum-induced hypomagnesemia and peripheral neuropathy. *Gynecol. Oncol.* 16:309, 1983.

Barach EM, Nowak RM et al: Epinephrine for treatment of anaphylactic shock. *J. Am. Med. Assoc.* 251:2118, 1984.

Barbieri RL, Evans S, Kistner RW: Danazol in the treatment of endometriosis: analysis of 100 cases with a 4-year follow-up. *Fertil. Steril.* 37:737, 1982.

Barrett AP: Oral mucosal complications in cancer chemotherapy. *Aust. N. Z. J. Med.* 14:7, 1984.

Bassett JM, Burks AH et al: Maternal and fetal metabolic effects of prolonged ritodrine infusion. *Obstet. Gynecol.* 66:755, 1985.

Bateman DN, Rawlins MD, Simpson JM: Extrapyramidal reactions with metoclopramide. *Br. Med. J.* 291:930, 1985.

Beller FK, Ebert C: Effects of oral contraceptives on blood coagulation: a review. *Obstet. Gynecol. Surv.* 40:425, 1985.

Benedetti TJ: Maternal complications of parenteral beta-sympathomimetic therapy for premature labor. *Am. J. Obstet. Gynecol.* 145:1, 1983.

Berkowitz RL, Coustan DR, Mochizuki TK: *Handbook for Prescribing Medications During Pregnancy.* Boston, Little Brown and Company, 1981.

Briggs GG, Bodendorfer TW: *Drugs in Pregnancy and Lactation: A Reference Guide to Fetal and Neonatal Risk,* Ed. 2. Baltimore, Williams and Wilkins Co., 1986.

Brocklebank J, Ray WA et al: Drug prescribing during pregnancy. *Obstet. Gynecol.* 132:235, 1978.

Brown NA, Fabro S: The value of animal teratogenicity testing for predicting human risk. *Clin. Obstet. Gynecol.* 26:467, 1983.

Burt RL, Leake NH, Dannenburg WN: Effect of synthetic oxytocin on plasma non-esterfied fatty acids, triglycerides and blood glucose. *Obstet. Gynecol.* 21:708, 1963.

Buttram VC Jr, Belue JB, Reiter R: Interim report of a study of danazol for the treatment of endometriosis. *Fertil. Steril.* 37:478, 1982.

Caritis SN, Lin LS, Wong LK: Evaluation of the phamacodynamics and pharmacokinetics of ritodrine when adminstered as a loading dose. *Am. J. Obstet. Gynecol.* 152:1026, 1985.

Carl W: Oral complications in cancer patients *Am. Fam. Physician.* 27:161, 1983.

Charles D: The use of metronidazole in Ob-Gyn infections. *Infect. Surg.* 3:769, 1984.

Chetkowski RJ, Meldium DR et al: Biologic effects of transdermal estrogen. *N. Engl. J. Med.* 314:1615, 1986.

Choo YC, Chan SYW et al: Ovarian dysfunction in patients

with gestational trophoblastic neoplasia treated with short intensive courses of Etoposide (VP-16-213). *Cancer* 55:2348, 1985.

Collaborative Group of Antenatal Steroid Therapy: Effects of antenatal dexamethasone administration in the prevention of respiratory distress syndrome. *Am. J. Obstet. Gynecol.* 141:276, 1981.

Corke BC, Spielman FJ: Problems associated with epidural anesthesia in obstetrics. *Obstet. Gynecol.* 65:837, 1985.

Cuellar FG: Bromocriptine mesylate (Parlodel) in the management of amenorrhea/galactorrhea associated with hyperprolactinemia. *Obstet. Gynecol.* 55:278, 1980.

Dalton ME, Jillson AE et al: Treatment of premature labor with the calcium antagonist nifedipine: a preliminary report. Personal communication.

Damewood MD, Grochow LB: Prospects for fertility after chemotherapy or radiation for neoplastic disease. *Fertil. Steril.* 45:443, 1986.

Datta S, Ostheimer GW: Neonatal effect of prolonged anesthetic induction for cesarean section. *Obstet. Gynecol.* 58:331, 1981.

Doering PL, Stewart RB: The extent and character of drug consumption during pregnancy. *J. Am. Med. Assoc.* 239:843, 1978.

Douglas JM, Critchlow C et al: A double-blind study of oral acyclovir for suppression of recurrences of genital herpes simplex virus infection. *N. Engl. J. Med.* 310:1551, 1984.

Druck MN, Gulenchyn KY et al: Radionuclide angiography and endomyocardial biopsy in the assessment of doxorubicin cardiotoxicity. *Cancer* 53:1667, 1984.

D'Souza SN, Black P et al: The effect of oxytocin in induced labor and neonatal jaundice. *Br. J. Obstet. Gynaecol.* 86:733, 1979.

Dudley DKL, Hardie MJ: Fetal and neonatal effects of indomethacin used as a tocolytic agent. *Am. J. Obstet. Gynecol.* 151:181, 1985.

Dunagin WG: Dermatologic toxicity. In Perry MC, Yarbro JW (Eds.) *Toxicity of Chemotherapy*. Orlando, Grune & Stratton, 1984.

Fekety R: Current approach to the treatment of antibiotic-associated diarrhea. *Infect. Surg.* 1:13, 1982.

Fester A: Provocative testing for coronary artery spasm with ergonovine maleate. *Am. J. Cardiol.* 46:338, 1980.

Francke E, Neu HC: Nephrotoxicity of aminoglycosides. *Infect. Surg.* 2:205, 1983.

Gala KV, Griffin TW: Hepatomas in young women on oral contraceptives: report of two cases and review of the literature. *J. Surg. Oncol.* 22:11, 1983.

Gambrell RD Jr: The menopause: benefits and risks of estrogen-progesterone replacement therapy. *Fertil. Steril.* 37:457, 1982.

Gambrell RD Jr, Bernard DM et al: Changes in sexual drives of patients on oral contraceptives. *J. Reprod. Med.* 17:165, 1976.

Geraci JE, Hermans PE: Symposium on antibiotics. Part II: vancomycin. *Mayo Clin. Proc.* 58:88, 1983.

Goldzieher JW, Moses LE et al: Nervousness and depression attributed to oral contraceptives: a double-blind placebo-controlled study. *Am. J. Obstet. Gynecol.* 111:1013, 1971.

Greenberg ER, Barnes AB et al: Breast cancer in mothers given diethylstilbesterol in pregnancy. *N. Engl. J. Med.* 311:1393, 1984.

Gross TL, Kuhnert BR et al: Maternal and fetal plasma concentrations of ritodrine. *Obstet. Gynecol.* 65:793, 1985.

Guillebaud J: Surgery and the pill. *Br. Med. J.* 291:498, 1985.

Hall B: Changing composition of human milk and the development of an appetite control. *Lancet* 1:779, 1975.

Hall DG, McGaughey HS et al: The effects of magnesium therapy on the duration of labor. *Am. J. Obstet. Gynecol.* 78:27, 1959.

Hammond CB, Jelovsek FR et al: Effects of long term estrogen therapy. *Am. J. Obstet. Gynecol.* 135:525, 1979.

Harwood KV, Aisner J: Treatment of chemotherapy extravasation: current status. *Cancer Treat. Rep.* 68:939, 1984.

Haspels AA, Andriesse R: The effect of large doses of estrogen post coitum in 2000 women. *Europ. J. Obstet. Gynecol. Reprod. Biol.* 3:113, 1973.

Hendricks CH, Brenner WE: Cardiovascular effects of oxytocic drugs used postpartum. *Am. J. Obstet. Gynecol.* 108:5, 1970.

Hensleigh, PA: Preventing rhesus isoimmunization: antepartum Rh immune globulin prophylaxis versus a sensitive test for risk identification. *Am. J. Obstet. Gynecol.* 146:749, 1983.

Herbst AL, Bern HA (Eds.) *Developmental Effects of Diethylstilbesterol (DES) in Pregnancy*. New York, Thieme-Stratton, 1981.

Hertz R, Lewis J Jr, Lipsett MB: Five years experience with the chemotherapy of metastatic choriocarcinoma and related trophoblastic tumors in women. *Am. J. Obstet. Gynecol.* 82:631, 1961.

Honore LH: Increased incidence of symptomatic cholesterol cholelithiasis in perimenopausal women receiving estrogen replacement therapy. *J. Reprod. Med.* 25:187, 1980.

Horwitz RI, Feinstein AR: Intravaginal estrogen creams and endometrial cancer; no causal association found. *J. Am. Med. Assoc.* 241:1266, 1979.

Ignoffo RJ, Friedman MA: Treatment of local toxicities caused by extravasation of cancer chemotherapeutic drugs. *Cancer Treat. Rep.* 7:17, 1980.

Ingemarsson I, Arulkumaran S, Ratnam SS: Single injection of terbutaline in term labor. 1. Effect on fetal pH in cases with prolonged bradycardia *Am. J. Obstet. Gynecol.* 153:859, 1985.

Ingemarsson I, Bengtsson B: A five year experience with terbutaline for preterm labor: low rate of severe side effects. *Obstet. Gynecol.* 66:176, 1985.

Jaffe W, Takane Y: Transient neurologic disturbances induced by high-dose methotrexate treatment. *Cancer* 56:1356, 1985.

Jeffcoate TNA, Miller J et al: Puerperal thromboembolism in relation to the inhibition of lactation of estrogen therapy. *Br. Med. J.* 4:19, 1968.

Johnson DE, Munson OP, Thompson TR: Effect of antenatal administration of betamethasone on hospital costs and survival of premature infants. *Pediatrics* 68:633, 1981.

Johnson JW, Mitzner W et al: Long-term effects of betamethasone on fetal development. *Am. J. Obstet. Gynecol.* 141:1053, 1981.

Juchau MR, Faustman-Watts E: Pharmacokinetic considerations in the maternal-placental-fetal unit. *Clin. Obstet. Gynecol.* 26:379, 1983.

Kasan PN, Andrews J: The effect of recent oral contraceptive use on the outcome of pregnancy. *Eur. J. Obstet. Gynecol. Reprod. Biol.* 22:77, 1986.

Kaufman DW, Miller DR et al: Noncontraceptive estrogen use and the risk of breast cancer. *J. Am. Med. Assoc.* 252:63, 1984.

Kay CR: Progestogens and arterial disease—evidence from

the Royal College of General Practitioners study. *Am. J. Obstet. Gynecol.* 142:762, 1982.

Kay CR: The Royal College of General Practitioners oral contraception study: some recent observations. *Clin. Obstet. Gynecol.* 11:759, 1984.

Kris MG, Gralla RJ et al: Improved control of cisplatin-induced emesis with high-dose metoclopramide and with combination of metoclopramide, dexamethasone, and diphenhydramine: results of consecutive trials in 255 patients. *Cancer* 55:527, 1985a.

Kris MG, Gralla RJ et al: Incidence, course, and severity of delayed nausea and vomiting following the administration of high-dose cisplatin. *J. Clin. Oncol.* 3:1379, 1985b.

Larson DL: Treatment of tissue extravasation by antitumor agents. *Cancer* 49:1796, 1982.

Lauersen NH, Merkatz IR et al: Inhibition of premature labor: a multicenter comparison of ritodrine and ethanol. *Am. J. Obstet. Gynecol.* 127:837, 1977.

Lawrence RA: *Breast Feeding: A Guide for the Medical Profession,* Ed. 2. St. Louis, C. V. Mosby Company, 1984.

Ledermann RP, Ledermann E et al: Anxiety and epinephrine in multiparous women in labor: relation to duration of labor and fetal heart rate pattern. *Am. J. Obstet. Gynecol.* 153:870, 1985.

Levitz RE, Mendelson LM: Managing patients with a history of penicillin allergy. *Infect. Surg.* 1:18, 1982.

Liggins GC: Premature delivery of fetal lambs infused with glucocorticoids. *J. Endocrinol.* 45:515, 1969.

Lipnick RJ, Buring JE et al: Oral contraceptives and breast cancer. *J. Am. Med. Assoc.* 255:58, 1986.

Lipshitz J, Klose CW: Use of tocolytic drugs to reverse oxytocin induced uterine hypertonus and fetal distress. *Obstet. Gynecol.* 66:165, 1985.

Lurain JR: Chemotherapy of gestational trophoblastic disease. In Deppe G (Ed.): *Chemotherapy of Gynecologic Cancer,* New York, Alan R. Liss, 1984.

Lyle KC: Female breast cancer: distribution, risk factors and effect of steroid contraception. *Obstet. Gynecol. Surv.* 35:413, 1980.

MacArthur BA, Howie RN et al: School progress and cognitive development of 6-year old children whose mothers were treated antenatally with betamethasone. *Pediatrics* 70:99, 1982.

Markman M, Cleary S et al: Intraperitoneal chemotherapy with high-dose cisplatin and cytosine arabinoside for refractory ovarian carcinoma and other malignancies principally involving the peritoneal cavity. *J. Clin. Oncol.* 3:925, 1985.

Mattia MA, Blake SL: Hospital hazards: cancer drugs. *Am. J. Nurs.* 83:759, 1983.

Meyer-Bahlburg HFL, Erhardt AA et al: Sexual activity level and sexual functioning in women prenatally exposed to diethylstilbesterol. *Psychosomat. Med.* 47:497, 1985.

Middleton J, Franks D et al: Failure of scalp hypothermia to prevent hair loss when cyclophosphamide is added to doxorubicin and vincristine. *Cancer Treat. Rep.* 69:130, 1985.

Miller SE: Effect of oral contraceptives on tryptophane and tyrosine availability: evidence for a possible contribution to mental depression. *Neuropsychobiol.* 7:192, 1981.

Morris NM, Udry JR: Depression of physical activity by contraceptive pills. *Am. J. Obstet. Gynecol.* 104:1012, 1969.

Morrow GR, Morrell C: Behavioral treatment for the anticipatory nausea and vomiting induced by cancer chemotherapy. *N. Engl. J. Med.* 307:1476, 1982.

Newton N, Foshee D, Newton M: Experimental inhibition of labor through environmental disturbance. *Obstet. Gynecol.* 27:371, 1966.

Nicosia SV, Matus-Ridley M, Meadows AT: Gonadal effects of cancer therapy in girls. *Cancer* 55:2364, 1985.

Nilsen PA, Meling AB, Abildgaard U: Study of the suppression of lactation and the influence on blood clotting with bromocriptine (CB 154) (Parlodel): a double blind comparison with diethylstilbestrol. *Acta Obstet. Gynecol. Scand.* 55:39, 1976.

Nusbacher J, Bove JR: Rh immune prophylaxis: is antepartum therapy desirable? *N. Engl. J. Med.* 303:935, 1986.

O'Dwyer PJ, Leylan-Jones B et al: Etoposide (VP-16-213): current status of an active anticancer drug. *N. Engl. J. Med.* 312:692, 1985.

Oster MW: Ocular side effects of cancer chemotherapy. Perry MC, Yarbo JW (Eds.): *Toxicity of Chemotherapy.* Orlando, Grune & Stratton, 1984.

Ovesen L: Drugs and vitamin deficiency. *Drugs* 18:278, 1979.

Pater JL, Willan AR: Methodologic issues in trials of antiemetics. *J. Clin. Oncol.* 2:484, 1984.

Petrie RH, Paul WL et al: Placental transfer of lidocaine following paracervical block. *Am. J. Obstet. Gynecol.* 120:791, 1974.

Phillipson EH, Kuhnert BR, Syracuse D: Maternal, fetal, and neonatal lidocaine levels following local perineal infiltration. *Am. J. Obstet. Gynecol.* 149:403, 1984.

Pike MC, Krailo MD et al: Breast cancer in young women and use of oral contraceptives: possible modifying effect of formulation and age at use. *Lancet* 2:926, 1983.

Pizzo PA: Granulocytopenia and cancer therapy: past problems, current solutions, future challenges. *Cancer* 54:2649, 1984.

Pizzo PA, Schimpff SC: Strategies for the prevention of infection in the myelosuppressed or immunosuppressed cancer patient. *Cancer Treat. Rep.* 67:223, 1983.

Porter JB, Hunter JR et al: Oral contraceptives and non-fatal vascular disease. *Obstet. Gynecol.* 66:1, 1985.

Poster DS, Penta JS et al: Delta-9-tetrahydrocannabinol in clinical oncology. *J. Am. Med. Assoc.* 245:2047, 1981.

Pritchard JA: The use of the magnesium ion in the management of eclamptogenic toxemias. *Surg. Gynecol. Obstet.* 100:131, 1955.

Ralston DH, Shnider SM: Fetal and neonatal effects of regional anesthesia in obstetrics. *Anesthesiol.* 48:34, 1978.

Rayburn WF, Wible-Kant J, Blebsoe R: Changing trends in drug use during pregnancy. *J. Reprod. Med.* 27:567, 1982.

Rayburn WF, Zuspan FP: *Drug Therapy in Obstetrics and Gynecology.* Ed 2. Norwalk, Conn., Appleton-Century-Crofts, 1986.

Reimer RR, Hoover R et al: Acute leukemia after alkylating-agent therapy of ovarian cancer. *N. Engl. J. Med.* 297:177, 1977.

Relini JP, Goldzieher JW: Oral contraceptives and cardiovascular disease: a critique of the epidemiologic studies. *Am. J. Obstet. Gynecol.* 152:729, 1985.

Resnik MC: Melasma induced by oral contraceptive drugs. *J. Am. Med. Assoc.* 199:601, 1967.

Richards SR, Chang FE, Stempel LE: Hyperlactacidemia associated with acute ritodrine infusion. *Am. J. Obstet. Gynecol.* 146:1, 1983.

Richman CM, Makii MM et al: The effect of lithium carbonate on chemotherapy-induced neutropenia and thrombocytopenia. *Am. J. Hematol.* 16:313, 1984.

Robbie MO, Sweet RL: Metronidazole use in obstetrics

and gynecology: a review. *Am. J. Obstet. Gynecol.* 145:865, 1983.

Robboy SJ, Noller KL et al: Increased incidence of cervical and vaginal dysplasia in 3,980 diethylstilbesterol-exposed young women. *J. Am. Med. Assoc.* 252:2979, 1984.

Rosen GF, Lurain JR et al: Hexamethylmelamine in ovarian cancer after failure of cisplatin-based multiple agent chemotherapy. *Gynecol. Oncol.* (In press).

Rosene KA, Featherstone HJ, Benedetti TJ: Cerebral ischemia associated with parenteral terbutaline use in pregnant migraine patients. *Am. J. Obstet. Gynecol.* 143:405, 1982.

Runowicz CD, Dottino PR et al: Catheter complications associated with intraperitoneal chemotherapy. *Gynecol. Oncol.* 24:41, 1986.

Russ JS, Rayburn WF, Samuel MJ: Uterine stimulants. In Rayburn WF, Zuspan FP (Eds.): *Drug Therapy in Obstetrics and Gynecology.* Ed. 2. Norwalk, Conn., Appleton-Century-Crofts, 1986.

Rustin GJS, Booth M et al: Pregnancy after cytotoxic chemotherapy for gestational trophoblastic tumours. *Br. Med. J.* 288:103, 1984.

Sabour MS, Fadel HE: The carpal tunnel syndrome—a new complication ascribed to the "Pill." *Am. J. Obstet. Gynecol.* 107:1265, 1970.

Saltiel E, McGuire W: Doxorubicin (Adriamycin) toxicity. *West. J. Med.* 139:332, 1983.

Scanlon JW: Effects of obstetric anesthesia and analgesia on the newborn: a select, annotated bibliography for the clinician. *Clin. Obstet. Gynecol.* 24:649, 1981.

Schilsky RL: Renal and metabolic effects of cancer treatment. In Perry MC, Yarbro JW (Eds): *Toxicity of Chemotherapy.* Orlando, Grune & Stratton, 1984.

Scialli AR: The reproductive toxicity of ovulation induction *Fertil. Steril.* 45:315, 1986.

Selevan SG, Lindbohm ML, Hornung RW: A study of occupational exposure to antineoplastic drugs and fetal loss in nurses. *N. Engl. J. Med.* 313:1173, 1985.

Shnider SM, Wright RG: Uterine blood flow and plasma norepinephrine changes during maternal stress in the pregnant ewe. *Anesthesiology* 50:524, 1979.

Sillman FH, Sedlis A, Boyce JG: A review of lower genital intraepithelial neoplasia and the use of topical 5-Fluorouracil. *Obstet. Gynecol. Surv.* 40:190, 1985.

Sillman RJ: In utero exposure to diethylstilbesterol: adverse effects on the reproductive tract and reproductive performance in male and female offspring. *Am. J. Obstet. Gynecol.* 142:905, 1982.

Slap GB: Oral contraceptives and depression: impact, prevalence and cause. *J. Adolesc. Health Care* 2:53, 1981.

Soltan MH, Hancock KW: Outcome in patients with post-pill amenorrhoea. *Br. J. Obstet. Gynaecol.* 89:745, 1982.

Speroff L, Glass RH, Kase NG: *Clinical Gynecologic Endocrinology and Infertility.* Ed. 3. Baltimore, Williams & Wilkins, 1983.

Stadel BV, Rubin GL et al: Oral contraceptives and breast cancer in young women. *Lancet* 2:970, 1985.

Stallworth JC, Yeh S, Petrie RH: The effect of magnesium sulfate on fetal heart rate variability and uterine activity. *Am. J. Obstet. Gynecol.* 140:702, 1981.

Stein RS, Howard CA et al: Lithium carbonate and granulocyte production. *Cancer* 48:2696, 1981.

Steir CM, Petrie RH: A comparison of magnesium sulphate and alcohol for the prevention of premature labor. *Am. J. Obstet. Gynecol.* 129:1, 1977.

Strauss SE, Takiff HE et al: Suppression of frequently

recurring genital herpes: a placebo-controlled double-blind trial of oral acyclovir. *New Eng. J. Med.* 310:1545, 1984.

Strickland DM, Leonard RG et al: Vaginal absorption of hexachlorophene during labor. *Am. J. Obstet. Gynecol.* 147:769, 1983.

Studd JWW, Crawford JS: The effect of lumbar epidural analgesia on the rate of cervical dilatation and the outcome of labor of spontaneous onset. *Br. J. Obstet. Gynaecol.* 87:1015, 1980.

Taylor GT, Cohen B: Ergonovine-induced coronary artery spasm and myocardial infarction after normal delivery. *Obstet. Gynecol.* 66:821, 1985.

Tayob Y, Adams J et al: Ultrasound demonstration of increased frequency of functional ovarian cysts in women using progestogen only oral contraception. *Br. J. Obstet. Gynaecol.* 92:1003, 1985.

Thompson RL, Wright AJ: Symposium on antibiotics. Part II: Cephalosporin antibiotics. *Mayo Clin. Proc.* 58:79, 1983.

Tindal VR: Factors influencing puerperal thromboembolism. *J. Obstet. Gynaecol. Br. Commonwlth.* 75:1324, 1968.

Tovey GH: Should anti-D immunoglobulin be given antenatally? *Lancet* 2:466, 1980.

Tsukamoto N, Matsukuma K et al: Cyclophosphamide-induced interstitial pneumonitis in a patient with ovarian carcinoma. *Gynecol. Oncol.* 17:41, 1984.

Turnbull AC: Puerperal thromboembolism and suppression of lactation. *J. Obstet. Gynaecol. Br. Commonwlth.* 75:1321, 1968.

Urban C, Nurenberg A et al: Chemical pleuritis as the cause of acute chest pain following high-dose methotrexate treatment. *Cancer* 51:34, 1983.

Van Barneveld PWC, Veenstra G et al: Changes in pulmonary function during and after bleomycin treatment in patients with testicular carcinoma. *Cancer Chemother. Pharmacol.* 14:168, 1985.

Vessey MP, Yeates D et al: Pelvic inflammatory disease and the intrauterine device: findings in a large cohort study. *Br. Med. J.* 282:855, 1981.

Von Hoff DD, Schilsky R et al: Toxic effects of cis-dichlorodiammineplatinum (II) in man. *Cancer Treat. Rep.* 66:1527, 1979.

Vorherr H, Vorherr UF et al: Vaginal absorption of povidone-iodine. *J. Am. Med. Assoc.* 244:2628, 1980.

Weir RJ, Briggs E et al: Blood pressure in women taking oral contraceptives. *Br. Med. J.* 1:533, 1974.

Weiss RB: The role of hexamethylmelamine in advanced ovarian cancer treatment. *Gynecol. Oncol.* 12:141, 1981.

Wilding G, Caruso R et al: Retinal toxicity after high-dose cisplatin therapy. *J. Clin. Oncol.* 31:683, 1985.

Wilson WR, Cockerill FR III. Symposium on antibiotics. Part II: Tetracyclines, chloramphenicol, erythromycin and clindamycin. *Mayo Clin. Proc.* 58:92, 1983.

Wynn V, Niththyananthan R: The effect of progestins in combined oral contraceptives on serum lipids with special reference to high-density lipoproteins. *Am. J. Obstet. Gynecol.* 142:766, 1982.

Zuspan FP, Arwood LL, Cordero L: Glucorticoids to enhance fetal lung maturity. In Rayburn WF, Zuspan FP (Eds.): *Drug Therapy in Obstetrics and Gynecology.* Ed. 2. Norwalk, Conn., Appleton-Century Crofts, 1986.

Zuspan FP, Talledo OE, Rhodes K: Factors affecting delivery in eclampsia: the condition of the cervix and uterine activity. *Am. J. Obstet. Gynecol.* 100:672, 1968.

RADIATION REACTIONS AND COMPLICATIONS: ETIOLOGY, PREVENTION, DIAGNOSIS AND MANAGEMENT

14

RAMANANDA M. SHETTY
TERRENCE J. BUGNO

Soon after the discovery of radiotherapy in the late 1890's, its usefulness for the management of gynecologic malignancies was recognized. Its therapeutic benefit, either alone or in combination with surgery, chemotherapy or immunotherapy, has continued to be redefined over the years as oncologists strive to select the best mode of therapy for each individual patient. Major advances in the understanding of the natural history of gynecologic tumors, better clinicopathologic staging, proper patient selection and technical advances have brought about a cautiously brighter outlook. The goal of any therapeutic approach is an uncomplicated cure. Fortunately, the anatomic arrangement of the female genital tract, the generally high tolerance to ionizing radiation of the tissues and the development of more sophisticated techniques to deliver cancericidal doses safely have allowed radiotherapists to function within an acceptable therapeutic ratio of cure to complication. For many malignancies, radiotherapy (RT) may be the treatment of choice, or it may provide an alternative to surgery (Table 14–1). Moreover, the role of RT in adjuvant or palliative settings must not be overlooked. The volume of patients requiring RT at some point in their treatment can be readily demonstrated by noting that in 1985 the American Cancer Society estimated that there would be 74,900 new invasive female tract cancers (Silverberg, 1985). It is estimated that 50 to 60% of patients will receive radiation during their clinical course, or nearly 40,000 women. Because of the number of women involved, a clear understanding of the effects of treatment and their management is in order.

This chapter will cover the prevention, diagnosis and management of acute reactions related to definitive RT. It will then focus on late sequelae from treatment in two major organ systems: the urinary and the gastrointestinal systems, since these are the areas to be most frequently reported to be at risk in patients treated for cure. Only a limited discussion of the sequelae related to combined treatment

Table 14–1. Treatment Strategies for Cure In Gynecologic Malignancies†*

Tumor Site	Surgery (S)	Radiotherapy (RT)	S + RT	S + Chemotherapy‡
Cervix	+	+	+	
Endometrium	+	+	+	
Fallopian tube	+		+	+ (+RT)
Gestational trophoblastic disease				+ (+RT)
Ovary	+		+	+ (+RT)
Uterine sarcoma	+		+	+ (+RT)
Vagina	+	+	+	
Vulva	+	+	+	

*In some instances, the stage of the disease will allow for only one form of definitive therapy, e.g., cervix, endometrium, vagina, and a second or third modality used as an adjuvant.

†Primary management approaches may differ with institution.

‡Various roles in combination management have yet to be clarified.

will be addressed here; additionally, advances in altered fraction schemes, radioprotectors/sensitizers, radiolabeled substances and high linear energy transfer (LET) radiations are beyond the scope of this text. Suffice it to say that selection of a single mode of therapy for the individual patient is usually preferable, since serious morbidity may be 2 to 10 times higher when, for example, surgery and RT are combined (Shingleton et al, 1969; Webb and Symmonds, 1979). However, this price may be justified in cure for locally advanced disease. Table 14–2 outlines the various factors influencing the appearance of complications in an irradiated field in terms of patient (host), disease (tumor) and treatment (technical or physician) parameters. Despite the best efforts and intentions of the physician, morbidity from therapy can occur, with serious complications generally occurring in 1 to 5% of patients. Though statistically valid, this sobering fact provides no comfort to the individual patient and physician

Table 14–2. Factors Influencing the Incidence and Severity of Reactions and Complications in an Irradiated Field

Patient (Host) Parameters
Current medical condition
  General: age; hydration and nutritional status; obesity; Karnovsky or activity scale
  Intercurrent illness: recovery from recent surgery or sequelae of chemotherapy; anemia; diabetes; hypertension; vascular disorders (atherosclerosis, collagen vascular disease); gastrointestinal disorders (ulcerative colitis, Crohn's disease, diverticulosis); genitourinary disorders (renal insufficiency, infection, incontinence, bladder dysfunction)
Past medical condition
  Previous intraabdominal or pelvic surgery: including type and radicality of procedure, evidence of pre- or postoperative morbidity, chronic stigmata and time course to the present problem
  Previous intraabdominal or pelvic infection: including PID, peritonitis, ruptured viscus and outcome
  Previous irradiation in the same area: total dose, method of treatment, indication and result, and time course to current problem
  Previous chemotherapy: drugs, doses and effects (acute and chronic)
Dose limiting structures, nearby areas at risk for disease
Overall host immunologic defense capacity
  Total protein/albumin stores
  Immunoglobulin distribution and lymphocyte subpopulations
  History of immunocompromised state(s)

Disease (Tumor) Parameters
Primary tumor location
True pathologic extent (local or regional vs. metastatic) and stage at the time of treatment
Primary tumor burden (volume)
Histopathology and grade; other prognostic factors
Areas at risk for subclinical disease
Natural history of the malignancy
Current status or presentation: primary-curative, recurrence (? disease free survival), or persistence (failure of previous modality)

Table continued on opposite page

Table 14–2. *Factors Influencing the Incidence and Severity of Reactions and Complications in an Irradiated Field* Continued

---

Treatment (Technical or Physician) Parameters
Accuracy of pre-treatment assessment of gross (clinical) and microscopic (subclinical) extent of disease
Role of radiotherapy in management
    Definitive
    Adjunctive
    Palliative
Combined modality approach
    Radiotherapy $\pm$ surgery, chemotherapy, hormonal therapy or immunotherapy
Place in treatment sequence
    Primary radiotherapy (RT)
    Sequential RT: before or after surgery, chemotherapy
    Concomitant RT with other modalities
Assignment of the target volume to be irradiated (tumor, risk areas, safety margin)
Assessment of anatomic variability
    Normal variants
    Iatrogenic variants secondary to surgical removal, sequelae of surgical manipulation, or antecedent infection
Type of ionizing radiation employed in treatment
    External beam radiation (EXT)
        Beam energy and characteristic: low (kilovoltage/orthovoltage); high (photon/gamma ray units, e.g., linear accelerators
            and Cobalt-60 units); electron beam; particles
        Field definition: opposing anterior/posterior ports (AP/PA); four field box techniques (AP/PA and opposing laterals);
            rotational or arc therapy; other customized field ports
        Dose (total) and dose per fraction scheme
        Treatment planning and dosimetry
        Quality assurance and reproducibility of daily treatment
        Completion of anticipated course of therapy
    Intracavitary radiation (IC)
        Type and characteristics of radioactive sources: Ra-226, Cs-137, Cf-252, Co-60
        Type of afterloading system: Fletcher-Suit, Bloedorn
        Proper placement of afterloading device
        Accurate localization of device into area to be treated relative to normal, adjacent strucures that may limit the dose
        Treatment planning and dosimetric analysis: dose and dose rates
        Completion of anticipated course of therapy
    Interstitial radiation (IS)
        Type and characteristics of radioactive sources: Ra-226, Ir-192 (seeds or wires), I-125
        System of placement and dosimetry: fixed or rigid, utilizing templates (Paris) or flexible system also with template
            (American)
        See also IC radiation
    Colloidal suspension radioiosotope therapy (CS)
        Type and characteristics of radioisotope or radiolabeled aggregates
        Assessment of dose to target structures, dose distribution
    Use of radiomodifiers
        Radiosensitizers: hydroxyurea, misonidazole, hyperbaric O_2
        Radioprotectors: WR-2721, penicillamine, radical scavengers
        Hyperthermia
    Combined modes of ionizing radiations
        Percentage of contribution from EXT, IC, IS or CS to total dose
Summary of total dose delivered: noted different radiobiologic consequences secondary to low dose continuous vs. high
    dose fractionated RT
Knowledge of normal tissue tolerances and necessary cancericidal doses for the malignancy in question
Any modifications or alterations required that deviate from standard therapy
Intangible factors including intrinsic radiosensitivity

Clinical Setting of a Suspected Reaction or Complication
Time of onset relative to therapy (during, zero to 3, 3 to 5, over 6 months)
Thorough review of patient/tumor/treatment parameters
Constellation of clinical signs and symptoms
Excluding recurrence or persistence of malignancy by appropriate diagnostic testing: re-biopsy suspicious areas when
    clinical symptoms exist
If test result is negative, proceed with clinical intervention
    Symptomatic therapy
    Active intervention: medical or surgical

involved. Further efforts are needed to optimize management, recalling the dictum *primum non nocere*.

PREVENTION, ANALYSIS AND MANAGEMENT OF CLINICAL PROBLEMS IN A PATIENT DURING A COURSE OF DEFINITIVE RADIOTHERAPY

The appropriately selected patient embarking upon definitive radiotherapy for her gynecologic malignancy may encounter a series of acute reactions and chronic complications that are dependent upon host, tumor and treatment factors (Table 14–2). Often these effects are magnified through ignorance and anxiety by the patient, and minimized by the treating physicians. Referring physicians tend to ascribe any change in the patient's clinical status to radiation, frequently without basis in fact. Knowledge of certain predisposing factors, attention to patient awareness and education and optimal technical execution of a radiation program can produce the desired result (cure), allay treatment fears, improve patient compliance and allow more rational management of impending side-effects. Common problems encountered during the often lengthy course of external beam and brachytherapy programs will be discussed. Proper understanding of therapeutic goals and objectives, preventive measures, assessment of high risk groups and optimal dose delivery methods by both patient and physicians is mandatory. Rationales for possible side-effects and the availability of typical symptomatic remedies must be openly discussed. In general, common sense based on the pathophysiologic changes induced by ionizing radiation will lead to the necessary recognition and management.

Ionizing radiation affects the treated tissues both directly and indirectly. Potential reactions can be predicted from the anatomy and physiology of the structures/organs exposed to the beam (Fig. 14–1). For most gynecologic tumors, various portions of the gastrointestinal tract, urinary tract, genital tract (including ovaries, tubes, uterus, cervix and portions of the vulvovaginal tissues), vascular and lymphatic structures, connective tissue (including peritoneum), bone and bone marrow, muscles, nerves (also spinal cord) and overlying dermis/epidermis are exposed to radiation. As radiation kills cells (a certain fraction each time: log cell kill), the effect is manifested as reproductive cell death, with probably intrinsic differences in cellular response, repair, repopulation, and regeneration kinetics for normal versus tumor systems (Ellis, 1978). Thus one exploits the selective effect of radiation to sterilize the tumor and leave the surrounding milieu with minimal permanent damage. This is essential for tumor radiocurability, and provides an acceptable therapeutic ratio. Structures and organ systems may differ widely in their sensitivities to radiation, as high as 20 fold (Rubin et al, 1975). See Table 14–3 for a comparative analysis.

Radiation produces no unique histopathologic effect on tissues; moreover, although a "radiation effect" can be demonstrated, clinical expression can only sometimes be predicted beforehand. In most cases, acute reactions have little prognostic influence on the appearance of late effects. The majority of acute reactions reflect the sensitivity of rapidly proliferating tissues, especially mucosal surfaces. Multiple variables, including time/dose/fractionation, anatomic constraints, precision and accuracy in dose delivery, may all impact on the development of a reaction. Resultant permanent damage to normal tissues may be a combination of progressively depleted populations of parenchymal cells coupled with altered vascularity (obliterative endarteritis) and stroma (connective tissue fibrosis). These processes always produce subclinical structural changes, which, on occasion, can lead to symptomatic functional compromise. For further information refer to Hall (1978), Rubin and Cassaret (1968) and Fajardo (1982).

External Beam Radiotherapy

PRETREATMENT EVALUATION AND PLANNING

Most treatment plans include a course of external beam pelvic RT either alone or in conjunction with intracavitary treatment. Pretreatment assessment begins with identifying specific host factors that may alter the response of the tumor and its surroundings (see Table 14–2). Local alterations in vascularity that influence outcome include atherosclerotic changes, hypertension, diabetes and previous surgical interventions that have produced devascularization. These recognized deficits in tolerance have prompted some institutions to reduce the total dose by 5 to 10% in affected patients. Previous surgical manipulation or a history of pelvic infection may predispose to adhesion

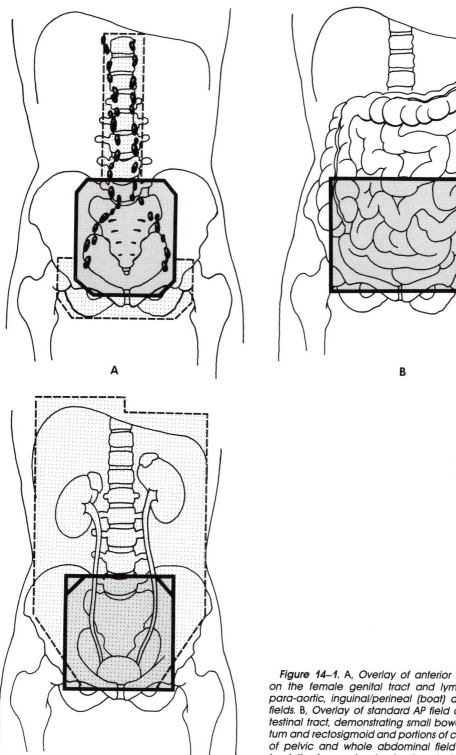

Figure 14–1. A, *Overlay of anterior treatment fields on the female genital tract and lymphatics; pelvic, para-aortic, inguinal/perineal (boat) and parametrial fields.* B, *Overlay of standard AP field on the gastrointestinal tract, demonstrating small bowel in pelvis, rectum and rectosigmoid and portions of colon.* C, *Overlay of pelvic and whole abdominal field on the urinary tract, the former showing treatment of one half to one third of the ureters, bladder and urethra.*

Table 14–3. Comparative Normal Tissue Tolerance to Ionizing Radiation vs. Cancericidal Doses for Structures at Risk in Gynecologic Malignancies*

Normal Female Genital Tract	Tissue† Class	Area/Volume	End Point	TD 5/5 Dose (Rad)‡	Comments
Ovary	I	whole	sterility	150–300§	650–2000 rad for permanent sterility
Fallopian tube	III	whole	stricture	unknown	? over 6000 rad
Uterus	III	whole	necrosis/perforation	over 10,000‖	10,000–20,000 rad tolerance without clinical sequelae
Cervix	III	whole	necrosis	unknown	? over 10,000 rad
Vulvovaginal tissues	III	whole	ulcer/fistula	9000‖	
Tissues at Risk					
Stomach	I	100 cm	perforation/ulcer/bleed	4500	
Intestine	I	100 cm	perforation/ulcer/bleed	5000	for 400 cm TD 5/5 = 4500 rad
Rectum	II	100 cm	ulcer/stenosis	6000‖	
Kidney	I	whole	nephrosclerosis	2000	
Ureter	II	5–10 cm	stricture	7500‖	
Bladder	II	whole	contracture/ulcer	6000‖	
Urethra	II	whole	stricture	unknown	? over 7000 rad
Bone marrow	I	segment	aplasia	3000	TD 50/5 = 4000 rad
Mature bone	II	10 cm	fracture/sclerosis/atrophy	6000	
Lymph node/ Lymphatics	III		sclerosis/atrophy	5000	? closer to 6000 rad
Skin	II	100 cm	dermatitis	5500	
Large artery/vein	III	10 cm	sclerosis	8000	
Connective tissue/ microvasculature	III	10 cm	fibrosis	6000	Reference tolerance¶
Spinal/peripheral nerves	II	10 cm	neuritis	6000	

Estimated Cancericidal Doses

    Subclinical disease: 4500–5000 rad (cGy) eradicates over 90%

    Microscopic disease: 5500–6000 rad (cGy)

    Gross/clinical disease: a function of volume (no. of clonogenic cells) e.g., early stage cervix cancer—8000 cGy to point A;

    Endometrial cancer: 10,000–20,000 rad surface

*Desired therapeutic ratio—comparison of dose-response curve for cure (eradication of tumor) vs. dose-response for limiting tissue tolerance resulting in, ideally, an uncomplicated cure. 1–5% severe morbidity may be the tolerated maximum.

†Tissue Class—developed by Rubin (1968, 1975) and others to rate organs in terms of dose/survival characteristics: Class I—ionizing radiation effects are fatal or have severe morbidity; Class II—radiation produces mild/moderate morbidity with permanent sequelae but compatible with survival; Class III—mild, transient, reversible effects.

‡TD 5/5—Dose exposure which results in 5% severe complication rate within a 5 year period; TD 50/5 is exposure resulting in 50% severe complications.

§Doses given are based upon standard fractionation 200 rad (cGy), 1000 rad/week, external beam radiation. One rad = 1 cGy.

‖Dose tolerances may vary when comparing high dose fractionated vs. low dose rate continuous brachytherapy; focal hot spots may occur but produce little clinical morbidity.

Reference Tolerance: describes dose to connective tissue or vascular tissues that are thought to be of intermediate radiation sensitivity and with which other tissues are compared.

formation, which alters structural anatomy by decreasing mobility within the peritoneal cavity. Pelvic shape and contour, as assessed by physical examination and radiography, help to define treatment borders. Age, thin or obese habitus, overall nutritional status, baseline hemoglobin concentration, and Karnovsky status may help pinpoint those patients requiring further supportive measures during and after radiotherapy.

The need for understanding the true clinicopathologic extent of disease cannot be empha-

sized enough; fortunately, thorough staging has been improved through the use of lymphography, IVP, CT scans with oral and intravenous contrast and MRI studies combined with a thorough physical examination. Clips marking the extent of tumor, if surgical staging is performed, can be invaluable. The radiotherapist must define the appropriate target volume for treatment (tumor volume and risk areas for subclinical disease) as well as the dose-limiting adjacent organs. Frequently, a standard pelvic field (12 to 15 cm.) is chosen. Inferior boundaries include the obturator foramen or the upper one half of the vagina, superiorly the L4 to L5 junction or the common iliac lymph nodes form the limits, and laterally the boundaries are 1 to 2 cm beyond the widest extent of the bony pelvis to encompass iliac drainage. Based on the radiotherapist's clinical judgment, modifications to this field are made; sometimes inguinal and perineal structures ("boat" shaped field), para-aortic lymphatics from T10 to L2 (panhandle or banjo field) or peritoneal contents (whole abdomen) are included in the treatment field. Either opposing anterior and posterior ports or a four field box technique are used to enclose this volume, with the lateral field extending anteriorly to the pubis to include the external iliac nodes, and posteriorly to the sacrum (S2) to cover the presacral nodes (10 cm × 12 to 15 cm).

Treatment planning techniques are indispensable to establish adequacy of tumor coverage and outline dose-limiting structures. Computer-assisted dosimetry, contours and orthogonal (AP or lateral) films with barium in the rectum, renografin in the bladder and the use of vaginal cylinders or markers for the cervix are standard techniques. Custom made blocks further optimize therapy. More recent attention has focused on the amount of small intestine in the pelvis. When surgical staging is undertaken, bowel can be excluded from the pelvis by omental interposition or use of a sling or mechanical devices (Russ et al, 1984; DeLuca and Ragins, 1985). At a minimum, pretreatment small bowel opacification studies in the prone, supine and decubitus positions can identify mobile small bowel that may be displaced outside the radiation field by positioning, possibly aided by a distended bladder (Green, 1983).

Advances in linear accelerator technology, especially the development of machines with energies well over 4 MeV, provide greater depth-dose characteristics to treat deep seated structures and spare skin, with improved therapeutic results and survival. However, internal organs may be exposed to higher radiation doses. Technical execution of planned RT should emphasize daily set-up reproducibility, skin markings and tattoos, immobilization devices where indicated and frequent monitoring of clinical response.

Once the overall individualized treatment plan has been finalized, preventive measures and patient education are given. Communication is crucial. We inform patients about the length of therapy, usually five to seven weeks, with treatments five days a week, and 180 to 200 cGy fractions to the treatment volume with all fields treated daily. We encourage them to carry on as normal activity as feasible. Anticipated side effects are outlined. Most patients frequently ask dietary questions. We advise a normal dietary intake, and if necessary, suggest high calorie, high protein supplements. A dietician specializing in cancer nutrition is an asset, and should be asked to counsel patients with significant weight loss (5 to 10%). More aggressive supplementation, such as enteral or parenteral nutrition, must be individualized. Weekly weights should be monitored and pretreatment total protein and albumin levels, lymphocyte counts and skin testing can indicate immune status and provide baseline values.

GASTROINTESTINAL TRACT

For most therapy, the gastrointestinal tract appears to be the major dose-limiting system in the pelvis, and symptoms often appear there. Irradiation of the small intestine (usually terminal ileum) and the large bowel (especially the colon and rectosigmoid regions) results in mucosal irritation, vascular congestion and edema. Increased smooth muscle contractility and peristalsis can lead to mild abdominal cramps, spasms and gas. When gastrointestinal symptoms occur, they usually begin by the latter half of treatment; careful questioning may reveal that as many as 50% of patients develop a change in bowel pattern. With hypermotility and decreased transit times, increased stool frequency and frank diarrhea may ensue. No evidence for a viral or bacterial gastroenteritis has been observed; this diarrhea is probably of multifactorial etiology and related to altered digestive enzyme and bile salt metabolism (Stryker and Demers, 1979). Symptomatic measures of graded intensity should be offered. Restriction of fiber and bulk-forming foods, gas producing foods, including dairy products (the brush border may be temporarily denuded of lactase and other enzymes) and bowel stimulants such as caffeine should be suggested. Often trial and error will show the effectiveness of these measures. Oral hydration, adequate protein intake and electrolyte replacement must continue. Judicious use of Kaopectate and, more importantly, antidiarrheal agents such as diphenoxylate and atropine (Lomotil), loperamide (Imodium) or opiate analogs will suffice. Recent experimental evidence on the loss of the cytoprotective prostaglandin barrier with radiotherapy has led to some encouraging results with buffered (enteric coated) aspirin

(Mennic and Dalley, 1973), other inhibitors (Stryker and Demers, 1979), and even bile salt agents (cholestyramine); however, further testing will be needed before general use is recommended. In our experience, these measures are sufficient to minimize symptoms and allow completion of treatment. In severe circumstances, a one to two week break or a dose fraction decrease sufficient for the mucosa and other tissues to regenerate may be necessary. An important point needs to be stressed. Because of the delayed onset and cumulative nature of intestinal irritation caused by RT, interruption of therapy will not immediately eliminate the reactions; they may persist for one to three weeks, and patients should be cautioned about this possibility.

In determining the prognosis, acute gastrointestinal reactions should be noted by the clinician since some evidence exists that with increasing severity of acute morbidity, an elevated late complication rate may appear. Studies by Bourne and co-workers (1983) and Buchler and co-workers (1971) suggest over a two- to threefold increase in late effects when serious acute sequelae were noted. On the other hand, most investigators find that late complications occur in patients who were relatively asymptomatic during treatment (Kline et al, 1972). Continued follow-up must be pursued. Optimized treatment plans should consider limiting the whole pelvic dose when possible and including midline shielding for treatment of parametrial tissues and lymphatics.

Treatment effects on the rectal mucosa mimic those on the small intestine, but also alter the rectum's storage function and capacity. Initially mucositis occurs, resulting in stool admixed with mucus, spontaneous passage of mucus or, if severe, symptomatic proctitis with pain and mild blood loss per rectum. The latter, though uncommon, can usually be handled well with local steroid suppositories or enemas. Analgesics or treatment interruption may rarely be required. Patients with advanced disease may experience more marked symptoms. Occasionally, severe bleeding may necessitate transfusion.' With time, as the rectal and perirectal tissues heal, the functional lumen is narrowed and becomes less distensible. Elimination may then become more frequent; a history of two to three movements over a short time in the morning as stool progresses downwards from the descending colon may be reported. A new bowel pattern may develop over the first six months after treatment.

Treatment of the perineal region or pelvis is often associated with diarrhea, and it may aggravate external or internal hemorrhoids. Symptomatic measures such as hemorrhoidal preparations with steroids for inflamed mucosa, sitz baths and perineal cleanliness are usually sufficient. Rarely is surgical intervention required.

In patients with specific intercurrent illnesses such as inflammatory disease of the bowel, spastic colon, diverticulitis or vascular disorders, a multidisciplinary management plan is best devised to address symptoms as they arise.

Treatment-induced nausea and vomiting are rare in conventional pelvic radiotherapy. When para-aortic nodal RT is necessary, these sequelae are more often encountered. Effects on the gastric mucosa, pyloric sphincter and proximal small bowel result in similar hypermotility and mucosal reactions. These reactions can accentuate diarrhea in the forward direction and produce nausea in reverse; the time course of the latter symptom is anywhere from one to eight hours after RT. Although it is not often recognized, the stomach may migrate inferiorly toward the pelvis and lie within the radiation beam. A review by Potish and co-workers (1983) of para-aortic RT showed a 47% incidence of nausea, nausea with emesis occurred in 20%, and 19% required treatment interruption. Factors that influenced the presence of symptoms included the volume treated (percentage of the stomach included in the port), the superior extent of the port (T10 versus T12) and the daily dose fraction (150 to 180 cGy versus 200 cGy). Antiemetic therapy with phenothiazines (e.g. prochlorperazine), given one-half to one hour prior to therapy and when needed offers symptomatic relief. Underlying systemic conditions, especially inadequate oral intake, should be monitored and corrected. Symptomatic gastritis can be managed with antacid therapy, although the clinical benefit of antacids is unclear since the mechanism of gastritis is not hyperacidity but mucosal ulceration and loss of cytoprotection.

URINARY TRACT

Urinary tract sequelae occur much less frequently than gastrointestinal complications during external radiation therapy, despite the bladder's close anatomic proximity to the uterus. Acute symptoms appear in approximately one of three patients. Pathophysiologic effects include mucosal irritation with fibrinopurulent exudate, submucosal edema and vascular congestion, which may appear as increased frequency, urgency, occasional bladder spasms and dysuria. Urodynamics are altered so that bladder capacity decreases, making urination more frequent. This can be aggravated by viral or bacterial colonization, cystitis, urethritis and, very rarely, pyelonephritis. The relationship of a history of asymptomatic bacteriuria or cystitis and the development of a reaction has not been sufficiently clarified. Baseline urinalysis prior to therapy can help identify pyuria or hematuria; IVP may disclose anatomic variants, as may cystoscopy if employed in staging. If symptoms arise, they usually appear by the latter half of therapy. History and physical examination should rule out obvious causes. Urinalysis will often reveal small numbers of white blood cells, amorphous crystals secondary to deposits formed on ulcerated mucosa, epithelial cells and debris. If bacteria are present, appropriate cultures should be obtained; if the cultures are positive, treatment should be given. Gross or microscopic hematuria (if not caused by the tumor) is unusual and more often represents an infectious rather than an inflammatory or ulcerative process. Previous or concomitant administration of chemotherapeutic agents such as cyclophosphamide must be noted and monitored. If cultures are negative, symptomatic measures are employed, including adequate fluid intake and bladder analgesics (pyridium) or antispasmodics (e.g., flavoxate or Urispas). Prophylactic antibiotics are not indicated. Good preventive measures have not been established, mostly because of anatomic constraints. Efforts to exclude portions of the bladder in the lateral field projection often fail because of the need to include the external iliac drainage. Specific methods to minimize anterior bladder wall radiation during intracavitary treatment have been more successful.

Bladder reactions appear to have no real prognostic significance for late effects in most series. The urinary tract's clinical tolerance to RT is higher; the vast majority of patients (over 75%) analyzed with late symptoms had no significant problems during the early course (Kline et al, 1972). Urethritis often presents in the same way as cystitis. Acute ureteral effects have not been described.

HEMATOPOIETIC SYSTEM

Hematologic effects are usually subclinical and reflect the degree of active bone marrow and lymphoid tissue exposed to radiation. Baseline factors may play a significant role. Marrow stem cell reserves are decreased in older women. Intercurrent illnesses, especially infection, may stress the marrow as will malnutrition, anemia due to blood loss or chronic disease, and chemotherapy. We routinely shape portals to exclude as much pelvic bone marrow as feasible. Generally, over 20% of active marrow may lie in the irradiated field, and the percentage rises with the use of para-aortic radiation (to about 30%) or with inguinal fields that may include the femoral head. Blood counts are monitored weekly, with expected changes usually occurring more often in the rapidly proliferating cell lines, white blood cells and platelets, than in the red cells. Hemoglobin should be maintained above 9 to 10 grams to maximize oxygen carrying capacity and to improve results. Transfusions are given when indicated without treatment interruption; iron replacement can also be used. Nadirs from concurrent chemotherapy must be anticipated and managed accordingly. Treatment interruption is usually necessary with significant neutropenia or thrombocytopenia (absolute neutrophil count < 750, total WBC < 1000 or total platelets < 50,000); delay may vary from a few days to a week. Overall recovery ensues after therapy, although the functional decrease in hemopoietic reserve in irradiated bone marrow may be long lasting. Fortunately, other areas increase their production of necessary cells to maintain adequate blood profiles. One population, the lymphocytes, may manifest a prolonged decrement years after RT, especially T cells (Onsurd, 1982). The clinical importance of this altered immune state has yet to be clarified.

SKIN AND SUBCUTANEOUS TISSUE

Acute skin reactions have been minimized because of the use of high energy photon beams with maximum dose delivery under the skin (0.5 to over 2 to 4 cm). Nonetheless, some patients may develop mild skin erythema and dry desquamation transiently late in treatment. It should be managed conservatively with baby oil, petroleum jelly or creams (without alcohol base or perfumes). Pruritus may be evident, reflecting decreased lubrication as sebaceous gland production stops. Areas with sloping contours or substantial tangential beam scattering effects such as the perineal or vulvar tissues tend to develop heightened reactions that require specific attention. In this regard, the female perineum appears to be less tolerant to ionizing radiation than the male counterpart. Intertriginous areas require constant local care to keep them clean and dry and to protect them from maceration and breakdown. Talcs or, preferably, cornstarch may be used after bathing. If wet desquamation occurs, washing with mild soap or the use of a solution of aluminum sulfate and calcium acetate (Domeboro) should help debride dead tissues; once the tissue is dry, either cornstarch or antibiotic ointments can be applied, according to preference. No doubt bacterial colonization occurs, but since this phase of skin reaction is self-limiting, clinical infection is rare. In the event frank ulceration or necrosis occurs (usually in the presence of gross tumor or node breakdown in the inguinal region), debridement and cleansing with peroxide solutions and then either iodoform gauze packing or bacteriostatic covering should be employed. Evidence for coexistent cellulitis or lymphangitis should be sought and appropriately managed by cultures and antibiotics. The use of analgesics for pain must be individualized. Healing may take one to two weeks or more, resulting in treatment delay; the patient should be frequently observed during this time.

Obese women with large panniculi may often feel a pulling or aching sensation in the anterior abdominal wall, related postoperatively to surgical healing and also to subclinical fat necrosis with fibrosis and hardening. These symptoms are often not predictable and should be managed with analgesia. Although it is not an acute reaction, subcutaneous fibrosis (lignification) may occur in pelvic tissues secondary to high dose RT, as a surgical sequela or as a result of replacement of the tumor by fibrosis. Though fibrosis is probably universally present microscopically, most areas remain asymptomatic except when there is encroachment on functionally active structures such as bowel or ureter. Impingement on nerves or muscles may produce ill-defined deep-seated perineal or low back pains, which may mimic recurrence. Careful diagnostic investigation using CT or MRI scanning may be helpful when the results are evaluated in conjunction with the clinical setting. Fibrosis usually stabilizes after a few years, and the rare symptomatic patient responds fairly well to analgesics as needed.

LYMPHATICS

Lower extremity edema as a manifestation of lymphatic obstruction is rarely if ever seen during or after definitive radiotherapy; if present, it is mild and typically bilateral. Almost invariably, lymphedema represents persistence or recurrence of disease, which requires specialized management. Unilateral swelling during or after RT may result from progressive disease, deep vein thrombosis, cellulitis or lymphangitis. Clinical examination along with flow studies or cultures may help to direct therapy. Lymphocysts are operative not radiation complications. Radiation can heighten surgical sequelae. If postoperative pelvic RT is given after intraperitoneal pelvic lymphadenectomy with gross disease, the risk of lymphedema may be increased two- to threefold. The onset may appear during or after completion of therapy, and may be slowly progressive over the next 6 to 12 months before stabilizing. Surgical support hose may help, or if lymphedema is intractable, surgical intervention may be required. Proper protection of the extremity from trauma and infection must be maintained. If combined dissection and radiotherapy is planned, an extraperitoneal approach to the lymphatics should be selected to lessen morbidity.

GENITAL

Ionizing radiation effects on normal or malignant gynecologic structures can also produce symptoms. High-dose fractionated RT that includes the ovaries in premenopausal females results in induced castration. Ovarian function will be permanently stopped by doses of 650 to 2000 cGy. The patient is likely to develop hot flashes, irritability, excessive perspiration and depression; separation of these symptoms from generalized RT effects may be difficult.

Acute uterine effects are subclinical, although endometrial slough may contribute to vaginal discharge. The cervix, especially if involved in the tumor, may generate a fibropurulent discharge with cell slough and debris. To prevent discomfort, vaginal douches may be prescribed (either vinegar and water or betadine) b.i.d. in addition to hot tub soaks. Bleeding from the tumor usually abates during RT, often after doses of 2000 cGy; radiation itself does not cause bleeding. The vaginal lining reacts similarly to other viscera. Vulvar tissues react like skin, with side effects accentuated by skin folds, glandular secretions, moisture and maceration. Potentially permanent epilation of pubic hair may result with high doses (over 5000 cGy). Given these complications, recommendations to sexually active women under treatment are for avoidance of intercourse until at least one month after therapy; at that time, intercourse may be resumed or a vaginal dilator may be prescribed to prevent stenosis.

GENERAL

Finally, constitutional factors such as fatigue or transient somnolence immediately after treatment are often described; their cause is not clear. Anxiety reactions to illness, shaken self-concept and psychologic overtones can be present and may require an understanding ear, support and encouragement from the patient's family and the treating physician. Support groups often provide an outlet for greater discussion among patients in similar situations (see Chapter 7). The radiotherapist must also identify patients who are not motivated to cooperate, especially those who are unable to accept the concept of tumor eradication without surgical removal; patient rapport is essential. In general, we subscribe to the concept of encouraging as normal a lifestyle as practical. The need for education as to the nature and consequences of RT cannot be overemphasized. As shown in the preceding discussion, a systematic approach that identifies the various "organ systems at risk" allows one to predict, prevent, or at least anticipate, and treat reactions.

Intracavitary and Interstitial Radiotherapy (Brachytherapy)

INTRACAVITARY RADIOTHERAPY

Acute reactions secondary to localized intracavitary vaginal insertion, typically of tandem/ovoid or vaginal cylinder devices, are of a more local nature. Irradiation injury in this setting is confined to the structures in immediate proximity: rectum and rectosigmoid, bladder and urethra, vagina and adjacent pelvic supporting tissues. Acute morbidity during treatment comes not so much from the treatment itself as from associated limitations on normal activity.

The rules outlined in Table 14–2 need to be recognized and applied in achieving a curative, uncomplicated outcome. Choice of an anesthetic becomes a key issue, since many women are elderly or have chronic illnesses. Most intracavitary insertions for cervical cancer need to be performed under general anesthesia, because of improved tumor localization and response to previous therapy and, more impor-

tantly, because of the necessary dilatation of the cervical os and manipulation of the afterloading device. If necessary, an epidural, spinal or local paracervical block can be substituted. For vaginal vault radiation after hysterectomy and bilateral oophorectomy for endometrial cancer, ovoids are routinely inserted under local analgesia with a pretreatment intramuscular injection of meperidine and hydroxyzine and intravenous diazepam in the radiotherapy suite.

Procedure. Pre-insertion studies include a complete blood count, electrolyte level determinations and urinalysis (with culture). The patient is prepared with cleansing enemas and vaginal douches. In the operating suite, the patient is carefully examined to assess residual tumor bulk and redefine any potentially difficult anatomic distortions that might alter the placement of afterloading devices. Once the sources are in place and secured with gauze packing and sutures, the patient recovers and remains at strict bedrest. Deep breathing exercises or incentive spirometry to improve respiratory function can help prevent atelectasis and fever. Since there will be a degree of vascular stasis imposed by bedrest, patients are instructed to exercise their legs frequently, in addition to receiving low dose subcutaneous heparin to decrease thromboembolic events. Continuous bladder drainage with a retention catheter is required for the duration of therapy, obviating the need to void around the packed vaginal vault and limiting distortion of the device owing to a distended bladder. Preoperative urinary tract infection is an indication for antibiotic therapy. Acidifying agents such as ascorbic acid, Mandelamine or cranberry juice (hippuric acid) may be given orally to minimize colonization by (usually) gram negative organisms. Some physicians prefer prophylactic antibiotics, usually Bactrim or Ampicillin, if instrumentation lasts over 24 hours. Intravenous fluids may be maintained not only for venous access, but to insure adequate fluid balance. Patients are placed at bowel rest through the use of low residue diets and antidiarrheal agents. These measures impede transit, keep the rectum from distending with stool and decrease the urge to defecate, which can influence the position of the device in the vagina.

Technical Complications. Attention must be given to proper technical placement to prevent geographic misses yet adequately deliver RT. Anatomic variants (e.g., retroflexed uterus, length of uterine canal, prolapsed cervix or uterus, narrow vaginal vault, obliteration of the fornices) must be assessed and accounted for in selecting the device and assigning the dose rate. Careful packing and angulation of the afterloading system must occur without distorting the relationships. Imperative to dosimetric planning and execution is the use of intraoperative orthogonal films for localization. Structures at risk must be radiographically identified, including the cervical os (metallic clips placed on the cervix), rectum and rectosigmoid (rectal probe or instillation of 50 to 100 ml of barium) and adjacent bladder and urethra (5 ml renografin in the catheter balloon or directly into the bladder). Additional markers can be placed or contrast material can be given to outline small bowel segments that may encroach upon the upper tandem. Visualization of the system in the supine position using dummy sources provides information crucial to calculating accurately the dose distribution to key points and risk regions, assuming the dummies are placed in the actual treatment position. Corrections in placement should be made at surgery.

Various loadings of active strength sources are tried by means of computer analysis and physician experience, choosing the optimal plan for delivering curative doses to target regions with spot analyses of average and maximal doses to the dose-limiting structures, the anterior rectal wall and posterior bladder wall (Kagan et al, 1976; Cunningham et al, 1981). Systems of analysis can correlate contributions to the total dose from combined therapy, dose and dose/rate effects (usually 60 to 80 cGy/hr to point A with higher doses to surfaces) to tumor control probability and complication rates. The review by Perez and co-workers (1984) highlights many of the technical difficulties encountered; the radiobiologic sequelae of low dose continuous versus high dose fractionated radiation, often summated, remains to be elucidated. General principles guiding therapy include delivery of high doses (total intracavitary [IC] + external beam therapy [EXT]) of 8000+ cGy to as small a target volume as necessary to encompass the tumor, and limit the high dose volume to normal tissues. If necessary, two intracavitary insertions may be preferred, to take advantage of further tumor shrinkage and reduce toxicity. Discussion of the choice of radioactive sources is beyond the scope of this chapter. Suffice it to say that currently most standard systems use Cesium-137, which has a half-life of 30 years, a photon energy maximum of 0.67 MeV, no alpha particle emission and lack of gaseous hazards with greater RT protection parameters than with its predecessor Radium.

Once sources are afterloaded at the bedside, appropriate radiation safety guidelines, as set by the National Council on Radiation Protection and Measurements (NCRP) and local hospital policy, need to be enforced. Patients should be in well-shielded private rooms with RT signs placed at designated areas. It should be re-emphasized that radiation is imperceptible to the senses, and thus no major change in the status of the patient should be anticipated. The room is monitored at predefined distances by the radiation safety officer. Moreover, instructions regarding visitation privileges by staff and relatives, use of film badges, and recommendations for exposure of nursing personnel should be clearly outlined. Familiarity with the inverse square law (dose rate inversely related to distance squared) should be put to practical use by all. For instance a patient with a total of 1g. Ra-equivalent Cesium-137 in a standard Fletcher-Suit tandem/ovoid placement would expose persons to approximately 100 mR/hr and 20 mR/hr at 0.5 and 5 feet from the bed. A typical nursing care situation of one-half hour at the patient's bedside (200 mR/hr) and one hour at 3 feet from the bed (50 mR/hr) would generate a total exposure of 150 mR. Radiation and nonradiation workers are allowed 5 Rem and 0.5 Rem, respectively, per year. Since exposure rate is proportional to activity, lesser exposure rates occur with smaller total activities. A calm, professional approach is required in handling patients during treatment. Once the sources are removed, the patient must be reassured that she is not radioactive and poses no threat to anyone.

Reactions During and After Insertion. Few overt side-effects occur during insertion. Symptomatic measures are all that are required; antiemetics are given when needed for occasional nausea, usually related to induced constipation and generalized discomfort; analgesics for pain; and sedatives or hypnotics for sleep. Perineal care should be limited so as not to disturb placement. Some discharge can be expected, but the only indications for premature removal of the device are persistent fever of >101 degrees F or frank vaginal bleeding, which are both very rare. Upon removal of the active sources and devices, progressive ambulation, enemas and douches are administered, and all prophylactic drug measures are discontinued. The patient undergoing a 24 to 72 hour insertion can be discharged on the day of removal.

The most obvious post-insertion side-effect is an acute fibropurulent discharge from the vagina, in addition to focal reactions in the urethra, bladder (especially posterior surface) and rectum (anterior aspects). Occasionally a transient blood-tinged discharge may result, but this and other secretions usually subside within a week. Daily vaginal douches and hot tub soaks are recommended to limit exudate from mucosal irritation and potential intravaginal adhesions. Mild labial swelling secondary to sutures and dependent posture is transient. Dysuria can occur secondary to instrumentation and often resolves spontaneously. By three to four weeks after treatment most acute reactions have abated.

INTERSTITIAL THERAPY

Interstitial therapy involves the same general guidelines for management. The clinical setting, either a booster dose in primary therapy or implantation for local recurrence alone or with external beam RT, must be analyzed to outline potential morbidity. Technical expertise is required, now often employing various rigid template designs for afterloading Iridium-192 ribbons or wires, or on occasion permanent Iodine-125 seeds, or Cesium-137 or Radium-226 needles. This type of therapy should be addressed as a local invasive surgical procedure and handled in that fashion.

ORTHOVOLTAGE THERAPY

A brief word about orthovoltage radiation therapy is appropriate. It is currently relegated to the treatment of emergency bleeding from the cervix, proximal or apical vault or cuff lesions, or as booster therapy after other external techniques. Other than therapeutic benefit few acute or chronic sequelae are seen, when it is used in this manner.

As discussed, acute and chronic sequelae from RT are largely predictable based upon anatomic and physiologic principles of host, tumor and treatment factors. Although inherent, they may remain subclinical. However, despite best efforts, some patients do develop overt clinical complications, and these will be the subject of the remainder of the chapter.

URINARY TRACT COMPLICATIONS

General Considerations

Four major areas in the urinary tract are at risk after definitive radiotherapy for gynecologic malignancies: kidney, ureter, bladder and urethra. Each has inherent relationships to genital structures or local-regional disease sites in commonly employed treatment regimens, as well as defined sensitivity to ionizing radiation. The kidney is the dose-limiting organ in the abdomen, whereas in the pelvis, apart from the fact that the small intestine is most vulnerable, anatomic proximity to the tumor necessarily results in cancericidal doses to neighboring urinary tract structures, including the lower one-third of the ureters, bladder and urethra. Indeed, the definition of point A not only relates to a volume of tissue 2 cm from the external os, but also defines the intersection of the uterine artery and ureter in the paracervical tissues. As the uterine corpus and cervix tolerate doses in excess of 10,000 cGy, tolerance of therapy and outcome lie in an adequate differential response between normal tissues and tumor. One must expect subclinical but real effects in the parenchyma and supporting tissues that create structural changes yet remain dormant; if the structures are significantly compromised, dysfunction will result.

The various urinary tract sequelae are listed by organ site in Table 14–4. Discussion in the literature of the true incidence and severity of complications after radiation therapy is ham-

Table 14–4. Urinary Tract Complications After Definitive Radiation for Gynecologic Malignancies*

Organ	Complication
Kidney	Acute radiation "nephritis" (sub)acute renal failure
	Radiation nephropathy with nephrotic syndrome
	Nephrosclerosis and chronic renal failure/insufficiency
	Hypertension: mild to malignant
	Hydronephrosis 2° to distal stenosis
Ureter	Transient or persistent hydroureter ± hydronephrosis
	Ureteral stricture: direct damage or secondary to periureteral fibrosis
	Ureterovaginal fistula ± vaginal necrosis; ± urosepsis/peritonitis
Bladder	Chronic cystitis
	Ulceration with focal necrosis
	Hemorrhagic cystitis
	Bladder contracture, atony, incontinence
	Vesicovaginal fistula ± vaginal necrosis; ± urosepsis/peritonitis
Urethra	Urethritis
	Urethral stricture/stenosis
	Urethral ulceration and necrosis
	Urethrovaginal fistula

*See text and Table 14–6 for grading systems.

pered by lack of consistency in reporting (1) proper staging and selection of patients, (2) extent of any surgical procedure (diagnostic or therapeutic) before or after radiation treatment, (3) inclusion of morbidity caused by combined therapy as having been caused by radiation alone, (4) selection of RT in more advanced or medically inoperable cases, (5) variety of treatment techniques utilized, (6) a decade of RT approaches analyzed, (7) inclusion of complications caused by recurrent disease and (8) the diligence with which side-effects are sought. Representative series will be quoted in each section, but no greater than 1 to 5% serious complication rates should be expected. Recent reports show grade 3 urinary tract morbidity to be as follows: 0.4% (Pourquier et al, 1982), 0.9% (Einhorn et al, 1985), 1.0% (Hamberger et al, 1983), 3.2% (Perez et al, 1984), 3.6% (Montana et al, 1985) and 4.2% (Hanks et al, 1983) (Table 14–5).

The first matter to be addressed when a woman presents with a clinical picture consistent with a urinary tract (or gastrointestinal tract) complication is to exclude the possibility of tumor recurrence. The literature notes that in the majority of women the tumor recurs within two to three years, an interval similar to that for treatment-related morbidity: one to two years for the gastrointestinal tract, and one to four years for the urinary tract (Hamberger et al, 1983). Recurrence of the disease in an advanced stage and significant sequelae will often appear earlier. A high index of suspicion is required, since the clinical pictures frequently overlap but the therapies are different. The classic picture of low back pain, lymphedema and hydronephrosis or fistula may signal recurrence in up to 80% of patients and yet mimic RT effects (Slater and Fletcher, 1971). One must not exclude the possibility of radiation effects, as Rotman and co-workers (1979) noted a significant incidence of obstructive uropathy (30%) and fistula formation (5%) in primarily irradiated patients. The radiation oncologist must critically review the selection and execution of the treatment strategy, focusing on portals for external beam and intracavitary radiation; dose reconstruction; contributions to various sites from local therapy, dose rate and anatomic peculiarities; tolerance and response to treatment, thus generating a likelihood index for complication formation. Nonetheless, after clinical and diagnostic studies, the patient may require biopsy or exploratory laparotomy to resolve the issue. The options available regarding recurrent disease management will not be discussed. Radiation sequelae will be considered later. Accurate assessment of the type and degree of functional impairment in the individual will help dictate a judicious selection of treatment measures.

Once a radiation complication has been documented, classification of its severity provides useful information for statistical analysis and guides the degree of intervention. Classification systems based on clinical, histologic or radiographic criteria have been developed (Table

Table 14–5. *Some Factors Correlated with an Increased Risk for Urinary (or GI) Tract Complications after Radiation*

Age (very young or > age 50)

Previous abdominal or pelvic surgery

Pelvic inflammatory conditions

Systemic illness (diabetes, hypertension, etc.) or intercurrent illness (infection, malnutrition, etc.)

Body habitus (thin or very obese)

Karnovsky or activity score

Previous renal dysfunction; underlying bowel disease(s)

Site of malignancy: increasing stage and tumor volume

Combined modality therapy (surgery, radiation, chemotherapy)

Total dose of ionizing radiation at designated points (e.g., central/lateral, surface, points A and B)

Increasing whole pelvic radiation dose (or as % of contribution to total dose)

For GI tract: small/large intestine in field

Para-aortic or whole abdominal radiation fields

Larger external beam field sizes or dose per fraction over 200 cGy vs. 150–180 cGy

Increasing high dose volume and dose contribution from intracavitary or interstitial radiation

Abnormal or distorted anatomy, e.g., narrow vagina, anteflexed or retroflexed uterus, obliteration of fornices

Type of intracavitary device, technique of placement, number and intensity of radioactive sources, precision in treatment planning and dose distribution/calculation

Dose rates to point A (cervix) over 80–100 cGy/hour

Dose rates to bladder/rectum over 60 cGy/hour

Total dose to bladder/rectum over 24 hour period

One vs. two intracavitary/interstitial insertions

Modification or deviation from standard methods

Choice and application of brachytherapy dosimetry methods

Any technical error in the execution of the treatment plan

Follow-up period of 1 to 4 years (then risk may decrease)

Biopsy of heavily irradiated tissues to exclude recurrence

Appearance of vaginal necrosis or rectovaginal fistula

Previous course of radiation

14–6). Most commonly used is some modification of the Kottmeier and Gray classification (1961).

In general, these systems imply that low grade (mild) problems require little or no intervention with an anticipated normal outcome, problems of intermediate (moderate) grade need some degree of medical intervention but minimal long-term dysfunction results, while those of high grade (severe) necessitate active measures and have the potential for serious long-term morbidity. In classifying severity and outcome of problems, analysis of causes has spawned prospectively employed methods to eliminate or lessen their impact. A good example is the grading system of Kagan and co-workers (1979). Retrospective analysis of 406 patients' course and outcome with respect to stage, dose, recurrence, performance status, survival and complications was undertaken. The premise was that injury, dose (especially from intracavitary RT) and anatomic factors were interrelated. Situations within the control of the oncologist in which optimization of techniques and recognition of certain parameters could be used constructively were identified. In over 70% of patients, a rational, potentially correctable explanation could account for the complication, without assuming "patient idiosyncrasy." The authors subsequently developed a therapeutic ratio of dose rates to critical points that would protect from excessive damage to normal tissue, yet not compromise cure. In general, departure from standard techniques (e.g., protruding vaginal sources), will often focally overdose areas at risk. Better attention to these and other anatomic variables decreased clinical manifestations (Bosch and Frias, 1977).

Another important issue is the effect of surgery upon late radiation injury. Boronow (1982) and T.H. Green (1981) discuss in their reviews the inherent differences in the etiology of complications. Surgical effects are felt less likely to be caused by intraoperative trauma, but more by devascularization, denervation or collections of serum or blood and infection, which heighten inflammatory reactions, influence structural healing and predispose to functional compromise. Ionizing radiations produce another constellation of pathophysiologic changes. Both surgical and radiation effects are magnified by systemic illness. Any combination therapy may increase complications, proportional to the radicality of either; statistically, the result is more than additive. Old and new data confirm a relative increase in complications of 2 to 10 times. These data have led to better preventive measures, patient selection and sequencing of therapies when a survival benefit has been proved. For instance, O'Quinn and co-workers (1980) showed a reduction in complications from 6 to 1.3% without a change in survival when less radical surgical measures were used. Green (1981) noted that greater attention to the intra-

Table 14–6. Representative Grading Systems for Radiation Complications

General (GI or urinary tract)
Gray-Kottmeier system (1961)
    Grade 1—mild symptoms, minimal mucosal change
    Grade 2—pain, mucous discharge, ulceration, hemorrhage, stenosis and necrosis, which may require hospitalization or medical management
    Grade 3—perforation, fistula formation or any process requiring hospitalization and surgery

Kagan et al system (1979)
    Grade R_1—complete recovery of signs/symptoms of complication; return to normalcy
    Grade R_2—incomplete recovery, requiring medical follow-up and management
    Grade S_1—one organ injury requiring surgical intervention $\pm$ complete functional recovery
    Grade S_2—multiple organ injuries requiring surgical intervention

Montana et al system (1983)
    Grade 1—symptom onset over 3 months after treatment, requiring medical management; complete recovery
    Grade 2—greater severity, selective surgical intervention, no significant permanent dysfunction
    Grade 3—surgical intervention necessary with the potential for fatal outcome

Specific (examples of urinary tract grading systems)
Bosch-Frias system (1977) (for clinical severity of bladder injury)
    Grade 1—one or more isolated episodes of cystitis
    Grade 2—intermittent hematuria/hemorrhagic cystitis of a persistent nature
    Grade 3—stenosis/hemorrhage requiring active intervention
    Grade 4—fistula

Leissner Kjellgren system (1959) (for cytoscopy graded bladder injury)
    Early—reddened mucosa and fibrinopurulent exudate
    Late—a. mild: local reaction on posterior wall above the interureteric fold, with increased vascularity, telangiectasias
          b. severe: stump-like elevation and hyperplasia of mucosa with swollen, furry red membrane, salt deposits ($\pm$ fistula formation)

Butcher et al system (1962) (for degree of urinary obstruction by IVP)
    Grade 1—minimal dilatation of the calyceal system
    Grade 2—moderate dilatation
    Grade 3—severe; radiographic evidence of decreased function
    Grade 4—nonvisualization of the urinary system

The above table is not meant to be comprehensive, but to offer some authors' approaches (e.g., clinical, histologic, or radiographic) to categorizing radiation complications. See references for complete citations.

operative approach alters morbidity. This includes atraumatic handling of tissues, preservation of vascularity, avoidance of postoperative hematoma or fluid collection by (suction) drains and postoperative bladder drainage and retraining. Attention to proper technique is particularly helpful for methods of reducing ureteral complications (see Chapter 7).

The management of any serious complication that leads to surgical intervention in a heavily irradiated field requires ingenuity and departure from standard techniques to be effective. The margin of safety is necessarily reduced, and any procedure can itself result in further morbidity. The interested reader should refer to the chapters by Green (1981) and Boronow (1982) and specific referenced literature on aspects of management. Libschitz's (1979) text on radiographic changes with discussion of clinical settings, and the descriptions of pathophysiologic changes by Rubin (1968; 1975), Fajardo (1982), Ellis (1978) and others are also useful. One must keep in mind that complications impact heavily on the quality of life in the cured patient and that treatment measures need to be individualized.

Kidney

The kidneys are retroperitoneal structures, situated posteriorly next to the transverse processes of the lower thoracolumbar vertebrae. The right kidney extends from T12 to L2, the left from T11 to L1 or L2. Anatomic variations such as duplication, pelvic or horseshoe kidneys (under 1%) can be seen during routine evaluation either with CT scans or intravenous pyelography (IVP) and subsequent iatrogenic injury can be minimized. Though the kidney is a dose-limiting tissue (along with liver and spleen), it is not included in conventional ports and thus is spared direct effects. Secondary hydronephrosis owing to a distal radiation site is a separate issue. The kidney, in part or whole, may be treated in the following settings: (1) whole abdominal RT; (2) palliative metastatic disease in lymphatics, the gastrointestinal tract or liver; (3) para-aortic RT (both medial aspects); (4) rare cases of unsuspected pelvic or horseshoe kidney. Rarely is any significant clinical insult noted, especially in whole abdominal RT and para-aortic RT, in which large patient populations have been followed. In whole abdominal therapy special precautions include localization of the kidney by an intravenous injection of

contrast material or by ultrasound followed by shielding, using custom made full posterior blocks at 1000 to 1500cGy, or transmission blocks to reduce the dose per treatment. In para-aortic fields, even if they extend to T10, only the medial aspects are exposed, the volume of which is not potentially great.

Acute radiopathologic changes from whole kidney radiation show direct tubular and glomerular damage, capillary obliteration, vasocongestion, interstitial fibrin deposits and edema, typically without symptoms. In the chronic reparative phase, a combination of parenchymal cell loss, vascular and fibrotic changes occur and appear to progress to nephrosclerosis and dysfunction. Chronic irradiated kidneys appear contracted, small and smooth; if untreated, the contralateral kidney will display compensatory hypertrophy. Radiosensitivity, according to Luxton's early orthovoltage data in seminoma, shows nephropathy and renal failure in those receiving 2800 cGy over a period of five weeks (Libschitz, 1979). Kim and co-workers reported on unavoidably irradiated kidneys in lymphoma; they showed that doses of 2450 cGy over a period of six weeks were associated with little impairment (1980).

The time course for radiation-induced "nephritis" is 6 to 13 months, with previous renal insufficiency or nephrotoxic chemotherapy lowering the threshold for damage and further accelerating the aging process. A compromised kidney may become manifest by hypertension or overt nephrotic syndrome. Individualized multidisciplinary management will be required, from supportive and medical approaches to hemodialysis, nephrectomy and rarely transplantation. If the acute insult is survived, chronic renal syndromes may appear with or without symptoms. Some patients will have malignant hypertension, others altered creatinine clearance and proteinuria, as well as other manifestations of renal insufficiency.

Renal insults are avoided through proper pretreatment planning. Should any portion of the kidneys be included in the field, selective baseline studies such as electrolytes, urinalysis, BUN/creatinine, creatinine clearance, IVP or renal scans should be performed.

Ureter

The ureters are urinary conduits lined by transitional cells, supported by smooth muscle walls with inherent peristaltic activity and suspended in retroperitoneal fibrous sheaths and adipose tissue. In their 25 to 30 cm retroperitoneal course from the renal pelvis to the ureterovesical junction they run anteromedially to the psoas and over the tips of the transverse processes. Many vessels and bowel segments overlie them. As they enter the pelvic confines, the left ureter bows out laterally to pass posteriorly to the sigmoid colon and its mesentery, crossing over the common iliac artery, then dipping posterolaterally and then medially at the level of the ischial spines. Finally it passes forward and medial to the uterine artery, crossing over at 2 cm from the lateral apsect of the cervix to enter the bladder. The right ureter follows a similar course, entering the pelvis by crossing over the external iliac artery. The vascular supply is segmental, formed by a plexus of vessels from multiple sources. The ureter may have intrinsically lowered oxygen requirements, with a less extensive blood supply in the mid-portion.

The ureters are treated in most conventional pelvic portals. The upper regions receive full doses in para-aortic ports. More significantly the lower one-half to one-third of the ureters are always included in external pelvic fields and intracavitary RT. The intimate relationship of the ureters to typical tumor sites demands that these segments receive cancericidal doses. Despite these circumstances, the lack of chronic complications is a testament to the inherent radioresistance of this organ (Moss et al, 1979).

Radiation injury to the ureter may be caused by direct damage to the mucosa with degeneration and slough of epithelial cells, smooth muscle atrophy and ischemia or altered peristalsis. In the majority of patients, repair is adequate and necrosis or functional compromise is absent. Most symptomatic effects are related to periureteral fibrosis, interstitial scarring and altered vascularity. These effects are further enhanced by pelvic inflammation, by surgical manipulation and, in cases in which the ureter passes through parametria involved with tumor, by becoming encased by fibrotic tissue during healing.

Stricture and stenosis are the commonest complications. Radiographic patterns include a long, thinned segment of pelvic ureter (unilateral or bilateral) or a focal area of stricture seen 4 to 6 cm above the ureterovesical junction where the ureter lies adjacent to the cervix (Libschitz, 1979). Other sequelae include hydronephrosis and fistula formation. The true incidence of ureteral complications is probably

less than 1 to 2%. Kaplan (1977) has reviewed in detail the older literature; Boronow's review (1982) quotes incidences from 0.4 to 4.0%. Occurrence is delayed, appearing one to four years after therapy in over 80% of patients (Perez et al, 1984); this delay may reflect the more indolent, progressive radiobiologic response of periureteral tissues. In other series, however, diligence in recording urinary tract sequelae was high. One older autopsy series showed pathologic evidence of hydronephrosis in 26.5% of patients without tumor after radiation treatment, and Rotman and co-workers reported a 30% incidence of obstructive changes, though with variable clinical expression (1979). Stricture or hydronephrosis often presents asymptomatically on a follow-up intravenous pyelogram or by blood chemical evidence of renal dysfunction. Another presentation may be ascending infection, flank pain, fever and active urosepsis secondary to urinary stasis. The clinical setting often indicates whether the cause is tumor recurrence or radiation sequelae. Antegrade or retrograde pyelography may disclose the site(s) of blockage, the presence of an obstructive mass or other signs. Obstruction on IVP without other symptoms may indicate that the stricture is benign if it is low, near the bladder, and no disease is found on palpation or CT scan or if it is higher, 4 to 6 cm above the ureterovesical junction, or medially displaced in the pelvis but within the high dose treatment region.

Management involves attempts to correct and preserve renal function usually by mechanically reopening the pathway and preventing recurrent blockage. Individualized assessment of the seriousness of the problem and personal philosophy must apply. T.H. Green (1981) and Boronow (1982) provide technical details and approaches to management. In general, immediate attention should be directed to correcting any active infectious process, and, if necessary, to performing percutaneous nephrostomy or internal stenting. If the patient is asymptomatic with minimal impairment, she may be observed and monitored by serial intravenous pyelograms, creatinine clearance determinations, ultrasound examinations or radionuclide scans, since a small minority of patients improve spontaneously. Under fluoroscopic guidance the ureter can be dilated if a focal stricture can be identified. A certain number of patients will require repeated procedures or progress to further renal compromise. At this point, surgical treatment may be appropriate if previous exploration to exclude recurrence has not already taken place. Exploration with lysis of adhesions and mobilization of the encased ureter may be sufficient to correct the deficit. Boronow (1982) expresses caution about this, feeling that this surgical manipulation, especially in the parametrial course of the ureter, may precipitate further cicatrix. Instead, he advocates a reimplantation procedure, the ureteroneocystostomy (see Chapter 4), which often results in long lasting function.

If these methods fail, a larger segment of ureter is blocked or bilateral obstruction is present, anastomosis above the radiation field may be preferable. Ureteroileoneocystostomy, transureteroureterostomy or if necessary a cutaneous ureterostomy may be indicated. If the situation warrants them, urinary diversion procedures that employ either an ileal or sigmoid loop can be successfully undertaken (see Chapter 4).

Ureterovaginal fistulas are virtually non-existent unless pelvic operations have also been performed. If present, as after combined treatment, they can be handled similarly to vesicovaginal fistulas (see later section and Chapter 4).

Bladder

GENERAL

The bladder is a hollow muscular reservoir with a capacity of 350 to 450 ml that lies behind the pubic symphysis and resides in the pelvis, unless maximally distended. Directly behind the posterior wall and trigone lie the uterus and vagina. Afferent (ureter) and efferent (urethra) connections complete the tract. The dome and posterior surfaces are lined by peritoneum, making contact with bowel likely. The bladder mucosa is transitional epithelium, whose deep basal layers provide regenerative cells. No limiting basement membrane exists, and capillaries penetrate the lining. Bladder thickness is a function of the degree of distension, with the mucosal surface supported by an array of submucosal connective and elastic stroma. The smooth muscle arrangement of the detrusor muscle is a random mixture of longitudinal and spiral fibers, all encapsulated by an adventitial layer. Rich arterial, venous and lymphatic pathways are evident.

The bladder is usually included in most conventional intracavitary and external fields. Specific risk areas include those near tumor, focal spots along the posterior bladder wall (especially the trigone) or, with whole pelvis RT, the entire organ.

After radiotherapy, the bladder undergoes a repair process, the extent of which may influence the subsequent development of late complications. As previously noted, the absence of acute symptoms does not predict eventual outcome (Kline et al, 1972). Although the urothelium is relatively radioresistant, the effect on the basal cell layer results in mucosal thinning and atrophy, often with superficial ulceration. The submucosal tissues heal by fibrosis with hyalinization and decreased elastin production. Smooth muscle effects are minimal, but altered blood flow in small vessels may result in induration, fibrosis and focal necrosis. Superficial telangiectasias and dilated, tortuous vessels throughout the wall often become exposed, with little protection from even minor trauma. The patient may be asymptomatic or may have acute urinary symptoms. Chronic irritation of the bladder can pose multiple clinical problems. A low-grade infectious process (usually gram negative or urea splitting bacteria) with disc-like salt deposits over focal ulcerations may be seen. The degree of ulceration will predict the consequences; large areas of focal necrosis may not heal well and may give rise to painful ulcers. If ulceration progresses with ischemic necrosis, rupture and perforation with fistula formation into the vagina can result. Often tumor and infection coexist with radiation effect. If mechanical trauma occurs, fragile vessels may rupture, resulting in hematuria and hemorrhagic cystitis. These conditions may be transient, microscopic findings on routine urinalysis, or gross hematuria with an eroded arteriole in a posterior ulcer crater may be found. Bladder wall thickening and fibrosis, decreased distensibility and reduced reservoir capacity can result in urinary frequency. If autonomic or sensory nerves are encased in fibrosis, deep-seated pelvic pain may result. On occasion, induration and swelling of the ureterovesical junction can promote reflux incontinence, obstruction or ascending infection.

CYSTITIS

Cystitis is probably the most common acute and chronic effect. The literature differs on the meaning of this term, as it often includes several interrelated symptoms. Usually excluded are gross hemorrhage, focal bladder ulceration and dysuria less than three months after RT. Cystitis has traditionally been categorized as of mild or grade one severity. It is the end result of progressive fibrosis and repair, with superficial ulceration and decreased bladder capacity sufficient to produce mild dysfunction.

The incidence of persistent cystitis is about 1 to 5.4%, subject to individual and treatment differences (Kottmeier, 1964). Minimal objective changes can be observed cystoscopically in over 80% of patients in the posttreatment period; the majority never develop clinical problems. Chau and co-workers (1962) and Perez and co-workers (1984) indicate that dysuria that produces lasting discomfort, spasm and frequency appears from one to five years later, lagging behind rectal changes. Most authors, both in the 1960's and in the 1980's, relate cystitis to high focal doses of intracavitary radium or cesium insertions; the risk is increased by altered anatomy, overexposure from deviated afterloading devices, or previous high dose external beam RT. The routine use of Fletcher-Suit applicator systems can probably provide better protection of the bladder through ovoid shielding. Studies that emphasize the role of external beam therapy show a rise in cystitis with doses over 5000 cGy (Hamberger et al, 1983; Chau et al, 1962).

The symptoms of dysuria, frequency and on occasion mild aching discomfort tend to be tolerable, but may wax and wane with bladder spasms. The major differential diagnoses include infection and early recurrence. A good general physical and pelvic examination plus urinalysis and culture is often sufficient to exclude infection. Often, the process is self-limiting and reassurance is adequate. If the symptoms persist and no other source is likely, cystoscopy may be valuable, if it is performed by an operator who is experienced in viewing the radiated bladder. Biopsy is rarely needed in this case unless an atypical lesion is noted. The literature is unclear on the exact effect of biopsy on subsequent fistula formation, but fistula occurrence is definitely increased, so it is wise to be cautious (Boronow and Rutledge, 1971).

Treatment is expectant and symptomatic. A combination of fluid management, mild analgesics and bladder anesthetics or antispasmodics can be prescribed, along with antibiotics if indicated. The symptoms will usually resolve without permanent functional deficit. Leissner and Kjellgren (1959) and others note that although cystoscopic regression occurs and symptoms abate with time, periodic microscopic hematuria may be found on routine urinalysis; additionally, desquamated transitional cells and amorphous crystals and sediment are observed.

ULCERATION

Focal ulceration may coexist with classic symptoms of cystitis and have a similar time course. Ulceration is a cystoscopic finding, usually on the posterior bladder wall or trigone adjacent to the primary tumor site and within the high dose/rate area. There may be slight hyperemic ulceration and elevation with telangiectasia, edema and a grayish, slough-covered but sharply limited ulcer crater. When severe, the ulcer crater has been likened to a coral reef (Kottmeier, 1964). Rarely are ulcers situated anteriorly if only a 4000 cGy whole pelvic dose is given, but anterior ulcers may appear after a dose of 5000 to 6000 cGy. Plain film radiography may show a dense shadow consistent with fibrotic calcifications speckled focally in the bladder wall. Intravenous pyelography can show thickening, loss of bladder capacity, rounding off and elevation off the pelvic floor and trabeculation (consistent with a contracted bladder) in addition to filling defects. These ulcers may be dormant, give rise to cystitis or produce significant hemorrhage. The incidence of ulcer formation approaches 3%, and the condition is often reported in conjunction with hemorrhagic cystitis.

HEMATURIA

After high dose radiotherapy a rare presentation is gross bleeding. It can be intermittent and painless, presenting one to two years after treatment. It is often associated with cystitis or bladder ulceration with rupture or erosion of a feeding arteriole in the crater (similar to duodenal ulcers that bleed). Bladder spasms may coexist and, at times, clot formation with urinary retention and obstruction result. This is considered a moderate to severe complication (grade 2 to 3), depending on the number of episodes, the method of treatment and the need for hospitalization, transfusion or a surgical procedure. Bosch and Frias (1977) noted that only 0.4% of patients had hemorrhagic cystitis, amounting to 14% of the total urinary complications. Others report incidences as high as 2.6% (IC + orthovoltage) and 7.8% (Villasanta, 1972), with a mean onset of 23.1 months and a an average duration of 9.7 months. Other contemporary series report that around 3% of patients show evidence of hematuria. Once again, infection, stone presence and recurrence have to be excluded.

If the hemorrhage is due to radiation changes, the first line of treatment is support with fluids, electrolytes and blood products. Antibiotics, analgesics and antispasmodics are given when indicated. Continuous bladder drainage and irrigation via a three-way catheter may prove beneficial; 0.5% acetic acid or potassium permanganate solution can be used for chemical coagulation. At cystoscopy, if a focal site can be located, fulguration can be attempted, although success rates and recurrent episodes may vary with the type of lesion and the operator's skill. A focal defect typically represents a problem related to intracavitary radiation therapy, whereas diffuse damage is unlikely to be related to intracavitary treatment alone, nor is it effectively treated with fulguration or laser therapy. Another approach offered by Green (1981) is intravesical tamponade using a transurethral balloon catheter inflated to compress the entire mucosal surface with a pressure equal to the diastolic blood pressure for 4 to 6 hours under regional (epidural) analgesia. Success rates were not reported for this technique.

A more recent approach is instillation of formalin; this technique was originally devised by Brown in 1968 and refined by various authors because of initially high rates of obstruction, papillary necrosis, ureteral fibrosis and intraperitoneal extravasation with 10% solutions. The mechanism of action lies in formalin's desiccating property, which hydrolyzes surface proteins and coagulates tissues. This action blocks leaky vessels in mucosal and in deeper areas. As tissues slough after this procedure, regeneration of the urothelium can be expected over the next month. Indications for formalin instillation include failure of conservative measures, persistent blood loss, fulguration failure, diffuse ulceration and concomitant cyclophosphamide-induced sequelae. Details of the procedure are outlined by Shrom and co-workers (1976) and Behnam and co-workers (1983) and include the following:

1. A pretreatment voiding cystometrogram is performed to establish any significant vesicoureteral reflux (relative contraindication).

2. With the patient under regional anesthesia and in a lithotomy position, a Foley catheter is snugly placed to prevent periurethral leakage.

3. A 1 to 5% formalin solution in sterile irrigant (usually physiologic saline) is instilled passively from about 15 to 25 cm above the symphysis for 10 to 20 minutes. If reflux is present, the catheter is not clamped, the patient is placed in a deep reverse Trendelenburg position and constant in-out irrigation of the entire volume (100 to 150 ml) with a maximum of 15 cm pressure is used.

4. The formalin is removed and the bladder is continuously irrigated over the next 24 to 48 hours.

Potential sequelae include suprapubic discomfort, dysuria, decreased bladder capacity and, rarely, incontinence, all echoing the presenting complaints but resolving in 7 to 10 days. Results are quite encouraging. In Behnam and co-workers' series, 9 of 10 problems were resolved by 72 hours, and all were resolved by five days; 10% recurred and all were successfully retreated. Shrom and co-workers reported an 86% initial success rate and an 83% retreatment success rate, stressing the efficacy and reliability of this program.

Other intravesical instillation methods, including the use of DMSO, silver nitrate and cortisone, have not achieved as reliable an effect and are not routinely recommended. In the fulminant, intractable case of hemorrhagic cystitis, arteriographic hypogastric artery embolization or surgical ligation, with or without urinary diversion or cystectomy, may be necessary to prevent exsanguination.

CONTRACTED BLADDER

Severe spastic or contracted bladder with a near complete loss of reservoir function may rarely be encountered. Painful micturition, pelvic pain, frequency and incontinence can accompany it. Green (1981) reviewed four methods of management from the literature. (1) Hydraulic dilatation under anesthesia can produce modest relief, although analgesia is required. (2) Cystoscopy with intramural injection of steroids has shown occasional benefit. (3) Augmentation cystoplasty by means of anastomosis of the bladder fundus to an ileal or colonic segment on its mesentery can increase bladder capacity and produce the need to void twice ("double void" phenomenon). (4) If the condition is truly intractable, denervation and complete urinary diversion, sometimes including cystectomy, can be considered.

VESICO-VAGINAL FISTULA

The most severe and potentially morbid complication results from progressive ulceration with loss of structural stability and rupture with fistulous tract formation. This may be enhanced by vaginal vault necrosis and is more frequent (up to 25 to 30%) with coexistent rectovaginal fistulas. Contemporary series report an incidence of under 2 to 3%; the M.D. Anderson Hospital and Tumor Institute reports a 1.2% incidence (Boronow and Rutledge, 1971), and the Mallinckrodt Institute reports an incidence of 1.1% (Perez et al, 1984). In the former series, of the 38 reported cases, 13 were caused by disease and 13 by a biopsy in an area of necrosis; only one was caused by radium needle placement. Strockbine and and co-workers (1970) observed that over 90% of fistulas occurred with massive central or vaginal disease that required more radical therapy for cure. Regardless of this, patients may present with watery, odoriferous vaginal discharge with varying degrees of pelvic discomfort or infection. Modifying Graham's approach (1965), diagnostic measures to identify the source of the fistula rely on the three cotton pledget test in the vagina (see Chapter 4). Instillation of methylene blue or indigo carmine into the bladder should identify the fistulous tract as being vesical or urethral in origin (distal or proximal coloring). If all sponges are dry, intravenous injection of indigo carmine can detect a ureterovaginal fistula. Intravenous pyelography may be useful as is information obtained by a CT scan of the pelvis with infusion of contrast material. Cystoscopy may permit visualization of the tract, and allow antegrade placement of stents for drainage.

Management, once recurrent disease is excluded, is long term, temporizing and not necessarily standardized. If drainage persists without infection or hydronephrosis, it can be permitted to continue, and perineal pads or a plastic vaginal cup receptacle draining to a thigh bag can be used. Continuous bladder drainage may be useful to decrease leakage, using a Foley catheter or a suprapubic tube. The patient's overall medical condition should be optimized, including correction of infection, anemia and malnutrition. Since the majority of vesico-vaginal fistulas are of large size with impaired vascularity and limited tissue mobility, spontaneous closure is rare (under 6%) (Strockbine et al, 1970). Continued perineal leakage of urine is poorly tolerated by most patients, but repair presents many difficulties, should not be immediate and should allow sufficient time for improvement in local tissue condition.

Surgical closure (primary) may be attempted in 30 to 50% of cases (Boronow, 1982). The rare, small fistula may be closed through a conventional vaginal approach. More frequently, partial (Latzko) or complete colpocleisis is useful. The complete procedure may be of the Twombly and Marshall type (selecting a posterior vaginal wall patch, resecting the significantly involved vaginal mucosa and covering the vesical defect) or by the Blaikley method (using the upper posterior vaginal wall to patch the defect). Success rates may be around 30 to 50%. Side-effects include incontinence, loss of coital function, stone formation, ascending infection or renal insufficiency. Some feel that the high complication and failure rates may not justify an attempt at primary closure. However, in selected cases it has proved beneficial.

Other methods of closure involve dissecting wide margins around the fistula so as to rejoin tissues without tension. Additionally, these techniques allow an improvement in vascularity in the heavily irradiated resected fistulous region by interposing a fresh pedicle of non-irradiated tissue and its blood supply. Thus a number of procedures employing pedicle grafts have been suggested, often with good results (Boronow, 1982). Muscle interposition techniques include the bulbocavernous muscle/fat pad method (Martius), leg muscle groups with gracilis (Ingelman-Sundberg and Graham and Kottmeier), sartorius, adductor longus or rectus abdominis muscle interposition. An omental interposition (Bastiaanse approach) has also been popularized. Individual preference and experience often dictate the selection.

Unfortunately, the majority (50 to 70%) of fistulas may come to permanent urinary tract diversion because of the massive defect and coexistent problems. Two major conduit sources for ureteral implantation can be chosen after consideration of the previous treatment ports. Bricker (1980) has had extensive experience with and refinement of the ileal conduit procedure, in which non-irradiated proximal portions of ileum are selected and the jejunum, with its attendant electrolyte and acid-base abnormalities, is avoided. Others advocate the use of either a sigmoid conduit, which is anatomically accessible, or a transverse colon conduit, which is potentially preferable since it is usually free from radiation effect. In either case, short segments (15 cm or less) should be chosen to avoid torsion, compromised vascularity and adhesion formation. Once the pouch has been created, viable ureteral segments outside the pelvis are isolated and end-to-side anastomoses made, either by spatulating and tunneling the ureter submucosally or by direct full thickness apposition. In this way permanent urinary diversion results, with a decrease in local symptoms at the actual fistula site. Side-effects may involve bowel necrosis, anastomotic stenosis or leak, hydronephrosis with a non-functional kidney, infection or ureterocutaneous fistula (Bricker, 1980).

Occasionally, in the carefully selected patient, urinary diversion may be temporary, not permanent. Kwon and Boronow (1979) describe a urinary undiversion procedure, akin to the diverting colostomy, staged resection and reanastomosis of the intestine. Urinary flow is diverted through an ileal or colon conduit. After several months delay, the fistula is closed. If closure is successful, the final stage is undiversion, taking down the conduit and creating a ureteroileoneocystostomy with return of a near normal and intact renal system. As experience is gained, the applicability of this approach will need to be evaluated (see Chapters 4 and 7).

Urethra

The intimate anatomic relationship between the female urethra, the anterior vaginal wall, the cervix and the bladder is well known. The urethra is 3 to 4 cm long and 8 mm in diameter. It is in proximity to the symphysis and just anterior to the vagina. Its lining consists of pseudostratified or transitional cell epithelium in the upper and middle parts, which changes to squamous cell epithelium at the external urinary meatus. The submucosa is made up of connective and elastic tissues and spongy venous spaces in addition to many periurethral glands. The submucosal tissues undergo significant RT-induced changes and often are responsible for the complications seen, which are, in fact, quite rare. The urethra may itself undergo degenerative sloughing of its mucosa, and its radiosensitivity is probably similar to that of the ureter.

Portions of the female urethra are often included in conventional treatments, the proximal portions in external therapy, and variable lengths in brachytherapy. These regions may experience acute mucosal irritation with frequency and dysuria similar to that in the bladder; this irritation tends to be mild and responds to conservative or non-specific measures. The treatment field for definitive radiotherapy of vulvovaginal carcinomas often includes the entire length of the urethra, as the field "spills" onto the perineal surface. Acute reactions, including edema, may persist for two to three weeks. During and immediately after brachytherapy procedures, the urethra and periurethral tissues may exhibit significant sequelae, since they are in such close proximity to the active sources. Attention to treatment detail can minimize focal overdoses in some cases, although high dose therapy must often be delivered to this area if curative intent is to be realized.

Fortunately, the urethra and submucosal supportive tissues repair RT damage like the ureter. Over the course of time local endarteritis, fibrosis and scarring will occur, the so-called periurethral fibrosis. The urethral lining may atrophy and become thin, mostly without overt functional deficit. If symptoms are present, the patient may complain of frequency, dysuria especially on starting micturition, occasional incontinence and a decrease in the urine flow. Physical examination may reveal areas of vaginal necrosis that are due to persistent or recurrent tumor; they are less likely to be the effect of radiation alone. There may be surrounding induration, pigment changes or telangiectasias, notably on the anterior vaginal surface. Biopsy is essential to differentiate tumor from necrosis, although the risk of fistula formation is always present. Urinalysis may help identify coexistent infection, which can be managed with antibiotics. If a diagnosis of urethral stricture or stenosis is strongly suggested because of intensive radiation doses given to that region, a urethrogram and voiding cystourethrogram can help define the anatomic relationships and determine the patency of the urethral canal. These procedures can also demonstrate potential fistulous tracts. Cystoscopy with directed biopsies may be required for pathologic assessment of areas of stenosis. The urethral dilatation that precedes visualization will often improve a benign obstruction to flow. Scant literature exists on the impact of stress incontinence.

The possible consequences of high dose radiotherapy include urethral stricture or ulceration, with its natural progression toward necrosis and subsequent fistula formation. These problems have been sporadically reported in the literature, but methods used for the management of ureteral and bladder complications often apply here. Most centers that treat large numbers of patients with vulvovaginal cancers report that complications, when present, occur primarily in those receiving combined external beam and brachytherapy programs, usually when vaginal doses have exceeded 8000 to 10,000 cGy (Prempree, 1982; Marcus et al, 1978; Boronow, 1982; Perez and Camel, 1982).

Generally speaking, urethral tolerance to high dose radiation remains quite high; most often mild and sometimes symptomatic stricture may result. Vaginal necrosis or ulceration, usually treated with hydrogen peroxide douches, may increase the subsequent development of a urethrovaginal fistula, especially in locally advanced disease (high volume of tumor that may become necrotic under therapy and leave a void in supportive tissues), or in anterior lesions to which high doses are necessarily delivered.

GASTROINTESTINAL TRACT COMPLICATIONS

General Considerations

The gastrointestinal regions at risk during definitive radiotherapy of gynecologic malignancies include the stomach, small and large intestines, rectum and, rarely, anal canal. Historically, intestinal damage was first reported soon after ionizing radiations were discovered; clinical abnormalities were being reported by the 1920's. Although the small intestine appears to be the most sensitive, earlier series of investigations, through the 1950's, focused on the complications of high dose intracavitary radium in the rectosigmoid region; included were reports of "pseudocarcinoma" and radiographic manifestations of rectal stricture, e.g., "hourglass" or "apple core" lesions. With the use of supervoltage radiation over the last 3 decades, a shift to greater skin sparing and increased depth dose characteristics has occurred and has allowed for improvements in dose distribution to the pelvic lymphatics and gynecologic organs; necessarily, gastrointestinal structures were targeted as well. Contemporary gastrointestinal sequelae are related to high dose external beam therapy alone or in combination with local brachytherapy programs. With heightened understanding of the mechanisms responsible for morbidity, emphasis has shifted to optimization of treatment approaches. Whether RT is used definitively or adjunctively, pretreatment identification of groups at increased risk (thin habitus, advanced age, prior surgery, inflammatory conditions, concurrent vascular diseases, or altered anatomy) allows a more rational use of potential prevention techniques during treatment. For a general discussion of these techniques, refer to the previous section on urinary tract complications.

Rubin and Cassaret (1968), Fajardo (1982) and Roswit and co-workers (1972) report that radiosensitivity decreases as follows: duodenum > jejunum > ileum > transverse colon > sigmoid > rectum. In 5% of patients, injury in the proximal region occurs at 4500 to 5000 cGy, and a dose of over 6000 cGy causes injury in the distal regions. A thicker walled, hollow viscus with a slower mucosal turnover rate can handle fractionated radiation with less morbidity and exhibit greater structural/functional reserve. Another crucial factor is the relatively fixed GI anatomic position of the gastrointestinal system (de novo or iatrogenic), which results in repeated daily exposures. Superimposed on these differences is individual sensitivity, such that a continuum of damage can exist for the same dose. Unquestionably, the dose per fraction (< or > 200 cGy), total dose (up to 10% reduction if standard therapy is poorly tolerated or if the patient is elderly) and total volume of tissue radiated are interrelated. As more aggressive therapeutic programs now include para-aortic or whole abdominal techniques, there is a trend toward pretreatment assessment of bowel immobility, percentage of volume irradiated and technique of delivery (four versus two fields, custom-designed portals, abdominal bath versus moving strip). Methods have focused on reducing the percentage of mobile bowel by placing the patient in the prone posture or in the Trendelenburg position, distending the bladder or, if feasible, surgically displacing structures out of pelvic portals. These and other methods are currently being explored and evaluated (see later discussion).

For the use of intracavitary/interstitial radiation therapy techniques, recognition of altered anatomic constraints and geometry created by the tumor or host, coupled with methods to assess doses to rectosigmoid structures (Kagan et al, 1979; Cunningham et al, 1981), has proved beneficial. Improvements include wider use of two intracavitary procedures, attention to dose rates (or ratios) to limiting structures and better knowledge of anatomic variables, which in over two thirds of cases can be predicted and remedied.

Overall gastrointestinal tract sequelae after definitive RT may range from 10 to 15% (Montana et al, 1985; Hanks et al, 1983). Table 14–7 lists the various complications. Grading sys-

Table 14–7. Gastrointestinal Tract Complications after Definitive Radiation for Gynecologic Malignancies*

Organ	Complication
Stomach	Pain and atrophic gastritis Non–acid-related ulceration Gastric outlet obstruction Perforation/hemorrhage

Small Intestine
  Duodenum
  Jejunum
  Ileum
  Associated mesentery
	Malabsorptive phenomena
	  (vitamin B$_{12}$, folate, fat,
	  protein, fluid and
	  electrolyte)
	Enteritis
	Ulceration (focal or segmental)
	  ± hemorrhage
	Obstruction (partial—
	  strictures, stenoses;
	  complete; intrinsic or
	  extrinsic
	Necrosis with fistula, ±
	  perforation ± peritonitis/
	  sepsis

Large Intestine
  Cecum and
    ascending colon
  Transverse colon
  Descending colon
    and sigmoid
  Rectum
	Proctitis, sigmoiditis or colitis
	  ± bleeding
	Focal ulceration
	Stricture or stenosis
	Obstruction
	Fistula ± perforation

Anus	Functional problems (usually
	  related to perianal skin
	  effects)
	Focal ulceration/necrosis

*See text and Table 14–6 for grading systems.

tems have been outlined previously, but one should expect contemporary series to report under 5% serious (grade 3) problems requiring surgical intervention; representative data are: 0.8 to 3.7% (Hanks et al, 1983), 2.4% (Porquier et al, 1982), 3.1% (Hamberger et al, 1983), 4.1% (Einhorn et al, 1985), 5% (Perez et al, 1984) and 7.6% (Montana et al, 1985). Complications, in order of increasing severity, include digestive abnormalities and malabsorption, grades of enteritis, stenosis/stricture or obstruction, perforation and fistula. They range from about 15% to less than 1 to 2%. The 2 to 10 times greater morbidity that is associated with combined surgery and radiation (which creates mechanical fixation and alters vascularity) must be remembered. Studies comparing RT alone with combination approaches that report grade 3 morbidity figures of 5 versus 15% (Rotman et al, 1979) 6 versus 15% (Weems et al, 1985) and 7 versus 21% (Perez et al, 1984) reinforce the notion that unless survival is enhanced, a single modality is preferred.

Complications usually develop in 6 to 24 months, although the risk period in the cured patient may be open-ended, since radiation effects may accelerate aging and other vascular disease states. The differential between recurrence and complications may not be straightforward in the clinical setting; this may be especially true when the disease is initially advanced, when a fistula forms or when evidence of mesenteric border (a common site for transperitoneal tumor spread) abnormalities appear on x-ray films. Documentation of distant disease or local recurrence may heighten suspicion. Judicious use of local biopsy, percutaneous CT-guided aspiration or biopsy or, if necessary, exploration may be indicated to resolve the dilemma.

Discussion of risks for the various regions will proceed from the stomach to the rectum. For further specific information, the reader should refer to the excellent histopathologic analyses of Fajardo (1982) and Rubin and Cassaret (1968); the radiographic studies by Libshitz (1979), Roswit and co-workers (1972). Roswit (1974), Rogers (1981) and Mendelson (1985); and the specific therapeutic interventions described by Wheeless (1981), Boronow (1982) and Smith (1982).

Stomach

The stomach is a peristaltic digestive organ that connects the esophagus to the duodenum. It is composed of an active secreting mucosal layer beneath which is a three-layer, overlapping, smooth muscular coat encased by serosa. The greater curvature attaches to the gastrosplenic ligament and greater omentum, and the lesser curvature attaches to the lesser omentum (hepatogastric ligament), which allows for support for vascular and lymphatic pedicles. The stomach is closely associated with all upper abdominal organs from the diaphragm to the colon at the pelvic brim. An arterial network from the celiac axis, with associated parallel lymphatics and corresponding venous drainage to the portal vein, straddles the stomach; innervation is primarily by the vagal and thoracic splanchnic nerves. The anatomic location of the stomach is from the level of T10 to L4, with restricted motion at the gastroesophageal junction and pylorus; fluoroscopy nicely demonstrates the mobility of the stomach and omentum inferiorly, toward the pelvis. Motion occurs with position changes (gravity) and in post-prandial states, especially in non-operated patients and thin elderly females. The cardiac (T10) pyloric and antral (T12 to L1) portions lie in the midline and are thus treated in para-aortic portals. The proliferative zone of mucosa in the isthmus of the glands and the base of the gastric pits is renewed at two- to six-day intervals, with acid and intrinsic factor parietal cells (body and fundus), pepsinogen chief cells (antrum) and mucous cells undergoing a slower turnover rate (Fajardo, 1982).

Because of these factors, one can anticipate acute and chronic sequelae from RT in the upper abdomen, either from whole abdominal therapy or from para-aortic lymphatic fields above L2 (note that high dose booster fields often employ AP/PA ports in addition to rotational or oblique techniques). The stomach is classified as a moderately radiosensitive organ; little long-term morbidity results from the use of fractionated doses of under 4500 cGy (Roswit et al, 1972; Jampolis et al, 1977; Potish et al, 1983), but morbidity rapidly escalates to about 50% when a dose of over 6000 cGy is given. As early as 1919, studies showed that doses under 2000 cGy often produced permanent reductions in acid and pepsinogen secretion in the absence of mucosal changes. With therapeutic doses, patchy edema, hemorrhage and exudates, which may heal incompletely and lead to chronic mucosal gland cell atrophy, telangiectasias, superficial erosions and vascular sclerosis, are seen. Acute changes in the muscular coat are absent; however, chronic atrophy, fibrosis, hyalinized arterioles, atypical fibroblasts and scarring occur, although less prominently than on the surfaces. Decreased gastric capacity can result. The interstitial fibrosis may involve nerve fibers or ganglia, which may affect peristalsis. Generally, these lesions remain subclinical, but, depending on the dose delivered to a relatively non-mobile or fixed structure, decreasing incidences of erosion (gastritis), focal ulceration (usually antral), hemorrhage (rupture of telangiectatic submucosal vessels in an ulcer crater or denuded atrophic mucosa) or, rarely, transmural perforation have been described. As opposed to the distal intestine, no clear effect of hypertension, diabetes or previous peptic ulcer has been implicated in increasing the probability of complications in the stomach.

Clinically, patients with gastric radiation effects typically present with slowly progressive upper abdominal pain or burning that is persistent and unrelated to meals. A more fulminant course may include anorexia with nausea and emesis (gastric outlet obstruction), weight loss and, rarely, hematemesis or perforation with peritonitis. The results of the physical examination may be within normal limits or may demonstrate epigastric tenderness, a palpable mass or peritoneal signs. After baseline tests, an upper gastrointestinal x-ray study with follow-through, with either dilute barium or Gastrografin or infusional methods, may disclose one of two common patterns (Rogers, 1981): either a solitary prepyloric or antral ulcer, 0.5 to 2 cm in diameter, usually on the posterior wall similar to the site of peptic ulcer, or a narrowed, deformed antral region without ulcer, which may mimic neoplasia. On fluoroscopic examination, there appears to be greater rigidity of the distal stomach, little peristaltic activity with variable smooth or irregularly thickened or effaced mucosal folds. Extrinsic abnormalities such as encasement by fibrosis or tumor can also be suspected. Associated duodenal narrowing may be present. Endoscopy, performed after the acute treatment period, may delineate a pale lining with fragile vessels, areas of atrophy or ulceration or extrinsic compression. Brush or biopsy specimens of suspicious areas can be examined. Gastric analysis may reveal a neutral pH, similar to that occurring in pernicious anemia. If stricture or focal narrowing is present, selective gentle dilatation can be attempted.

Management is a function of symptom severity. Since these ulcers are not acid related, unless they are due to hypersecretion in non-treated regions, they will not respond well to antacids, Cimetidine/Ranitidine, or cytoprotective agents, although these are often tried as first line therapy. A small number of ulcers may heal with the use of analgesics or antispasmodic or anticholinergic agents. Some authors have employed metaclopromide with success, mostly for the treatment of altered gastric motility. Unfortunately, many lesions may be slowly progressive and cause persistent pain; eventually, partial gastrectomy is required for adequate palliation. However, the anastomosis must be made in regions of otherwise normal, unirradiated bowel. More catastrophic events, such as hemorrhage, acute gastric outlet obstruction and perforation, should be swiftly managed with surgical intervention by those familiar with operating in irradiated fields. Better delineation of indications for treatment portals and the use of radioprotector agents may further alter the appearance and morbidity of gastric radiation.

Small Intestine

ANATOMIC AND PHYSIOLOGIC BACKGROUND

Though the small intestine is generally thought to be a mobile abdominal structure, the probability of radiation damage can be correlated with anatomic and physiologic properties. Acute effects have been covered previously. Of particular note in respect to chronic injury are mobility constraints: the duodenum and upper jejunum at the ligament of Treitz and the ileocecal region maintain relatively fixed positions, whereas the remaining small bowel can roam on its mesenteric pedicles in the abdominal cavity. For a given field size, fixed intestine, in both the prone and supine postures, is more likely then mobile intestine to receive full radiation doses during a course of external beam therapy. The area that most frequently shows clinical damage is terminal ileum. However, Roswit and co-workers (1972) note that sensitivity declines from the duodenum distally; consequently, the relatively infrequent treatment to the upper abdomen accounts for the uncommonly low incidence of injury to the upper small bowel. Dynamic free movement of bowel loops within the pelvic confines can be altered. Green (1975, 1983) demonstrated that 15% less volume was encompassed in the inferior peritoneal space and pelvis while one is prone, with over 50% of the volume showing upward displacement. The other major threat to small intestinal mobility is previous surgery or adhesions, with 65% of surgical cases, as compared with 18% of non-surgical cases, showing bowel fixed in the pelvis. Along with other risk factors and intrinsic sensitivity, this underscores the "innocent bystander" or "moving target" notions important in the development of injury when the patient undergoes daily radiation, as clear abscopal effects have not been documented.

Anatomically, the C-shaped, 25 cm long duodenum is nestled in the upper abdomen; it courses from the pylorus at the L1 level inferiorly along the right lumbar pedicles to L3 or L4, horizontally and slightly cephalad across L4, and finally it ascends to the paravertebral L2 region where it joins the jejunum. Covered by peritoneum and in proximity to all upper abdominal viscera, it is suspended along with the jejunum at the ligament of Treitz. This hollow viscus includes villi supported on submucosal circular projections (plicae). The 2.4 m jejunum begins at L2, has variable support from the dorsal body wall by reason of the mesentery and has a larger diameter with a thicker wall and more vascularity than the ileum. The 3.6 m ileum is thinner, has a smaller and shorter arcading arterial supply, is encased by more fat in the mesentery and contains Peyer's patches in the antimesenteric border. Perhaps 50% of this structure lies in the pelvis because of gravity or mechanical factors. The ileum terminates at the fixed ileocecal region in the right iliac fossa above the inguinal ligament. The various physiologic roles are too extensive to be reviewed here.

Histologically, the proliferative zone resides in the crypts of Lieberkühn, where tritiated thymidine studies show that cell division occurs every 24 hours in the undifferentiated cell pool and mucous glands. These cells undergo a series of divisions, differentiate, mature and migrate upward until they are extruded into the lumen; in steady states, the exfoliation rate equals the replication rate. Only endocrine cells migrate, and Paneth cells (granular secretory cells in glands) neither migrate nor mature (Fajardo, 1982; Rubin and Cassaret, 1968). Thus the mucosal turnover rate is three to six days, and the mucosa is predictably sensitive to acute radiation; however, if the radiation dose is fractionated, the surface integrity can be maintained. Significant stem cell depletion can translate into primary long-term parenchymal cell loss with subclinical dysfunction. The submucosal and mesenchymal tissues, smooth muscle and serosal tissues may display more permanent and progressive changes. Underlying vascular diseases, mechanical factors, inflammatory pelvic disorders, thin or obese habitus, age over 50, chemotherapy or radiation sensitizers may alter the tempo and clinical expression of damage.

RADIATION PORTS AND DOSE

Definitive radiotherapy ports for gynecologic malignancies with local extension or pelvic and para-aortic lymph drainage will necessarily cover all or a large part of the small intestine. Para-aortic fields up to L2 or L3 can be expected to cover the horizontal duodenum and varying amounts of jejunum and ileum. Classic, superiorly bordered pelvic fields up to L4 or L5 can encompass over 50% of the small intestine, unless methods to exclude it are undertaken. The volumes involved can be estimated by pretreatment opacification under fluoroscopic observation. Although the results are subject to host, volume and non-conventional treatment factors, most studies show that chronic clinical sequelae rise sharply with doses from 4500 to 6000 cGy. A 6000 cGy dose of external beam therapy delivered to the pelvis has a morbidity of 25 to 50%. Thus, a slim therapeutic window exists when cancericidal doses are given by external therapy, even in combination with intracavitary insertions, which can contribute high doses to the terminal ileum. With cautious treatment planning, serious sequelae occur in under 3% of cases.

PATHOLOGIC CHANGES FOLLOWING RADIATION

According to most histopathologists, the changes of progressive enteritis are variable, are pervasive, often show disparity with clinical or radiologic findings and are influenced by a non-quantifiable degree of individual sensitivity. The interval after radiation treatment is important; inflammation and edema occur earlier, and more fibrotic manifestations occur later. Irradiated bowel tends to appear mottled with pale red to gray peritoneal roughening and fibrinous deposits. The mesenteric fat is less prominent, thickened and shortened. The bowel itself may be narrowed in either long or short segments with gross induration in all layers. Inspection may show a pale mucosa with atrophy or frequent, focal shallow ulcers that may extend through the serosa as subclinical perforations with adhesions. Microscopically, villi are blunt with decreased surface areas, mucosal ulcers and inflammatory cells. The lamina propria and submucosa display the most progressive long-term changes; collagen replaces loose areolar tissues, and radiation fibroblasts, telangiectatic vessels, atrophic lymphatics and fibrosis of nerve fibers and ganglia are found. Perhaps the crucial radiopathologic finding is arteriolar obliterative endarteritis with recanalized fibrin thrombi. With time, worsening ischemia (like an accelerating aging process) may impede circulation and add its effects to those of underlying systemic illness, giving rise to a compromised splanchnic circulation. The muscularis is often thickened, somewhat fibrotic and distorted. Finally, the serosa, although thickened, may show fresh fibrin deposits years after radiation. The potential functional and anatomic side-effects from ionizing radiation are predictable based on dose and volumes. The appearance, texture and known functional compromise should also serve as a caution to the surgeon operating in the radiated abdomen or pelvis.

CLINICAL FINDINGS AND MALABSORPTION

Clinical manifestations of radiation effect range from those that are entirely asymptomatic to those of varying grades of enteritis, and those with overt, potentially catastrophic, complications requiring prompt surgical attention. Grading systems for injury have been outlined elsewhere. Chronic effects are not usually correlated with acute effects, though the former may coexist. The majority (75%) present within 6 to 24 months of treatment with earlier peak than for urinary problems, though sequelae may be observed over a long period as well (Boronow, 1982; Smith, 1982).

Duodenal side-effects present a similar clinical picture to those of the stomach, occurring with the use of para-aortic ports in the L1 to L4 region, and with doses in excess of 4500 cGy. Radiologic manifestations of ulcer, stricture or obstruction can be identified, especially in the second and third portions. Management options for the stomach apply.

The incidence of complications in the jejunum and partiularly in the ileum is 0.6 to 17% when fractionated total doses of over 4500 cGy are used; marked escalation in the complication rate occurs with whole pelvic doses of 5000 to 6000 cGy (Chau et al, 1962; Rogers, 1981). Also, one must not forget the contribution from intracavitary applications that occurs with the use of uterine tandem or Simon-Heyman capsules, which may deliver various amounts of radiation to the ileum, that often goes unrecognized in conventional treatment planning (Green, 1975; 1983). More recently, Gallagher and co-workers (1985) have shown a clear correlation between the pelvic small bowel volume, the total radiation dose and gastrointestinal toxicity. Once again, the patient's postoperative state, thin habitus, and combined pelvic and perineal procedures were important risk factors. With the use of sophisticated techniques, approximately 10% of patients will develop long-term overall side-effects; 2 to 3% of these will be of grade three toxicity.

The first major subdivision of injury includes patients who present with altered bowel peristalsis, degrees of loose stools (rarely bloody, but sometimes with steatorrhea), crampy pains, nausea and emesis. Malabsorption with anorexia, weight loss and dehydration may develop insidiously. Chronic mucosal atrophy, with the loss of functional enzymatic brush border activity and surface area, and altered reabsorption of nutrients can be found. Submucosal ischemia and fibrosis will be present. Symptoms may suggest regional enteritis, inflammatory or infectious conditions with diarrhea, or protein and bile salt or electrolyte losses. The results of the examination may be negative or palpable bowel loops and hyperperistalsis may be noted. A complete blood count may show anemia or an elevated mean corpuscular volume MCV. Long-term follow-up data by Lantz and Einhorn (1984) demonstrated low folate and vitamin B_{12} levels in 22% and 13%, respectively, by means of serum levels and Shilling's test. Fecal fat, protein, and bile salt analyses and D-xylose absorption studies can provide evidence of specific functional losses.

Radiographic findings will be reviewed below, but must exclude stasis, which may provide a nidus for bacterial overgrowth. Treatment varies with the level of dysfunction. The patient with occasional sporadic episodes should receive dietary counseling, and certain foods that exacerbate the bowel symptoms (i.e., bulk formers, caffeine and other stimulants and, on occasion, dairy products or those with high fat contents) should be restricted. Diphenoxylate or loperamide, given as needed, usually suffices, although a trial of clidinium bromide with chlordiazepoxide (Librax) may be useful. With more severe forms, consultation with a gastroenterologist versed in radiation-induced pathology should be obtained, so that intervention in the replacement of lost nutrients and medical stabilization of this enteropathy can be provided; vitamin B_{12}, folate, fluids, electrolytes and medium chain triglycerides may have to be supplied, and even total parenteral nutritional support may be indicated. If indicated, use of cholestyramine may limit bile salt sequelae and the secretory effects of bile on the colonic lining. Only in stasis caused by stricture and bacterial overgrowth that is unresponsive to broad spectrum antibiotics should surgical resection be entertained. If frank, persistent hematochezia that results from superficial ulcerations and vessel exposure does not resolve with conservative therapy, attempts at radionuclide or angiographic localization and selective embolization or resection should be considered.

INTESTINAL OBSTRUCTION

Partial (random focal or patchy strictures) or complete obstruction usually occurs in the mid to distal ileum. Two types are noted: (1) an intrinsic lesion, secondary to marked ischemic fibrosis, edema and thickening of the submucosal region with defunctionalized areas and a lack of normal motility, that causes mechanical obstruction; and (2) an extrinsic process, notably adhesions, that causes compression of bowel loops and blocks flow. Adhesions are rare in the absence of prior surgery, but previous operative manipulation will heighten the response to injury. Thus postoperative patients may have both problems superimposed on varying degrees of malabsorption. The incidence is less than 3% (Van Nagell et al, 1974; Swan et al, 1976). Although initially subacute, symptoms of pain, nausea, vomiting, obstipation and distension may rapidly progress to the familiar signs of acute bowel obstruction. One must be aware, however, that after pelvic radiation not all of the typical physical findings may be identified.

Once obstruction is diagnosed clinically, the patient should be hospitalized, placed on complete bowel rest and given intravenous fluids and nutrients, and pertinent investigations should be performed. Supine, upright and decubitus films may reveal air fluid levels, isolated loops with dilatation and staircase patterns and, potentially, free air. Bowel studies with either dilute barium or Gastrografin, if feasible, should be used to determine the cause of the obstruction. Underlying submucosal fibrosis, edema and ischemic effects can be visualized. X-ray signs include straightening and thickening of the valvulae conniventes, luminal narrowing and mural thickening of adjacent loops (> 2 mm), short segmental stenoses or long smooth strictures, nodal filling defects and thumbprinting, absence of mucosal pattern with barium pooling and sinus or fistula formation. Mucosal tacking and constant angulation of bowel loops increase the likelihood of adhesions. With experience, these findings can be distinguished from primary mucosal diseases such as inflammatory or infectious conditions or neoplasia. Mesenteric changes, consisting of adhesions and retraction with fixed, matted loops, are often noted. When viewed fluoroscopically, a pulling effect on the adjacent bowel with abnormal peristalsis can often mimic neoplasia. A mesenteric angiogram discloses tortuous, crowded and distorted vessels. It should be emphasized that many patients will also have changes in the colon or urinary tract, so supplementary studies will be necessary.

Management depends on the type of obstruction, partial or complete, simple or strangulating (see Chapter 4). When the obstruction may be related to radiation changes, except in cases of strangulation, most authors advocate a trial of bowel decompression using a long nasointestinal (Cantor) tube, hoping that motility is sufficient to permit the tube to advance past narrowed regions. If this conservative approach alleviates the symptoms and function returns, a medical regimen of an advancing low residue diet, psyllium mucilloid and, occasionally, anticholinergic or antispasmodic medication. Response to conservative measures is often temporary, and repeated episodes tend to culminate in surgical therapy.

Indications for surgery include repeated partial obstruction that does not respond to conservative measures, partial obstruction when the dose of pelvic radiation has been over 6500 cGy or complete obstruction with life-threatening symptoms (Smith, 1982). Three groups of radiation enteritis were described by Haddad and co-workers (1983): group 1, medical therapy for symptomatic relief; group 2, acute, life-threatening symptoms; group 3, long-standing intermittent obstruction or fistula. Only in the case of acute, life-threatening symptoms (group 2) should an operation be undertaken emergently, with acceptance of the attending acute morbidity and potential mortality. Neomycin and an erythromycin base should be used to clean the intestinal tract and to reduce the bacterial population before surgery and broad spectrum antibiotics should be given perioperatively.

Those patients coming to surgery should, if practical, have all medical parameters optimized prior to the planned procedure. Central venous total parenteral nutrition is important in reversing nutritional deficits (See Chapter 2). The surgical procedures recommended for the treatment of obstruction are, in part, functions of the training and perspective of the surgeon. Abdominal surgeons may favor resection over bypass, drawing an analogy to inflammatory bowel disease processes; conversely, many gynecologic oncologists favor bypass procedures with minimal operative manipulation. Qualified oncologic surgeons, versed in the nuances of the malignancy and its radiation treatment and expert in handling irradiated tissues, should be sought. In general, there is no substitute for choosing the simplest procedure that will relieve the injury. With significant, actual pathologic intestinal damage, a systematic approach that provides adequate exposure should be taken; cautious, meticulous handling of the often friable and thickened viscera is necessary. Lysis of adhesions and dissection should be limited. Necrotic intestine with fistula or perforation must be recognized, and the problem should be corrected.

Surgical options are described in Chapter 4, and techniques are described in Chapter 3.

Excision of isolated segments of diseased intestine may be appropriate (Lillemoe et al, 1983), but simple bypass procedures are indicated when widespread changes are evident. Regardless of the approach, surgical manipulation should be minimized.

After the operation, bowel decompression, hyperalimentation, antibiotics and stress ulcer prophylaxis should be maintained until the patient's clinical course improves. Postoperative morbidity and mortality are generally higher following anastomoses than after bypass procedures; morbidity includes dehiscence and leakage with intestinal dysfunction (Swan et al, 1976; Boronow, 1982; Lillemoe et al, 1983). Although management may be complicated, once the perioperative period passes, the patient can be offered significant long-term problem-free palliation. Close observation for a second gastrointestinal or urinary tract problem is essential, as repeated surgery further exacerbates the complications induced by devascularization and adhesions, up to 25% in one recent series (Perez et al, 1984).

FISTULA

A small intestinal fistula may show no clinical signs and be found at surgery, or it may produce symptoms related to adjoining organs. The types of intestinal fistula are illustrated in Figure 4–6. Fistulas may also involve the bladder and, rarely, the uterus, and multiple fistulas may occur. The differential diagnosis between fistulas of the small intestine and vagina and those of the large intestine can often be made on the basis of clinical signs. The ileum-related discharge is watery yellow and alkaline, producing excoriation and vulvar pain. The management of fistulas is covered earlier in this chapter and in Chapter 4.

Large Intestine and Rectosigmoid

GENERAL CONSIDERATIONS

Significant radiation changes in the colon, especially the rectosigmoid region, were more common through the 1950's, as noted previously. With current technologic advances, high dose radiation from either external beam therapy or brachytherapy can produce pathologic changes in the cecum, transverse colon (in para-aortic RT) and rectosigmoid (most common). These regions may routinely receive doses of over 4500 to 5000 cGy. Since there is less mobility of the large bowel, there is a greater opportunity for direct, repeated, daily exposure of the same anatomic region.

The large intestine is 1.5 m in length; anatomically, it is divided into segments based on position within the abdomen. The cecum lies beyond the ileocecal valve in the right iliac fossa in front and on the right side of the sacrum; although distensible, it remains relatively fixed. It joins the ascending colon and follows a course lateral to the right kidney until it abruptly angles (at the hepatic flexure) into the mobile transverse colon. The transverse colon crosses the umbilical zone; it is invested in peritoneum and suspended from the posterior body wall by a mesocolon at about the L2 to L4 level. From the splenic flexure, the descending colon runs lateral to the left kidney in a groove between the psoas and quadratus muscles into the left iliac fossa. The peritoneum-covered sigmoid with its mesocolon begins at the pelvic brim, crosses the sacrum and curves to the midline at S3, where it becomes the rectum. Grossly, the colon is distinguished by its taeniae, three longitudinal smooth muscle bands and epiploic appendages. Finally, the 12 cm rectum extends from the level of S3 to slightly below the coccyx, curving anteriorly to the right and then the left, where it terminates at the anus. Characteristic of the rectum are Houston's valves (rectal folds) with a complete outer longitudinal muscle coat.

Though similar histologically to small bowel, the active proliferative zone forms a higher proportion of the crypts with a slightly slower turnover of four to eight days. There is a smaller active cell cycle population, and because no villi are present, fewer cells/cm³ are at risk. The remaining layers experience similar radiation tolerance. These qualities make the colorectal region less susceptible to injury than the small intestine; tolerance increases from the transverse colon to the sigmoid to the rectum. Clinical manifestations of injury may reach 18% with doses of 5000 to 6000 cGy, and upward of one in three patients will show injury with doses of over 6000 cGy in conventional fractions (Roswit et al, 1972). The rectum commonly tolerates 5500 to 6000 cGy without incident. Above this, at 7000 to 8000 cGy, complications may rapidly escalate. These effects do not reflect varying contributions from external high dose rate fractionated radiation versus low dose rate intracavitary treatment; however, as early as 1961, Kottmeier and Gray stated that the maximal tolerable dose from intracavitary therapy should not exceed 2400 cGy/24 hours, nor should doses in excess of 5000 cGy be given to

the whole pelvis if complication rates are to remain small.

After therapeutic doses of radiation, mucosal alterations include crypt abscesses containing eosinophils (up to 3 months afterwards) and varying degrees of atrophy, goblet cell hyperplasia and superficial ulceration. Telangiectasias, hyaline fibrosis and edema may predispose to stricture formation. Obliterative endarteritis with ischemia may lead to late tissue necrosis, ulceration, fistula formation and perforation. As a result, in commonly treated gynecologic malignancies, the area that receives the highest dose and is most prone to injury is the rectosigmoid, which has an incidence of complications of 5 to 10%; complications consist of ulcer, bleeding, stenosis and, on occasion, fistulas.

PROCTO-SIGMOIDITIS

DeCosse and co-workers (1969), Chau and co-workers (1962), Villasanta (1972) and others describe procto-sigmoiditis, which usually appears 6 to 12 months after RT. It presents with tenesmus, mucus and blood admixed with stool and occasional constipation with decreased caliber of stool and a sensation of rectal fullness. Symptoms may be mild or prominent and often are self-limiting. A proctosigmoidoscopic examination may identify mucosal granularity, friability and telangiectasias with superficial ulceration throughout, although the anterior wall may show the most severe changes. A barium study usually shows spasm, smooth, thickened bowel and a narrowed rectal lumen. Management is conservative, as the great majority of cases resolve with time, and do not progress to ulceration. Methods to decrease mechanical abrasion of the lumen include prescription of low residue diets and mild sedation and judicious use of stool softeners, including psyllium mucocolloid or Colace, antispasmodic agents, cortisone enemas and sulfa drugs such as sulfasalazine (Azulfidine) in doses of 500 mg two to four times a day.

BLEEDING

In some patients, significant rectal bleeding will appear later, and be unresponsive to conservative measures. This is due more to a field effect than to a discrete ulcer crater. Wheeless (1981) notes that many patients with chronic bleeding received over 30 units of blood during the years prior to surgical intervention. In this rare case, mesenteric angiography can identify bleeding vessels in the rectosigmoid, and these can now be embolized successfully. Another option with a high success rate is a diverting colostomy, which can be closed six months later, after the hemorrhage resolves and rectal integrity has been restored.

ULCERATION

Symptoms of rectal ulceration usually appear 4 to 12 months after therapy, most commonly in those patients whose treatment had a large component of intracavitary therapy. These ulcers may be multiple or discrete. They are usually 4 cm in size and, typically, are located on the anterior rectal wall, transversely oriented at about 8 cm from the anus, which corresponds to the high dose region of the posterior vaginal fornix. These lesions appear against a gray, often telangiectatic, background as yellow, necrotic-based ulcers with flattened edges. Given the time course and the clinical situation, biopsy is not warranted, and management is conservative as in proctitis. Resolution can be demonstrated over time with serial proctoscopic examinations. These ulcers are not generally precursors of rectovaginal fistulas, unless persistent tumor exists or there is predisposing vaginal necrosis (DeCosse et al, 1969). Strockbine and co-workers (1970), Lee and co-workers (1976) and others have shown that the occurrence of many ulcers (over 70 to 80%) is predictable because of anatomic variation, a narrow vagina, or a radiation source that had been "hanging" or protruding into the vagina. Only in cases of very deep ulceration and necrosis with impending perforation should surgical management be considered.

STENOSIS AND STRICTURE

Significant stenoses or strictures that lead to partial obstruction occur less often in the rectosigmoid than in the small intestine. They may be the result of focally high doses to the rectosigmoid (e.g., at 12 cm from the anus, where the uterine tandem may deviate to the left). Rigid bowel with adhesions can also be implicated. Signs and symptoms are pain, rectal discharge and constipation or diarrhea. Radiologic studies show thickening and straightening of mucosal folds, submucosal thumbprinting, edema and hourglass, pipestem or apple core lesions that mimic carcinoma. A useful diagnostic clue can be the presence of a smooth,

elongated narrowing with elevation out of the pelvis and increased distance in the presacral space. Management depends on the time of the appearance of symptoms and the degree of luminal obstruction. Temporary relief by the use of mineral oil or manual dilatation in low anorectal strictures has been tried with some success. More frequently, the patient may come to permanent end colostomy, using the sigmoid if it was not significantly radiated or, more often, a left transverse colostomy outside the treatment portal. Some authors advocate permanent closure of the distal sigmoid (Hartmann's pouch).

FISTULA

Fistulas related to the rectum and sigmoid occur in less than 1 to 2% of patients in most series and are more common in previously operated patients. Symptoms of feculent vaginal discharge and direct or proctoscopic identification of a fistulous tract with anterior rectal wall necrosis confirm the diagnosis. As Graham (1965) noted, distinguishing tumor recurrence from complication is difficult and may require biopsy, but tumor tends to be nodular as opposed to the smooth, woody texture characteristic of radiation change. Treatment must be individualized; attention should be paid to the patient's overall medical condition and diversion of the fecal stream. A transverse colostomy is preferable, as it is outside the heavily irradiated region and dissection of the sigmoid region may be fraught with potential enterotomies and adhesions, especially if there are loculated abscesses or local peritonitis. If eventual closure of the fistula is anticipated, which may occur in 20 to 75% of cases (Wheeless, 1981; Graham, 1965), a double-barreled colostomy is advisable. Other patients may wish to accept permanent colostomy as long as the fistulous tract is not likely to heal. Coexistent vaginal necrosis and irritation are usually treated with hydrogen peroxide or Betadine douches, along with perineal soaks and analgesia. Once the acute problem has been resolved, vigilance must be maintained for additional complications.

SUMMARY

The objective of the preceding chapter has been to provide a framework for the understanding of complications sustained as a result of definitive radiotherapy for gynecologic malignancies. A logical, systematic approach based on host, tumor and treatment variables should allow one to: (1) improve patient selection for various therapeutic options; (2) predict and consequently prevent complications, based on known relationships within and outside fields of radiation; (3) recognize the clinical presentation of complications at the bedside; (4) understand the pathophysiologic changes that radiation produces in tissues, their probability of clinical expression, and differential diagnosis; and (5) develop some general guidelines for the management of the individual patient with a complication. As reiterated throughout, collaborative effort between gyncologic and radiation oncologists and practitioners of other disciplines should be fostered to offer the best care for such an individual. Continual support, both physical and emotional, for the cured patient with a radiation-related injury cannot be overemphasized. As new technology, especially more widespread use of chemoradiotherapy, implantation techniques, radiation protectors/sensitizers/modifiers, particle radiation, hyperthermia, intraoperative electron beam therapy and altered fraction schemes, moves into clinical use, critical analysis—using knowledge based on the pathophysiologic mechanisms of radiation changes—of efficacy with minimal attendant morbidity is essential. It is hoped that further advances will recognize and eliminate the iatrogenic complications and reactions that are under direct control of the therapist, refine risk assessments and optimize therapeutic measures for those patients with radiation-related injury.

REFERENCES

Behnam K, Path UB, Mariano, E: Intravesical instillation of formalin for hemorrhagic cystitis secondary to radiation for gynecologic malignancies. *Gynecol. Oncol.* 16:31,1983.

Boronow RC: Urologic complications secondary to radiation alone or radiation and surgery. In Delgado G, Smith JP (Eds.): *Management of Complications in Gynecologic Oncology*. New York, John Wiley and Sons, 1982.

Boronow RC: Management of radiation-induced vaginal fistulas. *Am. J. Obstet. Gynecol.* 110:1,1971.

Boronow RC, Rutledge F: Vesicovaginal fistula, radiation and gynecologic cancer. *Am. J. Obstet. Gynecol.* 111:85,1971.

Bosch A, Frias Z: Complications after radiation therapy for cervical carcinoma. *Acta Radiol. Ther. Phys. Biol.* 16:53, 1977.

Bourne RG, Kearsley JH et al: The relationship between early and late gastrointestinal complications of radiation therapy for carcinoma of the cervix. *Int. J. Radiat. Oncol. Biol. Phys.* 9:1445, 1983.

Bricker EM: Current status of urinary diversion. *Cancer* 45:2986, 1980.

Buchler DA, Kline JC et al: Radiation reactions in cervical cancer therapy. *Am. J. Obstet. Gynecol.* 111:745, 1971.

Butcher HR, Sugg WL et al: Ileal conduit method of ureteral urinary diversion. *Ann. Surg.* 156:682, 1962.

Chau PM, Fletcher GH et al: Complications in high dose whole pelvic irradiation in female pelvic cancer. *Am. J. Roentgenol. Radium Ther. Nucl. Med.* 87:22,1962.

Cunningham DE, Stryker JA et al: Routine clinical estimation of rectal, rectosigmoidal, and bladder doses from intracavitary brachytherapy in the treatment of carcinoma of the cervix. *Int. J. Radiat. Oncol. Biol. Phys.* 7:653,1981.

DeCosse JJ, Rhodes RS et al: The natural history and management of radiation induced injury of the gastrointestinal tract. *Ann. Surg.* 170:369, 1969.

DeLuca FR, Ragins H: Construction of an omental envelope as a method of excluding the small intestine from the field of postoperative irradiation to the pelvis. *Surg. Gynecol. Obstet.* 160:365, 1985.

Einhorn N, Patek E et al: Outcome of different treatment modalities in cervix carcinoma Stage IB and IIA. *Cancer* 55:949, 1985.

Ellis F: Tolerance of normal tissues and tumors to radiation. *Front. Radiat. Ther. Oncol.* 12:101, 1978.

Fajardo LF: *Pathology of Radiation Injury*. New York: Masson Publishing USA, Inc., 1982.

Fletcher GH: *Textbook of Radiotherapy*. Philadelphia: Lea & Febiger, 1980.

Gallagher MT, Brereton HD et al: A prospective study of 150 patients receiving pelvic irradiation correlating acute and late effects with dose of irradiation and volume of small bowel. *Int. J. Radiat. Oncol. Biol. Phys.* 11(1S):118, 1985.

Graham JB: Vaginal fistulas following radiotherapy. *Surg. Gynecol. Obstet.* 120:1019, 1965.

Green N, The avoidance of small intestine injury in gynecologic cancer. *Int. J. Radiat. Oncol. Biol. Phys.* 9:1385, 1983.

Green N, Iba G et al: Measures to minimize small intestine injury in the irradiated pelvis. *Cancer* 35:1633, 1975.

Green TH: Urologic complications of radical pelvic surgery and radiation therapy. In Coppleson M (Ed.): *Gynecologic Oncology: Fundamental Principles and Clinical Practice*. New York, Churchill Livingstone, 1981.

Haddad GK, Grodsinksy C et al: The spectrum of radiation enteritis: surgical considerations. *Dis. Colon Rectum* 26:590, 1983.

Hall EB: *Radiobiology for the Radiologist*. Philadelphia, Harper and Row, 1978.

Hamberger AD, Unal A et al: Analysis of the severe complications of irradiation of carcinoma of the cervix: whole pelvis irradiation and intracavitary radium. *Int. J. Radiat. Oncol. Biol. Phys.* 9:367, 1983.

Hanks GE, Herring DF et al: Patterns of care outcome studies: results of the national practice in cancer of the cervix. *Cancer* 51:959, 1983.

Jampolis S, Martin P et al: Treatment tolerance and early complications with extended field irradiation in gynecologic cancer. *Br. J. Radiol.* 50:195, 1977.

Kagan AR, DiSaia PJ et al: The narrow vagina, the antecedent for irradiation injury. *Gynecol. Oncol.* 4:291, 1976.

Kagan AR, Nussbaum H et al: A new staging system for irradiation injuries following treatment for cancer of the cervix uteri. *Gynecol. Oncol.* 7:166, 1979.

Kaplan AL: Post radiation ureteral obstruction. *Obstet. Gynecol. Surv.* 32:1, 1977.

Kim TH, Freeman CR et al: The significance of unilateral radiation nephropathy. *Int. J. Radiat. Oncol. Biol. Phys.* 6:1567, 1980.

Kline JC, Buchler DA et al: The relationship of reactions to complications in the radiation therapy of cancer of the cervix. *Radiology* 105:413, 1972.

Kottmeier HL: Complications following radiation therapy in carcinoma of the cervix and their treatment. *Am. J. Obstet. Gynecol.* 88:854, 1964.

Kottmeier HL, Gray MJ: Rectal and bladder injuries in relation to radiation dosage in carcinoma of the cervix. *Am. J. Obstet. Gynecol.* 82:74, 1961.

Kwon TH, Boronow RC: Undiversion: use in management of radiation induced bladder fistula. *Gynecol. Oncol.* 8:164, 1979.

Lantz B, Einhorn N: Intestinal damage and malabsorption after treatment for cervical carcinoma. *Acta Radiol.* [*Oncol.*] 23:33, 1984.

Lee KH, Kagan AR et al: Analysis of dose, dose-rate and treatment time in the production of injuries by radium treatment for cancer of the uterine cervix. *Br. J. Radiol.* 49:430, 1976.

Leissner H, Kjellgren O: Radium reactions in the bladder. *Acta Obstet. Gynecol. Scand.* 38:544, 1959.

Libshitz HI (Ed.): *Diagnostic Roentgenology of Radiotherapy Change.* Baltimore, Williams & Wilkins Company, 1979.

Lillemoe KD, Brigham RA et al: Surgical management of small bowel radiation enteritis. *Arch. Surg.* 118:905, 1983.

Marcus RB, Million RR et al: Carcinoma of the vagina. *Cancer* 42:2507, 1978.

Mendelson RM, Nolan DJ: The radiological features of chronic radiation enteritis. *Clin. Radiol.* 36:141, 1985.

Mennic AT, Dalley V: Aspirin in radiation induced diarrhea. *Lancet* 1:1131, 1973.

Montana GS, Fowler WC et al: Carcinoma of the cervix stage IB: results of treatment with radiation therapy. *Int. J. Radiat. Oncol. Biol. Phys.* 9:45, 1983.

Montana GS, Fowler WC et al: Analysis of results of radiation therapy for stage II carcinoma of the cervix. *Cancer* 55:956, 1985.

Moss WT, Brand WN et al: *Radiation Oncology: Rationale, Technique, Results.* St. Louis, C. V. Mosby Co., 1979.

O'Quinn AG, Fletcher GH et al: Guidelines for conservative hysterectomy after irradiation. *Gynecol. Oncol.* 9:68, 1980.

Onsrud M: Whole pelvic irradiation in stage I endometrial carcinoma: changes in members and reactivities of some blood lymphocyte subpopulations. *Gynecol. Oncol.* 13:283, 1982.

Perez CA, Breaux S et al: Radiation therapy alone in the treatment of carcinoma of the uterine cervix. Part II. Analysis of complications. *Cancer* 54:235, 1984.

Perez CA, Camel HM: Long term follow-up in radiation therapy of carcinoma of the vagina. *Cancer* 49:1308, 1982.

Potish R, Adcock L et al: The morbidity and utility of periaortic radiotherapy in cervical carcinoma. *Gynecol. Oncol.* 15:1, 1983.

Pourquier H, Dubois JB et al: Cancer of the uterine cervix: dosimetric guidelines for prevention of late rectal and rectosigmoid complications as a result of radiotherapeutic treatment. *Int. J. Radiat. Oncol. Biol. Phys.* 8:1887, 1982.

Prempree T: Role of radiation therapy in the management of primary carcinoma of the vagina. *Acta Radiol.* [*Oncol*]. 21:185, 1982.

Rogers LF: Radiation injury of the gastrointestinal tract. In Meyers MA, Ghahremani OG (Eds.): *Iatrogenic Gastrointestinal Complications.* New York, Springer-Verlag, 1981.

Roswit B: Complications of radiation therapy: the alimentary tract. *Semin. Roentgenol.* 9:51, 1974.

Roswit B, Malsky SJ et al: Severe radiation injuries of the stomach, small intestine, colon and rectum. *Am. J. Roentgenol.* 114:460, 1972.

Rotman M, John MJ et al: Limitations of adjunctive surgery in carcinoma of the cervix. *Int. J. Radiat. Oncol. Biol. Phys.* 5:327, 1979.

Rubin P, Cassaret GW (Eds.): *Clinical Radiation Pathology.* Philadelphia, W. B. Saunders Co., 1968.

Rubin P, Cooper R et al (Eds.): *Radiation Biology and Radiation Pathology Syllabus.* Chicago, American College of Radiology, 1975.

Russ JE, Smoron GL et al: Omental transposition flap in colorectal carcinoma: adjunctive use in prevention and treatment of radiation complications. *Int. J. Radiat. Oncol. Biol. Phys.* 10:55, 1984.

Shingleton HM, Fowler WC et al: Ureteral strictures following therapy for carcinoma of the cervix. *Cancer* 24:77, 1969.

Shrom SH, Donaldson MH et al: Formalin treatment for intractable hemorrhagic cystitis: a review of the literature with sixteen additional cases. *Cancer* 38:1785, 1976.

Silverberg E: Cancer statistics: 1985. *CA* 35:19, 1985.

Slater JM, Fletcher GH: Ureteral strictures after radiation therapy for carcinoma of the uterine cervix. *Am. J. Roentgenol.* 111:269, 1971.

Smith JP: Complications related to the radiated gastrointestinal tract. In Delgado G, Smith JP (Eds.): *Management of Complications in Gynecologic Oncology.* New York, John Wiley and Sons, 1982.

Strockbine MF, Hancock JE et al: Complications in 831 patients with squamous cell carcinoma in the intact uterine cervix treated with 3,000 rads or more whole pelvis irradiation. *Am. J. Roentgenol.* 108:293, 1979.

Stryker JA, Demers LM: The effect of pelvic irradiation on the absorption of bile acids. *Int. J. Radiat. Oncol. Biol. Phys.* 5:935, 1979.

Swan RW, Fowler WC, Boronow RC: Surgical management of radiation injury to the small intestine. *Surg. Gynecol. Obstet.* 142:325, 1976.

Van Nagell JR, Maruyama Y et al: Small bowel injury following radiation therapy for cervical cancer. *Am. J. Obstet. Gynecol.* 118:163, 1974.

Villasanta U: Complications of radiotherapy for carcinoma of the uterine cervix. *Am. J. Obstet. Gynecol.* 114:717, 1972.

Webb MJ, Symmonds RE: Wertheim hysterectomy: a reappraisal. *Obstet. Gynecol.* 54:140, 1979.

Weems DH, Mendenhall WM et al: Carcinoma of the intact uterine cervix, stage IB-IIA-B, ≥6 cm. in diameter: irradiation alone vs preoperative irradiation and surgery. *Int. J. Radiat. Oncol. Biol. Phys.* 11:1911, 1985.

Wheeless CR: Intestinal complications of radiation therapy of pelvic malignancy. In Coppleson M (Ed.): *Gynecologic Oncology: Fundamental Principles and Clinical Practice.* New York, Churchill Livingstone, 1981.

ANESTHESIA CONSIDERATIONS AND COMPLICATIONS IN OBSTETRIC AND GYNECOLOGIC SURGERY

15

RICHARD J. PEIRCE
HARRY COHEN

PREOPERATIVE EVALUATION

General

A major change has recently developed in the practice of obstetrics and gynecology; at least 50% of surgical procedures are performed either as outpatient admissions (ambulatory) or as "same day admissions." This has evolved as a result of attempts by Medicare/Medicaid and the insurance industry to contain rising medical costs as well as patient desire to minimize hospital stays and return to the home environment as soon as possible after surgery. This limitation on hospital stays poses a dilemma for the anesthesiologist, because the patients must be properly evaluated preoperatively. They may be seen either immediately before or several days prior to surgery. While seeing patients immediately before the operation is technically easy to do, there are several disadvantages. To conduct a full anesthesia interview, review laboratory work, give an explanation of anesthesia and its risks and have the patient sign consent forms generally requires 10 to 15 minutes. This delays the surgical schedule between cases and leads to poor utilization of operating room time. If the patient workup is incomplete, the anesthesiologist may be tempted to proceed with the anesthetic in order to save time and trouble. This may be detrimental to the patient's optimal management, and it may prove to be legally hazardous. The other alternative is to set up a facility with appropriate staffing to evaluate patients and perform whatever laboratory tests are necessary some time prior to the day of surgery. This method has several advantages. By seeing the patient beforehand, the anesthesiologist has more time available to discuss the patient's medical condition, the management of anesthesia and the patient's concerns and expectations for the perioperative period. This contributes to better rapport and should help to calm the patient and decrease her requirements for periop-

480

erative sedation. Medical problems can be recognized, and the appropriate workup can be instituted. Otherwise, if problems are not recognized until the day of surgery, cases may be cancelled until a satisfactory workup has been completed. This wastes time, increases health care costs and leads to poor utilization of operating room time. During the preliminary visit, the patient can be given necessary preoperative instructions, including dietary restrictions, use of preoperative medications and the need to arrange to have someone responsible accompany her home (postoperative sedation is a potential legal problem for the physician in third party lawsuits).

The preoperative evaluation should optimize the patient's medical conditions prior to surgery. A number of different medical problems and the medications used to treat them are of special concern to the anesthesiologist. For example, the evaluation and treatment of hypertension helps with intraoperative and postoperative control of blood pressure.

Cardiovascular System

Antihypertensive agents can be categorized into several groups: (1) central sympatholytic drugs, such as alpha methyldopa (Aldomet), reserpine and clonidine (Catapres); (2) beta adrenergic blocker drugs, such as propranolol (Inderal); and (3) vasodilating drugs, such as hydralazine (Apresoline) and minoxidil (Loniten) (Miller and Stoelting, 1981).

Alpha methyldopa may cause central nervous system (CNS) depression, augmentation of cardiovascular depression during general anesthesia, attenuation of the normal sympathetic response to surgery and hemorrhage and hepatic dysfunction, and it may result in a positive direct Coombs's test in 25% of patients, causing difficulty in cross matching blood.

Reserpine acts by depleting norepinephrine in nerve storage vesicles; in doing so it decreases the ability of the sympathetic nervous system to compensate for hemorrhage. Reserpine causes nasal congestion and interferes with nasal intubation; it also crosses the blood-brain barrier and may cause sedation, depression and reduction in the minimum alveolar concentration (MAC) for anesthetic agents.

Clonidine is an alpha adrenergic agonist that causes an initial vasoconstriction that decreases sympathetic outflow and increases the depressant effect of baroreceptors. Its plasma half-life is about 12 hours. If the medication is suddenly withdrawn, rebound hypertension may result. Therefore, this medication should either be continued before surgery and resumed shortly after surgery, or it should be slowly withdrawn before surgery to avoid perioperative hypertension.

Beta adrenergic blockers work by blocking beta-1 receptors which decreases cardiac output and myocardial contractility. Side-effects associated with beta blockers include a decrease in plasma renin, congestive heart failure, AV block, hypoglycemia, hyperkalemia, bronchoconstriction, precipitation of asthma attacks and decreased myocardial contractility. These side-effects limit the cardiovascular system's ability to cope with blood loss and stress. Also, the sudden withdrawal of this medication from a patient with coronary artery disease may induce signs and symptoms of myocardial ischemia.

Vasodilators such as hydralazine and minoxidil work by interfering with calcium transport in the smooth muscle of blood vessels, thus causing vasodilation. However, baroreceptors remain active, and this activity tends to increase sympathetic tone and cause tachycardia, offsetting the expected decrease in blood pressure from the vasodilation. To obtain maximum response, these agents are often combined with beta blockers, which minimize the tachycardia. In addition, minoxidil causes salt and water retention.

Diuretics are also commonly used by patients for control of hypertension or fluid retention. Diuretics may be associated with various electrolyte abnormalities. Accordingly, electrolyte levels must be measured preoperatively and regulated as necessary. The effects of electrolyte disturbances are covered in Chapter 2.

Prophylaxis for subacute bacterial endocarditis (SBE) includes a variety of antibiotics: penicillin or its derivatives, aminoglycosides, and intravenous vancomycin (Ueland, 1985) (see Chapter 2). These drugs should be given by protocol both preoperatively and postoperatively (which may be a problem in outpatients). The fact that these agents may cause allergic reactions is of major concern. Intravenous vancomycin has an allergic incidence of about 10%. It may also cause direct myocardial depression and hypotension. Should an allergic reaction become manifest, the antibiotic should be discontinued immediately, epinephrine, an antihistamine, or both should be administered (see Chapter 13) and the surgery should be deferred long enough to assure that the allergy has resolved and that no pulmonary complications have developed.

Hematologic System

Anticoagulants are not commonly used around the time of surgery (for reversal of effects, see Chapter 4), except for heparin in minidose form (usually 5000 units subcutaneously). Heparin may be safely used as prophylaxis for deep vein thrombosis during major surgery. Aspirin and the newer prostaglandin inhibitors are in very common use as analgesics and for relief of dysmenorrhea. They may be obtained over the counter (e.g., aspirin, Advil and Nuprin) or by prescription (e.g., Motrin, Anaprox, Naprosyn and Ponstel). These drugs inhibit platelet aggregation and may cause persistent bleeding at operative sites. Since this effect lasts about one week, these medications should be discontinued at least seven days before surgery; other analgesics, such as acetaminophen or codeine, may be substituted. If it is not possible to discontinue the use of these drugs, one should order a test of bleeding time in order to assess the effects of the drug.

Abnormal hemoglobin levels should be checked in black patients preoperatively. Approximately 10% of American blacks have sickle cell trait (heterozygous) and 0.2% have sickle cell disease (homozygous). The presence of this disease can be confirmed by a sickle cell preparation, and if the test result is positive, a hemoglobin electrophoresis test should be performed in order to determine the actual amount of hemoglobin S present. The trait, even with a hemoglobin level of 12 to 13 gms%, may be associated with a sickle cell crisis during stress. Perioperative management of patients with the trait or disease should include (1) avoiding hypoxemia by delivering high concentrations of inspired oxygen, (2) preventing blood stasis and sludging by providing adequate hydration, (3) avoiding hypothermia and (4) avoiding positions during surgery that predispose to peripheral blood stasis. One might also consider exchange transfusions to maintain hemoglobin A at a level greater than 40% to minimize morbidity; however, there are no well controlled studies to support use of this technique (Morrison et al, 1978).

Respiratory System

Asthma must be optimally controlled before the operation to minimize the possibility of a perioperative attack. Attacks during surgery may be very difficult to control, resulting in severe ventilatory problems and potentially disastrous consequences. If the patient is receiving theophylline, the level of theophylline may be checked to assure that the patient has therapeutic levels. Any patient on the equivalent of more than 15 mg/day of prednisone during the past year should receive steroids perioperatively (see Chapter 4). Anesthetic management of these patients can be difficult. There are no ideal agents for induction of anesthesia. Sodium thiopental may cause histamine release and precipitate an asthma attack; diazepam, because of its long half-life, may cause prolonged postoperative sedation; etomidate may cause myoclonic tremors on reduction; and ketamine, a bronchodilator, may cause hypertension, rigidity, and postoperative hallucinations, although these effects are minimized if the total dose is less than 1 mg/kg. Regional anesthesia is an excellent choice for patients with asthma, as it has no effect on ventilation and permits the use of their bronchodilating inhalers whenever necessary (including during surgery).

Central Nervous System

Treatment of migraine headaches may involve use of aspirin-containing compounds (e.g., Fiorinal) or beta blockers, the side-effects of which have been previously noted. However, some patients with migraine may also receive monamine oxidase (MAO) inhibitors (e.g., Nardil, Marplan or Parnate). These drugs cause an increase in the amount of norepinephrine stored in nerve terminals, and it may be released during times of stress, such as surgery. MAO inhibitors may cause extreme hypertension and lability of blood pressure during surgery. These drugs should be discontinued at least two weeks before surgery.

Psychiatric problems are treated with a variety of different medications. Sedatives may cause increased perioperative sedation and an increased tolerance to anesthetics. Tricyclic antidepressants (e.g., Tofranil, Elavil, Sinequan, amitriptyline) decrease catecholamine stores by blocking reuptake at nerve endings and may result in ECG changes; these changes include T wave changes, prolongation of the QRS complex, bundle branch block and ventricular premature contractions. Fatal arrhythmias may occur if tricyclic antidepressants are used in conjunction with halothane and pancuronium bromide. Phenothiazines and butyrophenones (e.g., Haldol) exhibit a dopamine receptor blocking action that results in a variable alpha adrenergic blocking effect and parasympathetic stimulation. They may also cause cholestatic jaundice and orthostatic hypotension, and they may decrease the body's ability to maintain temperature homeostasis, resulting in perioperative hypothermia. Lithium prolongs the effect of neuromuscular blocking agents and increases the MAC (minimum alveolar concentration) of anesthetic agents.

Thyroid Disorders

Thyroid disorders are commonly seen. Thyroid indices should be normal preoperatively. Hypothyroidism may result in hypotension, hypothermia and muscle weakness. Although thyroid supplemental drugs have long half-lives (1.4 to 10 days), one should still consider giving these agents on the morning of surgery in order to assure adequate thyroid levels. Hyperthyroidism may be aggravated during pregnancy or in association with trophoblastic disease. Hyperthyroidism may result in tachycardia, hypertension, hyperthermia and cardiac arrhythmias. It should be controlled preoperatively by whatever medical or surgical methods are necessary. When hyperthyroidism is controlled with medication, it should be given on the day of surgery. Symptoms of toxicity that occur during surgery can be managed with beta blockers, temperature maintenance, adequate hydration and electrolyte control.

Psychologic Aspects

The psychologic and emotional aspects of the care of both the obstetric patient, who is undergoing one of the most significant events in her life, and the gynecologic patient, who is undergoing surgery on her reproductive system, should be considered by the attending personnel. Either of these events is an emotionally profound experience for a woman. Because of the significance of these events, these patients may be more emotionally labile and more nervous about the planned procedures than other patients. In this regard, a pre-anesthetic visit may be extremely helpful, both for evaluating the patient's medical status as well as for developing an interpersonal relationship with the anesthesiologist, which will have calming and sedating effects. Studies have shown that patients who had a preoperative visit required less sedation than patients who were not visited. Taking whatever time is necessary to discuss the anesthetic and the patient's concerns will help to alleviate her anxieties and make the ordeal less stressful for the patient.

ANESTHESIA FOR GYNECOLOGIC SURGERY

Anesthesia for gynecologic operations may cause many unique problems for the anesthesiologist.

Laparoscopy

Laparoscopy may cause cardiac compromise during the intraperitoneal insufflation of gas or when the patient is in an extreme Trendelenburg position (Artusio and Sia-Kho, 1983). When carbon dioxide or nitrous oxide is insufflated at a pressure approaching 20 mm Hg, it can cause partial collapse of the vena cava, resulting in a decrease in cardiac preload and cardiac output. Patients who have borderline cardiac function have a propensity for congestive heart failure during laparoscopy. Complications are also reported following the use of the Verres needle (used for insufflation) and the sharp trocar (inserted prior to introduction of the optical instrument). There are case reports of perforation of the major arteries or the vena cava with major hemorrhage and circulatory collapse and of retroperitoneal gas insufflation, leading to pneumothorax and pneumomediastinum (see Chapter 6). The anesthesiologist must be vigilant in observing any remarkable changes in vital signs during laparoscopy. During carbon dioxide insufflation, inadequate ventilation via the endotracheal tube may result in hypercarbia, hypertension and tachycardia. The monitoring of end-tidal carbon dioxide by capnography will assist in the prevention of hypercarbia. In the unconscious patient (under general anesthesia), an endotracheal tube is mandatory if one is to prevent gastroesophageal reflux during the course of the laparoscopic procedure. If the surgeon plans to utilize electrocoagulation therapy via the laparoscope (for tubal sterilization or coagulation of endometriosis implants), carbon dioxide is the preferred agent for insufflation, since it will extinguish sparks. Nitrous oxide is to be avoided in this case, since it will support combustion and may lead to an extensive intraperitoneal burn.

Hysteroscopy and Dilatation and Curettage

Hysteroscopy and dilatation and curettage procedures are associated with several problems. First, the surgeon may perforate the uterus and traumatize adjacent structures. Resulting hemorrhage or trauma may require emergency laparotomy in the presence of hypovolemia and hypotension. Second, the anesthesiologist frequently encounters patients who have musculoskeletal problems such as osteoporosis, spinal deformities, disc disease or arthritis with limited motion. These patients require careful positioning on the operating table, preferably when they are awake, in order to assure personal comfort and to avoid further orthopedic damage during anesthesia and surgery. Third, hysteroscopy involves the use of insufflating agents (e.g., D5W, dextran 70, or carbon dioxide). These agents enter the peritoneal cavity via the fallopian tubes and can be absorbed. Dextran is a potential allergen and may produce an anaphylactic response, and carbon dioxide may cause hypercarbia.

Pregnancy Terminations (D & E) and Spontaneous and Missed Abortions

These procedures pose several problems. First, during spontaneous abortion, the cervix is usually dilated and completion of the abortion can be done with ease; intravenous sedation and, occasionally, a paracervical block will provide adequate analgesia. Evacuation of a missed abortion necessitates dilatation of the cervical canal, and hence requires either paracervical block, regional anesthesia or general anesthesia for patient comfort. Missed abortions are occasionally associated with a decrease in clotting factors that results in disseminated intravascular coagulation (DIC). Since DIC would be a contraindication to regional anesthesia, a coagulation profile should be done prior to surgery whenever a regional anesthetic is considered. Placental tissue may be organized to the extent that it is difficult to evacuate. Active bleeding may occur during curettage. Blood should be at least typed and screened prior to this procedure, as well as for other surgical procedures involving the pregnant uterus. Since general anesthesia with a potent inhalational agent may cause increased blood loss during curettage, a N_2O-narcotic technique is generally preferred. In the presence of pelvic infection, the patient may become acutely hyperthermic; appropriate intravenous antibiotic therapy should be administered prior to the procedure.

During a second trimester termination of pregnancy, one should anticipate the possibility of considerable blood loss; hence the patient should be cross-matched for a minimum of two units of blood. If a general anesthetic is chosen for a pregnancy beyond the 12th to 14th week, the anesthetic should be started with a rapid sequence induction with cricoid pressure or an awake intubation to prevent gastric aspiration. Again, the N_2O-narcotic technique, rather than a potent inhalational agent, will help avoid uterine relaxation and increased intraoperative blood loss. Regional anesthesia may also be considered for pregnancy termination. This technique has the advantage of minimizing the risk of gastric aspiration.

Although it is extremely rare, one may encounter a cervical pregnancy at the time of a dilatation and evacuation procedure. This presents the possibility of a major hemorrhage, necessitating either hypogastric artery ligation or hysterectomy to control the bleeding. The anesthesiologist must be fully prepared to provide major volume replacement and appropriate monitoring when this complication is encountered.

Trophoblastic disease, such as hydatidiform mole, may result in active blood loss during evacuation (up to 1 to 2 liters in less than one-half hour), depending upon the size of the uterus. A minimum of two large bore I.V. cannulas (preferably 14 or 16 gauge) should be placed preoperatively, four or more units of blood should be cross matched and available in the operating room (especially if the uterus is larger than 14 to 16 weeks' size) and N_2O-narcotic anesthetic should be used for the evacuation. The complications of trophoblastic disease may add to the anesthetic problems. Metastasis most frequently occurs (1) in the lungs (which decreases total lung capacity and the functional residual capacity), (2) in the brain (causing alterations in patient consciousness and increasing intracranial pressure) and (3) in the liver (causing alterations in liver function and in the ability to metabolize drugs). Human chorionic gonadotropin (HCG) chemically resembles thyroid stimulating hormone, and its increased level frequently results in a hyperthyroid state. If the patient has been receiving chemotherapy, myelosuppression and other systemic effects may be important.

Cervical Conization

Conization involves a potential for moderate to large blood loss at the time of surgery. Patients undergoing conization may also suddenly rebleed, usually one to two weeks after the initial surgery, presenting with hypovolemia, a full stomach and significant anesthetic risk.

Perineal Operations

Perineal operations include excision of condyloma, excision of Bartholin's cysts or abscesses and perineoplasty and are amenable to any type of anesthesia. The use of regional anesthesia may be advantageous if a patient presents with a full stomach.

Major Abdominal Operations

Major abdominal operations include a variety of procedures. Ovarian cystectomies are generally uncomplicated, short procedures. However, endometriosis may cause dense adhesions, requiring extensive dissection, and provide difficulty in obtaining hemostasis from raw surfaces. Ovarian tumors, both benign (e.g., Meig's syndrome), and malignant, may be associated with peritoneal and pleural effusions. Pleural effusion causes decreases in total lung capacity (TLC) and functional residual capacity (FRC), decreases in pulmonary compliance, and increases in shunting, all resulting in impaired oxygen delivery. If these changes are very marked, a thoracentesis should be done preoperatively to remove the fluid and improve pulmonary function.

Myomectomies involve a risk of extensive blood loss. The gynecologist may use a vasopressor (e.g., phenylephrine 1/100,000) locally in the uterus to aid in hemostasis. Vasopressors may cause systemic hypertension in a dose related fashion and predispose to arrhythmias if used in conjunction with halogenated anesthetics. Epinephrine administered in combination with halothane is more likely to cause an arrhythmia than when it is administered with enflurane or isoflurane. It is wise to avoid the use of epinephrine because of its arrhythmnogenic property. However, if the surgeon chooses to use it for hemostasis, the dose should be limited to less than 100 mcg/10 minutes and less than 300 mcg/hour.

Abdominal hysterectomy may result in bowel damage with peritonitis and bladder or ureteral injury. The anesthesiologist should observe the urine for blood and for any sudden decrease in volume. Frequently, there is blood-tinged urine, which may be produced by bladder trauma from the catheter or surgical retractors. This should be treated by diuresis and observation.

The diagnosis and management of bladder and ureteral injuries are covered in Chapter 3.

Ruptured ectopic pregnancy may result in hypovolemia. The extent of hypovolemia should be evaluated preoperatively by taking vital signs and examining the patient for evidence of orthostatic hypotension, cold skin, and pallor. If the patient is acutely volume depleted, aggressive crystalloid and blood replacement are recommended preoperatively, followed by a gentle induction of general anesthesia to avoid sudden decompensation. Induction of anesthesia is often carried out using the intravenous administration of ketamine or etomidate in preference to thiopental, which may cause more hypotension.

Hypogastric artery ligations are performed rather infrequently. They are used to attempt to preserve the uterus and childbearing function in the presence of uncontrollable uterine or pelvic hemorrhage. The patient will probably be hypovolemic, and general anesthesia must proceed with caution. Transvaginal bleeding during surgery may be assessed by using "lap" sponges in the vagina as a tampon; the sponges should be removed periodically to assess the continuing degree of bleeding. Bleeding may be exacerbated during the surgery if the adjacent hypogastric vein is injured. Since the ureter is also adjacent to the artery, the patient should be carefully observed for evidence of ureteral injury (e.g., hematuria or a sudden decrease in urine volume). The femoral and peripheral leg pulses should be checked preoperatively and postoperatively to assure that the external iliac artery was not ligated.

Tuboplasties usually involve minimal blood loss. However, they tend to be long procedures. The patient's core temperature should be monitored, and steps should be taken to maintain normothermia, such as keeping the operating room at 68 degrees F or warmer, using heated intravenous fluids, heating blankets and using low flow gas delivery in the anesthetic circuit. These steps minimize heat loss by reducing the heat of vaporization and by warming the inspired gases. Muscle relaxants are also utilized to prevent movement by the patient during microsurgery.

Minilap (abdominal) tubal ligations are much less stressful on the patient's cardiovascular and pulmonary systems than is laparoscopy, and thus may be indicated when the patient has significant cardiovascular or pulmonary disease. The incision is small, hence muscle relaxation is helpful for the surgeon. Since the operative procedure is brief, the new short-acting nondepolarizing muscle relaxants prove very useful in providing the necessary relaxation.

Vaginal Operations

Patients undergoing vaginal hysterectomies, repairs or tubal ligations do not require extensive muscle relaxation, and volatile agents seem to provide sufficient relaxation. Spinal and lumbar epidural blocks are particularly effective in providing surgical relaxation. Vasopressors, mentioned previously, are often used for local hemostasis. There is also a potential for bleeding if the surgeon loses control of the uterine or ovarian arteries from clamps or sutures as well as the potential for bladder and ureteral injury.

Radical Pelvic Operations

Radical procedures are usually performed for malignancy, and a number of features of these operations are pertinent for the anesthesiologist. The patients tend to be older, and they have a greater likelihood of having systemic disease (Miller, 1986). A review of organ system changes follows. Patients tend to have a decrease in cardiovascular reserve, in baroreceptor response, in liver function and in their ability to metabolize drugs. They undergo pulmonary changes, including a decrease in FEV (forced expiratory volume) and FVC (forced vital capacity), and the FEV_1 (amount of air expelled in the first second of forced expiration)/ FVC ratio decreases (the ratio is about 83% in a young adult versus about 60% at age 70). The arterial PO_2 decreases by 0.31 torr/year, although the alveolar PO_2 is constant. There is also a decrease in functional renal tissue, especially in the cortex. The renal physiology of these patients is altered; patients exhibit decreases of renal blood flow, glomerular filtration, creatinine clearance, response to sodium deficiency and to aldosterone excretion, with the attendant risk of hyperkalemia. Renin activity decreases by 30 to 50%.

Older patients also exhibit altered pharmacokinetics of drugs. The decreased renal function causes increased blood levels and prolongs the half-life of drugs. Decreased liver function retards the metabolic degradation of drugs. Decreased levels of plasma proteins, very common in cancer patients, tend to increase blood levels of the free, active drug. Decreases in the proportion of body water and lean body mass and an increase in the proportion of body fat change the characteristics of drug distribution in the body.

These patients must be seen before the operation to assure that their condition has been optimized. There are several common problems to assess. These include evaluating electrolyte losses after extensive bowel preparation, optimizing the patient's cardiovascular condition with medications as necessary, resolving anemia, using thoracentesis to remove significant pleural effusions and considering hyperalimentation in cachectic patients. During the evaluation, any arthritis of the jaw or neck that might cause problems during intubation should be noted.

There are also special intraoperative considerations. Patients undergoing radical pelvic surgery may need arterial lines to monitor blood pressure when significant blood loss is anticipated and to monitor blood gases when cardiorespiratory problems occur during surgery. Patients may need a central venous pressure (CVP) or pulmonary artery catheter in the presence of a compromised cardiovascular or pulmonary system, or if large fluid shifts (third spacing) are expected. There should be an adequate number of large I.V. cannulas, and blood should be typed and cross matched. Older patients require careful preoperative positioning to avoid pressure sores on their fragile skin and trauma to osteoporotic limbs. Rapid sequence induction of anesthesia should be considered to avoid aspiration if the patient has a bowel obstruction, a large amount of ascites or a hiatal hernia.

During abdominal procedures, one should anticipate considerable blood loss, particularly during extensive dissections for ovarian carcinoma or during radical hysterectomy. There will probably be major fluid shifts with bowel manipulation and dissection. There are also the risks of bladder or ureteral injury as well as a risk of air embolism with open pelvic veins while the patient is in the Trendelenburg position. Generally, these procedures are not amenable to regional anesthesia because of the length of surgery as well as the difficulty in achieving anesthesia for bowel manipulation and for para-aortic node and diaphragmatic biopsies. However, occasionally, a combination of regional anesthesia and a light general anesthetic (e.g., N_2O/O_2) given by endotracheal tube may be used to avoid some depressant side-effects of anesthesia, and this procedure has the additional advantage of providing postoperative analgesia with epidural narcotics.

Radical vulvectomy may be associated with

extensive bleeding. Also, these procedures are frequently done without placement of a Foley catheter, so urine output cannot be used as a sign of hydration. Regional anesthesia may be used during vulvar and vaginal surgery, and may be the method of choice in the presence of other systemic disease.

Postoperatively, patients who have had radical surgery require close monitoring, frequently in an intensive care unit. Fluid management is important because of the possibility of continuing fluid shifts and bleeding. The cardiovascular system and blood pressure control tend to be unstable in the immediate postoperative period. Also, pulmonary atelectasis is a significant problem, especially if the patient is weak and has had upper abdominal manipulation. These factors decrease the FRC and increase closing volume, which then cause atelectasis and associated hypoxemia. These patients frequently need at least incentive spirometry and, occasionally, mechanical ventilation to minimize atelectasis. Since these patients are debilitated, prophylactic minidose heparinization is advisable to avoid the complication of deep vein thrombosis and pulmonary emboli.

ANESTHESIA FOR OBSTETRICS

Obstetrical anesthesia presents a variety of special problems. Both the mother and the fetus are of concern to the anesthesiologist. In addition, the physiology of pregnancy causes the mother to react quite differently to drugs and anesthetic agents as compared with nonpregnant individuals. Virtually every organ system in the mother is subject to altered physiology.

Maternal Physiology

In the cardiovascular system, cardiac output increases about 30 to 40% during the first trimester; it continues to increase slightly during the second trimester and remains stable or decreases slightly during the third trimester (Shnider and Levinson, 1986). However, there may be a marked decrease at any time later in pregnancy if cardiac output is measured in the supine position. The pain and anxiety of labor increase cardiac output about 45% over prelabor values. Immediately after delivery, whether the patient has been delivered vaginally or by cesarean section, cardiac output increases about 80% over prelabor values because of the relief of aorto-caval compression and the contraction

of the uterus with expulsion of blood from the myometrium into the central circulation with an attendant increase in cardiac preload. These changes in cardiac output invoke considerable stress upon the myocardium. As a result, patients with pre-existing valvular or coronary artery disease may decompensate during pregnancy. The decompensation usually occurs early in the third trimester, during labor and immediately after delivery as these are times of maximum cardiac work.

Aorto-caval compression refers to compression of the aorta and inferior vena cava by the enlarging uterus when the mother is in the supine position (Phillips, 1983). Cardiac output and arterial blood pressure decrease because of (1) decreasing preload through compression of the vena cava and (2) increasing afterload by aortic compression, which causes a reflex decrease in cardiac output. The condition becomes progressively worse during the second and third trimesters and is aggravated by decreased maternal blood volume, positive pressure ventilation and sympathetic blockade. The compression may be minimized by having the patient assume either a sitting position or a pelvic tilt (lateral) position. Decreased blood flow to the uterus secondary to aorto-caval compression may cause or aggravate fetal distress; hence, any surgery during the second and third trimesters should be performed utilizing a pad under the right hip or a uterine displacing device, and the table should be tilted to the left.

Blood volume progressively increases about 35 to 40% during pregnancy. This consists of an increase in plasma volume from 40 to 70 ml/kg and an increase in blood cell volume from 25 to 30 ml/kg. A physiologic anemia of pregnancy occurs because the plasma volume increases relatively more than the RBC volume. However, the hemoglobin should remain greater than 10 gm%. The physiologic anemia reduces the oxygen carrying capacity of blood; this is compensated by (1) maternal hyperventilation, which increases the PaO_2; (2) increased cardiac output, which improves oxygen delivery to the various organs; and (3) a shift to the right of the oxyhemoglobin dissociation curve (the p50 changes from 26.7 mm to 30.2 mm), which allows greater extraction of oxygen from RBC by the tissues. The increases in blood volume and oxygen delivery help minimize changes in vital signs (e.g., pulse and blood pressure) despite large maternal blood loss of up to 1 to 2 liters. Therefore, these patients generally do not require blood transfusions as promptly as nonpregnant patients.

A number of changes occur throughout the respiratory system and in ventilation. As pregnancy progresses, a 3 to 4 cm elevation of the diaphragm occurs along with a compensatory 2 cm increase in the transverse diameter of the thorax. The net result is a less than 5% decrease in total lung capacity. The FRC decreases about 20%. This, combined with the increased minute ventilation causes rapid development of hypoxia and possible fetal distress during periods of apnea, such as at the time of intubation or when the mother holds her breath during pushing in the second stage of labor. This also increases the rapidity of induction and awakening from anesthesia. The expiratory reserve volume and the residual volume each decrease about 20%. Vital capacity and closing volumes remain unchanged.

A 10 to 20% increase in the maternal basal metabolic rate occurs during pregnancy, which is accompanied by a corresponding increase in oxygen uptake and utilization. Minute ventilation increases 50%, alveolar ventilation increases 70%, tidal volume increases 40%, the respiratory rate increases 15% and total compliance increases 30%. Pulmonary resistance decreases 50%, and diffusing capacity decreases 5%. FEV_1 is unchanged.

Because of the changes in ventilation, PCO_2 decreases to 30 to 33 torr, HCO_3 decreases by 4 mEq/l, pH remains either unchanged or slightly increased, and PO_2 increases by 10 torr.

Capillary engorgement and fragility occur throughout the body, including the respiratory tract. Because of this, women are prone to nosebleeds, bleeding gums and bruising during pregnancy. Capillary engorgement also considerably increases the risk of epistaxis during attempts at nasal intubation or passing nasogastric (NG) tubes.

The liver maintains a constant blood flow and serum bilirubin throughout pregnancy. Bromsulphalein (BSP) excretion, and the levels of aspartate aminotransferase (AST), lactate dehydrogenase (LDH), alkaline phosphatase, plasma proteins and serum cholesterol all slightly increase during pregnancy. Plasma cholinesterase activity decreases during pregnancy, although the decrease is generally not sufficient to affect the metabolism of usual clinical doses of succinylcholine or ester-linked local anesthetics.

Changes in the kidneys include increases in renal plasma flow, glomerular filtration rate and filtration fraction, and a 50% increase in creatinine clearance. Because of these changes, the BUN and serum creatinine levels decrease, and drugs that undergo renal clearance will have

shortened elimination half-lives. Also, due to increased serum progesterone levels, the renal collecting system dilates and muscular tone decreases, so patients are more prone to urinary tract infections.

Changes in the musculoskeletal system include a progressive lumbar lordosis and a propensity to acquire the carpel tunnel syndrome. Also, the vertebral ligaments undergo relaxation. This relaxation, combined with an enlarging uterus, tends to cause back pain. In the absence of neurologic deficit, in spite of back pain, regional anesthetics are acceptable when indicated.

The Fetal-Placental Unit

There are a number of factors that affect the transfer of drugs across the placenta (Devore, 1983). The placenta is a lipid membrane, and lipid soluble drugs cross the membrane readily, whereas water soluble and ionized drugs pass with difficulty. Drugs with a molecular weight of less than 300 daltons cross readily, whereas agents with a molecular weight of more than 1000 daltons cross with great difficulty. The binding of drugs to maternal proteins will reduce the amount of free drug. Since the transfer of free drug across a membrane is proportional to concentration gradient and follows Fick's Law of Diffusion, protein binding will reduce membrane transport or placental transfer from mother to fetus. All drugs used in anesthesia, with the exception of the depolarizing and nondepolarizing muscle relaxants in their usual clinical dosages, readily cross the placenta.

Following placental transfer, drugs proceed through the umbilical vein. The vein bifurcates, permitting part of the drug to pass directly into the fetal inferior vena cava and the remainder to enter the liver, where it undergoes biodegradation—this procedure is called the first pass effect. The free drug then enters the fetal right atrium where it is further diluted by blood from the superior vena cava. The drug is then transported through the foramen ovale and into the central circulation. However, there are several factors that tend to elevate fetal drug levels to amounts that are greater than would be expected. Fetal bood pH is normally 7.20 to 7.35 during labor, although it may decrease even more during fetal distress. The mother's pH, usually above 7.40 because of hyperventilation during labor, is alkaline compared to that of the fetus. When a drug with a pKa above 7.40 (i.e., most local anesthetics) is given to the mother, a certain amount will diffuse across the placenta into the fetal circulation. Here, the drug will further dissociate into its ionized form because of the relatively lower pH. Ionized agents cross the placenta with difficulty; hence, the ionized drug will be trapped in the fetal circulation. Since fetal hepatic enzymes are not fully developed, fetal metabolism of most drugs may be prolonged (Gregory, 1986). Drug excretion is delayed because fetal kidneys are not fully developed (the creatinine clearance at 28 weeks' gestation is only 25% of that expected at term). Even at term, the fetal kidney cannot concentrate urine and the glomerular filtration rate is less than that of an adult. The fetus also has a decreased level of serum albumin (3.5 gm/dl versus 4.5 gm/dl in a adult). This decreases protein binding in the fetus and permits more active, free drug to remain within the circulation. Finally, the blood-brain barrier is poorly developed in the fetus, especially if premature, and this permits higher brain levels of the drug.

There are also indirect maternal effects on fetal-placental perfusion. Oxygen delivery to the placenta and fetus depends on the oxygen content of the maternal blood as well as the maternal blood pressure. The uterine arteries are maximally vasodilated during pregnancy. Therefore, blood flow to the uterus is a pressure-dependent phenomenon. Any drug that causes vasoconstriction (e.g., alpha adrenergic vasopressors) or hypotension (e.g., antihypertensives) will decrease uterine perfusion and oxygen delivery to the placenta and fetus. Any drug that increases blood pressure by increasing myocardial contractility (e.g., beta adrenergic agents) should have a minimal affect on uterine perfusion. Hence, ephedrine is the vasopressor of choice, under most circumstances, to treat hypotension during pregnancy. Decreased intravascular volume following hemorrhage or severe pre-eclampsia may also be responsible for diverting blood flow from the uterus to other organs. Decreased oxygen content of maternal blood may also be caused by maternal hypoxia, apnea, anemia, and carbon monoxide poisoning. Decreased availability of oxygen from maternal blood to cross the placenta may be caused by a shift to the left of the oxyhemoglobin dissociation curve, as seen with maternal acidosis or hypothermia.

Special Anesthetic Considerations During Pregnancy

A number of medications used during pregnancy have implications in regard to the selection of anesthesia induction techniques and the dose of anesthetic used.

Magnesium sulfate, a therapeutic agent used in management of pre-eclampsia/eclampsia and a tocolytic agent for suppressing pre-term labor, may cause CNS depression, diuresis, mild vasodilation and neuromuscular blockade. Toxic levels of magnesium sulfate may interfere with ventilation and myocardial contractility. Therapeutic doses markedly potentiate the effects of depolarizing and non-depolarizing muscle relaxants. The dose of muscle relaxant administered concurrently with magnesium sulfate should be reduced and titrated with a blockade monitor in order to achieve the desired effect and to prevent over-dosage.

Beta mimetic agents such as ritodrine are used for uterine tocolysis. While these medications have principally an effect on beta$_2$ receptors, all have some effect on beta$_1$ receptors as well, and thus can cause tachycardia, increased myocardial contractility and increased myocardial oxygen consumption. An overdose of these agents may cause angina, even in young, healthy patients with no history of coronary artery disease. A baseline ECG may be advisable in patients receiving beta mimetic agents prior to the institution of therapy. Beta mimetic agents also cause hyperglycemia and hypokalemia. The hypokalemia is due to an intracellular shift of potassium. The total body potassium, however, remains normal. This hypokalemia should not be treated, unless it causes ECG changes, because the potassium will shift out of cells once therapy stops, and treatment may cause a rebound hyperkalemia.

Most anesthetic agents are teratogenic in some species if given at a particular time during pregnancy (Smith, 1983). Teratogenicity is difficult to study in the human because (1) there are different published rates of congenital anomalies, (2) it is difficult to set standarized controls during pregnancy and (3) these studies require a large population of patients. Only a few drugs have been shown to be definite teratogens in humans (see Chapter 13). Numerous studies of the teratogenic effects of inhaled anesthetics have been done; these studies have shown either no increase in risk or have had built in biases, poor controls or inadequate numbers to reach a final conclusion. However, to minimize risk to the fetus, elective surgery should be deferred until after pregnancy. Semi-emergency surgery should be deferred until after the first trimester, when possible.

Other drugs may be harmful when given during pregnancy, and should be used only when definitely indicated. Aminoglycosides and streptomycin may be ototoxic. Tetracyclines cause staining of the teeth. Antibiotics of these classes should be given after the umbilical cord is clamped during delivery. Thiazide diuretics may cause fetal thrombocytopenia. Sulfonamides and diazepam, if used shortly before delivery, displace fetal bilirubin from protein binding sites and may worsen kernicterus. In addition, diazepam in large doses (>30 mg) during labor may cause floppy, lethargic babies that do not feed well. The benefit to the patient from receiving one of these drugs should outweigh the potential risks involved. Whenever possible, a drug of the least potential toxicity should be used.

Surgical Procedures During Pregnancy

A number of surgical procedures may be performed during pregnancy. The procedures most often include cervical cerclage and exploratory laparotomies, usually for ovarian cysts or appendicitis, although almost any procedure, including open heart surgery, may be performed with reasonable safety for both mother and fetus.

During surgery, uterine blood flow should be maximized. This involves maintaining blood pressure and avoiding hypotension and hypovolemia. Perfusion can be best maintained by adequately replacing fluid and accurately gauging fluid and blood loss. Sponges should be weighed to estimate blood loss accurately, and the central venous pressure should be monitored as necessary. Vasoactive substances, especially alpha adrenergic and vasodilating agents, should be avoided as much as possible. Aorto-caval compression, which may occur any time after the first trimester, may be prevented by using table and left pelvic tilt with wedges or uterine displacing devices. In addition, fetal oxygenation must be maximized by using high maternal inspired oxygen concentrations and avoiding apnea, especially during intubation.

Fetal monitoring is advisable perioperatively. Continuous monitoring may not be possible during the first trimester or during lower abdominal procedures. In this case, the fetus may be monitored at least preoperatively and postoperatively by Doppler or ultrasound. During the second and third trimesters, continuous monitoring may be performed with external Dopplers. Some loss of beat to beat heart rate variability during general anesthesia should be

expected. Surgical manipulation that causes evidence of fetal distress, including bradycardia, tachycardia and late and variable decelerations should be avoided as much as possible. Of note, atropine and scopolamine cross the placenta and may cause fetal tachycardia and loss of heart rate variability. This can cause some difficulty in interpreting fetal heart rate changes. However, glycopyrrolate is a quaternary amine and does not cross the placenta readily; it is, therefore, the anticholinergic drug of choice. Beta mimetic agents, magnesium sulfate and adequate hydration are uterine tocolytics and will help prevent uterine contractions if the uterus becomes irritable in the perioperative period.

The anesthetic technique may be either regional or general. Even though no inhalational anesthetic has been definitely shown to be mutagenic in women, and no anesthetic technique has been shown to be clearly superior during pregnancy, most agents are mutagenic in some species. It would seem prudent to minimize doses of medication as much as possible and to consider using anesthetics that appear least toxic in laboratory animals. These include narcotics, muscle relaxants, and short-acting barbiturates. Regional anesthesia has several distinct advantages. The dose of drug for spinal anesthesia is so small that essentially none crosses to the fetus. For other regional techniques, such as epidural, caudal and axillary blocks, local anesthetics that are either highly protein bound (e.g., bupivacaine) or rapidly metabolized (e.g., 2-chloroprocaine) are useful. To avoid hypotension, fluid loading preoperatively and beta mimetic vasopressors should be used as necessary for control of blood pressure (except in patients with mitral or aortic stenosis or idiopathic hypertrophic subaortic stenosis).

Analgesia for Labor and Delivery

For most women, labor and delivery cause pain. Pain occurs principally during uterine contractions in the first stage of labor and at the time of delivery as the head passes through the introitus. Reasons for the variations in pain tolerance during labor are probably environmental and psychologic, but are not easily determined. Throughout recorded history, many methods have been used to relieve the pain. Psychologic and physical techniques (prepared childbirth) help many women, but with modern hospital deliveries, pharmacologic relief is frequently requested both during labor and at the time of delivery, even for spontaneous vaginal deliveries. Operative deliveries (forceps and episiotomy) and cesarean sections make some type of pain relief mandatory. Every anesthetic method available has certain benefits and potential complications. These will be further discussed in the following sections.

PREPARED CHILDBIRTH

Currently, there are several methods of prepared childbirth. These methods may be used to control the pain of labor as well as during uncomplicated, non-surgical deliveries. Natural childbirth or psychoprophylactic methods (e.g., Lamaze, Bradley) depend on patient conditioning, redirection of the patient's thought patterns away from herself and her pain to other focal points, plus support and reassurance from her labor coach. Using the McGill pain questionnaire, Melzack and co-workers (1981) noted that women who had taken prepared childbirth classes had lower pain scores during labor than women who had not had training. Scott and Rose (1976) noted that women prepared with the Lamaze method required less analgesia than those without training, although neonatal outcome was similar in the two groups. Hypnosis and acupuncture are not frequently used because they require very extensive preparation and have relatively poor success rates (see Chapter 10).

SEDATIVES

Systemic analgesia may be used for labor. As the name implies, this method does not afford complete pain relief, but does decrease the intensity of experienced pain and provides adequate pain relief for most labors and uncomplicated deliveries. Barbiturates are rarely used because of the prolonged fetal and neonatal sedation, which may persist for several days after delivery, and because of their possible antianalgesic effect (Bryant and Quirk, 1985). Phenothiazine derivatives, such as promethazine (Phenergan) and propiomazine (Largon), and a similar drug, hydroxyzine (Vistaril), are the most popular sedatives and antiemetics used during labor. It should be noted that promethazine may inhibit platelet aggregation and cause excessive bleeding during surgery (Thompson et al, 1973). Other phenothiazines, such as Thorazine, are not as popular because of the alpha adrenergic blocking potential with associated hypotension that may occur. Diazepam is infrequently used for several reasons. It achieves higher drug levels in the fetus than in the mother, and if it is used in doses exceeding 30 mg during labor, it may cause fetal effects, including hypotension, hypothermia, lethargy, hypotonia and poor feeding, that persist for several days after delivery. Doses of 5 to 10 mg decrease short-term variability of the fetal heart rate during fetal monitoring and interfere with interpreting the monitor. Diazepam also displaces bilirubin on neonatal albumin binding sites and places the neonate at risk for kernicterus. All of the aforementioned sedatives have the disadvantage that there is no specific antagonist drug for their effects. Should any of these drugs be used and cause excessive neonatal depression, the baby's cardiovascular system and ventilation must be supported until the baby can excrete or metabolize the drug to levels that cause no further depression.

AMNESICS

Scopolamine may be used to cause amnesia for the mother in labor. However, patients who receive scopolamine frequently become exceedingly restless and uncontrollable during the pain of labor. This drug also decreases mother-infant bonding by causing amnesia around the time of delivery. For these reasons, scopolamine is now used very rarely.

NARCOTICS

Narcotics are very popular and useful for providing systemic analgesia during labor and delivery (Albright et al, 1986). They have the advantage that their depressant effects, including respiratory depression of the newborn, can be promptly antagonized by naloxone (Narcan). In the newborn, the appropriate dose of naloxone is 10 mcg/kg, either I.M. or I.V. It is available for pediatric use in 2 ml ampules of 20 mcg/ml. Disadvantages of narcotics include hypotension, especially with morphine and meperidine (Demerol); bradycardia; respiratory depression and nausea and vomiting. Morphine, and to a lesser extent meperidine, may initiate histamine release, causing hives at the injection site, bronchoconstriction, especially in asthmatics, and contraction of the sphincter of Oddi, precipitating a gallbladder attack in patients with cholelithiasis and cholecystitis. Equianalgesic doses of the narcotics are: morphine, 10 mg; meperidine, 100 mg; fentanyl, 67 mcg; hydromorphone (Dilaudid), 2 mg and alphaprodine (Nisentil), 40 mg.

Morphine has a peak effect about 20 minutes after an intravenous injection and about one to two hours after an intramuscular injection. Its analgesic effect lasts four to six hours. Peak neonatal depression occurs about two hours after a maternal intramuscular dose, and it is associated with greater respiratory depression in the newborn than an equianalgesic dose of meperidine.

Meperidine's peak analgesic effect is 5 to 10 minutes after an intravenous dose and 40 to 50 minutes after an intramuscular dose. It provides three to four hours of analgesia. Fetal levels are highest two to three hours after maternal intramuscular administration and lowest if delivery occurs in less than one hour or more than four hours after a maternal intramuscular dose. Normeperidine is the principal metabolite of meperidine and has greater toxicity and less analgesia than meperidine (Miller and Anderson, 1954). Fetal concentration of normeperidine is highest four or more hours after a maternal dose of meperidine and is measurable in the neonatal urine for three days after delivery (Kuhnert et al, 1979a, b).

Alphaprodine (currently not available for clinical use) has a peak analgesic effect one to two minutes after an intravenous dose and 5 to 10 minutes after a subcutaneous dose. Its duration of analgesia is 45 minutes when given intravenously and one to two hours when given subcutaneously. Equianalgesic doses have more respiratory depression than either morphine or meperidine.

Fentanyl (Sublimaze) has a peak analgesic effect three to five minutes after an intravenous dose and seven to eight minutes after an intramuscular dose. Its duration of analgesia is 30 to 60 minutes when given intravenously and one to two hours when given intramuscularly. The rapid onset and short duration of the analgesic effect are advantageous in providing analgesia for short outpatient procedures such as a dilatation and curettage.

Butorphanol (Stadol) and nalbuphine (Nubain) have had limited use in obstetrics. They both possess agonist-antagonist properties. A dose of 2 mg of butorphanol or one of 10 mg of nalbuphine are equianalgesic to 10 mg of morphine. They both cause the same degree of respiratory depression in these doses, but there is a ceiling effect, and no further increase in respiratory depression occurs with additional dosage. Butorphanol has been associated with (1) greater patient sedation than that caused by other narcotics and (2) a sinusoidal fetal heart rate tracing, although there have been no adverse neonatal outcomes reported (Hatjis and Meis, 1986).

INHALATIONAL AGENTS

Inhalational analgesia, with agents such as N_2O or potent volatile agents (halothane or enflurane), is seldom used. This technique requires close supervision of the patient, and the maximal benefit is achieved only by continually varying the concentration of inspired gas, depending on the patient's changing alertness and depth of analgesia. Unless these agents are administered with an anesthesia circle system incorporating a scavenging system, contamination of the room with the gas will occur. Inadvertent overdosage may result in depression of the patient's cardiovascular system, depression of ventilation or gastric aspiration. In addition, higher doses of the halogenated agents may cause uterine relaxation and prolongation of labor.

Anesthesia for Labor and Delivery

Anesthesia for labor and delivery involves blocking the pain pathways of the involved nerves. The pain of the first stage of labor results from uterine contractions and from the response of stretch receptors to cervical dilation. Sensory fibers from the cervix, uterus and upper vagina coalesce in Frankenhaüser's ganglion on both sides of the cervix, travel to the pelvic plexus, and then to the middle and superior hypogastric plexus. The nerves accompany the sympathetic chain and enter the spinal cord at dermatome levels T10 through L1. The second stage of labor involves the pudendal nerve. The pudendal nerve originates as a coalescence of the nerve roots from S2 to S4 and travels just posterior to the junction of the ischial spine and sacrospinous ligament, at which point it fans out to innervate the labia, lower part of the vagina, perineal body and anus. A cesarean section requires the complete block of all nerve roots—T4 to S4—that innervate the abdominal wall, peritoneum and uterus.

LOCAL ANESTHESIA

Local perineal anesthesia is performed by the obstetrician immediately prior to delivery. The technique is quite simple, but provides anesthesia only to the perineal body for the episiotomy and repair. Potential complications include local anesthetic toxicity and, rarely, perineal hematoma formation. At times, an enlarging hematoma may require evacuation and placement of a drain. A local anesthetic field block, although rare, can be performed as a primary technique for cesarean section. The anterior abdominal wall and peritoneal surfaces are blocked in an emergency situation when anesthesia personnel are not immediately available to administer an anesthetic. Field block does not provide intense anesthesia, and the patient will experience some pain during the procedure. Once delivery has been accomplished, the anesthesiologist, upon arrival, will usually provide general anesthesia for completion of the surgery.

PUDENDAL NERVE BLOCK

Local anesthetic solution is deposited in the vicinity of the pudendal nerve as it passes just posterior to the junction of the ischial spine and sacrospinous ligament. The block, which may be done via a vaginal or a perineal approach, is simple to perform and provides anesthesia to the lower vagina, vulva and perineal body sufficient for an uncomplicated spontaneous or low forceps delivery. It does not provide anesthesia for labor or for other uterine surgical procedures such as a dilatation and curettage. The block will not cause systemic hypotension, since significant sympathetic block does not occur. The failure rate of the block depends upon user experience. Although the block does result in demonstrable maternal and fetal blood levels of the local anesthetic, anesthetic toxicity rarely occurs (Albright et al, 1986). As with any injection of local anesthetic, aspiration should always be done prior to injection of the anesthetic solution to minimize the risk of intravascular injection. There are also reported cases of rectal puncture, parametrial hematoma, inadvertent sciatic nerve block with possible neuritis (which may occur from the local anesthetic or needle trauma to the nerve) and paravaginal infections traversing fascial planes with resulting subgluteal abscess.

SYSTEMIC ANALGESIA FOR DELIVERY

Systemic analgesia with sedatives, narcotics or inhalational agents may be used to supplement local and regional anesthesia for delivery. While the obstetrician or nurse may administer injectable drugs, an anesthesiologist or CRNA (nurse anesthetist) is required to administer inhalational anesthetic agents. The dose of inhalational analgesia should be closely monitored both to provide maximum analgesia for the patient and to keep her awake and responsive enough to maintain her airway reflexes and prevent gastric aspiration, if she should vomit. Ketamine, a dissociative analgesic, may be used in small doses of approximately 0.25 mg/kg to provide profound analgesia for 5 to 10 minutes. The dose may be repeated for continued analgesia, although the risk of hallucinations or delirium will be minimized if the total dose is less than 1 mg/kg. Doses of less than 1 mg/kg have no appreciable fetal effect (normal Apgar scores) and are not associated with fetal chest wall rigidity, although fetal depression and chest wall rigidity may occur with larger doses (Akamatsu et al, 1974). Ketamine may also increase maternal heart rate and blood pressure. It is a bronchodilator and particularly useful for asthmatic patients.

PARACERVICAL BLOCK

Paracervical block, performed by the obstetrician during the first stage of labor, involves a submucosal injection of local anesthetic at 3 to 4 o'clock and 8 to 9 o'clock positions in the vaginal vault at the cervicovaginal junction. This will block Frankenhaüser's ganglia. The block is simple to perform, has a rapid onset of anesthesia, involves no sympathetic block and does not interfere with the maternal cardiovascular system. However, the block lasts no more than 60 minutes if mepivacaine is used and about 90 minutes if bupivacaine is used. No perineal anesthesia occurs following this block, and it is, therefore, of no use during vaginal delivery. The local anesthetic is injected in close proximity to the maternal uterine arteries, and provides opportunity for rapid maternal absorption. Hence, fetal local anesthestic toxicity and fetal bradycardia may occur. The reported incidence of fetal bradycardia ranges from 2 to 70%. Bradycardia is apparently caused by elevated fetal local anesthetic levels leading to myocardial and CNS toxicity and probable local uterine artery vasoconstriction with fetal hypoxia secondary to decreased placental perfusion. This may occur even when the local anesthetic solution does not contain a vasopressor. The bradycardia usually starts about 2 to 10 minutes after the injection and lasts about 5 to 10 minutes, although it may persist for up to 30 to 45 minutes. It is accompanied by decreased short-term variability and, occasionally, by late decelerations. This block should not be performed in patients with high risk pregnancies or if there is any evidence of fetal distress during labor. To prevent a fetal bradycardic episode following the block, small volumes and low concentrations of drug are used, with a pause for several minutes after blocking one side before proceeding to the other. Continuous fetal monitoring is mandatory during the block. If a bradycardic episode occurs, the mother is placed in the lateral position, intravenous fluids are increased to maximize uterine perfusion and oxygen is given to increase the fetal PO_2. If the bradycardia is not severe, time and drug redistribution will permit the effect to wear off before delivery. There is usually no effect on the Apgar scores if the bradycardia is corrected from one-half hour to one hour before delivery. For severe distress, an emergency delivery with a general anesthetic may be indicated, or if time permits, a spinal block, avoiding a high dose of local anesthetic may be used. There have also been case reports of inadvertent injection of the local anesthetic into the fetal scalp at the time of attempted paracervical block, leading to fetal death or brain damage.

CONTINUOUS LUMBAR EPIDURAL BLOCK

Epidural anesthesia can provide anesthesia for labor, operative delivery and cesarean section. Under most circumstances, it is probably the safest method of major anesthesia for labor and delivery. The block involves injection of a local anesthetic with a continuous catheter technique into the mid-lumbar area of the epidural space. It is possible to achieve a segmental block (T10 to L1) for labor, and by increasing the dose of anesthetic, extend the block to the sacral nerve roots for vaginal delivery or upward to the higher thoracic nerve roots to provide sufficient anesthesia for cesarean section. In addition to blocking the nerve roots, some of the local anesthetic diffuses across or through the dura into the spinal fluid, leading to a true spinal block. Peripheral or centrifugal diffusion of local anesthetic may also occur; the anesthesic solution passes beneath the dural collars of nerve roots as they exit from the spinal cord. Contraindications to the use of epidural (and spinal) anesthesia include: (1) blood dyscrasia or coagulopathy (with the risk of an epidural hematoma, requiring decompressive laminectomy), (2) local degenerative nerve disease, (3) local infection of skin over the proposed epidural injection site, (4) fetal distress, (5) hypovolemia and hemorrhage, (6) systemic infection with evidence of bacteremia and (7) patient refusal of regional block.

There are a number of factors that affect the level of anesthesia. The most important is the mass of drug injected, which is the product of the drug concentration and the volume. The patient's height is of some concern, particularly for a subarachnoid block. Taller patients tend to require a greater mass of drug than shorter patients to achieve the same dermatome level of the block. Patients between the ages of 16 and 20 require a maximum amount of drug for anesthesia. The amount needed then decreases progressively with age in a linear fashion. Atherosclerosis accelerates the aging process and tends to decrease the amount of drug necessary by up to 50%. Pregnancy and obesity are known to increase extradural venous pressure and cause further distension of the epidural veins. This venous distension will cause further spread of local anesthetic solution; hence, dose requirements under these circumstances are decreased. During pregnancy, the dose should be reduced by approximately one-third. The nerves immediately adjacent to the injection site have the shortest latent period; a rapid injection of drug will lead to greater spread of anesthesia, but the block will be less intense and there will be a greater risk of an inadequate block.

During labor small doses of local anesthetic are generally required. The usual recommended doses are 15 to 50 mg of bupivacaine or 120 to 200 mg of 2-chloroprocaine; the recommended perineal dose for vaginal delivery is 240 to 450 mg of 2-chloroprocaine, and for cesarean section 100 to 150 mg of bupivacaine or 600 to 900 mg of 2-chloroprocaine is appropriate. Epidural blocks have minimal fetal side-effects, provided maternal hypotension does not occur. The local anesthetic 2-chloroprocaine is hydrolyzed very rapidly in the maternal and fetal plasma. Bupivacaine is very highly protein bound in maternal plasma. These factors limit fetal exposure to the respective drugs. An epidural block may be administered once labor is well established or at any time following oxytocin augmentation of labor. Its effect on the progress of labor is uncertain (see Chapter 13). Anesthesia may be administered either intermittently or continuously by constant infusion pump. If the doses of medication are carefully titrated, an epidural block can povide segmental anesthesia of T10 to L1 during labor, allowing the parturient to move freely to comfortable positions in bed. Segmental lumbar and sacral anesthesia can be achieved for difficult vaginal deliveries, such as for twin or breech deliveries, while retaining the mother's ability to push effectively. Although the epidural anesthetic may diminish Ferguson's reflex, many women are able to push effectively during the second stage of labor. If the woman is unable to push and there is no fetal distress, the epidural may be permitted to "wear off" before any further "bearing down" is attempted. An epidural block also permits 100% oxygen administration to the mother during the delivery. Studies have shown that this results in higher Apgar scores and less fetal acidosis (Marx and Mateo, 1971; Ramanthan et al, 1982). An epidural block allows immediate mother-infant bonding and attempts at breast feeding.

Under most circumstances, an epidural block is safer than a general anesthetic for cesarean section (Spielman and Corke, 1985). One observes less neonatal depression following an epidural block, although a prolonged uterine incision to delivery time with either method is associated with fetal hypoxia and acidosis (Datta et al, 1981; Crawford et al, 1976). Maternal blood loss is less with an epidural block than with general anesthesia. Postoperatively, epidural anesthesia permits continuing pain control via epidural narcotics, a quicker return of intestinal function, less maternal stress as measured by plasma steroid levels and a decreased incidence of venous thrombosis.

The complications of epidural block are discussed in the following paragraphs.

Inadequate analgesic block may not relieve the pressure sensation of labor, and this is especially common during "back labor," which may occur in the presence of a vertex presentation with the occiput posterior.

The anesthetic may cause a sympathetic block, resulting in maternal hypotension and fetal bradycardia. The hypotension can be minimized by preloading the patient with 1 to 2 liters of isotonic crystalloid solution before starting the block.

Once an epidural anesthetic has been established, the patient should be confined to bed until it is no longer effective (the sympathetic block extends beyond the duration of the sensory block).

An epidural block will not relax the uterus and is of no use in situations that require uterine relaxation.

The reported incidence of "wet taps" or dural punctures following the attempted placement of an epidural needle is 0.5 to 2%. When this occurs, the probability of a post-puncture headache with a 16 or 17 gauge needle is said to be 60 to 80%. If a dural puncture occurs, the anesthetic may be discontinued and a different anesthetic planned, another attempt at epidural anesthesia may be made at a different interspace or the anesthetic may be continued as a continuous spinal anesthetic. A dural puncture may be treated initially with epidural saline injection, bedrest, analgesics, maternal hydration (either orally or intravenously) and an abdominal binder. If the headache persists, an epidural blood patch (epidural injection of autologous blood at the level of the dural puncture) is recommended on the second day or later after the dural puncture. A blood patch is 95 to 98% effective in relieving the headache. A blood patch is less effective when it is used earlier than the second day after the dural puncture.

Neurologic complications following epidural block include peripheral nerve damage and, very rarely, paralysis. Nerve damage may be either transient or permanent. It may be caused by needle trauma, direct injection of local anesthetic into the nerve roots or accidental injection of a neurotoxin into the epidural or intrathecal space with resulting neurotoxic effects on the spinal cord or nerve roots. For example, 2-chloroprocaine that contains the preservative bisulfite may cause adhesive arachnoiditis and nerve damage; other reported neurotoxins that have been injected are thiopental, alcohol and formaldehyde. Postoperative backaches have been reported following epidural anesthesia. Possibly, the backache results from relaxation of the muscles of the back with accompanying ligamentous strain. Backaches may be treated with heat and analgesics in the absence of neuropathy, subcutaneous hematoma or localized infection at the injection site.

Local anesthetic toxicity may occur after the administration of an exceedingly high dose of local anesthetic into the epidural space or after an inadvertent intravascular injection. Excessive levels of local anesthetic are present in the blood. Initial symptoms include tinnitus, a numb sensation around the mouth, an unusual taste in the mouth and dizziness. As blood levels progressively increase, manifestations of toxicity include somnolence, excitability, convulsion, coma and cardiac arrest. Patients who experience cardiac arrest from bupivacaine, which has a considerable capacity to bind to cardiac muscle, may be extremely difficult to resuscitate. If early signs of toxicity are noted, the seizure threshold may be increased by causing the patient to hyperventilate. If the signs continue to progress or if the patient begins to convulse, a small dose of thiopental (50 mg) or diazepam (2.5 to 5 mg) may be injected intravenously either to prevent or to shorten the seizure (De Jong, 1977). Larger doses of medication should be avoided because they may cause excessive respiratory depression in the post-ictal period. When a seizure occurs, the airway must be protected, the patient ventilated and the cardiovascular system supported as necessary.

"Bloody taps" occasionally occur during insertion of an epidural needle or catheter. This complication may be minimized by not proceeding with needle or catheter insertion during or immediately following a uterine contraction. At the time of a uterine contraction, venous pressure is elevated, with concomitant distension of the epidural venous plexus. In the presence of a "bloody tap," the epidural catheter may be partially withdrawn. However, if blood continues to be aspirated, the catheter should be completely withdrawn and reinserted at a different level or interspace. Subsequent injections of local anesthetic should be performed slowly and cautiously, since the epidural catheter may migrate into the vein once more.

In spite of negative aspiration, total spinal anesthesia may result from inadvertent intrathecal injection of local anesthetic. It may occur whenever a dose of anesthetic is injected into an epidural needle or catheter. The risk of total spinal anesthesia can be minimized by always starting with a test dose (2 to 3 ml) of anesthetic and waiting at least two to three minutes to observe for any intrathecal or intravascular effects. Single injections should be limited to 3 to 5 ml at a time, and an appropriate waiting period should be observed before additional anesthetic solution is given. Total spinal anesthesia, while frightening for the patient, may be easily treated by supporting ventilation and the cardiovascular system, by maintaining hydration and by administering vasopressors as necessary until the local anesthetic effect wears off. Epidural anesthetics require approximately 25 to 35 minutes from the time of initiation to the time of established blockade. Administration of epidural anesthetics should not be attempted during active labor when delivery is imminent nor when an immediate anesthetic effect is desired.

When sacral nerve roots are blocked following epidural anesthesia, the pelvic floor muscles may be sufficiently relaxed to interfere with internal rotation and descent of the presenting part. Maternal pushing may also be compromised. Pelvic floor relaxation, therefore, may

result in a higher incidence of forceps deliveries. To avoid this complication, the epidural anesthetic should not be administered until the fetal head is well engaged in the pelvis, and early doses of the medication should be of low concentration (e.g., 0.25% bupivacaine) in order to avoid the muscle relaxation that occurs with more concentrated doses.

CAUDAL BLOCK

Caudal anesthesia is an epidural anesthetic administered via the caudal canal. It has clinical applications for both labor and operative delivery. However, the dose of local anesthetic required for labor is two to three times that required with a lumbar epidural block. Although the caudal block technique has been utilized for cesarean section, it is not advised because of the large dose of local anesthetic solution necessary for upper thoracic anesthesia. A caudal block is technically difficult to perform, and has a failure rate of approximately 10 to 15%, either because of wide variations in sacral anatomy or difficulty in locating the sacral hiatus. Another disadvantage of this technique is the potential for fetal scalp puncture and injection of the local anesthetic into the fetal circulation, which may result in acute fetal local anesthetic toxicity, intrauterine convulsions, acidosis, hypoxemia, cerebral palsy and death. This complication may be prevented by performing a rectal examination prior to injection of the local anesthetic solution to rule out the presence of a needle or catheter traversing the rectum and entering the fetal scalp. The presence of a palpated epidural catheter in the rectum dictates its immediate removal. Other complications of the method are similar to those described for lumbar epidural blocks.

LUMBAR SYMPATHETIC BLOCKS

Lumbar sympathetic blocks are rarely performed for obstetric anesthesia because they are technically difficult to perform, are painful to initiate, involve multiple injections and offer no advantages over lumbar epidural blocks.

SPINAL BLOCK

Spinal anesthesia can provide profound anesthesia for vaginal delivery or cesarean section. It is generally not used for labor because it provides considerable muscle relaxation and is generally used as a single shot technique. Although spinal anesthesia may be used as a continuous technique, the incidence of dural puncture headache is very high with this technique. Failure to provide complete anesthesia is rare, less than 0.5%. Its effect is more rapid in onset than epidural anesthesia, requiring approximately 5 to 10 minutes to insert and establish anesthesia, versus about 25 to 35 minutes for an epidural block. The small dose of spinal anesthetic solution needed to establish the block will result in negligible maternal blood levels of local anesthetic. The recommended doses are 30 to 50 mg of lidocaine or 3 to 5 mg of tetracaine for perineal anesthesia and 50 to 100 mg of lidocaine or 8 to 10 mg of tetracaine for a cesarean section. The fetal effects of spinal anesthesia are negligible, providing maternal hypotension is avoided. However, a more abrupt onset of sympathetic blockade and hypotension, when compared with epidural anesthesia, can occur. The maternal blood pressure should be followed very closely after the subarachnoid injection. Methods to minimize the potential hypotension are similar to those used for epidural anesthesia and include preanesthetic hydration with 1 to 2 liters of isotonic crystalloid solution and left uterine displacement. Although it is controversial, many anesthesiologists recommend preanesthetic intramuscular ephedrine in doses of 25 to 50 mg. Ensuing hypotension should be immediately treated with uterine displacement, aggressive hydration, beta adrenergic vasopressors and oxygen. Spinal anesthesia is associated with a reported incidence of dural puncture headache from 0.5% with a 26 gauge needle to 60 to 80% with a 17 gauge needle.

General Anesthesia

General anesthesia is now rarely administered for an uncomplicated vaginal delivery, although it may be used if the patient is completely uncooperative to the point that the obstetrician cannot complete the delivery. The technique also may be indicated when uterine relaxation is required as for (1) delivery of an aftercoming head in a breech presentation, (2) the extraction of a second twin, (3) manual extraction of the placenta, or (4) to correct a complete or partial uterine inversion. General anesthesia, utilizing a rapid sequence induction technique, will ordinarily be selected when an obstetric emergency necessitates the immediate delivery of the infant. Induction of surgical anesthesia requires no more than 1 to 2 minutes and is accomplished by (1) pre-oxygenating the patient with 100% inspired oxygen, that is, having her deeply breathe three or four vital capacities in a rapid fashion, which results in nitrogen washout and saturation of the pulmonary functional residual capacity; (2) proceeding with cricoid pressure compression of the esophagus to prevent gastric reflux; (3) inducing sleep with any of a variety of intravenous agents, depending on the situation; (4) administering intravenous succinylcholine for rapid muscle relaxation; and (5) maintaining anesthesia of N_2O/O_2 and low doses of volatile agent to minimize the likelihood of maternal recall, and at the same time avoiding the possibility of uterine relaxation from larger doses of halogenated agents. Further muscle relaxants are provided as necessary, and supplemental narcotics are administered following the delivery to maintain the anesthesia. General anesthesia is claimed to maintain better maternal cardiac output, blood pressure and systemic vascular resistance when compared with regional anesthesia. It will not cause any degree of sympathetic blockade as occurs with regional anesthesia. These characteristics may make general anesthesia the method of choice for mothers with mitral or aortic stenosis or idiopathic subaortic stenosis (IHSS), and it is also preferred for maternal hypovolemia, as may occur following hemorrhage or other causes, or severe anemia. It is also recommended in mothers who have certain types of coagulopathy, since regional blocks are contraindicated, and in parturients who absolutely refuse regional anesthesia.

The major complications of general anesthesia are failed intubation and maternal pulmonary aspiration of gastric contents. The patient's airway and its adequacy for intubation should always be evaluated prior to induction of anesthesia. The airway may be further evaluated by applying topical anesthesia to the mouth and attempting to visualize the epiglottis or vocal cords by direct laryngoscopy. If the epiglottis or cords can be visualized, tracheal intubation should be successfully accomplished during a rapid sequence induction. If there is any doubt regarding the success of rapid induction, an awake oral intubation should be done after further topical anesthesia is applied. Small doses of fentanyl (50 to 100 micrograms) may provide adequate maternal sedation without associated fetal depression. Intubation may then be accomplished by direct laryngoscopy, or more comfortably for the patient, by oral fiberoptic intubation. The latter may be accomplished by use of a mouthpiece designed for the fiberoptic scope, which prevents the patient from biting down on the delicate fiberoptic bundle. Nasal intubation should be avoided primarily because epistaxis may result when the engorged, fragile capillaries in the nose are traumatized by attempts to pass the endotracheal tube.

Maternal pulmonary aspiration is a leading cause of maternal anesthetic morbidity and mortality. Statistics reported in the 1973–1975 "Confidential Inquiry" into morbidity and mortality from the United Kingdom reveal that 13.2% of maternal deaths were related to anesthetic causes, principally aspiration (Moir, 1980). During 1976 to 1978, 26 of 30 maternal anesthetic deaths were caused either by aspiration or by failed intubation (Hunter and Moir, 1983). The onset and severity of symptoms correlated with the volume and the pH of the aspirate, and with its nature (i.e., liquid or a mixture of liquid and solid) (Albright et al, 1986). Symptoms may begin immediately or up to 8 hours following the aspiration. A chemical pneumonitis will generally follow the aspiration of a substance with a pH of less than 2.5. The lower the pH beyond this point, the greater the severity of pulmonary complications (Teabeaut, 1952). The clinical picture is as follows: intense bronchospasm, increased lower airway resistance, decreased lung compliance, increased pulmonary artery pressure, decreased systemic blood pressure, decreased PO_2, increased PCO_2, pulmonary edema and decreased CVP (central venous pressure) secondary to massive fluid extravasation into the lungs. Particulate matter in the aspirate may obstruct the airway and cause pulmonary shunting.

Pregnant patients are predisposed to gastric aspiration for several reasons: (1) increased intra-abdominal pressure caused by the enlarging uterus, (2) increased plasma progesterone level during pregnancy, (3) use of narcotics for intrapartum analgesia, and (4) use of ethanol (occasionally used to stop labor). Each of these four will delay gastric emptying during labor. Also, hiatal hernias are present in approximately 20% of pregnant patients (Albright et al, 1986); during pregnancy an increase in gastric acid production may occur, with a lowering in pH of gastric contents.

The consequences of gastric aspiration can be prevented or minimized in several ways. (1) The use of regional anesthesia permits the patient to remain awake and use her own protective airway reflexes, thus eliminating the possibility of aspiration. (2) During labor, the patient should remain NPO or be given a minimal quantity of clear liquids. (3) The use of a nonparticulate, liquid antacid (e.g., 30 ml of 0.3 molar sodium citrate) before induction of anesthesia will raise the gastric pH above 2.5 and minimize pulmonary damage should aspiration occur. Gibbs and co-workers (1978) noted that particulate antacids (e.g., Maalox, Amphogel) may cause pulmonary damage if aspirated. H_2 receptor blockers (e.g., cimetidine and ranitidine) have not been approved by the FDA for use during pregnancy. Treatment with a nondepolarizing muscle relaxant before inducing anesthesia is controversial. These agents have been recommended to avoid the increase in intra-abdominal pressure that follows the muscle fasciculations caused by succinylcholine. However, this effect is not reliable. Also nondepolarizing muscle relaxants relax the cardiac sphincter of the stomach, which may predispose to regurgitation. Emptying of the stomach by nasogastric tube is not warranted, since it will not guarantee removal of the particulate food matter in the stomach and may cause epistaxis. The presence of a nasogastric tube also decreases the efficacy of cricoid pressure when one attempts to prevent reflux during induction, since it may prevent total occlusion of the esophagus. If general anesthesia is necessary, either a rapid sequence induction of anesthesia or an awake intubation is advisable; cricoid compression should not be released until proper placement of the endotracheal tube is confirmed and the cuff is inflated. If the attempt to intubate the patient fails, cricoid pressure should be maintained and the patient should be ventilated by mask until she is sufficiently awake to breathe spontaneously and protect her own airway. If the patient does vomit during anesthesia, the airway should be immediately suctioned with a large bore (e.g., Yankauer) catheter, and the patient should be placed in the Trendelenburg position to minimize aspiration into the lungs. The pH of the vomitus should be checked with pH paper or a blood gas machine. Liquid with a pH greater than 2.5 is less likely to cause severe pulmonary insufficiency than liquid with a lower pH. If particulate matter is present in the vomitus, bronchoscopy should be performed in an attempt to remove further particulate matter (food) from the trachea. Tracheal lavage should be avoided, as this may force particulate matter further down into the lungs. The use of steroids is controversial; studies have not substantiated their routine clinical use. The patient should be carefully observed, possibly in an intensive care unit, as symptoms may appear and worsen some hours after the initial insult. The progress of pulmonary dysfunction should be followed by chest x-rays and arterial blood gas determinations; adequate oxygenation should be maintained via intubation, positive end-expiratory pressure and mechanical ventilation as deemed necessary.

ANESTHESIA FOR OBSTETRIC EMERGENCIES

The problems and possible ill-effects of obstetric anesthesia are complicated by the sudden onset and serious nature of certain obstetric disorders. It is essential that the anesthesiologist be familiar with the clinical course of these conditions and that he discuss the obstetric situation and possible outcome with the obstetrician before starting the anesthesia.

Preeclampsia/Eclampsia

Pregnancy induced hypertension (PIH) occurs in about 3% of pregnancies. Preeclampsia consists of hypertension, proteinuria (>300 mg/day) and edema. Eclampsia includes the above triad of signs accompanied by seizures. In the presence of plasma fluid translocation and peripheral edema, one also observes intravascular fluid depletion and hemoconcentration. In severe PIH, volume replacement must be carried out with extreme care, utilizing central venous pressure or pulmonary capillary wedge pressure monitoring in an effort to promptly detect and prevent pulmonary edema. Albumin, when administered, may transudate into the lungs and exacerbate pulmonary edema by increasing the osmotic pressure in the alveolar spaces. A frequent complication of PIH is disseminated intravascular coagulation (DIC). For this reason, it is mandatory to obtain a platelet count and a fibrinogen level before attempting to give any regional anesthetic. Normally, platelet counts are unchanged during pregnancy; however, fibrinogen levels are approximately 50% greater when compared with those in the non-pregnant patient. A regional anesthetic given to a parturient with developing DIC may cause an epidural hematoma with complicating neurologic deficits. This will require an immediate decompressive laminectomy to avoid permanent deficit.

The most commonly administered drug in the treatment of PIH, and one that is likely to complicate anesthesia, is magnesium sulfate. It causes CNS depression, partial block of the neuromuscular junction, mild vasodilation and a decrease in blood pressure. An excessive dose may result in respiratory depression and cardiac arrest. Calcium is the specific antidote for neuromuscular blockade and should be readily available whenever magnesium sulfate is being administered (see Chapter 13). Magnesium sulfate also potentiates depolarizing and non-depolarizing neuromuscular blocking agents. The doses of these agents should be decreased appropriately and their effects carefully observed with nerve stimulators or blockade monitors. Mechanical ventilation and intubation should be continued until one is certain that the neuromuscular blocking agents have been sufficiently reversed and the patient has normal ventilatory parameters, indicating her ability to breathe adequately on her own.

Prior to and during anesthesia the blood pressure must be controlled to prevent maternal stroke and myocardial ischemia. However, uterine and placental perfusion are pressure dependent phenomena. Fetal distress may ensue if the material blood pressure is lowered either too rapidly or beyond a critical range. Generally, the maternal systolic pressure should be maintained at less than 160 mm Hg, and the diastolic pressure should be maintained at less than 110 mm Hg. The fetus should be closely monitored as the blood pressure is lowered to its desired range to assure that fetal distress does not develop.

Regional anesthesia may be utilized in mild to moderate disease during labor and delivery and for cesarean section. The intravascular volume should be optimized preoperatively in order to minimize the potential for hypotension and to maximize uterine perfusion. In performing an epidural block, one should administer small incremental doses of local anesthetic and allow time for the cardiovascular system to accommodate to the sympathetic blockade, thus avoiding profound changes in maternal blood pressure. In this regard, lumbar epidural blocks are superior to subarachnoid blocks because of the more gradual onset of sympathetic blockade.

For the patient with severe, uncontrolled PIH, a general anesthetic may be the preferred technique for operative delivery. There is no sympathetic blockade during general anesthesia. This permits better blood pressure control intraoperatively with appropriate doses of vasodilators. Intravenous nitroglycerine (Snyder et al, 1979) and nitroprusside have been safely administered for blood pressure control during induction of anesthesia to provide better control of the hypertension associated with intubation. However, nitroprusside is associated with the risks of fetal and maternal cyanide toxicity if it is used for prolonged periods or in high doses during pregnancy.

Placenta Previa

A patient with a placenta previa may be actively bleeding and in hypovolemic shock when she arrives at the hospital as an emergency admission; or she may not be bleeding at all and be hemodynamically stable. A cesarean section is commonly required. If the patient is bleeding actively, aggressive crystalloid and blood replacement must be carried out before the patient undergoes cesarean section. The main hemostatic mechanism of the uterus is myometrial contractility. The lower uterine segment, the site of placental implantation, contains a minimal amount of myometrium, and it contracts very poorly after the placenta has been delivered. Therefore, an increased potential for hemorrhage occurs during surgery, particularly when the placenta covers a large portion of the lower uterine segment. There is an even greater potential for intraoperative hemorrhage when placental implantation occurs on the anterior wall of the lower uterine segment and a vertical incision in the uterus may be necessary, leading to more blood loss. The location of the placenta can be accurately determined preoperatively by ultrasound scan. General anesthesia, which avoids sympathetic blockade and permits maximum control of vital signs, is the anesthetic technique of choice when the patient is actively bleeding or when there is a great potential for intraoperative hemorrhage at the time of cesarean section. However, in a stable non-bleeding, non-anemic patient, a regional anesthetic (preferably a lumbar epidural block) may sometimes be considered. When selecting a regional block for cesarean delivery in a patient with complicating placenta previa, a minimum of two veins should be cannulated (preferably with 14 or 16 gauge needles) preoperatively, the patient should be well hydrated, and a minimum of

four units of blood should be available in the operating room at the time of surgery.

Abruptio Placentae

Placental separation may be marginal, partial or complete. The parturient generally presents with hypertonic, painful uterine contractions; vaginal bleeding may be overt, or it may be concealed and sequestered behind the placenta. Thus, the degree of blood loss may be greater than is readily apparent. When retroplacental bleeding occurs, the blood may extravasate into the myometrium, causing a Couvelaire uterus, interfering with myometrial contractility and predisposing to increased uterine hemorrhage. These patients are likely to develop DIC; in preparing for possible induction of anesthesia, a coagulation profile must therefore be obtained. In the presence of placental abruption, the fetus is at increased risk, primarily because of disruption at the utero-placental interface that causes fetal oxygen deprivation. A marginal abruption may suddenly progress to a complete abruption, and fetal demise may occur at any time. In patients with abruptio placentae, regional anesthesia may mask the signs of increasing pain and abruption; use of an epidural block is contraindicated whenever the potential for a developing coagulopathy exists. An epidural hematoma and its neurologic sequelae may occur following a regional block in patients who are developing DIC. If the patient can successfully deliver vaginally, intravenous and inhalational analgesia supplemented by local anesthestic infiltration or a pudendal block will provide adequate pain relief. For cesarean section, a general anesthetic is undoubtedly the technique of choice.

Inversion of the Uterus

Uterine inversion may occur during the third stage of labor; it is often a consequence of traction on the umbilical cord. Occasionally, if the inversion is promptly recognized, the obstetrician may be able to replace the uterus in its normal position without benefit of anesthesia. However, a general anesthetic may be necessary to achieve relaxation. The early signs of acute inversion are (1) sudden severe hypotension in the absence of overt or extreme hemorrhage (probably vaso-vagal in origin), (2) severe hemorrhage from the open uterine venous sinuses with profound shock, and (3) a palpable mass in the vagina (the inverted uterine fundus). Until the uterus has been replaced in its normal position, oxytocic drugs are contraindicated because they make reduction more difficult. An anesthesiologist should be summoned as soon as uterine inversion has been diagnosed. Cardiovascular resuscitation should be initiated immediately, including aggressive fluid and blood administration via large bore intravenous cannulas. After rapid sequence induction of anesthesia, preferably starting with intravenous ketamine, oxygen, muscle relaxant and tracheal intubation, a potent inhalational anesthetic (e.g., halothane, enflurane or isoflurane) in an appropriate concentration will achieve uterine relaxation. Once adequate uterine relaxation occurs, the obstetrician should be able to re-invert the uterus into its normal position; the volatile anesthetic agent can then be discontinued and an oxytocin infusion started to promote uterine contractility.

Rupture of the Uterus

Uterine rupture rarely occurs spontaneously. In modern obstetric practice, it is more likely to occur (1) after a prior cesarean section, particularly as a result of a vertical uterine scar, (2) during active labor following previous uterine surgery (e.g., myomectomy), and (3) following a prolonged, obstructed second stage of labor. During labor, complete uterine rupture will generally result in cessation of all uterine activity. The patient may experience a ripping sensation in her lower abdomen at the time of the rupture, and fetal parts may then be readily palpated through the abdominal wall. Uterine rupture has been associated with a 1% maternal mortality and less than 1% fetal mortality in trial of labor. Treatment consists of placement of at least two large bore I.V. cannulas, aggressive replacement of fluid and blood and rapid administration of an anesthetic. There may be considerable hemorrhage during this laparotomy. Depending upon the extent and location of rupture, the uterus may occasionally be conserved. However, in most instances, a cesarean hysterectomy is required.

Cesarean Hysterectomy

A cesarean hysterectomy is occasionally an elective procedure. More often it is performed in an emergency situation when cesarean sec-

tion is complicated by severe bleeding. In the former case, the patient may be hemodynamically stable; if so, a general or regional anesthetic may be considered. In the latter, when the patient is hemodynamically unstable, general anesthesia, which will permit maximum control of vital signs, is the method of choice. However, if a regional block has already been administered, vital signs should be maintained by aggressive fluid and blood replacement.

ANESTHESIA IN THE POSTPARTUM PERIOD

A modern postpartum Recovery Room must have facilities and trained personnel equal to that of the general surgical Recovery Area, and the personnel must have the competence to care for the critically ill as well as the normal postpartum patient. The professional staff must have the ability to manage patients with common diseases associated with pregnancy and those who have invasive monitors, including arterial lines and pulmonary artery catheters. If these facilities are not available in the regular postpartum Recovery Room, the patient should be transferred to an Intensive Care Unit (ICU) with the necessary facilities. Unfortunately, Intensive Care Units frequently do not have personnel familiar with the special needs of the postpartum patient.

Physiologic and hormonal changes of pregnancy persist for up to six weeks postpartum. Surgery during the postpartum period involves many of the same risks that occur during pregnancy, including gastric aspiration and uterine hemorrhage. Both regional and general anesthesia can be used with appropriate precautions during surgery in the puerperium. To minimize the risk of aspiration, any elective surgical procedure, such as a tubal ligation, preferably should be deferred until at least eight hours after delivery; the patient should be maintained on intravenous hydration and remain NPO until the time of surgery. If a functioning regional anesthetic is already in place, elective surgery may be performed immediately following a vaginal delivery. The average blood loss during a vaginal delivery is about 500 ml, and about 1000 ml of blood is lost during an average cesarean section. The patient's hemoglobin should be checked before proceeding with elective postpartum surgery. In the event that the hemoglobin and hematocrit are less than 9.0 gms% and 28%, respectively, elective surgery should be postponed for several weeks, until the patient's hemoglobin has returned to a normal range following hematinic therapy. Meanwhile, many of the physiologic changes of pregnancy will have reverted to the non-pregnant state and this will permit a more liberal choice of anesthetic technique.

References

Akamatsu TJ, Bonica JJ et al: Experiences with the use of ketamine for parturition: primary anesthetic for vaginal delivery. *Anesth. Analg.* 53:284, 1974.

Albright GA, Ferguson JE et al: *Anesthesia in Obstetrics. Maternal, Fetal, and Neonatal Aspects*, Ed. 2. Boston, Butterworth Publishers, 1986.

Artusio JF, Sia-Kho E: Anesthesia. In Orkin FK, Cooperman LH (Eds.): *Complications in Anesthesiology*. Philadelphia, J. B. Lippincott Co., 1983.

Bryant CL, Quirk JG: Take advantage of barbiturates' many ob benefits. *Contemp. Ob/Gyn* 26:37, 1985.

Crawford JS, James FM, Crawley M: A further study of general anesthesia for Caesarean section. *Br. J. Anaesth.* 48:661, 1976.

Datta S, Ostheimer GW et al: Neonatal effect of prolonged anesthetic induction for Cesarean section. *Obstet. Gynecol.* 58:331, 1981.

De Jong RH: *Local Anesthetics.* Ed. 2. Springfield, IL, Charles C Thomas, 1977.

Devore JS: Fetal depression. In Orkin FK, Cooperman LH (Eds.): *Complications in Anesthesiology*. Philadelphia, J. B. Lippincott Co., 1983.

Gibbs CP, Schwartz DJ et al: Antacid pulmonary aspiration. In Abstracts of Scientific Papers, Annual Meeting Society of Obstetrical Anesthesia and Perinatology, Memphis, 1978.

Gregory GA: Pediatric anesthesia. In Miller RD (Ed.): *Anesthesia*. New York, Churchill Livingston, 1986.

Hatjis CG, Meis PJ: Sinusoidal fetal heart rate pattern associated with butorphanol administration. *Obstet. Gynecol.* 67:377, 1986.

Hunter AR, Moir DD: Confidential enquiry into maternal deaths. *Br. J. Anaesth.* 55:367, 1983.

Kuhnert BR, Kuhnert PM et al: Meperidine and normeperidine levels following meperidine administration during labor: I. Mother. *Am. J. Obstet. Gynecol.* 133:904, 1979a.

Kuhnert BR, Kuhnert PM et al: Meperidine and normeperidine levels following meperidine administration during labor: II. Fetus and neonate. *Am. J. Obstet. Gynecol.* 133:909, 1979b.

Marx GF, Mateo CV: Effects of different oxygen concentrations during general anesthesia for elective Caesarean section. *Can. Anaesth. Soc. J.* 18:587, 1971.

Melzack R, Taenzer P et al: Labour is still painful after prepared chldbirth training. *Can. Med. J.* 125:357, 1981.

Miller JW, Anderson HH: The effect of n-demethylation on certain pharmacologic actions of morphine, codeine, and meperidine in the mouse. *J. Pharmacol. Exp. Ther.* 112:191, 1954.

Miller RD: Anesthesia for the elderly. In Miller RD (Ed): *Anesthesia*, Ed. 2. New York, Churchill Livingstone, 1986.

Miller RD, Stoelting RK: Pharmacology of the autonomic nervous system. In Miller RD (Ed.): *Anesthesia*, Ed. 1. New York, Churchill Livingstone, 1981.

Moir, DD: Maternal mortality and anaesthesia. *Br. J. Anaesth.* 52:1, 1980.

Morrison JC, Whybrew WD et al: Use of partial exchange transfusion preoperatively in patients with sickle cell hemoglobinopathies. *Am. J. Obstet. Gynecol.* 132:59, 1978.

Phillips OC: Aorto-caval compression. In Orkin FK, Cooperman LH (Eds.): *Complications in Anesthesiology*. Philadelphia, J. B. Lippincott Co., 1983.

Ramanthan S, Gandhi S et al: Oxygen transfer from mother to fetus during Cesarean section under epidural anesthesia. *Anesth. Analg.* 61:576, 1982.

Roizen MF: Anesthesia implications of concurrent disease. In Miller RD (Ed.): *Anesthesia*, Ed. 2. New York, Churchill Livingstone, 1986.

Scott JR, Rose NB: Effect of psychoprophylaxis (Lamaze preparation) on labor and delivery in primiparas. *N. Engl. J. Med.* 294:1205, 1976.

Shnider SM, Levinson G: Obstetric anesthesia. In Miller RD (Ed.): *Anesthesia*, Ed. 2. New York, Churchill Livingstone, 1986.

Smith BE: Teratogenicity. In Orkin FK, Cooperman LH (Eds.): *Complications in Anesthesiology*. Philadelphia, J. B. Lippincott Co., 1983.

Snyder SW, Wheeler AS et al: The use of nitroglycerine to control severe hypertension of pregnancy during Cesarean section. *Anesthesiology* 51:563, 1979.

Spielman FJ, Corke BC: Advantages and disadvantages of regional anesthesia for Cesarean section. *J. Reprod. Med.* 30:832, 1985.

Teabeaut JR: Aspiration of gastric contents: an experimental study. *Am. J. Pathol.* 28:51, 1952.

Thompson C, Forbes CD, Prentice CRM: A comparison of the effects of antihistamines on platelet function. *Thromb. Diathes. Haemorrh.* 30:547, 1973.

Ueland K: Mitral valve prolapse: alleviating your pregnant patient's anxiety. *Contemp. Ob/Gyn* 26:47, 1985.

LEGAL AND ETHICAL COMPLICATIONS

16

MICHAEL NEWTON
ROBERT BOUER

LEGAL COMPLICATIONS

Historical Review and Current Status

The legal complications of operations and procedures consist of suits or threatened suits. Those who claim to be able to heal the sick have always been subject to lawsuits by patients or their families if the results of treatment were unsatisfactory. During the early growth of modern medicine (1860 to 1960), with its many technologic achievements, such suits were relatively infrequent. However, in the last 25 years (and particularly in the last 10 years) they have become almost an inevitable part of the practice of medicine. For example, before 1980 the frequency of claims per 100 physicians was 2.9, whereas from 1980 to 1984 it was 8.6—a 287% increase.

The reasons for this increase are complex. Up to 50 years ago physicians' opinions and advice were likely to be accepted without question. John Webster (1580 to 1625) remarked "physicians are like kings: they brook no contradiction." Relatively few explanations were given to patients, and complications were seldom discussed in detail. A bad result was usually considered by patient and physician alike to be an act of God, something unfortunate that just happened. Patients' understanding of the technical aspects of medicine was limited.

In the past 25 years, medicine has continued to become more technical, more complex and less personal. Patient care now depends on many ancillary professionals. In 1960 nurses and technicians were largely under physicians' orders and control. Now professional nurses, nurse clinicians, clinical nurse-specialists, social workers, dietitians, technologists and many others, while nominally part of the "medical team," have increased professional responsibility for the care of patients in the area of their expertise. Thus, the one-to-one relationship of trust between patient and physician is diluted,

503

and the physician's advice is often subject to the differing opinions of other professionals. Society, also, contributes to this change, at least in the United States. Information on the latest medical discoveries has been broadcast to the public first by books, then by radio and now by television, often without critical or informed comment on the value of these techniques. Physicians may be contacted by media representatives to comment on a new treatment even before an account of it has appeared in a scientific journal. Society has, in general, become more litigious and more aware of the possibility of recovering the cost of medical and related expenses through the courts. Respect for medical authority has greatly diminished as the consumer movement has grown. The physician has had to change with the times and provide advice on risks, benefits and alternatives, thus allowing and encouraging patients to participate in the decision making process. Finally, the medicolegal field is changing rapidly. Major changes may be anticipated in the next few years. The purpose of this section is to orient obstetrician-gynecologists to some of the current medicolegal complications and to indicate briefly some of the possible solutions.

Obstetrics and gynecology have been specially affected by the increase in litigation. A survey by the American College of Obstetricians and Gynecologists in the summer of 1985 showed that 71% of obstetrician-gynecologists in the United States had experienced liability claims. There are several reasons for this. First, of the ten most common surgical procedures performed in the United States, five are in the obstetric-gynecologic field: dilatation and curettage, hysterectomy, tubal ligation, cesarean section and oophorectomy. Second, women have become more conscious and concerned about their bodies and what may be done to them. Third, in obstetrics two individuals (and usually three if the father is included) are involved when a pregnant or delivering woman undergoes a procedure or an operation. Fourth, advanced technology and support equipment, as exemplified by neonatal intensive care units, have created an unacceptable level of expectation for parents, that all babies should be "perfect" and that the physician should be a guarantor of good results. Fifth, the statutes of limitation have now been extended in most states to cover a child for varying times after a medical procedure was performed on the mother or the infant. The tolling of the statutes of limitation in many jurisdictions begins at the age of majority; thus the obstetrician may be held responsible for delivery-related damages to a newborn for 20 years. The "usual" two year tort liability would begin to run at age 18 (majority). In the case of a child who is ruled incompetent, an obstetrician could be subject to suit during the life of the child.

Legal Aspects

A physician in a court of law is in the same position as a lawyer in the operating room. In each case the preliminary work, the actual trial or operation and the subsequent events are familiar to one and not the other. To be able to deal in a common sense fashion with legal complications the physician does not need to be a lawyer. But he should be familiar with the differences between law and medicine and with some of the common legal terms and procedures.

The physician's instinct and need are to solve a patient's medical problem as soon as possible. On the other hand, delays are intrinsic to the law; theoretically, delay is for the protection of all parties involved and to permit discovery of as many facts in the case as possible. Law is adversarial, medicine is not. The exchange of hostilities between opposing lawyers is essential to the Anglo-American system of justice; it is unfamiliar to the physician whose main objective is to help the patient and to enlist her cooperative aid in solving her health problems.

Legal Terms and Definitions

Problems that arise from the physician-patient relationship result from one of three principles: (1) the infringement of individual rights, (2) the contract between physician and patient and (3) the fiduciary or trust relationship between them in which the physician assumes responsibility for the patient. When a patient feels that the physician to whom she relates has not acted in accordance with her expectations, a legal complication may develop.

The following definitions may be helpful in understanding the processes involved in legal complications. For a more complete list see the book by Fineberg and co-workers (1984).

THE LAW ITSELF

Common Law. Common law is made by court decision.

Statutory Law. Law made by legislatures is statutory law.

Statute of Limitation. Statute of limitation is the time within which a person may assert a legal claim. This varies in different states and also relates to the time of discovery of the alleged injury.

RELATIONSHIPS BETWEEN PHYSICIANS AND PATIENTS

Lawsuits against physicians may be based on (1) assault and battery, (2) professional negligence or (3) breach of contract.

Assault and Battery. Assault and battery is the wrongful, harmful or offensive contact with another's body, or putting the other person in fear of such an attack, in other words, a deliberate contact of some type with a patient in a situation in which consent had not been granted.

A tort is a wrongful act to a patient or her property for which the law allows money damages. A tort is neither a crime nor a breach of contract. A tort may be intentional or unintentional. Assault and battery, defamation (libel or slander) and false imprisonment are examples of intentional torts. Surgery without informed consent, doing more than has been authorized (except in emergency situations or when the surgery is in the best judgment of the surgeon), operating on the wrong leg or on the wrong patient are situations in which the intentional torts of assault and battery can be alleged. An accusation of malpractice (professional negligence) is the form of tort that accounts for the great majority of litigation in obstetrics and gynecology.

Professional Negligence (Malpractice). This is the failure to exercise the degree of care that is used by reasonably careful physicians in the same or similar circumstances. Malpractice involves the omission of something that a reasonable and prudent person would do when guided by those considerations that ordinarily regulate human affairs or the commission of an act that such a person would not do. The failure to exercise "due care" must cause the patient injury. In a medical malpractice trial, the plaintiff's attorney must show that the physician's violation of the standard of care caused the patient's injury. The attorney can illustrate the violation in one of two ways, either through medical testimony establishing that the standards of the medical community were violated, thus effecting the patient's bad result, or by evoking the doctrine of *res ipsa loquitur* (see later discussion).

Contract. The agreement to care for a patient establishes a contract and creates duties for the physician and the patient. The physician seeking to terminate this contract must provide *notice* and an opportunity for the patient to obtain other care in reasonable time to avoid an accusation of "abandonment." A contract may be implied in law or implied in fact. A patient arriving in a delivery room in active labor creates a contract implied in fact, and obstetric delivery is a reasonable expectation. A patient brought to an emergency room in shock, suffering from a ruptured ectopic pregnancy and unaccompanied by a relative establishes a contract implied in law, and creates a duty on the part of the physician to meet the appropriate standard of care.

Standard of Practice. A term used in the legal definition of medical malpractice. A physician is liable only if the treatment, or the lack thereof, violates the standards of practice of reasonably competent physicians, in the same or similar circumstances, with comparable training and experience. Testimony establishing standard of care should be from qualified expert witnesses. Learned treatises are also permissible for this purpose. The locality rule, which limited the standard of care to those of the jurisdiction and region, is being replaced by a "national standard."

Vicarious Liability. A liability that the physician may have for the acts of someone else. For instance, the physician may be vicariously liable for the acts of the nurse in his office, since she is his employee. Vicarious liability will not extend to the acts of independent contractors such as anesthesiologists and consultants whose professional acts are not controlled by the physician. Hospital employees who act under the direction or the supervision of the physician may create a situation in which vicarious liability is a factor.

Informed Consent. A legal doctrine that requires that a physician obtain consent for treatment that is to be rendered or an operation that is to be performed. Without informed consent the physician may be held liable for a violation of the patient's rights, regardless of whether the treatment was appropriate and rendered with due care. Consent is "fully informed" only when the patient knows and understands all the factors that are material to making a decision as a reasonable person in the patient's position would do. In order to obtain fully informed consent, the physician must follow the listed steps:

1. Explain to the patient the diagnosis and nature of the condition or illness that calls for medical intervention.

2. Explain to the patient the nature and purpose of the treatment recommended.

3. Explain fully the known material risks and consequences associated with the recommended treatment.

4. Explain fully all feasible alternative treatments, including the option of taking no action, with a description of the risks and complications associated with the alternatives.

5. Explain in understandable terms the relative probability of success.

6. Allow the patient a reasonable amount of time to contemplate the information given, and encourage questions to ensure that the patient understands the information provided.

7. If possible, obtain the signature of the patient to indicate that the information was provided and understood.

8. Document in the patient's record that informed consent was obtained.

SPECIAL PRINCIPLES

Res ipsa loquitur. This is a legal doctrine that, when applicable, allows a patient to recover damages without the necessity of an expert witness to testify that the defendant physician violated the standards of practice. Generally, it is only applicable in situations in which negligence is clear and obvious, even to a layman, for example, foreign object cases in which a sponge is left in the abdomen, or when an unconscious patient falls off an operating table, bed or stretcher.

Captain of the Ship. This is a common law doctrine that makes the physician in charge of a medical team liable for the negligent acts of the members of the team. This doctrine is less applicable today. For example, in most jurisdictions a surgeon will no longer be considered responsible for a sponge count, since nurses employed by the hospital count the sponges and record the results.

Wrongful Birth. An action brought by the parents or parent of a child who is alleged to have been born as a result of negligence or breach of contract by the attendant physician.

Wrongful Life. The claim by a child to recover damages for being born because of the negligence of others.

Special Legal Complications in Obstetrics and Gynecology

LABOR AND DELIVERY

Several factors make the processes of labor and delivery particularly susceptible to legal complications. Statutes of limitations now extend the physician's liability for many years, because the full effect of a complication may not be assessable until the infant is fully grown or until society can appreciate that a birth injury may have occurred. Moreover, there is a tendency on the part of patients, their attorneys and the public to assume that the least irregularity in care during labor and delivery is responsible for the later development of cerebral palsy or mental retardation. This is far from the case (Illingworth, 1985). First, Paneth and Stark (1983) point out that (1) no more than 15% of cases of severe retardation can be attributed to perinatal events; (2) the majority of severely depressed babies suffer no detectable neurologic or intellectual sequelae; and (3) even in cases of cerebral palsy, at least 50% of all infants have no documented depression at the time of birth. Second, two individuals are involved, mother and child, at a crucial time in both their lives; the addition of the father as an interested third party compounds this. Third, labor and delivery may occur unexpectedly at any time of the day or night. Thus, the availability of the obstetrician and his ability to be present at the delivery or to provide an acceptable substitute is important. The danger is always present that a patient may claim that she has been abandoned. Fourth, much of the care of the patient during labor and delivery must, of necessity, be given by other professional personnel such as nurses, nurse-midwives, anesthesiologists and others for whom the physician may be responsible by the "Captain of the Ship" doctrine, even though they may have their own professional responsibilities.

GYNECOLOGY

Claims against physicians for errors in gynecologic management are most commonly related to the surgical aspects of the specialty and, therefore, are similar to those made against general and specialty surgeons. Such suits (and, indeed, many others) are likely to include claims against the hospital and other involved individuals. The difficulty about this from the defendant physician's position is that lawyers for other parties may defend the rights of their own clients with little regard to the effect of their efforts on other defendants. An example of this situation occurs in cases in which a sponge or instrument is left inside the peritoneal cavity after an operation. *Res ipsa loquitur* applies to such cases, since one does not normally expect to find a sponge in that location, and its mere presence may be considered prima facie evidence of malpractice. The physician may be involved as the "Captain of the Ship." However, if the circulating nurse reported the sponge count to be correct when it was not, the question may arise as to who is her superior and therefore responsible (besides her)—the physician or the hospital that pays her. Other acts that may give rise to claims in gynecology are common to other surgical procedures and include problems with anesthesia, blood transfusions (Jehovah's Witnesses) or recovery room mishaps.

During the last 10 years, hysterectomy (and oophorectomy) has been of particular concern to the public, because of the belief that this type of surgery may be performed unnecessarily. This public concern may have resulted in the decline in the rate of hysterectomy in the United States in the past three or four years from the very high levels previously reported; in fact, hysterectomy was and is more frequently performed in the United States than in any other country. Careful monitoring, in an attempt to limit the number of hysterectomies performed in the Canadian province of Saskatchewan, has apparently been successful (Dyck et al, 1977), but the introduction of second opinion programs has had an uncertain impact. However, patients have become more conscious of the effects of the operation and its complications. Among the complications are infection, hemorrhage, fistula formation and emotional and menopausal changes. Of special concern to gynecologists in this area, therefore, is the need to obtain informed consent from the patient before the procedure.

PREGNANCY: ITS TERMINATION AND PREVENTION

Termination of pregnancy (abortion) and of fertility (tubal ligation) have become legal and widely accepted in the United States during the last 20 years. Claims in regard to them relate to the surgical nature of the procedures and to informed consent. For instance, there is a small but definite chance of recanalization of the tubes after tubal ligation, and this possibility has to be explained to the patient in advance. Two additional concerns have arisen: wrongful birth and wrongful life. In wrongful birth suits the parents claim that if the physician had not been negligent, they would have been advised not to conceive or that if the woman were already pregnant, the physician failed to perform the necessary tests (i.e., amniocentesis, tests for Tay-Sachs disease) or to give advice

that would have shown the child to be defective (i.e., genetic counseling), thus denying the parents the option of abortion. In wrongful life suits a defective child (through the parents) may claim that owing to the physician's negligence the parents were denied the choice of not conceiving or of abortion after conception. Recent legal decisions indicate that claims for wrongful birth may in some instances raise relevant issues, whereas those for wrongful life may not be sustained.

Legal complications regarding contraception may involve the device that is used to prevent conception or the age and status of the woman given contraceptive advice. Among the intrauterine devices, the Dalkon shield has provided the most legal complications because of the serious infections associated with it. However, other IUDs may also be a problem because of the occurrence of perforation, pelvic infection and other complications. Informed consent and permission to insert IUDs are important, but less so now that IUDs have been largely withdrawn from the U.S. market. Recent concern about giving contraceptive advice to minors may also raise legal complications. It is essential that the obstetrician-gynecologist be familiar with state and local laws defining minors and how they may be given contraceptive counseling, i.e., with or without parental consent.

GENETICS AND RELATED PROBLEMS

Increases in knowledge about inherited diseases and the development of the fetus in utero have given rise to an entirely new set of possible medicolegal complications. Most of these are failures of omission, for example, the birth of a defective child because a diagnostic test such as chromosome analysis of amniotic fluid was not offered or performed. However, amniocentesis itself carries risks for both mother and fetus such as infection, injury to the fetus, hemorrhage, miscarriage or premature labor. Therefore, informed consent is essential prior to amniocentesis.

New diagnostic techniques have made invasive surgical management of fetal disease possible. Intrauterine transfusion for severe erythroblastosis fetalis has become an important part of obstetric management. Other fetal conditions that have been reported to be managed successfully include hydrocephalus and urinary tract obstruction. Further work with other fetal diseases can be anticipated. The legal and ethical issues raised by fetal surgery are discussed by Elias and Annas (1983). They point out that

some procedures must still be considered experimental and state specifically that "IRB (Institutional Review Board) review, detailed consent, an advocate for the fetus and a consent
auditor are all morally and legally appropriate."
Thus, fetal surgery performed without these
safeguards is open to serious legal complications.

SUBSTITUTE PARENTHOOD

Recent advances in knowledge of the physiology of fertilization and changes in social cus-
toms have permitted variations from the usual
method of conception, such as artificial insemination (including surrogate motherhood), in
vitro fertilization and genetic engineering. In
all of these except surrogate motherhood specific actions are performed by the physician that
may lead to medicolegal complications. The
overall legal and ethical aspects of these developments are discussed by Andrews (1986), and
the social policy considerations are reviewed by
Elias and Annas (1986).

The birth of a child with physical or mental
defects following artificial insemination may
present major litigation problems for the partic-
ipating physician. These problems are summarized by Hirsh (1983). Detailed informed consent is essential prior to insemination.

In vitro fertilization has stirred popular interest and concern. Apart from the ethical issues
(see later discussion), there are many ways in
which the physician or his associates can be
involved in legal complications, for example, if
pregnancy does not result, if abortion occurs or
if a defective child is born. In spite of the fact
that the motivation of most couples seeking in
vitro fertilization is very high and the limited
chance of success is well recognized, there is
considerable potential for claims. Gene manipulation is in part a by-product of in vitro fertilization and in part a result of studies on bacterial
genes. At present, it is primarily an ethical
dilemma and strictly experimental.

BREAST DISEASE

Since breast cancer is the second most common cancer in women and since breast disorders are largely related to reproduction, the
diagnosis of breast disease properly lies within
the obstetrician-gynecologists's purview. A major cause of legal actions is failure to diagnose
cancer. The fact that in most parts of the United
States obstetrician-gynecologists do not provide
surgical treatment for breast diseases, benign

or malignant, does not detract from the responsibility for diagnosis, particularly since obstetrician-gynecologists are often the only physicians
to examine women regularly. Omission, therefore, of recognized diagnostic procedures or of
recommendations that the patient seek them
elsewhere may lead to claims of malpractice.
Recommendations for consultation should be
documented. A similar risk occurs if studies
such as cytologic examination of the aspirate of
a cyst or needle or open biopsy do not lead to
a diagnosis of a cancer that is later found, or if
such procedures result in an infection or unsightly scars.

PROLONGATION OF LIFE AND RESUSCITATION

Except for gynecologic oncologists, obstetrician-gynecologists seldom have to deal with
dying adult patients, although stillbirth and
early neonatal death fall within their province.
In acute situations, it is clearly a physician's
duty to do all that he can to preserve life. When
all attempts to cure have been unsuccessful and
death is imminent (sooner or later), the question
of life-prolonging treatment remains under discussion. Both legal and ethical questions are
involved.

Since the ethical questions (see later discussion) are not easy to decide, parties with differing interests in particular cases have had recourse to the law in attempts at resolution.
These cases have generally occurred in other
than obstetric-gynecologic situations, but a brief
account of the problems involved is appropriate
here because of the occasional case that involves
the obstetrician-gynecologist.

In many instances, the initiation or continuation of cardiopulmonary resuscitation (CPR)
is in question. Present-day CPR usually means
that (in a hospital) a special team is summoned
to apply resuscitative measures and that these
measures are continued until the patient is
clearly brain dead. The measures include transfer to and maintenance of the patient in an
intensive care unit.

It is difficult to decide whether or not CPR
should be started in a patient who has no chance
of eventual survival. At the present time a nurse
or other professional cannot make this decision;
it is the physician's responsibility. He dis-
charges it by writing or not writing a DNR (do
not resuscitate) order on the patient's chart.
How the physician arrives at that decision is an
ethical and practical matter and is discussed
later. Legally the physician is on relatively safe
ground if his decision follows accepted medical

standards, either devised by the institution concerned or, in the absence of such guidelines, developed from generally accepted principles (Greenlaw, 1982).

The Process of a Legal Complication

ORIGINS

Complications of the doctor-patient relationship result from (1) alleged infringement of the basic rights of the individual (patient), (2) breach of contract between physician and patient or (3) betrayal of the trust placed by the patient in the physician. Infringement of the rights of a patient is present if (1) there is a duty that the physician owes to the patient, (2) there is a dereliction or breach of that duty, (3) damage results, and (4) damage is directly caused by the dereliction. An agreement between physician and patient is similar to a commercial contract. If the outcome of the agreement is not what the patient expected, she may complain that the physician broke the contract. The trust placed by a patient in her physician is exemplified by her consent to examinations and procedures. Therefore, such consent must be explicit and defined.

Some clues to the likelihood of a claim against the physician may be obtained if the procedure or operation did not turn out as expected, or if the patient and her family appear dissatisfied. If such clues are absent, a request for or subpoena of the records by the patient's attorney is the first sign of an impending legal complication.

LITIGATION

The resolution of a medicolegal complication involves litigation by the adversary system. This process may vary in different jurisdictions, but, in general, consists of the following steps.

The Complaint. The plaintiff* files a written complaint in court. The complaint states the relevance of the plaintiff's claims and demands judgment for an amount equal to or greater than the jurisdictional amount required for admission to the desired court. The defendant receives notice of the complaint by means of a summons served by an officer of the court.

Motions. The defendant may file motions contending that the plaintiff's claims are not recognized by the law as being compensable.

---

*"Plaintiff" and "defendant" imply "or her/his attorney" in each case.

The Answer. If there are no motions by the defendant or if the motions are denied, the defendant next must file (by a specific date) an answer responding to the allegations made by the plaintiff. The answer may deny the allegations and include certain "affirmative" defenses such as contributory negligence, expiration of the statute of limitations or the existence of a release by the plaintiff.

The Reply. In some jurisdictions the plaintiff is permitted to reply to any affirmative defenses; in others, they are simply assumed to be denied.

Issues. Complaint, Answer and Reply (if permitted) constitute the issues upon which the trial will be based. Only evidence related to these issues (or an amendment to them approved by the court) will be permitted at the trial.

Pre-trial Discovery. The pre-trial discovery covers investigation of the facts by the plaintiff and the defendant. Formal methods of doing this include orders to produce records and documents, requests for physical examinations, written interrogatories and oral depositions. In written interrogatories the defendant or the plaintiff can require the adversary to answer, in writing and under oath, relevant questions. In oral depositions the involved parties or others related to the case (such as expert witnesses) can be required by subpoena to answer all questions formally and under oath. Questions and answers are taken down verbatim and transcribed by a court reporter. Depositions taken for discovery provide information for both sides so that there will be no surprise testimony at the trial. They are available for impeachment during court testimony. Evidentiary depositions may be read at trial, after review by the judge, if the witness cannot be present. If such depositions are recorded on videotapes, they can be shown in court under the same conditions.

Pre-trial Conference. At such conferences the judge may convene the opposing parties or their lawyers and explore the possibilities for settlement or methods of simplifying or shortening the trial.

The Trial. It is beyond the scope of this chapter to give the details of a trial. The elements are: selection of the jury (unless the right to a jury has been waived), opening statements by the plaintiff's and the defendant's lawyers, evidence given by witnesses for the plaintiff and for the defense, closing arguments by the opposing attorneys, the judge's instructions to the jury on the law and, finally, deliberation and a verdict by the jury. The usual burden of proof is that the preponderance of evidence favors the plaintiff. At any point the judge may dismiss the case and enter a summary judgment. This does not prevent further action by the plaintiff, since there is no double jeopardy in civil cases.

The progress of litigation may be delayed at many points. The discovery phase may be prolonged because of the difficulty of coordinating the schedules of attorneys and witnesses or for many other reasons. The trial may be put off because of the pressure on the court, or it may be delayed (continued) by either side in order to complete its investigations. Litigation may also be halted by settlement. This is a negotiated agreement between the parties with specific regard to monetary awards and definition of responsibility. Since a settlement depends in large part on the legal strength of the opposing cases, it is largely a matter to be determined by the attorneys, although the principals (plaintiff and defendant) must agree to the terms. A settlement has the effect of a verdict. It is approved by the court and is binding on all parties.

If either party is dissatisfied with the results of a trial, he or she may ask the judge to overturn the verdict or permit a new trial. If these motions are denied, the dissatisfied party has the option of appealing to a higher court. A description of the procedures for this is beyond the scope of this chapter.

Prevention of Legal Complications

MEDICAL ASPECTS

For the obstetrician-gynecologist a serious legal complication is at best an unfortunate and expensive consequence of medical practice and at worst a professional and financial disaster. If he wins or settles the suit, some publicity, if not in the media then among colleagues, inevitably results, and this is almost always to his detriment. Apart from this, review of records, conferences with lawyers, depositions and court appearances divert important time from practice and therefore from income. The emotional aspects of being a defendant are an added burden. It behooves the physician, therefore, to do everything he can to reduce legal complictions to a minimum, although there are undoubtedly some that cannot be prevented in the present litigious climate. It is helpful to recognize the reasons for medicolegal complications. Table 16–1 gives examples of allegations against physicians and their frequency.

Table 16–1. Physician Malpractice Allegations (1978–1982)*

Primary Allegation	No. of Claims	Percent
Lack of informed consent	185	32
Emotional trauma	134	23
Abandonment	89	15
Billing problems	85	15
Failure to refer	45	8
Failure to disclose, inform patient of condition	43	7

*From St. Paul Fire and Marine Insurance Co. *Medical World News* Feb. 27, 1984. Adapted with permission.

The cardinal principles for avoiding suits are discussed in the following paragraphs.

Knowledge. Learning does not stop at the end of medical school or residency. It is a physician's duty to remain abreast of recent developments in his field of medical care. Moreover, he should remain technically skillful in those areas in which he practices and should recognize that consultation with an appropriate expert is necessary when he encounters a condition or a complication that is outside his usual area of expertise and that may constitute a danger to the patient's life or her future well-being.

Good Patient Care. Good patient care is hard to define. But, in essence, it means treating the patient with kindness, courtesy and concern; discussing her problems with her as an individual; and explaining carefully any planned treatment, its alternatives, effects and possible complications. This, indeed, is the basis for informed consent.

Consideration of the Patient's Family. It is important to treat the patient's immediate family with the same consideration as the patient herself. They deserve to know what is going on with their relative, what to expect and what they can do to help.

Records. A physician's records are the main basis upon which his treatment is subsequently judged. A case may not come to discovery or trial for years. Memories fade, witnesses are lost, and a well-written legible contemporaneous record may establish the physician's thinking and credibility and show that the appropriate standard of care was met. Check list forms are helpful for recording basic histories and physical examinations. However, there is no substitute for a narrative account of the patient's primary problem and an outline of the planned treatment. When this account is more than a few words in length, dictated, transcribed and signed notes are far superior to written notes. Legible handwriting may be used for very brief notes. Once written, records should not be erased or corrected; if correction is absolutely necessary, the revision should be initialed and dated. If possible, the results of all contacts with the patient by the physician or his staff, even by telephone, should be recorded. Attempts to trace a patient or to persuade her to return for follow-up should also be recorded, and any evidence of her non-compliance with instructions or recommendations should be included in the record.

Physicians' Associates and Assistants. Medical care no longer takes place in the context of a one-to-one relationship between physician and patient. Many other professionals and paraprofessionals are now involved in patient care. Their connection with the physician may be as close as the single office assistant who is personally employed by the physician or as distant as the technician who draws the patient's blood for chemical tests in the hospital. Yet, on the basis of the "Captain of the Ship" doctrine, the physician may be held liable for these agents' acts of omission or commission. More recent decisions may make the more distant agents, such as operating room nurses and physical therapists, the responsibility of those to whom they report, for example, the Director of Nursing or the Head of the Physical Therapy Department. But this uncertainty makes it all the more important that the physician carefully discuss with and instruct his associates in what he wants them to do and why and when he wants them to do it. Generally, he has to leave the technical aspects of their tasks up to them, with the expectation that they have been properly trained. However, if they are employed by the physician, it is his responsibility to have checked on their training and experience. Another important aspect of the multiplicity of caregivers is that communication must be maintained between primary and consulting or substitute physicians and between the physician(s) and other members of the health care team. It is important to avoid making derogatory comments about other physicians and the care they have given the patient. Such remarks are often the first stage in the development of a lawsuit.

Physicians' Responses to Legal Complications. The first actions taken when a suit begins may make a difference in its outcome and its effect on the physician's professional standing and activities. Basic precepts are to call the insurance company promptly, discuss the matter fully and frankly with the insurance company and the attorney and to avoid talking to a patient's attorney. If records are requested or subpoenaed, copies should be sent and the originals should be retained. If the suit proceeds to the point where the obstetrician-gynecologist is required to give a deposition or testify in court, it is important to be as well prepared as possible by thoroughly reviewing the records and consulting with the attorney. Assisting the attorney in preparing the case may be very helpful. Advice on physicians' courtroom behavior can be obtained from the Department of Professional Liability of the American College of Obstetricians and Gynecologists.

Responsible Participation as an Expert Witness. Irrespective of the litigant on whose behalf he has been asked to testify, the expert witness should regard his testimony as a consultation in which he attempts, in good faith, to clarify a difficult situation. Thus, he should support his opinion by references and limit his testimony to fields in which he can reasonably claim expertise. Moreover, the expert witness has a duty to help to maintain the quality of care and to give a clear and understandable explanation of complex medical terms and treatments (Brent, 1982; Kunin, 1984).

LEGAL ASPECTS

Contributions that the the legal profession can make to decreasing the legal complications of obstetric-gyncologic procedures are less obvious. Any changes are antithetical to the practice of law, since the professional activity of the lawyer is to represent an injured client and see that the physician who errs does not go without detection or penalty if what he has done involves suffering or expense to the patient. However, five legal problems that cause concern are (1) the lack of careful review of the case by an expert to establish the likelihood of a real cause of action prior to filing the complaint and setting the legal system in motion; attorneys should be reponsible for capricious and frivolous lawsuits; (2) the delay in bringing a case to trial or settlement; (3) contingency fees; (4) solicitation (advertisement) by lawyers for malpractice cases; and (5) the importance of obtaining recognized medical experts to testify in legal cases.

Delays are the concern of the courts, which are often constricted by the number of cases to be tried; however, the courts are also wary of overstepping the rights of the litigants to prepare their cases fully. Contingency fees ostensibly permit those who are without substantial resources to obtain the services of a lawyer. However, they have probably contributed to the many excessive monetary sums awarded in recent years by juries in personal injury cases. Also, it seems likely that the possibility of very large awards or settlements in favor of plaintiffs encourages advertising of legal services for malpractice cases. The use of appropriate expert witnesses by the legal profession is most important. A good expert witness can contribute greatly to the determination of a fair solution to the dispute and that, in a democracy governed by law, is of fundamental importance.

COMBINED MEDICAL AND LEGAL ASPECTS

Combined efforts by medicine and law to prevent or mitigate legal complications take two forms: pragmatic and educational. To date, the former have included arbitration, the no-fault approach and a clearer definition of informed consent, whereas the latter have included various educational techniques to involve both physicians and lawyers and to improve communication and understanding between members of each field.

A variety of arbitration strategies have been suggested. Acceptance of arbitration in case of future injury as a part of consent to hospitalization or procedures has been tried, but it was found to be impractical because patients cannot be expected to sign away their rights to make a claim for injury before the event. On the state level, the requirement that review or arbitration panels examine the evidence has had some success. Usually such panels include legal representatives of the plaintiff and of the defendant physician, a judge and, possibly, expert witnesses selected by the panel. Decisions by the panel are usually not binding on the parties, since that would jeopardize the plaintiff's right to a jury trial. However, such decisions may, in some instances, be introduced into any subsequent trial, and, in such a situation, these decisions obviously have weight.

A number of proposals have been advanced to designate an agreed set of events as compensable. In studies done on this subject in the fields of general surgery and orthopedic surgery, it was possible for experts to agree on certain adverse outcomes that were unavoidable or relatively infrequent. If similar studies could be performed for obstetrics and gynecology, the problem of compensation in this field might be simplified. In reviewing the situation, Tancredi (1982) states, "When one considers all of the economic factors that enter into compensation for injured patients, the DCEs (designated compensable events) may not only be more equi-

table but also more economically efficient." Of course, if an event falls outside the list of DCEs, the current tort system would apply.

An attempt was made by the Texas legislature to codify the risks that a physician is required to disclose to a patient prior to an operation. The purpose of this was to simplify what the patient needs to be told. However, the rigidity of the system may be self-defeating, and general agreement on such risks is difficult to reach.

In the educational area, several developments give promise of lessening legal complications. First, there is an increasing number of individuals with both medical and legal degrees; these individuals should provide a broader view of the problems. Second, more seminars on medicolegal problems are being presented for both physicians and lawyers. Third, increased time in medical school devoted to the consideration of risk factors may alert young practitioners to the prevention of legal complications. This is particularly applicable to residents and students in departments of obstetrics and gynecology; unfortunately, very few departments cover this subject in anything more than a casual manner. Finally, specific education of lawyers and physicians in the proper responsibilities, motivation and behavior of expert witnesses should help to illuminate problem cases and bring them to a swifter conclusion (Brent, 1982).

FUTURE DEVELOPMENTS

For the physician, and especially for the obstetrician-gynecologist, the current (1986) medicolegal situation is of great concern because of the likelihood of suits and the high cost of Professional Liability Insurance (up to $50,000 a year or more). In some areas, a significant number of obstetrician-gynecologists have given up the practice of obstetrics for these reasons. Many solutions have been proposed. They fall into three groups: (1) continuing education in risk management and improved peer review for physicians; (2) legislative reform; and (3) public education. The first is fundamental and of primary importance. The second and third solutions are closely linked.

Legislative changes have received much attention from physicians, less from lawyers and some from the public. They include such proposals as (1) development of screening panels that might eliminate frivolous cases, (2) limitation of the amounts of awards and the requirement of periodic rather than large lump sum payments, (3) establishment of a sliding scale for contingency fees, (4) early dismissal of cases against uninvolved physicians and others, (5) elimination of punitive damages, (6) permission for physicians wrongfully accused of malpractice to seek recourse and (7) establishment of standards for expert witnesses. The enthusiasm of legislatures for any or all of these concepts is likely to be limited, unless public awareness and concern reaches a higher point than at present. Failing legislative remedies, there is likely to be a further increase in Professional Liability Insurance premiums for physicians. This will have to be paid by specific charges to the patients for such insurance, increased fees or state or federal contributions from tax monies. None of these solutions is entirely satisfactory.

Legislative changes will not be possible without public expression of concern about the situation, since legislators respond to this stimulus. Currently, more information is being given by knowledgeable physicians and the media. If this information remains truly educational and its broadcast is sustained, it is likely to result in legislative discussion of the issues and, possibly, some constructive changes. A significant contributory issue is the increasing number of liability suits involving private and public firms and organizations outside medicine and their resultant difficulty of obtaining adequate insurance coverage.

ETHICAL COMPLICATIONS

The Nature of Ethical Complications

Ethical complications of an obstetric or gynecologic procedure arise when there is a conflict as to the right course of action to take. Such a conflict may occur before, during or after a procedure. It may be a conflict of responsibilities for the physician alone or may involve the physician, other professional personnel, the patient, the patient's family, the hospital, other patients or one or more branches of government. It may be a simple dilemma such as the appropriateness of continuing postoperative pain relief or a complex problem such as the decision to use or not use major resuscitative measures for a patient with terminal cancer. It is often associated with a legal complication.

Every ethical dilemma is unique. But to treat it as unique and to approach it de novo would cause endless and repetitious labor. It is helpful, therefore, to have some basic knowledge of the principles that have been developed by students of ethics over the years and that are still evolving. Some of the theoretic considerations are discussed by Beauchamp and Childress (1983). They include:

1. Are the consequences of a specific act good or bad (utilitarianism), and for whom are such consequences good or bad?

2. How do principles such as truth-telling, promise-keeping or justice relate to the issue? If they are important, are they based on theologic, empiric or intuitive reasons?

3. What is the duty of the physician (or other professional)? Normally, the physician's duty is to the patient, as outlined in the various physician's oaths and codes. For example, one of the most potent duties is to do no harm (*non nocere*). But the physician also has duties to the patient's family, to society as a whole and to the law.

Recognition and Diagnosis of Ethical Problems

Difficult ethical problems have increased in the past few years. Among the reasons for this are the complexities of modern medical techniques, the increasing number of professionals concerned with patient care who have their own standards and duties and the decrease in the physician's authority in patient management. It is important, therefore, to recognize what is an ethical issue and what is not. To take a simple example, the prescription of a specific antibiotic for the management of a urinary tract infection is a matter of knowing or discovering the available information on the effectiveness of various drugs on the organisms involved and choosing the best. It is a medical and not an ethical decision. If, however, a patient is found to have trichomoniasis, it is an ethical question to decide if her partner(s) should be treated without him/them first having been examined. There are many such ethical dilemmas in obstetrics and gynecology, some of which are detailed later in the discussion. However, the ethical problem is almost always associated with other problems, which may be of overriding concern and may need resolution before the ethical core is uncovered. For example, giving contraceptive advice to minors may be forbidden without parental consent in the state in which a particular physician practices. If the physician recognizes that a specific 16-year-old patient is especially likely to become pregnant if she does not receive proper contraceptive advice, the ethical question for him is whether he should inform the parents and get their consent at the expense of divulging his knowledge or fears about his patient.

An ethical problem may not be recognized as such. Often there appears to be merely a difference of opinion as to the right action to take. This may involve an internal dilemma for the physician or other professionals; sometimes the conflict may arise because of external factors such as the law or the public good; and sometimes the patient or her family may disagree with the proposed course of action or treatment for reasons that are not related to the medical aspects of the situation.

Whether a conflict of rights or duties is identified as ethical or not may be irrelevant so long as it is recognized as something beyond a strictly medical, nursing or other technical question. Some persons are better able to appreciate the importance of such difficulties than others. But familiarity with the analysis of situations for their ethical content makes them easier to recognize. Recognition makes for clarification and may help to define the right course to take. Also, it is helpful to understand those areas in obstetrics and gynecology in which ethical issues are especially likely to arise.

Ethical Complications in Obstetrics and Gynecology

GENERAL PROBLEMS

General ethical problems are common to all branches of medicine. Examples of those that have particular relevance to obstetrics and gynecology are refusal of treatment, confidentiality, human experimentation and delegation of responsibility.

Refusal of Treatment. Refusal of treatment by a patient presents the physician with an ethical (and legal) conflict when he feels that the recommended treatment is medically appropriate. Should he accept the patient's statement, attempt to overpersuade her or withdraw from the case? The answer depends on the urgency and severity of the patient's illness and the possible reason for the refusal (Applebaum and Roth, 1983). Supplying the patient with more information, including family members in the decision and obtaining a consultation with another qualified physician are all helpful approaches. If, finally, the patient continues to refuse the important part of the treatment, it is essential to document this in the record.

Confidentiality. Codified principles of medical ethics have stressed the importance of confidentiality. Thus, the oath of Hippocrates states "What I may see or hear in the course of treatment or even outside of the treatment in regard to the life of men, which on no account may be spread abroad, I will keep to myself, holding such things shameful and not to be spoken about." The American Medical Association's 1971 Principles of Medical Ethics somewhat circumscribe this broad statement, stating "A physician may not reveal the confidences entrusted him in the course of medical attendance or the deficiencies he may observe in the character of patients, unless he is required to do so by law or unless it becomes necessary to protect the welfare of the individual or the society." By 1980 the Principles were modified to read "A physician . . . shall safeguard patient confidences within the constraints of the law." The International Code of Medical Ethics adopted in 1949 makes an uncompromising statement: "A doctor owes to his patient absolute secrecy on all which has been confided in him or which he knows because of the confidence entrusted in him" (Veatch, 1977; Beauchamp and Childress, 1983).

Confidentiality has been eroded in the past few decades (and will be further eroded in the future) by the ready availability on computers of personal and medical data about patients (Hiller and Seidel, 1982). In obstetrics and gynecology confidentiality becomes an issue in relation to prescribing contraceptive advice to minors, in communicating plans for or results of operations or procedures to the patient's family and friends and in reporting the results of examinations to third parties. In two instances the physician's duty is clear, when he is authorized to release information by a competent patient or when he is required by law to do so. Ethical questions arise when the physician's own conscience is opposed to the law in question or when he has doubts about the competence of the patient. There may be no easy solution, particularly in the era of computerization. When in doubt, however, the physician has to assemble the data on the possible breach of confidentiality and do what he believes to be in the patient's best interest. If such action goes against his own conscience, he must decide whether to take it or withdraw from the situation with appropriate safeguards so that the patient continues to receive care. With regard to competence, a patient has to be regarded as competent unless she has been declared incompetent, is unconscious or is under the effect of mind-altering medication.

Human Experimentation. Human experimentation raises important ethical issues in obstetrics and gynecology, particularly in regard to studies performed in pregnancy, in which the interest of the fetus and, to some extent, of the fetus' father as well as those of the mother are important. These issues include fetal surgery and the study of abortuses and placentas. Published guidelines for human experimentation such as the Nuremberg Code (1948), the Declaration of Helsinki (1964 and 1975) and the AMA Ethical Guidelines for Clinical Investigation (1971) have not been very explicit (Beauchamp and Childress, 1983). The Declaration of Helsinki touches on the problem of minors in Article XI, which states that "In case of legal incompetence informed consent should be obtained from the legal guardian in accordance with national legislation. When physical or mental incapacity make it impossible to obtain informed consent or when the subject is a minor, permission from the responsible relative replaces that of the subject in accordance with national legislation." The AMA statement further clarifies this under Section 4C.

"Minors or mentally incompetent persons may be used as subjects only if:

1. The nature of the investigation is such that mentally competent persons would not be suitable subjects.

2. Consent, in writing, is given by a legally authorized representative of the subject under circumstances in which an informed or prudent adult would reasonably be expected to volunteer himself or his child as a subject."

The U. S. Department of Health and Human Services has promulgated regulations for the protection of human subjects, including fetuses in utero. These place a duty on the physician or investigative scientist to obtain the mother's (and the father's, if appropriate and available) consent to experiment on the fetus. Moreover, they state clearly that studies may be done if they pose minimal risk to the fetus and if the purpose of the activity is to meet the fetus' health needs. However, they do not address (and could not do so even if they completely forbad such studies) the rights of the fetus as compared with those of the mother or father or of the advancement of knowledge. The question of whose rights take precedence is not easily answered for two reasons. First, it is not clear whether a developing fetus, totally dependent on its mother until it reaches the age of viability,

has rights similar to those of a mature adult or even of a newborn separated from its mother. Second, if such a fetus has rights, who can speak for it? Should the spokesperson be its mother or an adult advocate? Or can guidelines be drawn for its emotions and thoughts? A special facet of studies involving human subjects is the randomized trial. Is it ethically sound to undertake it? If so, how should the patient be informed and how long should the study continue. These and other ethical questions are discussed by Schafer (1982).

Delegation of Responsibility. Delegation of responsibility is particularly relevant in obstetrics and gynecology because of (1) the increasing participation in patient care by nurse-midwives, clinical nurse specialists, nurse clinicians, specialized nurses and other professionals and (2) the involvement, in teaching institutions, of housestaff in gynecologic and obstetric operations and procedures. In the first case, an ethical question may arise because the various professionals disagree (and make known their disagreement) about the right treatment. Such instances might include, for example, continuation of uncomfortable chemotherapy for a patient whose chance of cure is nil and of survival is small, administration of pain relief in labor, which involves a conflict between mother and fetus, or the performance of difficult radiologic or other studies in debilitated patients. In the second case, the problem of delegation of operative or procedural care to a house officer in training presents ethical difficulties in discussions with the patient and in gaining informed consent. This question has recently been discussed by Thomasma and Pickleman (1983). It is essential that (1) close supervision by the attending obstetrician-gynecologist be provided in all cases; (2) that the patient understand that she is in a teaching institution and that housestaff will participate in her care; and (3) that any operative or other procedure will be managed by a team, with the attending obstetrician-gynecologist directing the procedure and appropriate parts being played by the various members of the team.

SPECIFIC OBSTETRIC AND GYNECOLOGIC ETHICAL PROBLEMS

The following are examples of specific ethical problems that may confront the obstetrician-gynecologist.

Conception and Fetal Development. The last

three decades have seen the development of several techniques of conception other than coitus between two adults anxious to produce an offspring. These include artificial insemination (by husband, donor or frozen sperm), in vitro fertilization (IVF), embryo transfer and surrogate motherhood. Apart from the legal problems of such conceptions, i.e., the rights of mother, father, child and others involved and the related contracts, ethical questions are common. For example, a sperm donor has a personal ethical problem about responsibility for his possible, unknown child, especially if he is married. In Great Britain the legislative and ethical problems of the newer methods of fertilization have been addressed, and recommendations have been made by the Warnock Committee (1984). The ethical aspects of in vitro fertilization have been the subject of much discussion, and a statement on this subject was made by the American Fertility Society in 1984. Surrogate motherhood and, by analogy, embryo transfer raise ethical questions for all parties involved. These were addressed by the American College of Obstetricians and Gynecologists in 1983 in a policy statement, "Ethical Issues in Surrogate Motherhood." The related problem of artificial insemination of the single woman raises personal ethical issues for the physician; it is discussed by Strong and Schinfield (1984).

Genetics. Modern genetics poses some ethical problems and is likely to pose more. When the geneticist diagnoses a condition with potential problems for a family, what are his duties to third-party relatives to whom the information might be valuable, when his patient demands that it be kept confidential? Potential ethical problems related to genetics include gene manipulation and duplication.

Pregnancy: Prevention and Termination. The ethical conflicts presented by the prevention of pregnancy (contraception) and by pregnancy termination by abortion or permanently by sterilization arise in large part from the conflict between theologically based principles and the rights of the individual. Previously, in the United States, the law provided a deterrent. That is no longer so, and, in spite of possible legal changes in the future, the legal aspects of any action taken are bound by current conditions. If the ethical conflict lies within the physician himself or herself, he is certainly not required to act contrary to his beliefs. A "conscience clause," protecting the right of a physician or hospital to follow ethical or religious convictions in denying abortion and sterilization

has been affirmed by the United States Supreme Court.

Labor and Delivery. In the past 30 years the increasing concern of women and their husbands for active participation in labor and delivery has posed problems for physicians and other professionals that have been, in part, ethical in nature. Such concerns have included preparation for childbirth, which is often outside the physician's control, the presence of fathers or other close relatives and friends during labor and in the delivery room and the interest in mothers and babies (and fathers) being close together after delivery to enhance breastfeeding and facilitate bonding between infants and parents. The ethical problems (camouflaged by matters of confidentiality, privacy and legal concerns) have involved conflicts between the physician's notion that what he was accustomed to do was best for his patient and his desire to have satisfied, happy patients. Most often the conflict has been successfully resolved by a negotiated, though not necessarily written, contract between the physician and the patient as to what is to be done in a variety of circumstances.

A second problem bordering on ethical issues has been the induction of labor. Here, conflict has been between the convenience of the physician, the convenience of the patient and the possible risks of induction. It has become clear that the last of these factors is paramount, particularly since injury occurring to mother or baby as a possible result of induction may be compensable in a legal sense.

A third question, both ethical and legal, has recently arisen in obstetrics. Can and should a woman be forced to submit to a cesarean section against her will if a physician determines the necessity for the operation to save the life of the unborn fetus (Annas, 1982)?

A fourth conflict, clearly ethical and widely discussed, has been the management of the very premature baby. While this is more properly the concern of the neonatologist, there may be places and times when a major decision, ethical in nature, has to be made by the obstetrician at the time of delivery. A physician's duty, according to all codes of ethics, is to preserve life. But the question is: At what age or size is it appropriate to use extraordinary (or optional) methods to do this when the use of extraordinary methods means that scarce financial and hospital resources are preempted and when the chance of success and the chance of serious complications from the methods used are similar?

Gynecology. Ethical problems in gynecology are very similar to those in other surgical specialties. Obtaining informed consent prior to an operation or procedure was discussed earlier. Although the more recent focus on this issue has been legal, it may present an ethical problem in several ways (and similar situations may arise when the patient is being informed of the results of the operation). First, how completely should the truth be told? Does the omission of some truths, because a physician believes it to be in his patient's best interest for her not to know everything, violate the principle of truth-telling? Are there conflicts of interest between the patient and her family with regard to the physician's recommendations? How should these be resolved? What is the physician's position if the patient decides to seek other advice, particularly if she plans to use an unorthodox treatment that has no proved chance of success?

The use of blood or blood products in women belonging to religious groups such as the Jehovah's Witnesses presents another dilemma. In obstetrics the conflict is even more acute because the fetus is involved and cannot speak for itself. The conflict lies between the patient's religious belief that she should not receive blood or blood products and the physician's belief that her life may be in danger if such products are not used. When the conscious adult patient alone is involved, her autonomy is paramount. A more difficult question arises if she is unconscious or unable to decide. In this case, the physician's duty to save life becomes more insistent, and the courts have excused him from penalty in these circumstances. The fetus, on the other hand, has no advocate and, therefore, a response from the courts has been sought and successfully so on his behalf. The management of Jehovah's Witnesses is discussed by Bonadkar and co-workers (1982).

Terminal Care. The final set of ethical complications arises in patients with terminal illness after gynecologic (or obstetric) operations or procedures. These relate to the continuation of therapeutic measures, the relief of pain and resuscitative efforts. The ethical problems are interrelated. A well stated principle has been the general rule since 1914; this is that every human being of adult years and sound mind has a right to determine what shall be done with his own body. A physician's duty, as most conceive it, is to continue treatment while there is any chance of success, however remote, to relieve suffering, without causing such complications as respiratory depression or possibly habituation to the drugs used, and to resuscitate those who have acute respiratory or cardiac arrest. On the other hand, especially in terminal cancer, the patient, her family or, indeed, other professionals may feel that complicated resuscitative efforts that may eventually turn out to be unsuccessful are not justified in expense or suffering, especially when death is imminent.

These conflicting views lead to ethical and legal dilemmas involving two important practical problems in management. First, how much life support, for example, intravenous fluids, antibiotics or other medication should be given? Such situations should probably be treated on an individual basis, depending on what is necessary to prevent pain and emotional distress (Micetich et al, 1983). Recent legal aspects of this question are discussed by Paris and Reardon (1985). Second, the physician, other supporting personnel, patient and family must decide what to do if the patient's heart or respiration stops suddenly. When this happens, nursing staff are obliged to call for the cardiopulmonary resuscitation team if it is available. If the decision is made not to use extraordinary resuscitative measures, the attending physician must order this and record on the chart that no treatment is available for the patient's disease, that he has discussed the situation with the patient (if she is able to do this) and her family, and that all are agreed that only ordinary resuscitative measures are to be used, i.e., the CPR unit is not to be called. This is widely known as a DNR (do not resuscitate) order. There may be opposing views about DNR orders among family members or, less commonly, among members of the health care team. It is important, when possible, to resolve these differences without resort to a referee who may not be aware of all the relevant factors in the situation.

Management of Ethical Complications

THE INDIVIDUAL CASE

Many ethical issues remain concealed because of the participants' uncertainty as to their exact nature or unwillingness to express contrary opinions, their lack of sensitivity to ethical issues or their feeling that the problems are insoluble. Differences between professional caregivers, especially between nurses and physicians, are probably more common than is generally recognized (Gramelspacher et al, 1986). However, recognition, discussion and an honest attempt to answer the questions should, in the long run, benefit the patient and her family and at least bring understanding of the dilemma to all involved in the patient's care.

Ethical dilemmas cannot be solved like a crossword puzzle, although detailed analysis may be helpful in some instances (Candee and Puka, 1984). The problems are sometimes acute, but often they can be addressed in a leisurely fashion. All that one can hope for is a full expression of views and adoption of what seems to be the best course of action under the circumstances. This can be achieved in several ways.

Individual Consideration. Since the possible courses of action are usually a major concern of the physician, he should, in many cases, be the primary organizer of meetings between himself and others who are uncertain about the right thing to do.

Group Discussions. If a team of professionals is taking care of a patient, it is essential that significant ethical questions be discussed by the group, particularly among those individuals who have had closest contact with the patient. In any such meeting, the patient and her family should be represented in some fashion. It is often not easy to have them present in person; therefore, it may be desirable to have the staff member who has the best relationship with the patient represent her at the meeting and serve as her advocate. The presence of someone (such as a chaplain or other counselor) who has a special interest in ethical problems can be very helpful, especially if he is able to pinpoint the rights and duties involved.

Committees on Ethics. Increasing interest has been shown recently in hospital Committees on Ethics. Although such committees may be of value in education (see later discussion), there is danger of their becoming formal regulatory or even disciplinary bodies, when the ethical problems involved are often a matter for mutual resolution of the various individual consciences, beliefs and duties. Ethics committees are discussed in detail by Crawford and Doudera (1984).

GENERAL ISSUES

Issues such as prolongation of life, refusal of treatment, or resuscitation of the small newborn are of general interest. In a teaching hospital that has a Committee on Ethics, a departmental or a hospital-wide conference can be held, based on a particular case but permitting broad discussion of all the issues involved. One or more members of the Ethics Committee can

serve as moderator(s) or resource person(s) for such meetings or workshops.

Prophylaxis of Ethical Complications

The complexity of modern obstetric-gynecologic operations and procedures is such that ethical dilemmas will continue and will increase. Since they can have a disturbing, even devastating effect on medical personnel, patients and families, it is better to try to forestall them. The following methods may be of help.

UNDERGRADUATE AND GRADUATE EDUCATION OF PHYSICIANS

Exposure to basic ethical theories in high school or college is an important part of general education and an invaluable background for consideration of ethical problems in clinical medicine. Most medical schools offer some exposure to medical ethics. Often the subject is taught as an elective course, apart from the clinical situations that the student encounters. The teaching of ethics is usually regarded as a secondary or tertiary educational function. Correlations of ethics with actual cases as they occur would emphasize the importance of the subject to the student and open his mind to the possibility of ethical conflicts in the future.

GRADUATE EDUCATION IN OBSTETRICS AND GYNECOLOGY

Graduate education is largely technical in nature. Problems in ethics occur frequently, as illustrated earlier, but the ethical problem is often not mentioned in an otherwise complicated situation. The introduction of ethical questions and the use of guest speakers on ethical topics would do much to orient the young specialist to ethical problems. A program for teaching bioethics during an obstetric-gynecologic residency has recently been described by Elkins and co-workers (1986).

CONTINUING EDUCATION

A hospital-wide ethics committee with broad membership is a valuable resource. It should include physicians, nurses, social workers, administrators and interested others. It can sponsor hospital conferences or supply expertise for specific departmental workshops on problems arising from a particular case or cases.

References

American College of Obstetricians and Gynecologists: Professional liability insurance and its effect: report of a survey of ACOG's membership. *American College of Obstetricians and Gynecologists*, Washington, D. C., 1985.

Andrews LB: Legal and ethical aspects of new reproductive technologies. *Clin. Obstet. Gynecol.* 29:190, 1986.

Annas GJ: Forced cesarean section: the most unkindest cut of all. *Hasting Center Reports* 12(3):16, 1982.

Applebaum PA, Roth LH: Patients who refuse treatment in medical hospitals. *J. Am. Med. Assoc.* 250:1296, 1983.

Beauchamp TL, Childress JE: *Principles of Biomedical Ethics*, Ed. 2. New York, Oxford University Press, 1983.

Bonadkar MI, Eckhous AW et al: Major gynecologic and obstetric surgery in Jehovah's Witnesses. *Obstet. Gynecol.* 60:587, 1982.

Brent RL: The irresponsible expert witness: a failure of biomedical graduate education and professional accountability. *Pediatrics* 70:754, 1982.

Candee D, Puka B: An analytic approach to resolving problems in medical ethics. *J. Med. Ethics* 10:61, 1984.

Crawford RE, Dondera AE: *Institutional Ethics Committees and Institutional Health Care Decision Making*. Ann Arbor, Michigan, Health Administration Press, 1984.

Dyck FJ, Murphy FA et al: Effect of surveillance on the number of hysterectomies in the province of Saskatchewan. *N. Engl. J. Med.* 296:1326, 1977.

Elias S, Annas GJ: Perspectives on fetal surgery. *Am. J. Obstet. Gynecol.* 145:807, 1983.

Elias S, Annas GJ: Social policy considerations in noncoital reproduction. *J. Am. Med. Assoc.* 255:62, 1986.

Elkins TE, Strong C et al: Teaching of bioethics within a residency program in obstetrics and gynecology. *Obstet. Gynecol.* 67:339, 1986.

Fineberg KS, Peters JD et al: *Obstetrics/Gynecology and the Law*. Ann Arbor, Michigan, Health Administration Press, 1984.

Fost N, Crawford RE: Hospital ethics committees: administrative aspects. *J. Am. Med. Assoc.* 253:2687, 1985.

Gramelspacher GP, Howell JD, Young MJ: Perceptions of ethical problems by nurses and physicians. *Arch. Intern. Med.* 146:577, 1986.

Greenlaw J: Orders not to rescuscitate: dilemma for acute care as well as long-term care facilities. *Law, Medicine, Health Care* 10:29, 1982.

Hiller MD, Seidel LF: Patient care management systems, medical records, and privacy: a balancing act. *Public Health Rep.* 97:332, 1982.

Hirsh BD: Parenthood by proxy. *J. Am. Med. Assoc.* 249:2251, 1983.

Illingworth RS: A Paediatrician asks—why is it called birth injury? *Br. J. Obstet. Gynaecol.* 92:122, 1985.

Kunin CM: The expert witness in medical malpractice litigation. *Arch. Intern. Med.* 100:139, 1984.

Micetich KC, Steinecker PH, Thomasma DC: Are intravenous fluids morally required for a dying patient. *Arch. Intern. Med.* 143:975, 1983.

Paneth N, Stark RL: Cerebral palsy and mental retardation in relation to indicators of perinatal asphyxia. *Am. J. Obstet. Gynecol.* 147:960, 1983.

Paris JJ, Reardon FE: Court responses to withholding or withdrawing artificial nutrition and fluids. *J. Am. Med. Assoc.* 253:2243, 1985.

Schafer A: The ethics of the randomized clinical trial. *N. Engl. J. Med.* 307:719, 1982.

Strong C, Schinfeld JS: The single woman and artificial insemination by donor. *J. Reprod. Med.* 29:293, 1984.

Tancredi LR: Designated compensable events: a no-fault approach to medical malpractice. *Law, Medicine, Health Care* 10:200, 1982.

Thomasma DC, Pickleman J: The ethical challenges of surgical training programs. *Bull. Am. Coll. Surg.* 68:18, 1983.

Veatch RM: *Case Studies in Medical Ethics*. Cambridge, Massachusetts, Harvard University Press, 1977.

The Warnock Committee: *Br. Med. J.* 289:238, 1984.

Note: Numbers in *italics* refer to illustrations; numbers followed by t indicate tables.